DIET AND NUTRITION IN ORAL HEALTH

D1622853

SECOND EDITION

DIET AND NUTRITION IN ORAL HEALTH

Carole A. Palmer, EdD, RD
Professor and Head, Division of Nutrition
 and Oral Health Promotion
Department of Public Health and Community Service
Tufts University School of Dental Medicine

Professor, Gerald J. and Dorothy R. Friedman
 School of Nutrition Science and Policy
Tufts University
Adjunct Professor, Tufts University School of Medicine
Boston, Massachusetts

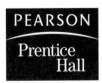

PEARSON

Prentice
Hall

Upper Saddle River, New Jersey 07458

Library of Congress Cataloging-in-Publication Data

Palmer, Carole A.
    Diet and nutrition in oral health / Carole A. Palmer. — 2nd ed.
       p. cm.
    Includes bibliographical references and index.
    ISBN 0-13-171757-X
       1. Nutrition and dental health.   I. Title

RK281.P35 2007
617.6′01—dc22   2006049808

Notice: The author and the publisher of this volume have taken care that the information and technical recommendations contained herein are based on research and expert consultation, and are accurate and compatible with the standards generally accepted at the time of publication. Nevertheless, as new information becomes available, changes in clinical and technical practices become necessary. The reader is advised to carefully consult manufacturers' instructions and information material for all supplies and equipment before use, and to consult with a healthcare professional as necessary. This advice is especially important when using new supplies or equipment for clinical purposes. The author[s] and publisher disclaim all responsibility for any liability, loss, injury, or damage incurred as a consequence, directly or indirectly, of the use and application of any of the contents of this volume.

Publisher: Julie Levin Alexander
Executive Editor: Mark Cohen
Associate Editor: Melissa Kerian
Editorial Assistant: Nicole Ragonese
Managing Editor for Production: Patrick Walsh
Production Liaison: Christina Zingone
Manufacturing Manager: Ilene Sanford
Manufacturing Buyer: Pat Brown
Design Director: Maria Guglielmo
Cover Designer: Maria Vicareo

Interior Design: GGS Book Services
Formatting: GGS Book Services
Director of Marketing: Karen Allman
Senior Marketing Manager: Harper Coles
Marketing Coordinator: Michael Sirinides
Marketing Assistant: Wayne Celia
Printer/Binder: Bind-Rite Graphics
Cover Printer: Phoenix Color Corporation
Cover Image: Getty Images/Digital Vision

Credits and acknowledgments borrowed from other sources and reproduced, with permission, in this textbook appear on appropriate pages within text.

Pearson Education LTD., London
Pearson Education Singapore, Pte. Ltd.
Pearson Education, Canada, Ltd.
Pearson Education–Japan
Pearson Education Australia PTY, Limited

Pearson Education North Asia Ltd.
Pearson Educación de Mexico, S.A. de C.V.
Pearson Education Malaysia, Pte. Ltd.
Pearson Education, Upper Saddle River, New Jersey

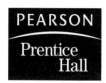

10 9 8 7 6 5 4 3 2 1
ISBN 0-13-171757-X

Contents

Preface

WHAT'S NEW IN THIS EDITION OF *DIET AND NUTRITION IN ORAL HEALTH?*

In recent years, the importance of oral health has received increasing recognition as research has defined relationships between oral and systemic diseases, and the surgeon general of the United States has focused much needed attention on a national crisis in oral health.

Nutrition plays many important roles in oral health promotion and disease prevention. Good nutrition provides the foundation for good oral health. Diet plays a major role in the etiology or prevention of dental caries, and is an important supporting factor in other oral infections. Conversely, oral health is a major determinant of good nutrition. Disturbances in the oral cavity can profoundly affect diet and ultimate nutritional status.

Dentistry today is changing to meet the needs of a changing population. Life expectancy continues to increase, and the nature and demographics of oral diseases are changing. Associated oral conditions such as coronal caries, root caries, periodontal disease, edentulism, cancer, AIDS, and oral infections all have nutritional implications.

The American Dental Association and the American Dental Hygienists' Association recommend that dental professionals "maintain current knowledge of nutrition recommendations as they relate to general and oral health and disease," and that they "effectively educate and counsel their patients about proper nutrition and oral health." The American Dietetic Association concurs by stating that "nutrition is an integral component of oral health" and supports "collaboration between dietetics and dental professionals . . . for oral health promotion and disease prevention and intervention."

Yet, even with the knowledge of the relationships that exist between nutrition and oral health, many dental health professionals are still hesitant to give nutrition guidance to their patients. The reason most often given for their reluctance to incorporate nutrition into their practices is their feeling of unpreparedness in both the science of nutrition and how to apply it effectively to assist dental patients. This book is specifically designed to help overcome these obstacles by providing:

- Current *information* about the many relationships between nutrition, oral health, and general health
- *Models and guidelines* for implementing diet screening and guidance into clinical practice
- *Practical suggestions* to help patients with various oral conditions improve their diets.

In this second edition, we have made a variety of additions and improvements. There are three entirely new chapters: Chapter 7, "How the Body Uses Fluids"; Chapter 10, "Dietary Supplements"; and Chapter 20, "Oral and Nutritional Concerns for People with Special Health Care Needs." We have also restructured several of the chapters as a result of valuable feedback from our users. We have included a section on diabetes mellitus in Chapter 4, "Carbohydrates," and have moved the information on cardiovascular diseases to Chapter 6, "Lipids in Health and Disease." We then consolidated chronic health conditions, immune-compromising conditions, and oral infections into Chapter 11, "Nutritional and Oral Implications of Common Chronic Health Conditions."

Particularly important, we have included additional information in an Instructor's Manual and CD-ROM. This support package has four distinct components:

- An Instructor's Manual with lecture outlines and topics for discussion
- Examination questions for each chapter
- PowerPoint lectures for each chapter
- Video presentations to demonstrate applied nutrition and counseling skills

We hope that these changes will improve student understanding and provide instructor assistance.

The book is still divided into four sections:

- **Part 1** provides the core information on the basic concepts of human nutrition and their relevance to oral health and dental practice.
- **Part 2** focuses on specific nutrition issues of dental patients and oral conditions.
- **Part 3** provides oral health nutrition information from a lifecycle perspective.
- **Part 4** provides the "nuts and bolts" of integrating meaningful nutrition care into dental practice.

How to Use This Second Edition

This book can serve as a quick reference or as a clinical manual to enable you to answer patient questions and to integrate nutrition into clinical practice as comfortably as you would fluoride and other preventive modalities.

You can use this book as a *text* by reading the chapters and answering the questions posed in the case studies to test understanding.

You can use the book as a *"how-to" manual* for diet screening and guidance by reading Part 4 and adapting the guidelines and materials provided in the Appendices and CD-ROM to your own clinical setting.

You can use this book as a *reference* by referring to those chapters relating to specific nutrition topics, life-cycle groups, or health-related conditions, and referring to the last chapter and the Appendices for helpful resources.

We hope that you find this book useful and informative, and that you will share any knowledge gleaned with your patients and your colleagues toward the goal of achieving better oral health for all.

ACKNOWLEDGMENTS

The second edition of this book required the dedication of many individuals, some who updated their chapters from the first edition, and some who joined us for the first time to write or update chapters. Once again, I thank all of our authors for their contributions and promptness in submitting their work.

Once again, I thank all of those colleagues, friends, and family who provided support while I was developing this edition of the text, especially the dean of Tufts University School of Dental Medicine, Dr. Lonnie Norris, and my department chair Dr. Catherine Hayes. Of course, I must again thank my close friend and mentor Johanna Dwyer for always being there for me as supporter, cheerleader, and wise counselor.

Finally, again I thank my husband Dr. Charles Zumbrunnen who provided unstinting support and kept me laughing with his asides, such as "they never taught me any of this in dental school. I want my money back." He continues to be selfless in his support for me and this work, and I cannot thank him enough.

Contributors

Linda Boyd, RDH, RD, EdD
Associate Professor
Director, Division of Graduate Studies
Department of Dental Hygiene
Idaho State University
Boise, Idaho
Chapters 4, 6, 11, 14

Glenda Butt, MS, RDH
Director, School of Dental Hygiene
Dalhousie University
Halifax, Nova Scotia, Canada
Chapter 21

Mary Cooper, RDH, MSEd
Professor, Dental Hygiene
Purdue University
Fort Wayne, Indiana
Chapter 2

R. Rebecca Couris, PhD, RPh
Associate Professor of Nutrition Science
and Pharmacy
Massachusetts College of Pharmacy
Boston, Massachusetts
Chapter 16

Dominick DePaola, DMD, PhD
President
Forsythe Dental Research Center
Boston, Massachusetts
Chapter 1

Johanna T. Dwyer, DSc, RD
Professor, Tufts University Schools of
Nutrition Science & Policy & Medicine
Director, Frances Stern Nutrition Center,
New England Medical Center Hospital
Boston, Massachusetts
Chapter 3

Lisa F. Harper, BSDH, MPH, RD
Assistant Professor
Baylor College of Dentistry
The Texas A&M University System
Health Science Center
Dallas, Texas
Chapters 15 and 17

Catherine Hayes, DMD, DMSc
Professor and Chair
Department of Public Health and Community Service
Tufts University School of Dental Medicine
Boston, Massachusetts
Chapter 12

Michelle Henshaw, DDS, MPH
Assistant Professor
Director of Community Health Programs
Department of Health Policy & Health Services
Research
Goldman School of Dental Medicine
Boston University
Boston, Massachusetts
Chapter 19

Karen Schroeder Kassel, MS, MEd, RD
Registered Dietician
Freelance Medical Writer
Medway, Massachusetts
Chapter 23

Elizabeth A. Krall, MPH, PhD
Associate Professor and Director
Epidemiology Division
Department of Health Policy & Health Services Research
Goldman School of Dental Medicine
Boston University
Boston, Massachusetts
Chapter 19

Katherine Kwon, MS
Tufts–New England Medical Center
Frances Stern Nutrition Center
Boston, Massachusetts
Chapter 20

George M. Lessard, PhD
Professor of Biochemistry and
Dental Sciences
Schools of Medicine and Dentistry
Loma Linda University
Loma Linda, California
Chapter 5

William W. McCloskey, Pharm D
Chair, Department of Pharmacy Practice
Associate Professor of Clinical Pharmacy
Massachusetts College of Pharmacy
Boston, Massachusetts
Chapter 16

Teresa Marshall, PhD, RD, LD
Visiting Assistant Professor
Department of Preventive and
Community Dentistry
College of Dentistry
University of Iowa
Iowa City, Iowa
Chapter 18

Connie Mobley, PhD, RD
Professor, Nutrition
School of Dental Medicine
University of Nevada Las Vegas
Las Vegas, Nevada
Chapter 13

Athena S. Papas, PhD, DMD
Professor and Co-Head
Division of Geriatric Dentistry
Department of General Dentistry
Tufts University School of Dental Medicine
Boston, Massachusetts
Chapter 8

Kathryn Thornton, DMD
Maumee, Ohio
Chapter 12

Stacy A. Weill, MS, RD
Project Manager, Clinical Research
PPD Development
Austin, Texas
Chapter 4

Jennifer Weston, MS, RD, LDN
Clinical Dietitian
Tufts School of Medicine & Nutrition Science
Boston, Massachusetts
Chapter 3

Reviewers of the Second Edition

Joyce C. Hudson, RDH, MS
Clinical Assistant Professor
Indiana University School of Dentistry
Indianapolis, Indiana

Nancy L. Shearer, RDH, BS, MEd
Coordinator, Dental Hygiene
Cape Cod Community College
West Barnstable, Massachusetts

Donal Scheidel, DDS
Associate Professor/Attending Dentist, Dental Hygiene
University of South Dakota
Vermillion, South Dakota

Patricia S. Wellner, RDH, MSHS, CC
Assistant Professor and Coordinator, Dental Hygiene
College of DuPage
Glen Ellyn, Illinois

Reviewers of the First Edition

Eugenia Bearden, RDH, MEd
Assistant Professor, Dental Hygiene
Clayton College and State University
Lilburn, Georgia

Marlene A. DeFeo, RDH, MS
Associate Professor, Dental Hygiene
Hudson Valley Community College
Troy, New York

Jan Mengle
Assistant Professor, Dental Hygiene
Armstrong Atlantic State University
Savannah, Georgia

Nancy L. Shearer, RDH, BS, MEd
Coordinator, Dental Hygiene
Cape Cod Community College
West Barnstable, Massachusetts

Chapter **1**

Nutrition as the Foundation for General and Oral Health

Carole A. Palmer and Dominick DePaola

OUTLINE

OBJECTIVES

The student will be able to:

- Explain why nutrition is important in dentistry.
- Describe the general relationships between diet and nutrition, and oral health and disease.
- Define common nutritional terms.
- Differentiate between essential and nonessential nutrients.
- List the classes of nutrients.
- Differentiate between primary and secondary malnutrition.
- Discuss how digestion occurs along the gastrointestinal tract.
- Describe how nutrients are absorbed.
- Discuss the process of utilization and storage of nutrients.
- Discuss how the oral cavity is the gatekeeper to nutrition.
- Detail how taste and smell affect nutrition.

INTRODUCTION TO NUTRITION IN DENTISTRY

From the earliest time, the relationship between what people ate and the health of their teeth has been recognized. Cave dwellers had severe dental erosion as a result of their highly fibrous diet, mixed with sand and dirt. As civilization progressed, upper-class citizens were distinguished from those of lower classes by the rotten teeth that were associated with their use of costly refined sugars (Wynbrandt, 1998). Yet it wasn't until the 1950s that the exact mechanisms that link sugars with caries were delineated. Since then, many increasingly complex relationships between foods and nutrients, and oral health and disease have been researched and delineated. It is now recognized that diet and nutrition play important roles in oral health and disease. The Surgeon General of the United States, in his landmark report *Oral Health in America*, emphasized the crucial but often overlooked fact that one cannot be healthy without a healthy mouth.

Diet and nutrition affect and are affected by the condition of the oral cavity. Good nutrition is the foundation for oral and general health. Conversely, the oral cavity is the pathway to the rest of the body, so any problems in the oral cavity can profoundly affect appetite, diet, and ultimately, nutritional status. Figure 1–1 diagrams the relationship between nutrition and oral health.

Dentistry is changing today to meet the needs of a changing population. Life expectancy continues to increase. In 1950 about 15 million people in the United States were over age 65 and few people were older than 85. By 2050 the number of adults over 65 is expected to reach 80 million, and the number over the age of 85 is expected to reach 20 million (Bahls, 2002).

The nature and demographics of oral diseases are also changing. Edentulism and partial tooth loss have diminished in the United States, and dental caries is now the principal cause of tooth loss in all but the oldest citizens (Burt & Eklund, 1999). Dental caries is the most common chronic condition of childhood. It is five times more prevalent than childhood asthma and seven times more prevalent than hay fever. Five to 10%

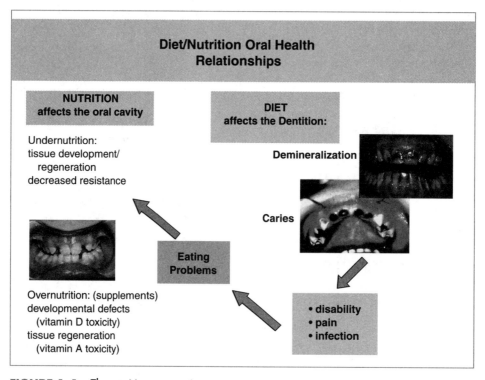

FIGURE 1–1 The nutrition connection.

of preschool-age children suffer from early childhood caries and almost 20% of all children aged 2–5 have untreated caries in primary teeth. (These figures are much higher for children in lower income families.) Over 45% of school children and 94% of adults have experienced caries in permanent teeth.

Periodontal disease also continues to be a significant problem, with 70% of adults worldwide having some degree of gingivitis or periodontitis (*Oral Health in America*, 2000). Other major health issues such as cancer, AIDS, oral infections, and the aging process have oral implications. All of these oral conditions have nutritional implications.

The American Dental Association (ADA, 1996) "encourages dentists to maintain current knowledge of nutrition recommendations as they relate to general and oral health and disease" and encourages them to "effectively educate and counsel their patients about proper nutrition and oral health." Other health professional organizations have similar recommendations (American Dental Hygienists Association [ADHA], 1998; American Dietetic Association, 1996).

Yet, even as more relationships are shown between nutrition and oral health, dental health professionals are often hesitant to give nutritional guidance to their patients. The reason given most often is the dental team's feeling of unpreparedness in both the content of nutrition information and how it should be applied in patient care (Palmer, 1990).

The mission of the modern dental team is to promote oral health via the treatment of oral disease, restoration of oral function, and implementation of strategies to prevent further disease and promote oral health. This means an active focus on the biological bases of oral diseases and conditions, their management, and their prevention. Nutrition affects and is affected by all of these.

This book is designed to provide the background information and applications that health professionals need to provide meaningful dietary guidance as part of total oral health promotion for all patients. Topics will include:

- The basics of nutrition today
- The roles of diet and nutrition in oral conditions
- How to recognize and diagnose relevant dietary and nutritional conditions in clients
- How to manage dietary and nutritional issues either by direct patient guidance or appropriate referral

THE UNIQUE ORAL CAVITY: GATEKEEPER TO NUTRITION

The oral cavity is often referred to as the "mirror of overall health" because the earliest clinical signs of nutritional or other health disorders are first seen in the oral cavity. The reason is that the oral soft tissues have a more rapid turnover time (3 to 7 days) than other tissues in the body (DePaola, Faine, Palmer, 1999). This is thought to be an adaptation over time to the many assaults that the oral cavity is subjected to on a daily basis (e.g., hot foods, cold foods, eating utensils). Anyone who has mistakenly sipped coffee that is too hot will realize that although the tissue sloughs off immediately, it is back to normal in a couple of days; but if he or she burned an arm or leg, it would take weeks to heal. Because of this rapid tissue turnover, immediate tissue needs for nutrients are greater in the oral cavity and deficiencies or toxicities will be clinically evident in the oral cavity sooner than in other parts of the body. Indeed, most of the clinical signs of nutritional deficiencies and toxicities are seen in or around the mouth.

The Importance of the Senses (Taste and Smell) to Nutrition

The senses of taste and smell play important roles in nutrition and health (Figure 1–2). In prehistoric times, people used their ability to taste and smell food as a guide to whether food was safe to eat or was spoiled or poisonous. Today, the senses of taste and smell contribute significantly to appetite and the ability to

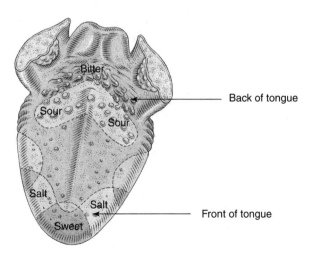

FIGURE 1–2 How the tongue senses taste.
Source: John Woodcock © Dorling Kindersley.

enjoy food. Conversely, decreased ability to taste or smell food can cause major declines in appetite and ultimately to malnutrition.

Taste is the only sensory system—with the exception of pain—that is fully developed at birth. Humans are born with about 10,000 taste buds, which turn over approximately every 10 days (Schiffman, 1997). This continuous renewal process makes the sense of taste particularly vulnerable to malnutrition.

Taste buds are found on the dorsal surface of the tongue, tongue–cheek margin, base of the tongue near sublingual gland ducts, the soft palate, pharynx, larynx, epiglottis, uvula, and first third of the esophagus. There are four different kinds of papillae on the tongue. The most common, the filliform papillae, are not involved with taste, but rather are thought to exist to provide a rough surface to help propel food in the mouth.

The papillae on the anterior two-thirds of the tongue are called fungiform papillae and usually have one to eighteen taste buds. Each fungiform papilla has about six small taste pores, with clusters of specialized taste buds below them. During the chewing and swallowing process, food chemicals reach the taste bud, and different cells are stimulated, depending on the type of taste stimulus. It is generally accepted that the five taste sensations are sweet, sour, salt, bitter, and umami (glutamate). Tongue movements prolong and improve taste sensations on the soft palate. The papillae on the posterior lateral sides of the tongue are foliate papillae and consist of vertical folds. The foliate papillae have more taste buds than the fungiform papillae. In the very middle of the tongue in the back are the circumvallate papillae. There are fewer than a dozen, but they are dense with taste buds (Schiffman, 1997). Taste buds are also found on the roof of the mouth. Taste is the primary dimension by which young children decide upon food acceptance or rejection. The responses of children to tastes differ markedly from those of adults. In general, children have a greater preference for sweet-tasting foods, and a greater rejection of bitter-tasting foods than adults. It may be that genetic variations in taste receptor genes as well as cultural differences also are major determinants of the differences in sensitivity to bitter and sweet tastes in both children and adults (Mennella, Pepino, Reed, 2005).

Taste is often mistaken for smell. Humans can detect from 10,000 to over 100,000 different odors. They can also detect pheromones, which are chemicals released from members of the same species that stimulate hormonal or behavioral responses. The sense of smell is facilitated by millions of olfactory sensory neurons located in the olfactory epithelium lining the nasal cavity. The neurons transmit sensory signals to the olfactory bulb in the brain. The olfactory bulb sends signals to the olfactory cortex, which then sends olfactory information to those higher cortical areas where the conscious perception and discrimination of odors is thought to occur (Buck, 2004). Olfactory receptors die and regenerate every few months. Odors can be detected only if the flavor molecules are in vapor form (Hess, 1992). Cold foods cannot be smelled until they warm up. The trigeminal system of nerve branches running between the brain and the nose and mouth detects irritants such as hot chili, pepper, mint, and carbonation (Accounting for taste, 1990). Taste, smell, reaction to irritants, texture, temperature, color, and appearance all work together to determine total flavor.

Taste and smell decline significantly with age; sense of smell declines faster than taste. Medications, health conditions, and radiation therapy can all decrease (hypogeusia) or alter (dysgeusia) taste perception. Impaired taste perception can increase risk of food poisoning when the ability to discern spoilage by taste is impaired. People vary in their taste perception ability within age groups. Some are very sensitive to food factors such as the bitterness of saccharine or other artificial sweeteners, whereas others are unable to detect these same factors.

As taste sensitivity diminishes people may compensate by increasing their use of salt and sugar. This could result in increased risk of hypertension and root caries in older patients. Thus, anything that affects the sense of smell or taste can impact nutrition via appetite and food choices. Upper dentures can blunt taste sensation by covering taste buds. Oral infections can also affect taste buds. Head and neck radiation and certain medications can radically affect how foods taste and can result in radical changes in appetite and diet.

WHAT DOES NUTRITION REALLY MEAN TODAY?

Of the ten leading causes of death today, five have poor diet as a risk factor: heart disease, stroke, diabetes, liver disease, and some cancers. These account for two-thirds of all deaths in North America (National Center for Health Statistics, 1997).

Associations between foods and disease have been recognized and reported for centuries, but it was not until the 20th century that most nutrients were isolated and their functions and mechanisms of action determined.

The science of nutrition has also evolved in its focus. In past years, the primary goal was to determine what and how much of various nutrients and foods the body needs to prevent nutritional deficiencies. For example, although the importance of citrus fruits in preventing scurvy has been recognized for centuries, vitamin C (ascorbic acid) was not isolated, named, and synthesized until the 1930s. As a result, earlier dietary recommendations were designed with the goal of helping populations prevent nutritional deficiencies. By the 1950s, dietary deficiency diseases were largely eradicated in developed countries. Today's nutrition research is focusing upon determining other health effects of food components beyond just the nutrients themselves. A major goal is to determine how nutrition can help prevent chronic diseases and prolong life. Foods and food components that can help prevent cancers, heart disease, and other degenerative conditions are all being actively researched. Research is targeting known nutrients such as vitamins; other food constituents such as phytochemicals; social factors such as eating habits and patterns (e.g., frequency of eating); and food balance (percentage of various types of foods consumed) in an attempt to use food to help meet contemporary health goals.

Advances in food engineering and technology have also resulted in greater potential to manipulate foods to meet nutritional goals. Genetic engineering has resulted in lower fat meats, tomatoes with good flavor year-round, and virus-resistant squash. Fortification can be used to boost the amount of nutrients normally found in foods and to add nutrients to foods that do not usually contain them. Good examples might be the fortification of orange juice with calcium and the fortification of milk with vitamin D. Synthetic foods such as nonfat fats and nonsugar sweeteners are coming to market at a rapid pace.

Nutritional supplements have grown from encompassing primarily vitamins and minerals, including herbals, phytochemicals, diet drugs, and other such supplements. As a result, the line between nutrients as foods and nutrients as pharmaceuticals or medicine is becoming blurred.

THE LANGUAGE OF NUTRITION

Although the terms *diet* and *nutrition* are often used interchangeably, in fact they have important differences that are particularly significant in the practice of dentistry. Table 1–1 shows definitions of common nutrition terms.

What Are Essential Nutrients?

The essential nutrients are those necessary for body function. The term arose in the twentieth century when it was observed that some human and animal diseases were associated with poor diets and could be prevented or cured by adding food constituents to the diet. These were termed *essential* nutrients. Nutrients that can be eliminated from the diet with no adverse health consequences are termed *nonessential* nutrients. Essential nutrients are those that the body cannot synthesize, so they must be provided by the diet (with a few exceptions). There are about 45 essential nutrients. The concept of essentiality is species specific; within species, nutrients may be deemed essential or nonessential depending on stage of development or health condition. For example, vitamin C is essential to humans but not to most other animals. Certain amino acids are essential to infants but not adults.

In summary, today, traditional nutrition concepts are being revised in light of new knowledge on the benefits foods, nutrients, nonnutrient food components, and diet in reducing the risk of some degenerative diseases provide and improving immune function and longevity throughout life.

What Are the Nutrient Classes?

Food is defined as "that which is eaten to provide necessary nutritive elements" (Dirckx, 2001). (This narrow definition ignores the importance of food to enjoyment and quality of life, however.) Foods have many components: water, fiber, phytochemicals, essential and nonessential nutrients, and so on. The nutrients are traditionally divided classified into six classes:

- carbohydrates (carbon, hydrogen, and oxygen)
- protein (carbon, hydrogen, oxygen, and nitrogen)
- fat (carbon, hydrogen, and oxygen)
- vitamins (organic compounds: carbon, hydrogen, oxygen, sometimes nitrogen, sometimes minerals)

TABLE 1-1 Definitions

Nutrition	• The science of how the body uses food to meet its requirements for growth, development, repair, and maintenance. • *Nutritional status* is the condition of health as it relates to food and nutrient intake, absorption, and utilization. It is an important factor in immunity and resistance to oral infection.
Diet	• The pattern of individual food intake, eating habits, and kinds and amounts of foods eaten. • Affected by a host of psychosocial factors such as ethnic background, tradition, religion, lifestyle, peer influence, personal attitudes, and health condition. • Major risk factor for dental caries development. • Can also affect general health as in cardiovascular disease or diabetes mellitus. In turn, medical conditions such as diabetes mellitus can affect the oral condition and affect diet choices. • A healthful diet contains all of the necessary nutrients in amounts needed to meet individual needs.
Nutrients	• The chemical components of foods, which are needed by the body. • Found in various amounts and combinations in foods; more than 50 known nutrients.
Foods	• Substances that are consumed and provide nutrients to the body. • Few foods contain only one nutrient. An exception is table sugar, which is only sucrose. • There is no perfect food (with the exception of mother's milk for babies).
Malnutrition	• Impaired health related to nutritional status. • Can be due to nutrient or caloric deficiency, excess, or imbalance. • Caused by problems with food intake, absorption, utilization, or excretion. • Loss of teeth is a predictor of malnutrition in adult patients. In turn, oral impairment such as ill-fitting dentures or oral cancer can affect ability and desire to eat and subsequent nutritional status.
Overnutrition	• Excess of calories or essential nutrients above known requirements for health.
Undernutrition	• Deficiency of calories or essential nutrients below known requirements for health.

• minerals (inorganic compounds, free ions)
• water (hydrogen and oxygen)

Nutrients are required on a consistent basis and serve a variety of essential functions such as:

• providing energy sources for body work (carbohydrate, protein, fat).
• maintaining a constant internal environment (water, minerals, protein, fat).
• providing structural components for growth, development, and maintenance of body tissues and fluids (protein, fat, water).
• regulating metabolic processes (carbohydrate, protein, fat, vitamins, minerals, water).

Thus, nutrients can be thought of as compounds consumed in foods that are required for health. The traditional concept of nutrient definition is currently undergoing major reassessment with the growth of research in nonnutrient food components, such as phytochemicals, now in progress. Phytochemicals are biologically active compounds found in food, but not considered to be essential to life using current nutrient criteria. Many of these compounds, however, have been shown to have significant protective effects in the body. It may be that the definition of *essential* will change to encompass such food constituents as phytochemicals. It may then mean that the functions of nutrients may expand in scope as well. In recent years, the adequacy of this current classification system has been called into question (Harper, 1999).

What Is Malnutrition and What Causes It?

The term *malnutrition* is often misused and narrowly defined (Figure 1–3). Malnutrition merely means bad nutrition. The term is often used primarily to describe the undernutrition seen in nutrient and calorie deficiencies. Starving groups and individuals are most commonly referred to as malnourished; however, any aberrations from optimal nutriture can rightfully be called malnutrition. Obesity is also a form of malnutrition (i.e., overnutrition). Nutrient deficiency anemias are forms of malnutrition. Excessively high-fat diets leading to elevated serum lipids and heart disease risk also qualify as malnutrition. Nutrient excesses can lead to

toxicities and other side effects and equally qualify as forms of malnutrition. Thus, in order for the term *malnutrition* to have meaning, it must be further defined and specified. Without explanation, it means about as much as the term *American*.

Primary malnutrition results from inadequate food intake. The etiology is usually socioeconomic. For example, adequate food may be unavailable or inaccessible, the cost may be prohibitive, lack of knowledge may lead to improper food choices, or preparation techniques may result in nutrient destruction.

Secondary (or conditioned) malnutrition occurs when there is interference with adequate digestion, absorption, or utilization of foods. In secondary malnutrition, the diet chosen is adequate, but physiological factors interfere with proper nutrient utilization. Contributors to secondary malnutrition can include dental problems, drug–nutrient interactions, digestive disturbances, and malabsorption syndromes. For example, an elderly patient with xerostomia and ill-fitting dentures may avoid fresh fruits and vegetables and meats that need to be chewed. Instead, she may gravitate to soft or liquid food choices such as coffee, tea, toast and jam. These foods will satisfy her appetite but will provide very little in nutritional value. Malnutrition may be the result.

The development of a nutritional deficiency or toxicity is a gradual and progressive process (Figure 1–4). Problems begin with inappropriate food intake. This leads to decrease or increase of nutrients throughout the body. At some point, the deficiency or excess impairs body functioning such as enzyme activity, growth, and development. Finally, in the most advanced stages, there may be clinically observable signs and symptoms, and eventually disability and death. It is important to note that clinical signs and symptoms are evident only in the more advanced cases. The major impairments in development and function caused by nutritional excesses or deficiencies are not clinically visible. This is why it is *never* appropriate to use clinical signs as the sole criterion for determining nutritional status.

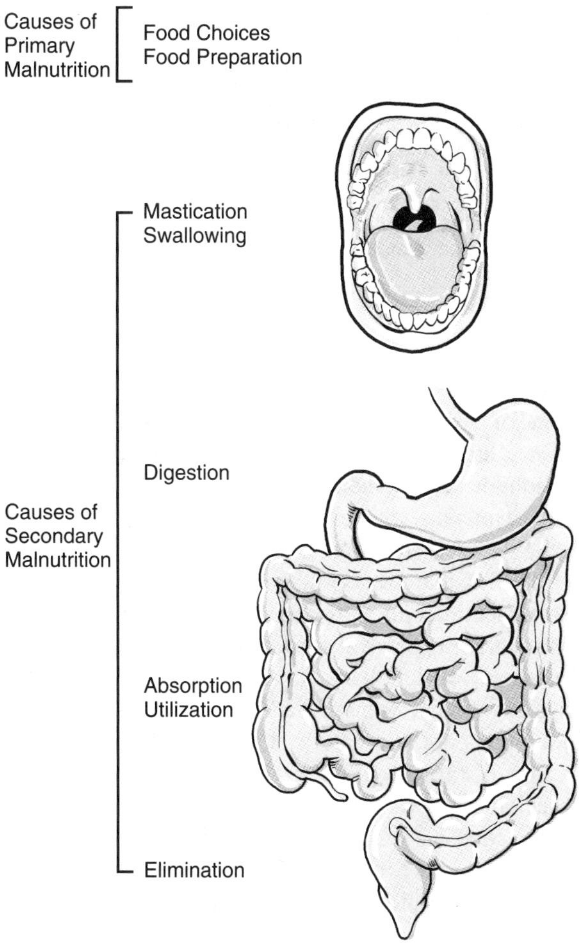

HOW DOES FOOD BECOME US?

The Nutrients and Body Composition

Good nutrition is essential to the development of a healthy oral cavity. All structures depend on adequate and consistent supplies of nutrients for their development and continued integrity.

Causes of Primary Malnutrition
— Food Choices
— Food Preparation

Causes of Secondary Malnutrition
— Mastication / Swallowing
— Digestion
— Absorption / Utilization
— Elimination

FIGURE 1–3 The nutrition spectrum.
Source: Darisse Paquette, CMI.

Process of Nutritional Deficiency or Toxicity

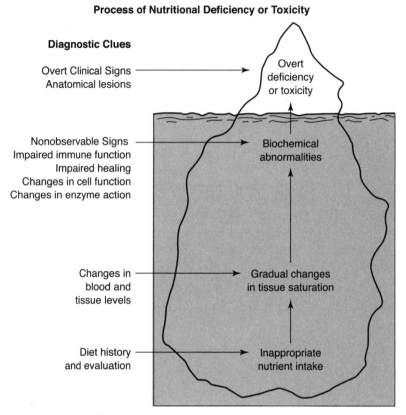

FIGURE 1–4   Like an iceberg.
Source: Adapted from Darisse Paquette, CMI.

TABLE 1–2   Body Composition

Nutrient	Approximate % of Body Weight
Water	60%
Fat	10–50% (optimal 15% men, 28% women)
Protein	12%
Minerals	5%
Carbohydrate	Negligible

Source: From Forbes GB: Body composition: Influence of nutrition, physical activity, growth, and aging. In Shils M, Olsen J, Shike M, Ross AC (eds): *Modern Nutrition in Health and Disease,* 9th ed. Baltimore: Williams & Wilkins, 1999.

The body is composed of elements derived from nutrients (Table 1–2). More than 95% of body weight is made of nonmetallic elements: carbon, hydrogen, oxygen, and nitrogen. The remainder is made up of mineral elements, with calcium and phosphorus being most highly represented. The body is composed of four types of compartments: cells, mineralized skeleton, extracellular fluid, and adipose or fat tissue. Protein, carbohydrate, fat, and the minerals are detailed in later chapters.

Water is responsible for about 60% of body weight. The majority is intracellular, with the remainder as extracellular in serum, cerebrospinal fluid, tissue spaces, and saliva. Water is essential to body function. The normal weight human can live without food for 60 days but can live without water for only 14 days. Older individuals are at greater risk for dehydration, which can be life threatening, so sufficient fluid intake is especially important in older people. The body's fluid composition can vary greatly from day to day depending on intake, kidney function, and diet. High-protein diets lead to early fluid losses, which diet adherents often mistake for actual body fat reduction. They are most dismayed when the weight returns as rapidly as it is lost.

THE PROCESS OF NUTRITION

The Oral Cavity and Esophagus

Digestion of food begins in the oral cavity, where both physical and chemical digestion begins (Figure 1–5). Oral digestion is short (about 30 seconds) as compared to gastric and intestinal digestion (1 to 10 hours), so its importance is often overlooked and neglected. However, oral digestion has an important impact on overall digestion and may influence the entire digestive process, including the metabolic response to starches (Hoebler, Karinthi, Devaux, 1998). Mechanical digestion begins with the process of biting and chewing food. Breaking foods into particles ensures that pieces will be small enough to be swallowed safely. In addition, the smaller pieces of food provide more surface area for saliva to aid in propelling food to the esophagus and for digestive enzymes to function (Table 1–3). In the

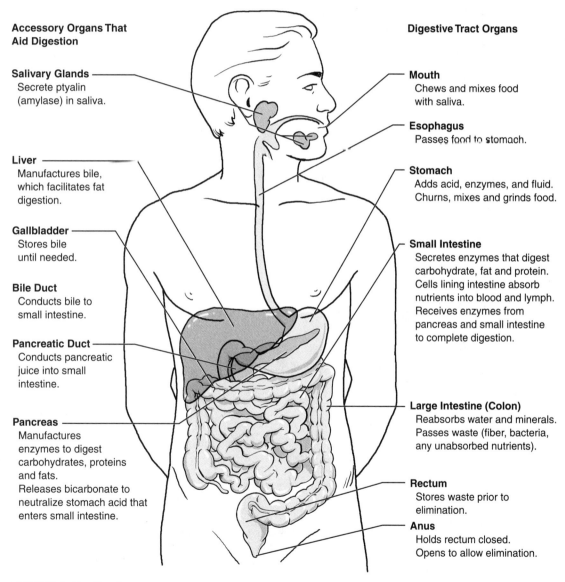

FIGURE 1–5 The digestive process.
Source: Darisse Paquette, CMI.

TABLE 1–3   Enzymes Complete the Digestive Process

Mouth

Chews and mixes food with saliva

Starch $\xrightarrow{\text{Ptyalin}}$ Dextrins

Stomach

Adds acid, enzymes, and fluid

Churns, mixes, and grinds food to a liquid mass

Protein $\xrightarrow{\text{Hydrochloric Acid Pepsin}}$ Polypeptides

Liver

Manufactures bile, which facilitates fat digestion

Fats $\xrightarrow{\text{Bile}}$ Emulsified fat

Small Intestine

Enzymes from pancreas and small intestine complete digestion

Carbohydrates

Pancreas

Starch $\xrightarrow{\text{Amylase}}$ Maltose and Sucrose (disaccharides)

Intestine

Lactose $\xrightarrow{\text{Lactase}}$ Glucose and Galactose (monosaccharides)

Sucrose $\xrightarrow{\text{Sucrase}}$ Glucose and Fructose

Maltose $\xrightarrow{\text{Maltase}}$ Glucose and Glucose

Protein

Pancreas

Proteins $\xrightarrow{\text{Trypsin}}$ Dipeptides

Polypeptides

Proteins $\xrightarrow{\text{Chrymotrypin}}$ Dipeptides

Polypeptides

Polypeptides $\xrightarrow{\text{Carboxypeptidase}}$ Amino Acids
Dipeptides

Intestine

Polypeptides $\xrightarrow{\text{Aminopeptidase}}$ Amino Acids

Dipeptides

Dipeptides $\xrightarrow{\text{Dipeptidase}}$ Amino Acids

Fat

Pancreas

Fats $\xrightarrow{\text{Lipase}}$ Glycerol, Glycerides (di–, mono–), Fatty acids

Intestine

Fats $\xrightarrow{\text{Lipase}}$ Glycerol, Glycerides (di–, mono–), Fatty acids

Source: Darisse Paquette, CMI.

mouth, the only chemical digestion is the action of amylase on starches. This mechanism is particularly important to dentistry in that it allows large molecule starches, which are not fermentable by plaque acids, to be hydrolyzed into shorter chain carbohydrates that are fermentable. This mechanism accounts for the cariogenic potential of starches.

The actions of the tongue in concert with saliva, teeth, and palate propel food to the back of the mouth where it is swallowed and passes through the esophagus to the stomach. No digestive activity occurs in the esophagus. Several sphincters along the gastrointestinal tract modulate the flow of food in response to various physical and chemical stimuli.

The Stomach

In the stomach, the cardiac sphincter modulates the entrance of food into the stomach. Goblet cells produce mucus to protect stomach lining from the acid. Chief cells produce pepsinogen, which helps initiate the hydrolysis of protein with the aid of hydrochloric acid (HCl). Parietal cells in the stomach wall release HCl to make gastric content acidic. Parietal cells also secrete intrinsic factor, the protein that facilitates the absorption of vitamin B_{12}. This stomach acid also halts the action of amylase on starches. The acidic food mass that moves on to the small intestine is called chyme.

The Small Intestine

The majority of food digestion occurs in the duodenum of the small intestine, from which nutrients are absorbed. The pyloric valve moderates the entry of chyme into the duodenum. There digestive enzymes from the intestinal cell wall and some from the pancreas act to hydrolyze foods into absorbable nutrients. Three classes of enzymes—carbohydrases, lipases, and proteases—catalyze the hydrolysis of the energy-providing nutrients. Bile from the gallbladder emulsifies fat and makes it accessible to lipase. As chyme moves along the small intestine, nutrients are hydrolyzed to their final absorbable components: monosaccharides, amino acids, fatty acids, and glycerol. By the time it reaches the end of the small intestine, it has been exposed to more than 200 meters squared (m^2) of intestinal surface area where all nutrients with the exception of water and some minerals are absorbed.

The small intestine is lined with four to five million fingerlike projections called villi. Each villus has a layer of epithelium over a layer of connective tissue (lamina propria), which is supplied with capillaries for blood circulation and lacteals for lymph circulation. On the surface of each villus is the brush border, which is composed of 500 to 600 microvilli. The result is an enormous surface area available for absorption activity. Absorption can be either active or passive. Active absorption requires carriers to help move nutrients across the brush border. Passive absorption occurs when nutrients move from an area of greater concentration in the intestine to an area of lesser concentration in the circulation without the assistance of carriers. Absorption is a selective process by which the body can help protect itself from deficiencies (by absorbing more) or excesses (by absorbing less). Once absorbed, nutrients move to the liver and then to all cells. The water-soluble substances (water-soluble vitamins, minerals, amino acids, glucose) enter the bloodstream directly. Fat-soluble substances (fatty acids, cholesterol, fat-soluble vitamins) enter the lymphatic system and then move to the blood from which they move to the liver and then the cells.

Nutrient Utilization (Cellular or Intermediary Metabolism)

Within cells, nutrients function to supply energy, build or maintain tissues, or regulate body metabolism with the aid of specific enzymes that facilitate these processes. Examples are the conversion of amino acids to new tissue, hormones, or enzymes; the conversion of stored glycogen into fat; the conversion of fatty acids into cell membranes; and the incorporation of calcium, phosphorus, and magnesium into bone.

The energy requirements of the body take priority over all other functions. Glucose, glycerol, and fatty acids produce most body energy; but if the supply is inadequate, amino acids will be used as well. Energy is derived from carbohydrates (4 calories per gram [cal/g]); proteins (4 cal/g); fat (9 cal/g); and alcohol (7 cal/g). Carbohydrates, proteins, and fats for the most part are transformed into the common denominator acetyl coenzyme A (CoA). The CoA then enters the tricarboxylic acid cycle (TCA cycle, also known as the citric acid cycle, or the Krebs cycle). This process of energy release from food is shown in Figure 1–6.

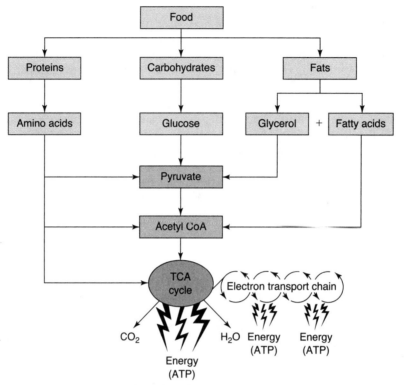

FIGURE 1–6   Energy release from food.
Source: From *Robinson's Basic Nutrition and Diet Therapy:* 8/E, by Weigley/Mueller/ Robinson, © 1997. Reprinted with permission.

Nutrient Storage

Energy derived from food is stored for the short term as adenosine triphosphate (ATP) in cells, intermediately as glycogen in the liver, and long term as fat in adipose tissue. Fat-soluble vitamins are stored in adipose tissue as well. Protein, iron, and vitamin A are stored in the liver. Many of the minerals are stored in bone. Water-soluble vitamins are not stored, per se, but are found in greater amounts in depots throughout the body. All nutrients are undergoing active metabolism. Even "stored" nutrients are constantly being used up and replenished.

The Large Intestine

The large intestine encompasses the cecum, colon, rectum, and anal canal. By the time the food reaches the large intestine, most digestion and absorption have been completed. Undigested food components move on to the large intestine, where water and minerals are reabsorbed. No digestive activity takes place in the large intestine. However, bacteria attack undigested residues to assist in elimination. Solid waste is formed into feces and excreted via the rectum and anus.

Waste Excretion

Excretion is the elimination of undigested by-products of food and other substances such as toxins, bacteria, and sloughed-off body cells. There are four organs of excretion:

- Skin: eliminates water via perspiration, and small amounts of some minerals and nitrogenous wastes
- Lungs: eliminate carbon dioxide and water
- Kidneys: eliminate most nitrogenous waste, water, minerals, excess water-soluble vitamins, and detoxified substances
- Bowel: eliminates undigested food and indigestible fiber, bile pigments, intestinal bacteria, and other metabolic by-products

SUMMARY AND IMPLICATIONS FOR DENTISTRY

Nutrition is the foundation for the oral cavity and the entire body. Nutritional problems can affect the oral cavity directly and indirectly. Conversely, problems of the oral cavity can have a major impact on eating and subsequent nutritional status. The challenge for the dental team is to be able to recognize nutritional problems when they exist and to help patients optimize their nutritional status for the sake of their oral health and their total health.

REFERENCES

Accounting for taste. *University of California Berkeley Wellness Letter*. November 1990:7.

Joint Report of the American Dental Association Council on Access, Prevention and Interprofessional Relations and Council on Scientific Affairs to the House of Delegates: Response to Resolution 73H-2000, October 2001.

American Dental Hygienists Association: *Policy on Prevention of Dental Caries and Food Programs* 13-98/15-94/30-75. 16-64. 14-94/26-74, 1998.

American Dietetic Association; ADA reports; Position of the American Dietetic Association: Oral health and nutrition. *J Am Diet Assoc* 1996; 96:184–89.

Bahls C: Alzheimer research joins the mainstream. *The Scientist* 2002; 16:2.

Buck, LB: Olfactory receptors and odor coding in mammals. *Nutr Rev* 2004; 62(11):S184–S188.

Burt B, Eklund S: The professions of dentistry and dental hygiene. In Burt B, Eklund S: *Dentistry, Dental Practice, and the Community*, 5th ed. Philadelphia: WB Saunders, 1999.

Combs GF Jr: Should intakes with beneficial actions, often requiring supplementation, be considered for RDAs? *J Nutr* 1996; 126:2373s–76s.

DePaola D, Faine M, Palmer C: Nutrition in relation to dental medicine. In Shils M, Olsen J, Shike M, Ross AC (eds): *Modern Nutrition in Health and Disease*, 9th ed. Baltimore: Williams & Wilkins, 1999.

Dirckx JH, ed: *Stedman's Concise Medical Dictionary for the Health Professions*, 4th ed. Philadelphia: Lippincott Williams & Wilkins, 2001.

Forbes GB: Body composition: influence of nutrition, physical activity, growth, and aging. In Shils M, Olsen J, Shike M, Ross AC (eds): *Modern Nutrition in Health and Disease*, 9th ed. Baltimore: Williams & Wilkins, 1999.

Harper AE: Defining the essentiality of nutrients. In Shils M, Olsen J, Shike M, Ross AC (eds): *Modern Nutrition in Health and Disease*, 9th ed. Baltimore: Williams & Wilkins, 1999.

Hess MA: Taste: The neglected nutritional factor. *Top Clin Nutr* 1992; 7:1–6.

Hoebler C, Karinthi A, Devaux MF: Physical and chemical transformations of cereal food during oral digestion in human subjects. *Br J Nutr* 1998; 80:429–36.

Lachance P, Langseth L: The RDA concept: time for a change? *Nutr Rev* 1994; 52:266–70.

Mennella J, Pepino MY, Reed DR: Genetic and environmental determinants of bitter perception and sweet preferences. *Pediatrics* 2005; 115(2):e.216–e22.

National Center for Health Statistics: Births and deaths: Preliminary data for 1997. *National Vital Statistics Reports* 1998; 47(4).

Oral health in America: A report of the Surgeon General. Washington, DC: U.S. Department of Health and Human Services, 2000.

Palmer C: Nutrition counseling in dental education: Issues and challenges. *J Dental Ed* 1990; 54:513–18.

Schiffman SS: Taste and smell losses in normal aging and disease. *JAMA* 1997; 278:1357–62.

U.S. Department of Commerce, Bureau of the Census: *U.S. Population Estimates by Age, Sex, Race, and Hispanic Origin: 1993–2050.* Series P-25, No. 1104. Washington, DC: Government Printing Office, 1994.

Wynbrandt, J: *The Excruciating History of Dentistry.* New York: St. Martin's Press, 1998.

Chapter **2**

What Is an Adequate Diet?

Carole A. Palmer, Mary Cooper, and Riva Touger-Decker

OBJECTIVES

The student will be able to:
- Discuss the standards for assessing nutritional adequacy of diets.
- Discuss the guidelines to be used in planning nutritionally adequate diets.
- List basic diet and nutrition guidelines to use in diet education of patients.
- Discuss the proper interpretation of food labels.
- Discuss the implications of new and future food issues in the economy including functional foods and genetically engineered foods.
- List and describe the functions of antioxidants in the body.
- Distinguish between vitamins and phytochemicals, and functional foods.
- Discuss some of the major functions of food phytochemicals.
- Explain the potential benefits of nutritional genomics research.

INTRODUCTION

A healthful diet is essential to overall good health and to help prevent and control chronic diseases such as diabetes, hypertension, hypercholesterolemia, and obesity. Yet, achieving a nutritionally adequate diet can be a challenge for many consumers. Despite the abundance of food choices available today, people often have a difficult time making healthful food choices, especially when eating away from home.

In the past two decades, the number of meals and snacks eaten away from home has increased by more than two-thirds. Busy lives, families with both parents employed, and more affordable and convenient fast-food outlets all contribute to this trend. Americans eat approximately 2.7 meals per day, a number that has remained fairly stable. However, snacking has increased to 1.6 times per day with 22% of snacks eaten away from home. As a result, almost a third of total caloric intake occurs away from home. Foods consumed away from home generally contain more of the nutrients overconsumed by Americans (fat, saturated fat, cholesterol, and sodium) and fewer of the nutrients underconsumed (fiber, calcium, and iron) (Lin, Frazão, Guthrie, 1999). On a positive note, many restaurants have taken steps in recent years to improve their offerings by targeting low-fat, low-carbohydrate, and "heart healthy" food choices. Fast-food restaurants have also responded by offering lower fat choices and providing nutrient information on their offerings.

Health professionals need to be able to help consumers choose healthy diets by being familiar with the dietary recommendations and guidelines for health and reinforcing them in clinical settings. Dental team members are in an excellent position to conduct diet and nutrition risk assessment relative to general and oral health, provide and reinforce diet information relative to oral disease management, and refer patients to registered dietitians (RDs) for more in-depth care. Registered dietitians are important allies in assisting clients with their nutritional needs because they are the only health professionals credentialed to provide medical nutrition therapy.

This chapter reviews the various standards and guidelines for planning an adequate diet. Chapter 22 details the process of patient assessment essential to determining dietary adequacy and the risk factors that may predispose an individual to nutritional or other problems.

PLANNING NUTRITIONALLY ADEQUATE DIETS

There are no "good" or "bad" foods. All foods can fit into a healthful diet. Planning an adequate diet requires making food choices that include the types and amounts of nutrients needed daily to maintain health and to prevent disease and disability. The keys to a healthy diet are:

- *Adequacy:* sufficient foods to meet caloric and nutrient needs.
- *Variety:* selecting a wide variety of foods to ensure a breadth of nutrient intake.
- *Moderation:* to avoid excess calories and reduce dietary risks for chronic diseases.

A variety of science-based dietary guidelines and food guides are available to assist in the nutrition education process. The primary guidelines are detailed below.

Human Nutritional Requirements

Dietary Reference Intakes (DRIs) (Institute of Medicine, 1997, 1998, 2005)

The Recommended Dietary Allowances (RDAs) document the state of the knowledge of human nutrient requirements (National Research Council [NRC], 1989). "RDAs are the levels of intake of essential nutrients that, on the basis of scientific knowledge, are judged (by the Food and Nutrition Board of the Institute of Medicine) to be adequate to meet the known nutrient needs of practically all healthy persons" (NRC, l989). RDAs provide "safe and adequate" amounts of nutrients needed by individuals on a daily basis.

The first RDAs were published in 1942 and listed nutritional requirements for only seven nutrients, and consisted of a single value for nutrient needs for various age groups. To keep abreast with emerging research, these standards have been reevaluated and reissued approximately every 4 years. The latest version of these standards, renamed the Dietary Reference Intakes (DRIs), is the most detailed document to date and includes several important innovations.

The DRIs (Institute of Medicine [IOM], National Academy of Sciences, 1997, 1998) provide guidelines for determining general nutrient needs of healthy individuals, and detail the amounts of nutrients recommended to help reduce risk of chronic disease and prevent deficiencies and toxicities. Nutritional deficiencies or toxicities may result from inappropriate intake, or decreased or increased nutrient absorption, utilization, metabolism, or excretion. The risks of nutrient toxicities also rise with the increased use of supplements in the population.

DRIs exist for vitamins, minerals, and trace elements (IOM, 1997, 1998). DRIs for antioxidants are currently being developed (Rock, 1998). In 1998, the IOM released *Dietary Reference Intakes: Proposed Definition and Plan for Review of Dietary Antioxidants and Related Compounds* (Standing Committee, 1998). This report defines dietary antioxidants as "a substance in foods that significantly decreases the adverse effects of reactive oxygen species (ROS), reactive nitrogen species (RNS) or both on normal physiological function in humans" (Standing Committee, 1998).

The DRIs offer four different reference values depending on the amount of information available:

The **Recommended Dietary Allowance (RDA)** is the amount of a nutrient needed for healthy people (differing by age group). The RDA for most nutrients is based on the determined average requirement for health *plus* a margin of safety set at a level that will meet the needs of nearly all of a healthy population. Thus, the RDA is *not* the minimum nutrient requirement to prevent deficiency, but rather is the optimum intake judged to promote health.

The **Estimated Average Requirements (EARs)** describe the nutrient intake that is estimated to meet specific acceptability requirements in 50% of people within a specific age or gender group.

Adequate Intake (AI) applies to nutrients for which insufficient data exist to support a specific RDA.

The **Tolerable Upper Levels (ULs)** is the newest category and resulted from increasing evidence of detrimental effects of high intakes of some nutrients. The UL sets a level of intake above which there is evidence of dangerous health effects (NRC, 1989).

Figure 2–1 describes the criteria for the different standards. Tables 2–1 to 2–6 provide the DRI tables and they are in the Appendix as well.

The DRIs provide the foundation for building a healthy diet by detailing human nutritional requirements. For this data to be applicable to diet planning, these nutrient recommendations must be translated into consumer-friendly diet guidelines. These guidelines are also important to highlight food choices that can help promote health and prevent chronic disease.

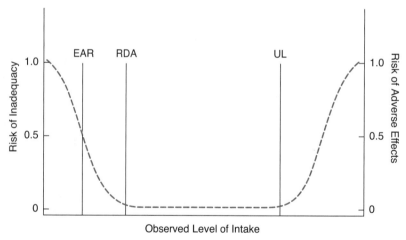

FIGURE 2–1 Dietary Reference Intakes. The Estimated Average Requirement (EAR) is the intake at which the risk of inadequacy is 0.5 (50%) to an individual. The Recommended Dietary Allowance (RDA) is the intake at which the risk of inadequacy is very small—only 0.02 to 0.03 (2–3%). The Adequate Intake (AI) does not bear a consistent relationship to the EAR or the RDA because it is set without being able to estimate the average requirement. It is assumed that the AI is at or above the RDA if one could be calculated. At intakes between the RDA and the Tolerable Upper Level (UL), the risks or inadequacy and of excess are both close to 0. At intakes above the UL, the risk of adverse effect may increase.
Source: Reprinted with permission from *Dietary Reference Intakes for Calcium, Phosphorus, Magnesium, Vitamin D, and Fluoride.* Copyright © 1997 by the National Academy of Sciences. Courtesy of the National Academy Press, Washington, D.C.

TABLE 2–1 Dietary Reference Intake (DRIs): Recommended Intake for Individuals, Vitamins

Life Stage Group	Vit A (µg/d)a	Vit C (mg/d)	Vit D (µg/d)b,c	Vit E (mg/d)c	Vit K (µg/d)	Thiamin (mg/d)	Riboflavin (mg/d)	Niacin (mg/d)e	Vit B6 (mg/d)	Folate (µg/d)f	Vit B12 (µg/d)	Pantothenic Acid (mg/d)	Biotin (µg/d)	Choline g (mg/d)
Infants														
0–6 mo	400*	40*	5*	4*	2.0*	0.2*	0.3*	2*	0.1*	65*	0.4*	1.7*	5*	125*
7–12 mo	500*	50*	5*	5*	2.5*	0.3*	0.4*	4*	0.3*	80*	0.5*	1.8*	6*	150*
Children														
1–3 y	300	15	5*	6	30*	0.5	0.5	6	0.5	150	0.9	2*	8*	200*
4–8 y	400	25	5*	7	55*	0.6	0.6	8	0.6	200	1.2	3*	12*	250*
Males														
9–13 y	600	45	5*	11	60*	0.9	0.9	12	1.0	300	1.8	4*	20*	375*
14–18 y	900	75	5*	15	75*	1.2	1.3	16	1.3	400	2.4	5*	25*	550*
19–30 y	900	90	5*	15	120*	1.2	1.3	16	1.3	400	2.4	5*	30*	550*
31–50 y	900	90	5*	15	120*	1.2	1.3	16	1.3	400	2.4	5*	30*	550*
51–70 y	900	90	10*	15	120*	1.2	1.3	16	1.7	400	2.4i	5*	30*	550*
>70 y	900	90	15*	15	120*	1.2	1.3	16	1.7	400	2.4i	5*	30*	550*
Females														
9–13 y	600	45	5*	11	60*	0.9	0.9	12	1.0	300	1.8	4*	20*	375*
14–18 y	700	65	5*	15	75*	1.0	1.0	14	1.2	400i	2.4	5*	25*	400*
19–30 y	700	75	5*	15	90*	1.1	1.1	14	1.3	400i	2.4	5*	30*	425*
31–50 y	700	75	5*	15	90*	1.1	1.1	14	1.3	400i	2.4	5*	30*	425*
51–70 y	700	75	10*	15	90*	1.1	1.1	14	1.5	400	2.4h	5*	30*	425*
>70 y	700	75	15*	15	90*	1.1	1.1	14	1.5	400	2.4h	5*	30*	425*
Pregnancy														
14–18 y	750	80	5*	15	75*	1.4	1.4	18	1.9	600i	2.6	6*	30*	450*
19–30 y	770	85	5*	15	90*	1.4	1.4	18	1.9	600i	2.6	6*	30*	450*
31–50 y	770	85	5*	15	90*	1.4	1.4	18	1.9	600i	2.6	6*	30*	450*

(continued)

TABLE 2–1 Dietary Reference Intake (DRIs): Recommended Intake for Individuals, Vitamins (Continued)

Lactation													
14–18 y	1,200	115	5*	19	75*	1.4	1.6	17	2.0	500	2.8	7*	35*	550*
19–30 y	1,300	120	5*	19	90*	1.4	1.6	17	2.0	500	2.8	7*	35*	550*
31–50 y	1,300	120	5*	19	90*	1.4	1.6	17	2.0	500	2.8	7*	35*	550*

Note: This table (taken from the DRI reports, see www.nap.edu) presents Recommended Dietary Allowances (RDAs) in **bold type** and Adequate Intakes (AIs) in ordinary type followed by an asterisk (*). RDAs and AIs may both be used as goals for individual intake. RDAs are set to meet the needs of almost all (97 to 98 percent) individuals in a group. For healthy breastfed infants, the AI is the mean intake. The AI for other life stage and gender groups is believed to cover needs of all individuals in the group, but lack of data or uncertainty in the data prevent being able to specify with confidence the percentage of individuals covered by this intake.

[a] As retinol activity equivalents (RAEs). 1 RAE = 1 μg retinol, 12 μg β-carotene, 24 μg α-carotene or 24 μg β-cryptoxanthin. The RAE for dietary provitamin A carotenoids is twofold greater than retinol equivalents (RE), whereas the RAE for preformed vitamin A is the same as RE.

[b] As cholecalciferol, 1 μg cholecalciferol = 40 IU vitamin D.

[c] In the absence of adequate exposure to sunlight.

[d] As α-tocopherol. α-tocopherol includes *RRR*-α-tocopherol, the only form of α-tocopherol that occurs naturally in foods, and the 2*R*-stereoisomeric forms of α-tocopherol (*RRR*-, *RSR*-, *RRS*-, and *RSS*-α-tocopherol) that occur in fortified foods and supplements. It does not include the 2*S*-stereoisomeric forms of α-tocopherol (*SRR*-, *SSR*-, *SRS*-, and *SSS*-α-tocopherol), found in fortified foods and supplements.

[e] As niacin equivalents (NE). 1mg of niacin = 60 mg of tryptophan; 0–6 months = preformed niacin (not NE).

[f] As dietary folate equivalents (DFE). 1 DFE = 1 μg food folate = 0.6 μg of folic acid from fortified food or as a supplement consumed with food = 0.5 μg of a supplement taken on an empty stomach.

[g] Although AIs have been set for choline, there are few data to assess whether a dietary supply of choline is needed at all stages of the life cycle, and it may be that the choline requirement can be met by endogenous synthesis at some of these stages.

[h] Because 10 to 30 percent of older people may malabsorb food-bond B_{12}, it is advisable for those older tha 50 years to meet their RDA mainly by consuming foods fortified with B_{12} or a supplement containing B_{12}.

[i] In view of evidence linking folate intake with neutral tube defects in the fetus, it is recommended that all women capable of becoming pregnant consume 400 μg from supplement or fortified foods in addition to intake of food folate from a varied diet.

[j] It is assumed that women will continue consuming 400 μg from supplements or fortified food until their pregnancy is confirmed and they enter prenatal care, which ordinarily occurs after the end of the periconceptional period—the critical time for formation of the neutral tube.

Source: Reprinted with permission from *Dietary Reference Intakes for Water, Potassium, Sodium, Chloride, and Sulfate.* Copyright © 2004 by the National Academy of Sciences. Courtesy of the National Academy Press, Washington, D.C.

TABLE 2-2 Dietary Reference Intake (DRIs): Tolerable Upper Intake Levels (UL[a]), Vitamins

Life Stage Group	Vitamin A (μg/d)[b]	Vitamin C (mg/d)	Vitamin D (μg/d)	Vitamin E (mg/d)[c,d]	Vitamin K	Thiamin	Ribo-flavin	Niacin (mg/d)[d]	Vitamin B6 (mg/d)	Folate (μg/d)[d]	Vitamin B12	Pantothenic Acid	Biotin	Choline (g/d)	Carotenoids[e]
Infants															
0–6 mo	600	ND[f]	25	ND	ND	ND	ND	ND	ND	ND	ND	ND	ND	ND	ND
7–12 mo	600	ND	25	ND	ND	ND	ND	ND	ND	ND	ND	ND	ND	ND	ND
Children															
1–3 y	600	400	50	200	ND	ND	ND	10	30	300	ND	ND	ND	1.0	ND
4–8 y	900	650	50	300	ND	ND	ND	15	40	400	ND	ND	ND	1.0	ND
Males, Females															
9–13 y	1,700	1,200	50	600	ND	ND	ND	20	60	600	ND	ND	ND	2.0	ND
14–18 y	2,800	1,800	50	800	ND	ND	ND	30	80	800	ND	ND	ND	3.0	ND
19–70 y	3,000	2,000	50	1,000	ND	ND	ND	35	100	1,000	ND	ND	ND	3.5	ND
>70 y	3,000	2,000	50	1,000	ND	ND	ND	35	100	1,000	ND	ND	ND	3.5	ND
Pregnancy															
14–18 y	2,800	1,800	50	800	ND	ND	ND	30	80	800	ND	ND	ND	3.0	ND
19–50 y	3,000	2,000	50	1,000	ND	ND	ND	35	100	1,000	ND	ND	ND	3.5	ND
Lactation															
14–18 y	2,800	1,800	50	800	ND	ND	ND	30	80	800	ND	ND	ND	3.0	ND
19–50 y	3,000	2,000	50	1,000	ND	ND	ND	35	100	1,000	ND	ND	ND	3.5	ND

[a] UL = The maximum level of daily nutrient intake is likely to pose no risk of adverse effects. Unless otherwise specified, the UL represents total intake from food, water, and supplements. Due to lack of suitable data. ULs could not be established for Vitamin K, thiamin, riboflavin, vitamin B12, pantothenic acid, biotin, carotenoids. In the absence of ULs, extra caution may be warranted in consuming levels above recommended intakes.

[b] As preformed vitamin A only.

[c] As α-tocopherol; applies to any form of supplemental α-tocopherol.

[d] The ULs for vitamin E, niacin, and folate apply to synthetic forms obtained from supplements, fortified foods, or a combination of the two.

[e] β-Carotene supplements are advised only to serve as a provitamin A source for individuals at risk of vitamin A deficiency.

[f] ND = Not determined due to lack of data of adverse effects in this age group and concern with regard to lack of ability to handle excess amounts. Source of intake should be from food only to prevent high levels of intake.

Source: Reprinted with permission from *Dietary Reference Intakes for Water, Potassium, Sodium, Chloride, and Sulfate.* Copyright © 2004 by the National Academy of Sciences. Courtesy of the National Academy Press, Washington, D.C.

TABLE 2-3 Dietary Reference Intakes (DRIs): Recommended Intakes for Individuals, Elements

Life Stage Group	Calcium (mg/d)	Chromium (µg/d)	Copper (µg/d)	Fluoride (mg/d)	Iodine (µg/d)	Iron (mg/d)	Magnesium (mg/d)	Manganese (mg/d)	Molybdenum (µg/d)	Phosphorus (mg/d)	Selenium (µg/d)	Zinc (mg/d)	Potassium (g/d)	Sodium (g/d)	Chloride (g/d)
Infants															
0–6 mo	210*	0.2*	200*	0.01*	110*	0.27*	30*	0.003*	2*	100*	15*	2*	0.4*	0.12*	0.18*
7–12 mo	270*	5.5*	220*	0.5*	130*	11	75*	0.6*	3*	275*	20*	3	0.7*	0.37*	0.57*
Children															
1–3 y	500*	11*	340	0.7*	90	7	80	1.2*	17	460	20	3	3.0*	1.0*	1.5*
4–8 y	800*	15*	440	1*	90	10	130	1.5*	22	500	30	5	3.8*	1.2*	1.9*
Males															
9–13 y	1,300*	25*	700	2*	120	8	240	1.9*	34	1,250	40	8	4.5*	1.5*	2.3*
14–18 y	1,300*	35*	890	3*	150	11	410	2.2*	43	1,250	55	11	4.7*	1.5*	2.3*
19–30 y	1,000*	35*	900	4*	150	8	400	2.3*	45	700	55	11	4.7*	1.5*	2.3*
31–50 y	1,000*	35*	900	4*	150	8	420	2.3*	45	700	55	11	4.7*	1.5*	2.3*
51–70 y	1,200*	30*	900	4*	150	8	420	2.3*	45	700	55	11	4.7*	1.3*	2.0*
>70 y	1,200*	30*	900	4*	150	8	420	2.3*	45	700	55	11	4.7*	1.2*	1.8*
Females															
9–13 y	1,300*	21*	700	2*	120	8	240	1.6*	34	1,250	40	8	4.5*	1.5*	2.3*
14–18 y	1,300*	24*	890	3*	150	15	360	1.6*	43	1,250	55	9	4.7*	1.5*	2.3*
19–30 y	1,000*	25*	900	3*	150	18	310	1.8*	45	700	55	8	4.7*	1.5*	2.3*
31–50 y	1,000*	25*	900	3*	150	18	320	1.8*	45	700	55	8	4.7*	1.5*	2.3*
51–70 y	1,200*	20*	900	3*	150	8	320	1.8*	45	700	55	8	4.7*	1.3*	2.0*
>70 y	1,200*	20*	900	3*	150	8	320	1.8*	45	700	55	8	4.7*	1.2*	1.8*
Pregnancy															
14–18 y	1,300*	29*	1,000	3*	220	27	400	2.0*	50	1,250	60	12	4.7*	1.5*	2.3*
19–30 y	1,000*	30*	1,000	3*	220	27	350	2.0*	50	700	60	11	4.7*	1.5*	2.3*
31–50 y	1,000*	30*	1,000	3*	220	27	360	2.0*	50	700	60	11	4.7*	1.5*	2.3*
Lactation															
14–18 y	1,300*	44*	1,300	3*	290	10	360	2.6*	50	1,250	70	13	5.1*	1.5*	2.3*
19–30 y	1,000*	45*	1,300	3*	290	9	310	2.6*	50	700	70	12	5.1*	1.5*	2.3*
31–50 y	1,000*	45*	1,300	3*	290	9	320	2.6*	50	700	70	12	5.1*	1.5*	2.3*

Note: This table presents Recommended Dietary Allowances (RDAs) in **bold type** and Adequate Intakes (AIs) in ordinary type followed by an asterisk (*). RDAs and AIs may both be used as goals for individual intake. RDAs are set to meet the needs of almost all (97 to 98 percent) individuals in a group. For healthy breastfed infants, the AI is the mean intake. The AI for other life stage and gender groups is believed to cover needs of all individuals in the group, but lack of data or uncertainly in the data prevent being able to specify with confidence the percentage of individuals covered by this intake.

Source: Reprinted with permission from *Dietary Reference Intakes for Water, Potassium, Sodium, Chloride, and Sulfate.* Copyright © 2004 by the National Academy of Sciences. Courtesy of the National Academy Press, Washington, D.C.

TABLE 2-4 Dietary Reference Intakes (DRIs): Tolerable Upper Intake Levels (UL^a), Elements

Life Stage Group	Arsenic^b	Boron (mg/d)	Calcium (g/d)	Chromium	Copper (µg/d)	Fluoride (mg/d)	Iodine (µg/d)	Iron (mg/d)	Magnesium (mg/d)	Manganese (mg/d)	Molybdenum (µg/d)	Nickel (mg/d)	Phosphorus (g/d)	Potassium	Selenium (µg/d)	Silicon^d	Sulfate	Vanadium (mg/d)^e	Zinc (mg/d)	Sodium (g/d)	Chloride (g/d)
Infants																					
0–6 mo	ND^f	ND	ND	ND	ND	0.7	ND	40	ND	ND	ND	ND	ND	ND	45	ND	ND	ND	4	ND	ND
7–12 mo	ND	ND	ND	ND	ND	0.9	ND	40	ND	ND	ND	ND	ND	ND	60	ND	ND	ND	5	ND	ND
Children																					
1–3 y	ND	3	2.5	ND	1,000	1.3	200	40	65	2	300	0.2	3	ND	90	ND	ND	ND	7	1.5	2.3
4–8 y	ND	6	2.5	ND	3,000	2.2	300	40	110	3	600	0.3	3	ND	150	ND	ND	ND	12	1.9	2.9
Males,																					
Females																					
9–13 y	ND	11	2.5	ND	5,000	10	600	40	350	6	1,100	0.6	4	ND	280	ND	ND	ND	23	2.2	3.4
14–18 y	ND	17	2.5	ND	8,000	10	900	45	350	9	1,700	1.0	4	ND	400	ND	ND	ND	34	2.3	3.6
19–70 y	ND	20	2.5	ND	10,000	10	1,100	45	350	11	2,000	1.0	4	ND	400	ND	ND	1.8	40	2.3	3.6
>70 y	ND	20	2.5	ND	10,000	10	1,100	45	350	11	2,000	1.0	3	ND	400	ND	ND	1.8	40	2.3	3.6
Pregnancy																					
14–18 y	ND	17	2.5	ND	8,000	10	900	45	350	9	1,700	1.0	3.5	ND	400	ND	ND	ND	34	2.3	3.6
19–50 y	ND	20	2.5	ND	10,000	10	1,100	45	350	11	2,000	1.0	3.5	ND	400	ND	ND	ND	40	2.3	3.6
Location																					
14–18 y	ND	17	2.5	ND	8,000	10	900	45	350	9	1,700	1.0	4	ND	400	ND	ND	ND	34	2.3	3.6
19–50 y	ND	20	2.5	ND	10,000	10	1,100	45	350	11	2,000	1.0	4	ND	400	ND	ND	ND	40	2.3	3.6

^{a} UL = The maximum level of daily nutrient intake that is likely to pose no risk of adverse effects. Unless otherwise specified, the UL represents total intake from food, water, and supplements. Due to lack of suitable data, ULs could not be established for arsenic, chromium, silicon, potassium, and sulfate. In the absence of ULs, extra caution may be warranted in consuming levels above recommended intakes.

^{b} Although the UL was not determined for arsenic, there is no justification for adding arsenic to food or supplements.

^{c} The ULs for magnesium represent intake from a pharmacological agent only and do not include intake from food and water.

^{d} Although silicon has not been shown to cause adverse effects in humans, there is no justification for adding silicon to supplements.

^{e} Although vanadium in food has not been shown to cause adverse effects in humans, there is no justification for adding vanadium to food and vanadium supplements should be used with caution. The UL is based on adverse effects in laboratory animals and this data could be used to set a UL for adults but not children and adolescents.

^{f} ND = Not determinabe due to lack of data of adverse effects in this age group and concern with regard to lack of ability to handle excess amounts. Source of intake should be from food only to prevent high levels of intake.

Source: Reprinted with permission from *Dietary Reference Intakes for Water, Potassium, Sodium, Chloride, and Sulfate.* Copyright © 2004 by the National Academy of Sciences. Courtesy of the National Academy Press, Washington, D.C.

TABLE 2–5A   Dietary Reference Intakes (DRIs): Acceptable Macronutrient Distribution Ranges

	Range (percent of energy)		
Macronutrient	Children, 1–3y	Children, 4–18y	Adults
Fat	30–40	25–35	20–35
n-6 polyunsaturated fatty acids[a] (linoleic acid)	5–10	5–10	5–10
n-3 polyunsaturated fatty acids[a] (α-linoleic acid)	0.6–1.2	0.6–1.2	0.6–1.2
Carbohydrate	45–65	45–65	45–65
Protein	5–20	10–30	10–35

[a] Approximately 10% of the total can come from longer-chain n-3 or n-6 fatty acids.

TABLE 2–5B   Dietary Reference Intakes (DRIs): Recommended Intakes for Individuals, Macronutrients

Life Stage Group	Total Water[a] (L/d)	Carbohydrate (g/d)	Total Fiber (g/d)	Fat (g/d)	Linoleic Acid (g/d)	α-Linolenic Acid (g/d)	Protein[b] (g/d)
Infants							
0–6 mo	0.7*	60*	ND	31*	4.4*	0.5*	9.1*
7–12 mo	0.8*	95*	ND	30*	4.6*	0.5*	**11.0**[c]
Children							
1–3 y	1.3*	**130**	19*	ND	7*	0.7*	**13**
4–8 y	1.7*	**130**	25*	ND	10*	0.9*	**19**
Males							
9–13 y	2.4*	**130**	31*	ND	12*	1.2*	**34**
14–18 y	3.3*	**130**	38*	ND	16*	1.6*	**52**
19–30 y	3.7*	**130**	38*	ND	17*	1.6*	**56**
31–50 y	3.7*	**130**	38*	ND	17*	1.6*	**56**
51–70 y	3.7*	**130**	30*	ND	14*	1.6*	**56**
>70 y	3.7*	**130**	30*	ND	14*	1.6*	**56**
Females							
9–13 y	2.1*	**130**	26*	ND	10*	1.0*	**34**
14–18 y	2.3*	**130**	26*	ND	11*	1.1*	**46**
19–30 y	2.7*	**130**	25*	ND	12*	1.1*	**46**
31–50 y	2.7*	**130**	25*	ND	12*	1.1*	**46**
51–70 y	2.7*	**130**	21*	ND	11*	1.1*	**46**
>70 y	2.7*	**130**	21*	ND	11*	1.1*	**46**
Pregenancy							
14–18 y	3.0*	**175**	28*	ND	13*	1.4*	**71**
19–30 y	3.0*	**175**	28*	ND	13*	1.4*	**71**
31–50 y	3.0*	**175**	28*	ND	13*	1.4*	**71**
Lactation							
14–18 y	3.8*	**210**	29*	ND	13*	1.3*	**71**
19–30 y	3.8*	**210**	29*	ND	13*	1.3*	**71**
31–50 y	3.8*	**210**	29*	ND	13*	1.3*	**71**

Note: This table presents Recommended Dietary Allowances (RDAs) in **bold** type and Adequate Intakes (AIs) in ordinary type followed by an asterisk (*). RDAs and AIs may both be used as goals for individual intake. RDAs are set to meet the needs of almost all

(continued)

TABLE 2–5B   Dietary Reference Intakes (DRIs): Acceptable Macronutrient Distribution Ranges (Continued)

(97 to 98 percent) individual in a group. For healthy infants fed human milk, the AI is the mean intake. The AI for other life stage and gender groups is believed to cover the needs of all individuals in the group, but lack of data or uncertainty in the data prevent being able to specify with confidence the percentage of individual covered by this intake.
[a] *Total* water includes all water contained in food, beverages, and drinking water.
[b] Based on 0.8g/kg body weight for the reference body weight.
[c] Change from 13.5 in prepublication copy due to calculation error.

TABLE 2–5C   Dietary Reference Intakes (DRIs): Additional Macronutrient Recommendations

Macronutrient	*Recommendation*
Dietary cholesterol	As low as possible while consuming a nutritionally adequate diet
Trans fatty acids	As low as possible while consuming a nutritionally adequate diet
Saturated fatty acids	As low as possible while consuming a nutritionally adequate diet
Added sugars	Limit to no more than 25% of total energy

Source: Tables 2–5a, b, and c reprinted with permission from *Dietary Reference Intakes for Energy, Carbohydrate, Fiber, Fat, Fatty Acids, Cholesterol, Protein, and Amino Acids (Macronutrients)*. Copyright © 2002 by the National Academy of Sciences. Courtesy of the National Academy Press, Washington, D.C.

Guidelines for Planning Nutritionally Adequate Diets

Dietary Guidelines for Americans 2005

The *Dietary Guidelines for Americans* are a joint effort of the U.S. Department of Health and Human Services (USDHHS) and the U.S. Department of Agriculture (USDA) to provide science-based advice for planning healthful diets (USDHHS and USDA, 2005). A basic premise of the *Dietary Guidelines* is that nutrient needs should be met primarily through consuming foods. Foods provide an array of nutrients and other compounds that may have beneficial effects on health. The 2005 edition of the USDHHS *Dietary Guidelines* makes dietary recommendations in nine general areas. In each area, there are key recommendations and more detailed recommendations for specific population groups. Taken together, they encourage most Americans to eat fewer calories, be more active, and make wiser food choices. These categories are listed below and detailed in Table 2–7:

- Adequate nutrients within calorie needs
- Weight management
- Physical activity
- Food groups
- Fats
- Carbohydrates
- Sodium and potassium
- Alcoholic beverages
- Food safety

The 2005 edition places a stronger emphasis than did past editions on calorie control and increasing physical activity. See Figure 2–2 for a history of USDA's food guidance. This is a result of the growing weight problem in the United States. Almost two-thirds of Americans are overweight or obese and more than 50% do not obtain the physical activity needed to control their weight. The *Dietary Guidelines* also are recommending consumption of more nutrient-dense foods such as fruits, vegetables, and whole grains, and low-fat and fat-free milk and milk products. In addition to the government-issued *Dietary Guidelines for Americans*, complementary dietary guidelines have also been developed by private agencies such as the American Heart Association (AHA) and American Cancer Society (American Cancer Society, 1996).

TABLE 2-6 Dietary Reference Intakes (DRIs): Estimated Average Requirements for Groups

Life Stage Group	CHO (g/d)	Protein (g/d)[a]	Vit A (µg/d)[b]	Vit C (mg/d)	Vit E (mg/d)[c]	Thiamin (mg/d)	Riboflavin (mg/d)	Niacin (mg/d)[d]	Vit B6 (mg/d)	Folate (µg/d)[e]	Vit B12 (µg/d)	Copper (µg/d)	Iodine (µg/d)	Iron (mg/d)	Magnesium (mg/d)	Molybdenum (µg/d)	Phosphorus (mg/d)	Selenium (µg/d)	Zinc (mg/d)
Infants																			
7–12 mo		9*									0.7			6.9					2.5
Children																			
1–3 y	100	11	210	13	5	0.4	0.4	5	0.4	120	0.7	260	65	3.0	65	13	380	17	2.5
4–8 y	100	15	275	22	6	0.5	0.5	6	0.5	160	1.0	340	65	4.1	110	17	405	23	4.0
Males																			
9–13 y	100	27	445	39	9	0.7	0.8	9	0.8	250	1.5	540	73	5.9	200	26	1,055	35	7.0
14–18 y	100	44	630	63	12	1.0	1.1	12	1.1	330	2.0	685	95	7.7	340	33	1,055	45	8.5
19–30 y	100	46	625	75	12	1.0	1.1	12	1.1	320	2.0	700	95	6	330	34	580	45	9.4
31–50 y	100	46	625	75	12	1.0	1.1	12	1.1	320	2.0	700	95	6	350	34	580	45	9.4
51–70 y	100	46	625	75	12	1.0	1.1	12	1.4	320	2.0	700	95	6	350	34	580	45	9.4
>70 y	100	46	625	75	12	1.0	1.1	12	1.4	320	2.0	700	95	6	350	34	580	45	9.4
Females																			
9–13 y	100	28	420	39	9	0.7	0.8	9	0.8	250	1.5	540	73	5.7	200	26	1,055	35	7.0
14–18 y	100	38	485	56	12	0.9	0.9	11	1.0	330	2.0	685	95	7.9	300	33	1,055	45	7.3
19–30 y	100	38	500	60	12	0.9	0.9	11	1.1	320	2.0	700	95	8.1	255	34	580	45	6.8
31–50 y	100	38	500	60	12	0.9	0.9	11	1.1	320	2.0	700	95	8.1	265	34	580	45	6.8
51–70 y	100	38	500	60	12	0.9	0.9	11	1.3	320	2.0	700	95	5	265	34	580	45	6.8
>70 y	100	38	500	60	12	0.9	0.9	11	1.3	320	2.0	700	95	5	265	34	580	45	6.8
Pregnancy																			
14–18 y	135	50	530	66	12	1.2	1.2	14	1.6	520	2.2	785	160	23	335	40	1,055	49	10.5
19–30 y	135	50	550	70	12	1.2	1.2	14	1.6	520	2.2	800	160	22	290	40	580	49	9.5
31–50 y	135	50	550	70	12	1.2	1.2	14	1.6	520	2.2	800	160	22	300	40	580	49	9.5
Lactation																			
14–18 y	160	60	885	96	16	1.2	1.3	13	1.7	450	2.4	985	209	7	300	35	1,055	59	10.9
19–30 y	160	60	900	100	16	1.2	1.3	13	1.7	450	2.4	1,000	209	6.5	255	36	580	59	10.4
31–50 y	160	60	900	100	16	1.2	1.3	13	1.7	450	2.4	1,000	209	6.5	265	36	580	59	10.4

Note: This table presents Estimated Average Requirements (EARs), which serve two purposes: for assessing adequacy of population intakes, and as the basis for calculating Recommended Dietary Allowance (RDAs) for individuals for those nutrients. EARs have not been established for vitamin D, vitamin K, pantothenic acid, biotin, choline, calcium, chromium, fluoride, manganese, or other nutrients not yet evaluated via the DRI process.

[a] For individual at reference weight (Table 1–1).

[b] As retinol activity equivalents (RAFs). 1 RAE = 1 µg retinol, 12 µg β-carotene, 24 µg α-carotene, or 24 µg β-cryptoxanthin. The RAE for dietary provitamin A carotenoids is two-fold greater than retinol equivalents (RE), whereas the RAE for preformed vitamin A is the same as RE.

[c] As α-tocopherol, α-Tocopherol includes *RRR*-α-tocopherol, the only form of α-tocopherol that occurs naturally in foods, and the *2R*-stereoisomeric forms of α-tocopherol (*RRR*-, *RSR*-, *RRS*-, and *RSS*-α-tocopherol) that occur in fortified foods and supplements. It does not include the *2S*-stereoisomeric forms of α-tocopherol (*SRR*-, *SSR*-, *SRS*-, and *SSS*-α-tocopherol), also found in fortified foods and supplements.

[d] As niacin equivalents (NE). 1 mg of niacin = 60 mg of tryptophan.

[e] As dietary folate equivalents (DFE). 1 DFE = 1 µg food folate = 0.6 µg of folic acid from fortified food or as a supplement consumed with food = 0.5 µg of a supplement taken on an empty stomach.

*indicates change from prepublication copy due to calculation error.

Source: Copyright © 2002 by the National Academy of Sciences. All Rights Reserved.

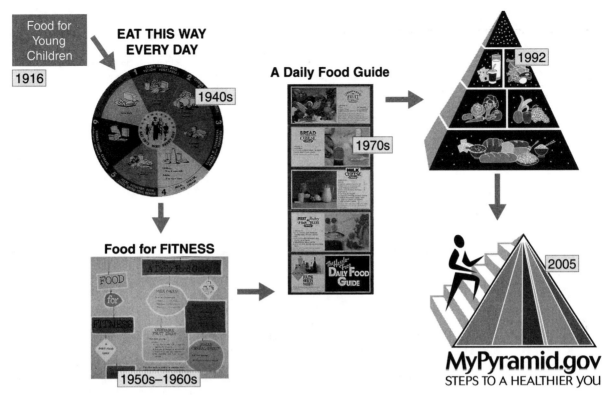

FIGURE 2-2 History of the USDA's food guidance system.
Source: From the USDA website, http://www.mypyramid.gov/downloads/MyPyramid.

TABLE 2-7 *Dietary Guidelines for Americans 2005*

Adequate Nutrients Within Calorie Needs	**Key Recommendations** • Consume a variety of nutrient-dense foods and beverages within and among the basic food groups while choosing foods that limit the intake of saturated and *trans* fats, cholesterol, added sugars, salt, and alcohol. • Meet recommended intakes within energy needs by adopting a balanced eating pattern, such as the USDA food guide (MyPyramid) or the DASH eating plan. **Key Recommendations for Specific Population Groups** • *People over age 50:* Consume vitamin B_{12} in its crystalline form (i.e., fortified foods or supplements). • *Women of childbearing age who may become pregnant:* Eat foods high in heme-iron or consume iron-rich plant foods or iron-fortified foods with an enhancer of iron absorption, such as vitamin C-rich foods. • *Women of childbearing age who may become pregnant and those in the first trimester of pregnancy:* Consume adequate synthetic folic acid daily (from fortified foods or supplements) in addition to food forms of folate from a varied diet. • *Older adults, people with dark skin, and people exposed to insufficient ultraviolet band radiation (i.e., sunlight):* Consume extra vitamin D from vitamin D-fortified foods or supplements.
Weight Management	**Key Recommendations** • To maintain body weight in a healthy range, balance calories from foods and beverages with calories expended. • To prevent gradual weight gain over time, make small decreases in food and beverage calories and increase physical activity.

(continued)

TABLE 2-7 *Dietary Guidelines for Americans 2005* (Continued)

Key Recommendations for Specific Population Groups
- *Those who need to lose weight:* Aim for a slow, steady weight loss by decreasing caloric intake while maintaining an adequate nutrient intake and increasing physical activity.
- *Overweight children:* Reduce the rate of body weight gain while allowing growth and development. Consult a health care provider before placing a child on a weight-reduction diet.
- *Pregnant women:* Ensure appropriate weight gain as specified by a health care provider.
- *Breastfeeding women:* Moderate weight reduction is safe and does not compromise weight gain of the nursing infant.
- *Overweight adults and overweight children with chronic diseases or on medication:* Consult a health care provider about weight-loss strategies prior to starting a weight-reduction program to ensure appropriate management of other health conditions.

Physical Activity

Key Recommendations
- Engage in regular physical activity and reduce sedentary activities to promote health, psychological well-being, and a healthy body weight.
  - To reduce the risk of chronic disease in adulthood, engage in at least 30 minutes of moderate-intensity physical activity, above usual activity, at work or home on most days of the week.
  - For most people, greater health benefits can be obtained by engaging in physical activity of more vigorous intensity or longer duration.
  - To help manage body weight and prevent gradual, unhealthy body weight gain in adulthood, engage in approximately 60 minutes of moderate- to vigorous-intensity activity on most days of the week while not exceeding caloric intake requirements.
  - To sustain weight loss in adulthood, participate in at least 60 to 90 minutes of daily moderate-intensity physical activity while not exceeding caloric intake requirements. Some people may need to consult with a health-care provider before participating in this level of activity.
- Achieve physical fitness by including cardiovascular conditioning, stretching exercises for flexibility, and resistance exercises or calisthenics for muscle strength and endurance.

Key Recommendations for Specific Population Groups
- *Children and adolescents:* Engage in at least 60 minutes of physical activity on most, preferably all, days of the week.
- *Pregnant women:* In the absence of medical or obstetric complications, incorporate 30 minutes or more of moderate-intensity physical activity on most, if not all, days of the week. Avoid activities with a high risk of falling or abdominal trauma.
- *Breastfeeding women:* Be aware that neither acute nor regular exercise adversely affects the mother's ability to successfully breastfeed.
- *Older adults:* Participate in regular physical activity to reduce functional declines associated with aging and to achieve the other benefits of physical activity identified for all adults.

Food Groups to Encourage

Key Recommendations
- Consume a sufficient amount of fruits and vegetables while staying within energy needs. Two cups of fruit and 2 ½ cups of vegetables per day are recommended for a reference 2000 calorie intake, with higher or lower amounts depending on the calorie level.
- Choose a variety of fruits and vegetables each day. In particular, select from all five vegetable subgroups (dark green, orange, legumes, starchy vegetables, and other vegetables) several times a week.
- Consume 3 or more ounce-equivalents of whole grain products per day, with the rest of the recommended grains coming from enriched or whole grain products. In general, at least half the grains should come from whole grains.
- Consume 3 cups per day of fat-free or low-fat milk or equivalent milk products.

Key Recommendations for Specific Population Groups
- *Children and adolescents:* Consume whole grain products often; at least half the grains should be whole grains. Children 2 to 8 years should consume 2 cups per day of fat-free or low-fat milk or equivalent milk products. Children 9 years of age and older should consume 3 cups per day of fat-free or low-fat milk or equivalent milk products.

Fats

Key Recommendations
- Consume less than 10% of calories from saturated fatty acids and less than 300 mg/day of cholesterol, and keep *trans* fatty acid consumption as low as possible.

- Keep total fat intake between 20 to 35% of calories, with most fats coming from sources of polyunsaturated and monounsaturated fatty acids, such as fish, nuts, and vegetable oils.
- When selecting and preparing meat, poultry, dry beans, and milk or milk products, make choices that are lean, low fat, or fat free.
- Limit intake of fats and oils high in saturated or *trans* fatty acids, and choose products low in such fats and oils.

Key Recommendations for Specific Population Groups
- *Children and adolescents:* Keep total fat intake between 30 to 35% of calories for children 2 to 3 years of age and between 25 to 35% of calories for children and adolescents 4 to 18 years of age, with most fats coming from sources of polyunsaturated and monounsaturated fatty acids, such as fish, nuts, and vegetable oils.

Carbohydrates

Key Recommendations
- Choose fiber-rich fruits, vegetables, and whole grains often.
- Choose and prepare foods and beverages with little added sugars or caloric sweeteners, such as amounts suggested by the USDA food guide (MyPyramid) and the DASH eating plan.
- Reduce the incidence of dental caries by practicing good oral hygiene and consuming sugar- and starch-containing foods and beverages less frequently.

Sodium and Potassium

Key Recommendations
- Consume less than 2300 mg (approximately 1 teaspoon) of sodium (salt) per day.
- Choose and prepare foods with little salt. At the same time, consume potassium-rich foods, such as fruits and vegetables.

Key Recommendations for Specific Population Groups
- *Individuals with hypertension, blacks, and middle-aged and older adults:* Aim to consume no more than 1500 mg of sodium per day, and meet the potassium recommendation (4700 mg/day) with food.

Alcoholic Beverages

Key Recommendations
- Those who choose to drink alcoholic beverages should do so sensibly and in moderation—defined as the consumption of up to one drink per day for women and up to two drinks per day for men.
- Alcoholic beverages should not be consumed by some individuals, including those who cannot restrict their alcohol intake, women of childbearing age who may become pregnant, pregnant and lactating women, children and adolescents, individuals taking medications that can interact with alcohol, and those with specific medical conditions.
- Alcoholic beverages should be avoided by individuals engaging in activities that require attention, skill, or coordination, such as driving or operating machinery.

Food Safety

Key Recommendations
- To avoid microbial foodborne illness:
  - Clean hands, food contact surfaces, and fruits and vegetables. Meat and poultry should not be washed or rinsed.
  - Separate raw, cooked, and ready-to-eat foods while shopping, preparing, or storing foods.
  - Cook foods to a safe temperature to kill microorganisms.
  - Chill (refrigerate) perishable food promptly and defrost foods properly.
  - Avoid raw (unpasteurized) milk or any products made from unpasteurized milk, raw or partially cooked eggs or foods containing raw eggs, raw or undercooked meat and poultry, unpasteurized juices, and raw sprouts.

Key Recommendations for Specific Population Groups
- *Infants and young children, pregnant women, older adults, and those who are immunocompromised:* Do not eat or drink raw (unpasteurized) milk or any products made from unpasteurized milk, raw or partially cooked eggs or foods containing raw eggs, raw or undercooked meat and poultry, raw or undercooked fish or shellfish, unpasteurized juices, and raw sprouts.
- *Pregnant women, older adults, and those who are immunocompromised:* Eat only deli meats and frankfurters that have been reheated to steaming hot.

MyPyramid

MyPyramid (Figure 2–3) was released by the USDA in April 2005 to replace the earlier Food Guide Pyramid, in a continuing effort to provide consumer-friendly diet-planning guidelines (USDA MyPyramid). The earliest of these guidelines were the Basic Four or Basic Seven Food Groups first released in the 1940s. All of these graphic-based guidelines were designed to help consumers choose daily food intake patterns that continue to meet current nutritional standards. MyPyramid

provides a basic guide to selecting a healthful diet based on the *Dietary Guidelines for Americans 2005* (USDHHS and USDA, 2005). Its key concepts combine moderate consumption of calories in addition to incorporating physical activity, which is the newest element in the symbol. Thirty minutes of physical activity is recommended for most days. In addition, more specific guidelines are noted regarding the types and amounts of foods to eat. In MyPyramid, there are 12 different pyramids recommending amounts to consume from each food group based on age, gender, and physical

Anatomy of MyPyramid

One size doesn't fit all
USDA's new MyPyramid symbolizes a personalized approach to healthy eating and physical activity. The symbol has been designed to be simple. It has been developed to remind consumers to make healthy food choices and to be active every day. The different parts of the symbol are described below.

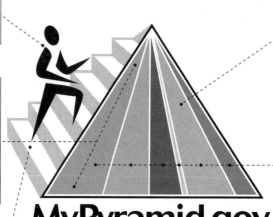

Activity
Activity is represented by the steps and the person climbing them, as a reminder of the importance of daily physical activity.

Moderation
Moderation is represented by the narrowing of each food group from bottom to top. The wider base stands for foods with little or no solid fats or added sugars. These should be selected more often. The narrower top area stands for foods containing more added sugars and solid fats. The more active you are, the more of these foods can fit into your diet.

Personalization
Personalization is shown by the person on the steps, the slogan, and the URL. Find the kinds and amounts of food to eat each day at MyPyramid.gov.

Proportionality
Proportionality is shown by the different widths of the food group bands. The widths suggest how much food a person should choose from each group. The widths are just a general guide, not exact proportions. Check the Web site for how much is right for you.

Variety
Variety is symbolized by the 6 color bands representing the 5 food groups of the Pyramid and oils. This illustrates that foods from all groups are needed each day for good health.

Gradual Improvement
Gradual improvement is encouraged by the slogan. It suggests that individuals can benefit from taking small steps to improve their diet and lifestyle each day.

MyPyramid.gov
STEPS TO A HEALTHIER YOU

USDA
U.S. Department of Agriculture
Center for Nutrition Policy
and Promotion
April 2005 CNPP-16

USDA is an equal opportunity provider and employer.

GRAINS   VEGETABLES   FRUITS   OILS   MILK   MEAT & BEANS

FIGURE 2–3   MyPyramid.
Source: From the USDA website, http://www.mypyramid.gov.

activity. Consuming the recommended amount from each food group provides most of the nutrients required daily.

The MyPyramid symbol is a simple triangular shape that additionally emphasizes the importance of physical activity in daily life by showing the person climbing the steps of the pyramid. There are also six color bands that represent the fat, sugar, and salt category, as well as the five food groups—grains are orange, vegetables are green, fruits are red, milk is blue, and meat and beans are purple. As the steps reach the top of the pyramid, the bands narrow, emphasizing the importance of eating in moderation. The wider part of the bands represents foods with little or no solid fats, added sugars, or caloric sweeteners. These foods should be selected more frequently to obtain the most nutrition from calories. Individuals can also receive personalized recommendations through the interactive technology provided on the MyPyramid.gov website. When consumed in the recommended amounts, the food groups represented in the pyramid provide almost all of the nutrients required for good health.

As an example, the following recommendations are based on a 2000 kilocalorie (kcal) diet (Table 2–8). How much from each food group do you need? The grain group represents breads, pasta, cereals, and rice. The recommended consumption is 6 ounces (six servings) every day from this group, with at least half from whole grains. This food group provides sources of simple and complex carbohydrates, trace elements, dietary fiber (in whole grain sources), and B vitamins. Enriched grain and cereal products provide consumers with a significant proportion of their B vitamin and trace element intake. Figure 2–4 shows sample MyPyramid recommendations for adults.

The fruits and vegetables groups likewise provide excellent sources of dietary fiber (if high-fiber sources are selected) as well as vitamin C, vitamin A, fiber, phytochemicals, and other nutrients. MyPyramid recommends consuming 2 1/2 cups of vegetables and 2 cups of fruit daily. It is also recommended to consume a variety

TABLE 2–8   *Standard Serving or Portion Sizes*

Food Group	*Amount Equaling 1 Serving*
Grain group	1 slice of bread $1/2$ bagel, English muffin 1 ounce of cold cereal $1/2$ cup of cooked cereal, rice, pasta 4 crackers
Vegetable group	1 cup of raw leafy greens 1 cup of cooked vegetables $1/2$ cup of vegetable juice 1 medium piece of vegetable (e.g., carrot)
Fruit group	1 medium piece of fruit (e.g., apple, pear) $1/2$ cup chopped or canned fruit $1/3$ cup of fruit juice
Milk, cheese group	1 cup of milk, yogurt 1 $1/2$ ounces cheese 1 $1/2$ cups of ice cream
Meat, poultry, fish, dried beans, eggs, nuts	2–3 oz cooked meat, fish, poultry 1 oz meat $1/2$ cup of cooked dry beans 1 egg 2 Tbsp. peanut butter

My Pyramid Plan

Based on the information you provided and the average needs for your age, gender and physical activity [Age: 25, Sex: female, Physical activity: Less than 30 Minutes] your results indicate that you should eat these amounts from the following food groups daily.

Your results are based on a 2000 calorie pattern*.

▶ Grains[1]	6 ounces
▶ Vegetables[2]	2.5 cups
▶ Fruits	2 cups
▶ Milk	3 cups
▶ Meat & Beans	5.5 ounces

[1] Make Half Your Grains Whole
Aim for at least 3 whole grains a day

[2] Vary Your Veggies
Aim for this much every week:

Dark Green Vegetables = 3 cups weekly
Orange Vegetables = 2 cups weekly
Dry Beans & Peas = 3 cups weekly
Starchy Vegetables = 3 cups weekly
Other Vegetables = 6 1/2 cups weekly

Oils & Discretionary Calories
Aim for 6 teaspoons of oils a day

Limit your extras (extra fats & sugars) to 265 Calories

*This calorie level is only an estimate of your needs. Monitor your body weight to see if you need to adjust your calorie intake.

FIGURE 2–4 Sample MyPyramid recommendations for adults.
Source: From the USDA website, http://www.mypyramid.gov.

of fruits and vegetables, especially dark green and orange vegetables, to receive all necessary nutrients. This food group also tends to be lower in caloric density than the other groups.

The dairy product group provides an excellent source of protein as well as calcium. Fortified dairy products may also contain added vitamins A and D. Individuals who are lactose intolerant can use lactose-reduced milk and cheese products. Newer products such as soy milk and cheese also fall into this group. The recommendation in MyPyramid is 3 cups of low-fat or fat-free milk, yogurt, and other milk products daily.

The meat and bean group includes animal and vegetable sources. Animal sources include meat, fish, poultry, game, and eggs. Vegetarian sources include nuts, beans, and tofu. This group provides essential protein as well as other nutrients, such as iron and zinc, depending on the source chosen. Animal protein products also provide vitamin B_{12}. Recommended consumption for a 2000 calorie diet is 5 $^1/_2$ ounces from the meat and bean group.

Fats, sugars, and salt, the final group, should be used only in limited amounts. This group includes fats such as margarine, butter, oil, cream cheese, and cream. It also includes ice cream, cakes, cookies, candy, and other snack foods, and baked products rich in fat and sugar. Consumers should try to obtain their fats primarily from fish, nuts, and vegetable oils, and to use sugars, fats, and salt judiciously in food preparation.

Eliminating one or more food groups, such as breads, grains, and cereals, as well as fruits and some vegetables to limit carbohydrate intake (e.g., as a weight-loss strategy) is inappropriate because each group provides certain essential nutrients not consistently available in the other food groups. Selection of lower calorie foods from all groups, in amounts necessary to meet each individual's needs, is the best strategy for any diet, weight management or otherwise. Figures 2–5 and 2–6 show how the U.S. actual consumption compares to recommendations for foundation foods and extras.

Food guide pyramids have been developed for a variety of special groups such as older adults

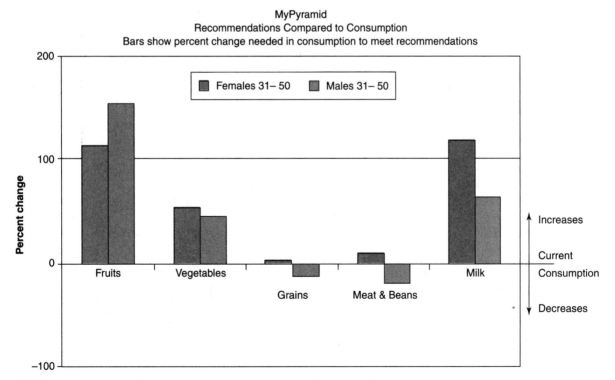

FIGURE 2–5   MyPyramid recommendations compared to U.S. consumption of food groups.

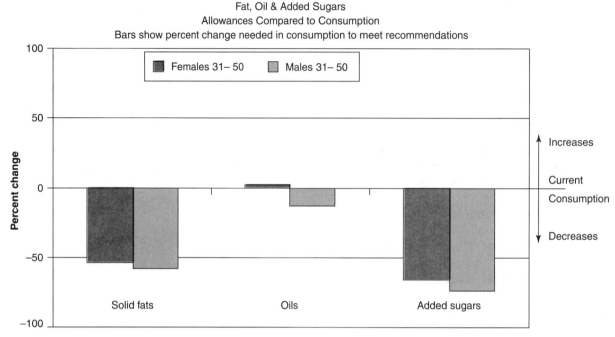

FIGURE 2–6 Recommendations of MyPyramid compared to consumption: fats, oils, added sugars.

(Chapter 19), children (Chapter 17), vegetarians (Chapter 5), and for a variety of ethnic groups.

The Canadian equivalent of MyPyramid is a crescent or rainbow (Figure 2–7). Canada also has food guides for children and older adults. Despite the way that the guidelines are graphically represented, all have the same purpose: they are to be used by the general public to provide nutrition education and diet guidance in terms that are understandable to most consumers.

Food pyramids provide not only a means for planning adequate diets with individuals and groups but also a quick assessment tool for health professionals and consumers to use to assess diet adequacy. Recalls of previous days' intake can be compared with the food pyramid. A pyramid-based diet evaluation can provide the practitioner and the patient with a broad qualitative assessment of diet adequacy or diet risk (see Chapter 22). Individuals lacking in any food groups (with the exception of fats, sweets, and oils) should be counseled to increase intake of that particu-

lar group. Those consuming large or frequent servings of foods from the fats, sugars, and salt group should be advised to increase their intake from the other, more nutritional groups, and decrease intake of foods from this group.

What Is a Serving?

MyPyramid recommends specific numbers of servings from each food group for various consumer age groups, and uses standardized portion sizes. This is important because the concept of a "serving" can have very different meanings from person to person. To a young weightlifter, a serving of steak may mean 16 ounces. To an older person with a declining appetite, a serving may mean one bite of hamburger. The portion sizes recommended in the pyramid are *standardized* portion sizes used universally in nutrition education, assessment, and labeling. Table 2–9 details the standard portion sizes. It is important that those using MyPyramid understand what "portion" or

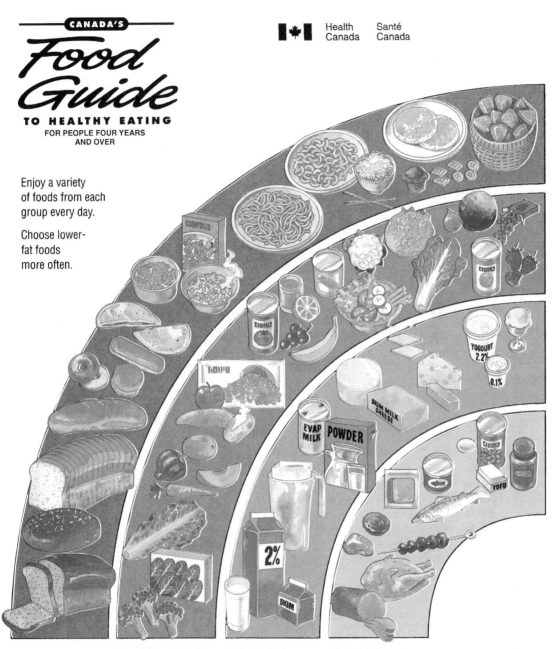

Health Canada   Santé Canada

Canada's Food Guide

TO HEALTHY EATING
FOR PEOPLE FOUR YEARS
AND OVER

Enjoy a variety
of foods from each
group every day.

Choose lower-
fat foods
more often.

Grain Products
Choose whole grain
and enriched
products more
often.

Vegetables & Fruit
Choose dark green and
orange vegetables and
orange fruit more often.

Milk Products
Choose lower-fat
milk products more
often.

Meat & Alternatives
Choose leaner meats,
poultry and fish, as well
as dried peas, beans and
lentils more often.

Canada

FIGURE 2–7 Canadian food guide.
Source: From Health Canada website, http://www.hc-sc.gc.ca.

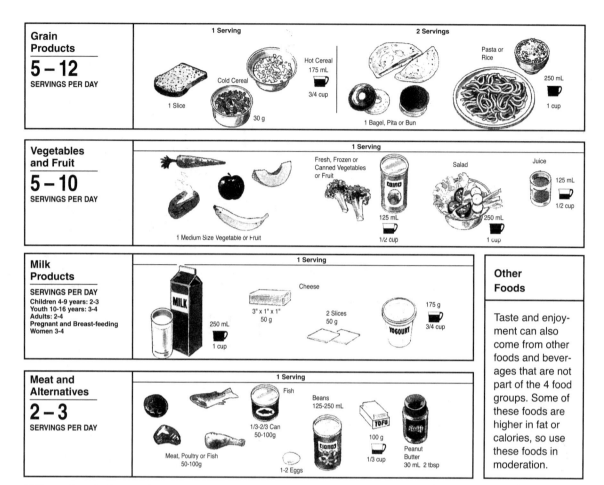

Grain Products

5 – 12 SERVINGS PER DAY

1 Serving — 1 Slice, Cold Cereal 30 g, Hot Cereal 175 mL 3/4 cup

2 Servings — 1 Bagel, Pita or Bun, Pasta or Rice 250 mL 1 cup

Vegetables and Fruit

5 – 10 SERVINGS PER DAY

1 Serving — 1 Medium Size Vegetable or Fruit; Fresh, Frozen or Canned Vegetables or Fruit 125 mL 1/2 cup; Salad 250 mL 1 cup; Juice 125 mL 1/2 cup

Milk Products

SERVINGS PER DAY
Children 4-9 years: 2-3
Youth 10-16 years: 3-4
Adults: 2-4
Pregnant and Breast-feeding Women 3-4

1 Serving — MILK 250 mL 1 cup; Cheese 3" x 1" x 1" 50 g; 2 Slices 50 g; Yogourt 175 g 3/4 cup

Meat and Alternatives

2 – 3 SERVINGS PER DAY

1 Serving — Meat, Poultry or Fish 50-100g; Fish 1/3-2/3 Can 50-100g; 1-2 Eggs; Beans 125-250 mL; Tofu 100 g 1/3 cup; Peanut Butter 30 mL 2 tbsp

Other Foods

Taste and enjoyment can also come from other foods and beverages that are not part of the 4 food groups. Some of these foods are higher in fat or calories, so use these foods in moderation.

Different People Need Different Amounts of Food

The amount of food you need every day from the four food groups and other foods depends on your age, body size, activity level, whether you are male or female, and if you are pregnant or breast-feeding. That's why the Food Guide gives a lower and higher number of servings for each food group. For example, young children can choose the lower number of servings, while male teenagers can go to the higher number. Most other people can choose servings somewhere in between.

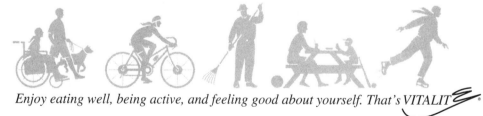

Enjoy eating well, being active, and feeling good about yourself. That's VITALIT®

FIGURE 2–7 (Continued)

TABLE 2–9   How Much from Each Food Group Do You Need?

MyPyramid recommends the amount of food to be consumed from each food group based on kilocalories needed for nutrition, physical activity, and lifestyle behavior. The energy required by the demands of the body depends on age, gender, weight, and physical activity level.

Based on a 2000 kilocalorie intake per day, the following are recommendations from each food group.

- Fruits—2 cups of fresh, canned, or frozen
- Vegetables—2$\frac{1}{2}$ cups of raw or cooked
- Dairy—3 cups of fat-free or low-fat milk or equivalent milk products
- Grains—6 oz (3 oz from whole grain products and the remaining amount from enriched or whole grain products)
- Meat and beans—5$\frac{1}{2}$ oz from lean meats and poultry; also attempt to eat more fish, beans, peas, nuts, and seeds

"serving" means, so that they do not misinterpret their own diet quality. For example, one slice of bread is considered a serving so a sandwich would contain *two servings* of the bread group. The weightlifter's portion of steak would be four 4 oz. servings of meat. Table 2–10 shows sample calories provided by food group choices.

Dietary Guidelines to Address Specific Conditions or Health Risks

American Heart Association Dietary Guidelines

The American Heart Association (AHA) has published dietary guidelines that are designed to help consumers eat a heart-healthy diet. The AHA guidelines are more specific than the *Dietary Guidelines for Americans* in terms of amounts and types of foods that will reduce risk of heart disease. These guidelines recommend that:

1. Total fat intake should be no more than 30% of total calories.
2. Saturated fatty acid intake should be 8 to 10% of total calories.
3. Polyunsaturated fatty acid intake should be up to 10% of total calories.
4. Monounsaturated fatty acids should make up to 15% of total calories.
5. Cholesterol intake should be less than 300 milligrams (mg) daily.
6. Sodium intake should be less than 2400 mg daily, which is about 1-$\frac{1}{4}$ teaspoons of salt.
7. Carbohydrates should make up 55 to 60% or more of total calories, with emphasis on increasing sources of complex carbohydrates.
8. Total calories should be adjusted to achieve and maintain a healthy body weight.

TABLE 2–10   Sample Calories Provided from MyPyramid Food Choices

Sample Calories in Recommended Servings from MyPyramid	
Recommended Servings	*Average Calories and Range of Possible Calories Depending on Choices*
2 cups fruit	240 calories (100–300)
2$\frac{1}{2}$ cups vegetables	125 calories (60–400)
5 servings of whole grains	420 calories (420–660)
3 servings of low-fat dairy products	300 calories (240–360)
5 ounces of lean meats, fish, beans, nuts	300 calories (200–510)
5 teaspoons oils	200 calories (160–215)
	Total Calories: 1585 (1180–2445)

Source: Adapted from Ayoob KT: Presentation to the New Hampshire Dietetic Association Annual Meeting, February 9, 2005, Rochester, NH.

The following calculations demonstrate how to use these guidelines to design a heart-healthy diet.

Assume the total day's calorie requirement is 2000 kcals:

$$60\% \text{ of kcal from CHO} = .60 \times 2000$$
$$= 1200 \text{ kcal from CHO or}$$
$$300g \text{ of CHO } (1200 \text{ kcal/4 kcal/g})$$

$$30\% \text{ of kcal from fat} = .30 \times 2000$$
$$= 600 \text{ kcal from fat or}$$
$$67g \text{ of fat } (600 \text{ kcal/9 kcal/g})$$

$$10\% \text{ of kcal from protein} = .10 \times 2000$$
$$= 200 \text{ kcal from protein or}$$
$$50g \text{ of protein } (200 \text{ kcal/4 kcal/g})$$

Consumers can then use food composition tables or diabetic-type exchange lists to determine what food choices and portions fit into this pattern.

American Cancer Society Diet Guidelines

The American Cancer Society offers four basic nutrition guidelines designed to reduce the risk of various forms of cancer (American Cancer Society, 1999). They are:

- **Choose most of the foods you eat from plant sources**. Fiber-rich foods such as fruits, vegetables, whole grains, and legumes are loaded with antioxidants, phytochemicals, vitamins, and minerals known to reduce the risk of cancer.
- **Limit your intake of high-fat foods, particularly from animal sources**. High-fat diets have been associated with an increased risk of cancers of the colon, rectum, prostate, and endometrium.
- **Be physically active: achieve and maintain a healthy weight**. Research confirms that small spurts of activity can add up to real health benefits.
- **Limit consumption of alcoholic beverages, if you drink at all**. Alcohol consumption increases the risk of cancer of the mouth, esophagus, pharynx, larynx, and liver in men and women, and breast cancer in women, according to the guidelines. A new general recommendation within the guidelines says reducing alcohol consumption is a good way for women who drink regularly to reduce their risk of breast cancer.

Dietary Approaches to Stop Hypertension (DASH) Eating Plan

The DASH eating plan was devised by the National Heart, Lung, and Blood Institute (NHLBI) of the National Institutes of Health (NIH) to help people reduce their blood pressure. The DASH diet plan was tested in a multicenter clinical trial and was found to result in significant reductions in blood pressure in the group who followed the eating plan. The DASH eating plan contains about 3000 mg of sodium a day (about half of average American intake), is low in saturated fat, cholesterol, and total fat, and emphasizes fruits, vegetables, and low-fat dairy foods. It is also low in red meat, sweets, and sugar-containing beverages, and high in magnesium, potassium, calcium, protein, and fiber. The DASH daily diet plan for a 2000 calorie diet is as follows:

Grains and grain products	6–8 servings/day
Vegetables	4–5 servings/day
Fruits	4–5 servings/day
Low-fat dairy foods	2–3 servings/day
Meat, poultry, fish	2 or fewer servings/day
Fats and oils	2–3 servings/day
Nuts, seeds, dry beans	4–5 servings/week
Sweets	5 servings/week

The Concept of Nutrient Density

The concept of nutrient density is useful in diet planning because it highlights the nutritional value of foods in relationship to the calories provided. Some foods such as salad greens are packed with vitamins and minerals, but provide few calories. These foods are considered high-nutrient-density, low-calorie foods. Other foods such as candy bars or pie have relatively few nutrients in relation to the calories they provide. These are categorized as low-nutrient-density, high-calorie foods. Compare a piece of custard pie to a half-ounce of cheddar cheese. A piece of custard pie provides 110 mg of calcium and 250 calories, whereas a half-ounce of cheddar cheese provides 102 mg of calcium and only 60 calories. The cheddar cheese provides about the same calcium, but only a quarter the calories of the pie.

When trying to maintain a nutritious diet within reasonable calorie limits, individuals should choose primarily high-nutrient-density, low-calorie foods and avoid foods that are calorie packed and provide little nutritional value. Individuals with limited appetites, such as some elderly and cancer patients, also need to learn to consume the greatest nutritional value into the smallest food volume. "Empty calorie" foods that may satisfy their appetite should be avoided because they provide calories but little, if any, nutritive value (e.g., cakes, cookies, candy). Figure 2–8 shows how foods can differ in nutrient density versus caloric density.

The nutrient content and nutrient density of many foods eaten away from home may not be evident to consumers who fail to consult restaurant food information materials. For example, in some fast-food restaurants the chocolate shake contains more sodium than french fried potatoes. A fish sandwich may be quite high in fat and calories because the fish is breaded and fried.

Food Composition Tables

Standardized food composition tables have been developed by many organizations from data provided by industry, universities, and governmental agencies. These tables are available in the form of written manuals (Pennington, Spungen, 2004), on the Internet (USDA Nutrient Database), and by contract (University of Minnesota Nutrient Database) using standardized nutrient profiles of large numbers of fresh and packaged foods. Such tables do not take into consideration nutrient bioavailability, however. *Bioavailability* refers to the absorption of consumed nutrients by the body. Bioavailability can be affected by a large number of factors including individual nutrient status, presence of inhibitors or enhancers of absorption, and other health-related factors. The new computer diet assessment programs such as MyPyramid provide personalized diet assessment based on such data.

Food Labels: Aids to Wise Food Choices

The U.S. Food and Drug Administration (FDA) has taken some of the mystery out of planning a healthful diet by requiring detailed food labels on foods and beverages (Figure 2–9), and maintaining strict

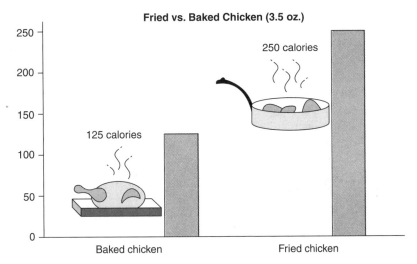

FIGURE 2–8 How foods differ in caloric density.

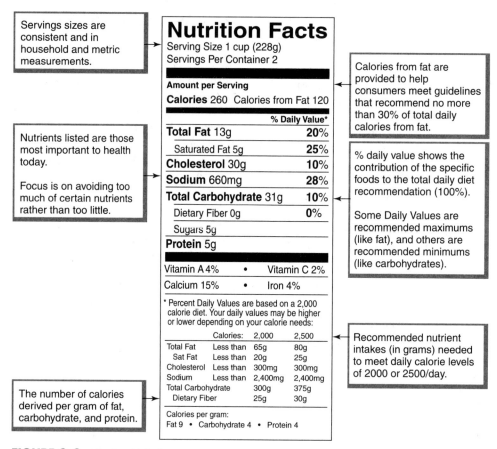

Servings sizes are consistent and in household and metric measurements.

Nutrients listed are those most important to health today.

Focus is on avoiding too much of certain nutrients rather than too little.

The number of calories derived per gram of fat, carbohydrate, and protein.

Nutrition Facts

Serving Size 1 cup (228g)
Servings Per Container 2

Amount per Serving

Calories 260 Calories from Fat 120

	% Daily Value*
Total Fat 13g	**20%**
Saturated Fat 5g	**25%**
Cholesterol 30g	**10%**
Sodium 660mg	**28%**
Total Carbohydrate 31g	**10%**
Dietary Fiber 0g	**0%**
Sugars 5g	
Protein 5g	

Vitamin A 4%	•	Vitamin C 2%
Calcium 15%	•	Iron 4%

* Percent Daily Values are based on a 2,000 calorie diet. Your daily values may be higher or lower depending on your calorie needs:

		Calories:	2,000	2,500
Total Fat	Less than		65g	80g
Sat Fat	Less than		20g	25g
Cholesterol	Less than		300mg	300mg
Sodium	Less than		2,400mg	2,400mg
Total Carbohydrate			300g	375g
Dietary Fiber			25g	30g

Calories per gram:
Fat 9 • Carbohydrate 4 • Protein 4

Calories from fat are provided to help consumers meet guidelines that recommend no more than 30% of total daily calories from fat.

% daily value shows the contribution of the specific foods to the total daily diet recommendation (100%).

Some Daily Values are recommended maximums (like fat), and others are recommended minimums (like carbohydrates).

Recommended nutrient intakes (in grams) needed to meet daily calorie levels of 2000 or 2500/day.

FIGURE 2–9 The food label.

Source: From http://www.cfsan.fda.gov/~dms/foodlab.html#twoparts.

guidelines over the use of health claims and terms such as "light," "natural," and "fat free" (U.S. FDA website). If the manufacturer wishes to label a product "light" or "low fat," for example, the product must meet specific content requirements. These are shown in Figure 2–10. If the product meets the criteria for low fat, the label may state "this product is low in fat. A diet low in fat may reduce the risk of some cancers." Certain health claims are also allowed on food labels if the product meets specified criteria. Table 2–11 lists the currently authorized health claims. Both the Food Safety and Inspection Service (FSIS), a part of the USDA, and the FDA, a part of the USDHHS, oversee food labeling. The FSIS regulates meat and poultry labeling, whereas the FDA regulates all other labeling of food products and ingredients added to foods. Under this last

category are foods with added nutrients or botanicals, such as products with added vitamins, minerals, or herbs.

Foods exempt from nutrition labeling include plain coffee, tea, most spices, restaurant foods, foods prepared in food stores and restaurants and sold to consumers (e.g., bakery, deli, and fast-food products), as well as foods in very small packages. However, they must include the manufacturer phone number for product information.

All food product labels must include:

* product name, net contents, name and address of manufacturer, ingredient labeling and the "Nutrition Facts" panel (nutrient content) on the label (Clydesdale, 1999).

REDUCED – LESS – FEWER...

Foods labeled with these claims must contain at least 25 percent less of the nutrient than the reference food. This applies equally to calories, sodium, fat, saturated fat, cholesterol, and total sugars.

HIGH

Calls attention to the beneficial nutrients found in foods.

The nutrient must make up 20% or more of the Daily Value of a single reference serving.

LIGHT

Allowed on foods that have been reduced in fat by at least 50% when compared to a reference food that derives 50% or more of its calories from fat
– or –
Allowed on foods that have been reduced in fat by 50% or in calories by 1/3 when compared to a reference food that derives fewer than 50% of calories from fat.

Light in sodium.............. 50% reduction in sodium
Light in color....... permitted if adequately described

FREE

Nutritionally insignificant, can be labeled as zero

Sodium free........................... less than 5mg
Calorie free...................... less than 5 calories
Sugar free................. less than 0.5g total sugars
Fat free............................... less than 0.5g
Saturated fat free*...................... less than 0.5g
Cholesterol free**......... 2mg or less of saturated fat

*not more than 1% of grams of total fat from trans fatty acids.
**foods containing more than 13g total fat per reference amount must show fat content per serving.

LOW

Allows frequent consumption of a food w/o exceeding recommended dietary guidelines

Low sodium..................... not more than 140mg
Low calorie................. not more than 40 calories
Low fat.............................. not more than 3g
Low saturated fat........... not more than 1g and not more than 15% calories from saturated fat
Low cholesterol............. not more than 20mg per 50g if serving size is small

---

FIGURE 2-10 Criteria for using certain terms on labels.

TABLE 2-11 FDA-Authorized Health Claims on Labels

* Calcium and osteoporosis
* Sodium and hypertension (high blood pressure)
* Dietary fat and cancer
* Dietary saturated fat and cholesterol and the risk of coronary heart disease
* Fiber-containing grain products, fruits, and vegetables, and cancer
* Fruits, vegetables, and grain products that contain fiber, particularly soluble fiber, and risk of coronary heart disease
* Fruits and vegetables and cancer
* Folate and neural tube birth defects
* Dietary sugar alcohol and dental caries (cavities)
* Dietary soluble fiber, such as that found in whole oats and psyllium seed husk, and coronary heart disease
* Soy protein and coronary heart disease
* Plant sterols and plant stanol esters and coronary heart disease

- ingredients listed in descending order of content in the product (by ingredient weight from greatest to least). Ingredient lists must include contents of color additives, sources of protein hydrolysates, casienate (a milk product in products that may be nondairy), and the percentage of juice in products claiming to have vegetable or fruit juice.

A Nutrition Facts panel is required on food labels and provides specific nutrient data based on a mean of the DRIs for adults with calorie requirements of 2000 calories per day. Information required on the Nutrition Facts panel includes:

- nutrient information for a typical serving of the product (including portion size) and number of servings for the package (serving sizes are standardized).
- calories per serving.
- calories per serving from fat followed by grams of fat (total and saturated), and of carbohydrate (grams of sugar), dietary fiber, and protein.
- sodium and cholesterol in milligrams (mg) per serving.

The percent daily value for 2000 calorie reference diets is listed for vitamins A and C, calcium, and iron, as well as fat, cholesterol, sodium, total carbohydrate, and dietary fiber. The percent daily value can be used to compare food products to one another to determine how the food serving fits into the reference diet based on its nutrient content (Clydesdale, 1999).

Here are a few key pointers about what you'll find under **Nutritional Information:**

INGREDIENTS: WHOLE WHEAT, WHEAT BRAN, SUGAR, SALT, MALT, THIAMIN HYDROCHLORIDE, PYRIDOXINE HYDROCHLORIDE, FOLIC ACID, REDUCED IRON, BHT.

NUTRITION INFORMATION
PER 30G
SERVING CEREAL
(175mL, 3/4 CUP)

ENERGY	Cal	100
	kJ	420
PROTEIN	g	3.0
FAT	g	0.6
CARBOHYDRATE		24.0
SUGARS	g	4.4
STARCH	g	16.6
FIBRE	g	3.0
SODIUM	mg	265
POTASSIUM	mg	168

PERCENTAGE OF RECOMMENDED DAILY INTAKE

THIAMIN	%	46
NIACIN	%	6
VITAMIN B6	%	10
FOLACIN	%	8
IRON	%	28

- **Serving Size** tells you the size of serving for which the nutrition information is given. If you eat more or less than this amount, remember that the calories and the content of other nutrients like fat and sodium increase or decrease as well!

When food is packaged as a single serving, the nutrition information is given for the single serving portion.

- **Energy** is the calories (Cal) per serving. Energy is also given in kilojoules (kJ).

- **Fat** shows the total amount of fat in food. Some products also give the content of various kinds of fat: polyunsaturates, monounsaturates, saturates and cholesterol. However, to choose lower fat foods more often, the most useful information is the grams of total fat.

- **Carbohydrate** includes the content of sugars, starch and fibre. In this example you get a complete breakdown of carbohydrate. Sometimes you get information on one type of carbohydrate only.

- **Sodium** is a measure of the amount of salt in a food.

- **Percentage Recommended Daily Intake** is the way which vitamins and minerals are listed. If you are interested in any one nutrient, the information may be useful to you.

FIGURE 2-11 Canadian food label.
Source: From http://www.hc-sc.gc.ca/fn-an/alt_formats/hpfb-dgpsa/pdf/label-etiquet/cr_tearsheet-cr_fiche_e.pdf.

A major value of food labels is that the consumer can read the label and determine how the particular food product fits into overall diet recommendations. This is particularly useful when attempting to stay within specific limits for calories, fat, or sodium. For example, if only one serving of a food contains 50% of the daily recommendation for fat, the rest of the day's intake will have to be very low in fat or risk being in excess of the recommendation. The Canadian food label also has set requirements (shown in Figure 2–11). As of 1994, the FDA set requirements for food supplement labels as well

(Figure 2–12)(USDHHS and FDA, 2005). These are detailed in Chapter 10.

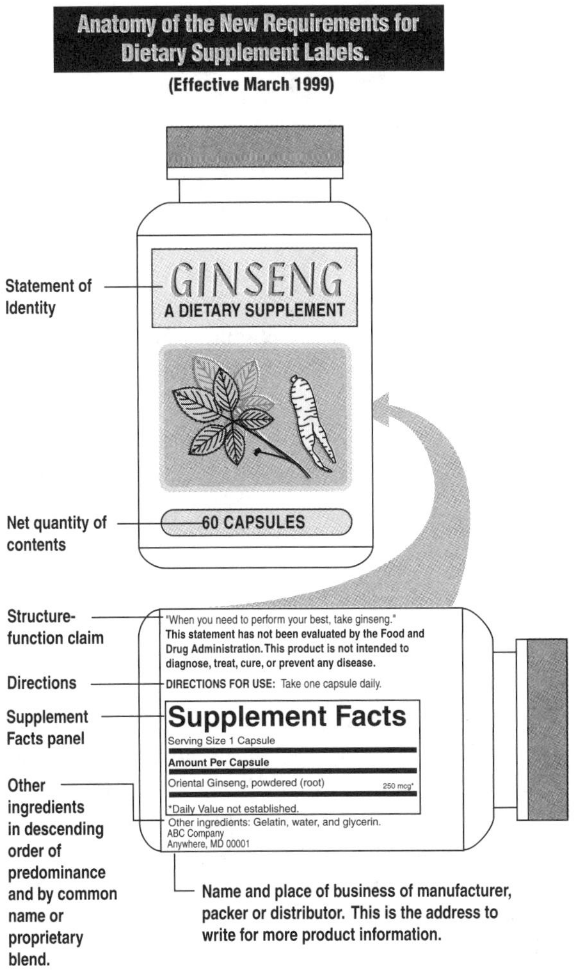

BEYOND NUTRIENTS: EMERGING SCIENCE ON FOODS AND HEALTH

Hippocrates said, *"Let food be thy medicine and medicine be thy food."* Recent years have seen an explosion of research on health effects of foods that go beyond the effects of the traditional macro- and micronutrients required for basic health. Areas of research range from basic research on the effects of phytochemicals and antioxidants in health promotion and disease prevention, to the manipulation of food composition via genetic engineering, to the personalization of foods and diets to meet individual needs. These new areas of nutrition science are reviewed below.

Antioxidants

Antioxidants are compounds that protect cells from excessive oxidation, and include Vitamins C and E, beta-carotene, copper, manganese, and selenium. Oxygen is essential for life; more than 95% of the majority of the oxygen we breathe is used by mitochondria for energy production. However, a small percentage of oxygen taken in (1 to 3%) is used to synthesize "reactive oxygen species" or "free radicals." These free radicals are generated as part of oxygen metabolism, and also can result from exogenous sources such as smoking, radiation, and air pollution. These include superoxide radical (O_2), and hydrogen peroxide (H_2O_2). Free radicals are reactive chemical species with one or more unpaired electrons. When they come into contact with metal ions like iron and copper, they become a highly reactive free radical, the hydroxyl radical (OH^-), which will attack and damage all areas of the human body, altering their structure or function. The body makes some free radicals for useful purposes, such as to kill bacteria and funguses (Halliwell, 2002).

Oxidative Stress

In the healthy human body, the production of free radicals is carefully controlled. Antioxidants function to deactivate these free radicals. The body has built-in

Anatomy of the New Requirements for Dietary Supplement Labels.
(Effective March 1999)

GINSENG — A DIETARY SUPPLEMENT

- Statement of Identity
- Net quantity of contents — 60 CAPSULES
- Structure-function claim
- Directions
- Supplement Facts panel
- Other ingredients in descending order of predominance and by common name or proprietary blend.
- Name and place of business of manufacturer, packer or distributor. This is the address to write for more product information.

FIGURE 2–12 U.S. supplement label.
Source: From http://vm.cfsar.fda.gov/~acrobat/fdsuppla.pdf.

antioxidant defense systems, such as superoxide dismutase enzymes. In addition, antioxidants are available in the diet. However, when there are defects in this protective process such as in disease or aging, the free radicals may overwhelm the normal protective mechanisms and cause great damage. The imbalance between free radicals and antioxidant protective mechanism is often termed "oxidative stress." Oxidative stress can result from increased production of free radicals such as from toxins, cigarette smoke or disease, or from decreased availability of antioxidants such as in malnutrition.

Oxidative stress can result in oxidative damage to all cells and can interfere with cell metabolism. Particularly severe oxidative stress can cause cell death. Although there is a question whether oxidative stress is an early or late event in degenerative conditions, there is good evidence that it is an early event in atherosclerosis and some cancers, and is a key player in the tissue injury of chronic inflammatory disease. It has been suggested that the aging process is involved with the deterioration of cell mitochondria, some of which involves oxidative damage.

In addition to O_2, nitric oxide (NO) is also a free radical, which has useful roles in the body. However, when overproduced, it can cause tissue damage. Overproduction has been implicated in chronic inflammatory diseases, septic shock, and neurodegenerative diseases. When nitric oxide and O_2 are overproduced, they can interact. The O_2/NO interaction is considered an explanation of the low-density lipoprotein (LDL) oxidation seen in early atherosclerotic lesions.

Thus, oxidative stress results from the production of harmful free radicals from exposure to environmental factors such as sunlight, pollution, and smoking, or from the body itself. When stress overcomes the body's defense mechanisms, the resulting cell damage is thought to contribute to chronic conditions of aging such as cancer, infections, heart disease, cataracts, and macular degeneration.

How Antioxidants Work

Antioxidants attack and scavenge the free radicals, protecting cellular components from being destroyed. The body's antioxidant system is made of enzymes (superoxide dismutase, glutathione peroxidase), vitamins, minerals, and other compounds. Several vitamins and minerals have proven antioxidant abilities either directly or as a component of antioxidant enzyme systems. Vitamins C and E, and beta-carotene are independent antioxidants. The trace minerals copper, manganese, and selenium are essential components of protective antioxidant enzyme systems. These antioxidants not only function directly as antioxidants, but they also work with each other. Vitamin C helps reactivate vitamin E after it has neutralized free radicals. Selenium is a backup for vitamin E in scavenging free radicals. High dietary consumption of polyunsaturated fats increases the requirement for antioxidants to protect the fat from free radical damage. Diets high in polyunsaturated fats and low in antioxidants may result in increased cancer risk caused from increased free radical formation.

The epidemiologic links between antioxidant nutrients and disease are based primarily upon dietary intakes or blood levels that result from food choices rather than supplements (Rock et al.). A major problem in interpreting the epidemiologic data is that foods rich in antioxidants, such as fruits and vegetables, also have other constituents such as phytates, flavenoids, and some carotenoids, which may also exert effects (Halliwell, 2002).

Several major chemopreventive trials using antioxidant micronutrients have been completed and *do not* support the widespread use of antioxidant nutrient *supplements* to prevent cancer. In one large Finnish trial of male smokers averaging in their 50s, intake of 20 mg/day of synthetic beta-carotene over 5 to 8 years was associated with an 18% *increase* in lung cancer, and vitamin E supplements had no effect. However, serum and dietary alpha-tocopherol (vitamin E) and beta-carotene at baseline were inversely related to risk of lung cancer during the trial (Virtamo et al., 2003). The Carotene and Retinol Efficacy Trial (CARET) was halted when the cancer incidence in the treatment group was 28% higher than in controls (Goodman et al., 2004). In Linxian, China, combinations of 15 mg synthetic beta-carotene, 50 micrograms (μg) of selenium, and 30 mg of vitamin E daily for 5 to 6 years resulted in reduced incidence of cancers of the upper gastrointestinal (GI) tract in undernourished adults. Cancer mortality and total mortality were both reduced by 10 to 13% in the study population (Blot et al., 1993).

In summary, the evidence to date indicates a protective effect of a variety of food antioxidants. However, there is a lack of good, randomized, controlled clinical trials on the effects of supplements. Thus, the recommendation should be to increase dietary intake of antioxidants via antioxidant-rich foods. Eating high-antioxidant-containing foods or merely doubling the intake of fruits and vegetables can raise the antioxidant power of the blood from 13 to 25% (Cao, Booth, Sadowski, Prior, 1998).

Phytochemicals

In addition to the usual nutrients known to be involved in normal metabolism, plant foods contain many other natural, nonnutritive compounds, some of which have newly recognized health effects. These compounds are called phytochemicals. There are hundreds or even thousands of phytochemicals found in fruits, vegetables, and some herbs. Phytochemicals are biologically active substances in plants that give plants their color, odor, flavor, and defense systems. They have also recently been associated with protection against chronic diseases such as heart disease, cancer, diabetes, and hypertension. Research on these food components is in its infancy, but many of these compounds show great promise in enhancing the value of certain foods beyond just their nutrient composition. Most phytochemicals are heat-stable and not lost by cooking in water. The majority of active phytochemicals in grain products are in the bran and germ, so whole grains should be consumed. The best way to get the protective benefits of the myriad food phytochemicals is to eat a diet rich in fruits, vegetables, and whole grains. Scientists believe that it is the combined effects of phytochemicals in whole food that provides the most benefit. This synergism does not take effect when one phytochemical is isolated and provided in supplement form. Consuming concentrated extracts of fruits and vegetables containing very high levels of phytochemicals is not recommended because activity and side effects of these forms are not known.

Functional Foods

Alfred E. Newman stated, *"We are living in a world today where lemonade is made from artificial flavors and furniture polish is made from real lemons."* *Functional food* is a generic term for any food, modified food, or food ingredient that may provide a health benefit beyond the traditional nutrients it contains (Backgrounder, 1998; Clydesdale, 1999). These foods have also been called *nutraceuticals, pharmafoods*, and *designer foods*. See Tables 2–12 and 2–13. Even natural foods could be considered functional foods because they contain phytochemicals. For example, broccoli, carrots, and tomatoes are rich in physiologically active components such as sulforaphane, beta-carotene, and lycopene, respectively. Herbals, and foods that have been modified or fortified with additional nutrients, phytochemicals, and/or herbals, would also be considered functional foods. In addition, functional foods include foods fortified and marketed as dietary supplements such as cereal bars with added gingko biloba and candies with added zinc and echinacea. Food biotechnology will continue to provide new venues for functional food development (American Dietetic Assoc., 2004).

Because *functional foods* is not a legal term, many of the so-named products have sprung merely from marketing ingenuity (American Dietetic Assoc., 2000). The unprecedented increase in consumer interest in the health benefits of foods and their components has often outpaced the scientific evidence to support many of the claims made (Anderson, Milner, 2004). Today, the nutraceutical market is approximately $86 billion and growing steadily (International Food Information Council [IFIC], 2004).

Functional foods may be categorized as:

* Whole foods that have been associated with reduced risk of disease.
* Food components for which there is evidence of a diet–disease relationship.
* Foods that have been fortified to increase the level of a specific nutrient or food component that has been associated with prevention or treatment of a disease or other clinical condition.

Functional foods were introduced earlier in the 20th century, when iodine was added to salt to prevent

TABLE 2-12 Categories of Functional Foods

Category	Examples
Whole foods that have been associated with reduced risk of disease	• Fruits and vegetables and reduced risk of certain cancers • Fermented dairy products with bacteria (probiotics) that improve gastrointestinal health • Cruciferous vegetables (cabbages, brussels sprouts, broccoli) and reduced cancer risk • Cranberry juice and reduced risk of bacteriuria
Food components for which there is evidence of a diet–disease relationship	• Lycopene in tomatoes and reduced risk of cancers • Polyphenols in tea, associated with cancer prevention and reduced serum cholesterol • Soluble fiber and reduced risk of heart disease • Sterol and stanol esters and reduced risk of heart disease • Omega-3 fatty acids in fatty fishes and reduced serum cholesterol
Foods that have been fortified to increase the level of a specific nutrient or food	• Calcium-fortified orange juice for bone health • Fiber-supplemented snack bars for GI health • Folate-enriched grain products to help prevent neural tube defects and high homocysteine levels • Stanol or sterol-enriched margarine for heart health

Source: Adapted from Functional Foods; Policy statement of the American Dietetic Association, 2004.

TABLE 2-13 Sample Functional Food Components, Their Potential Benefit, and the Strength of the Supporting Evidence

Class/Components	Srength of Evidence	Food Source*	Potential Benefit
Carotenoids			
Beta-carotene	Strong	Carrots, various fruits	Neutralizes free radicals that may damage cells; bolsters cellular antioxidant defenses
Lutein, Zeaxanthin	Weak to moderate	Kale, collards, spinach, corn, eggs, citrus	May contribute to maintenance of healthy vision
Lycopene	Moderate	Tomatoes and processed tomato products	May contribute to maintenance of prostate health
Dietary (functional and total) Fiber			
Insoluble fiber	Strong	Wheat bran	May contribute to maintenance of a healthy digestive tract
Beta glucan**		Oat bran, rolled oats, oat flour	May reduce risk of coronary heart disease (CHD)
Soluble fiber**		Psyllium seed husk	May reduce risk of CHD
Whole grains**		Cereal grains	May reduce risk of CHD and cancer; may contribute to maintenance of healthy blood glucose levels
Fatty Acids			
Monounsaturated fatty acids (MUFAs)	Moderate	Tree nuts	May reduce risk of CHD
Polyunsaturated fatty acids (PUFAs)—Omega-3 fatty acids—ALA	Moderate	Walnuts, flax	May contribute to maintenance of mental and visual function
PUFAs—Omega-3 fatty acids—DHA/EPA	Strong	Salmon, tuna, marine and other fish oils	May reduce risk of CHD; may contribute to maintenance of mental and visual function

PUFAs—Conjugated linoleic acid (CLA)	Weak	Beef and lamb; some cheese	May contribute to maintenance of desirable body composition and healthy immune function
Flavonoids			
Anthocyanidins		Berries, cherries, red grapes	Bolster cellular antioxidant defenses; may contribute to maintenance of brain function
Flavonols	Moderate	Onions, apples, tea, broccoli	Neutralize free radicals that may damage cells; bolster cellular antioxidant defenses
Proanthocyanidins		Cranberries, cocoa, apples, strawberries, grapes, wine, peanuts, cinnamon	May contribute to maintenance of urinary tract health and heart health
Isothio`cyanates			
Sulforaphane	Weak to moderate	Cauliflower, broccoli, broccoli sprouts, cabbage, kale, horseradish	May enhance detoxification of undesirable compounds and bolster cellular antioxidant defenses
Plant Stanols/Sterols			
Free Stanols/Sterols[**]	Strong	Corn, soy, wheat, wood oils, fortified foods and beverages	May reduce risk of CHD
Stanol/Sterol esters[**]		fortified table spreads, stanol ester dietary supplements	May reduce risk of CHD
Polyols			
Sugar alcohols—xylitol, sorbitol, mannitol, lactitol	Strong	Some chewing gums and other food applications	May reduce risk of dental caries
Prebiotic/Probiotics			
Inulin, Fructo-oligosaccharides (FOS), Polydextrose	Moderate	Whole grains, onions, some fruits, garlic, honey, leeks, fortified foods and beverages	May improve gastrointestinal health; may improve calcium absorption
Lactobacilli, Bifidobacteria		Yogurt, other dairy and non-dairy applications	May improve gastrointestinal health and systemic immunity
Phytoestrogens			
Isoflavones—Daidzein, Genistein	Moderate	Soybeans and soy-based foods	May contribute to maintenance of bone health, healthy brain and immune function; for women, maintenance of menopausal health
Lignans		Flax, rye, some vegetables	May contribute to maintenance of heart health and healthy immune function
Soy Protein			
Soy Protein[**]	Strong	Soybeans and soy-based foods	May reduce risk of CHD
Sulfides/Thiols			
Diallyl sulfide, Allyl methyl trisulfide	Weak to Moderate	Garlic, onions, leeks, scallions	May enhance detoxification of undesirable compounds; may contribute to maintenance of heart health and healthy immune function
Dithiolthiones		Cruciferous vegetables	Contribute to maintenance of healthy immune function

[**]Examples are not an all-inclusive list.
[**]FDA approved health claim established for component.
Source: Adapted from http://ific.org © 2005 International Food Information Council Foundation and Functional Foods: Position of the American Dietetic Association, 2004.

goiter, vitamin D was added to milk to prevent rickets, and refined white flour was "enriched" with some of the vitamins and minerals removed during processing.

In 1993, when the FDA ruled that foods high in certain nutrients, such as calcium, could put health claims on their labels, manufacturers began increasing these beneficial nutrients in their products. They added nutrients to products that did not normally contain them (e.g., calcium in orange juice, calcium-fortified waffles, psyllium-fortified grain products, antioxidant-fortified juices, and vitamin-fortified candy). Researchers are also developing more potentially healthful foods through genetic engineering (e.g., high-phytochemical broccoflower and tomato products with more beta-carotene). However, there are no special labeling laws for these products and they merely must abide by the FDA's food and supplement labeling laws. Recently, some food-specific health claims have been allowed. Oat cereal may state that "soluble fiber from oatmeal, as part of a low saturated fat, low cholesterol diet, may reduce the risk of heart disease." Cranberry juice may state the ability of cranberries to "combat urinary tract infections." The claims allowed by the FDA are strictly controlled. However, in 1994, when Congress allowed structure or function claims for dietary supplements, food manufacturers also started making such claims. So instead of making a health claim, functional food makers make claims that a food can affect body structure or function, which do not have to be approved by the FDA.

Some of these products have sound scientific foundation (calcium-fortified orange juice to help prevent osteoporosis, and folate-fortified flour to help prevent birth defects). However, others are misleading in their purported benefits (orange drinks with calcium provide only sugar, water, and calcium), unproven (many of the herbs), or potentially harmful (again, some herbs). Unlike drugs or food additives, the ingredients in functional foods do not have to be tested to prove if they are safe. Also, adding a healthful ingredient does not make a good food out of a poor one, especially if the same or equal ingredients can be obtained at less cost from foods that are full of other nutrients as well. For example, fortified potato chips are still high in salt and fat.

Also, each food is a unique system with nutrients and other components in specific relationship to one another. When the components of the whole foods are isolated and provided individually and in different doses, they may not have the same effects. Additionally, it is impossible to tell the quality and standardization of the active ingredients in the product, the form of the ingredients, or their actual efficacy.

Food Biotechnology: Genetically Engineered Foods

The latest in food biotechnology represents an evolution in agricultural methods. Genetically engineered food sources include select potatoes, tomatoes, and some soy and rapeseed (canola) oil foods. Future technology crops may include other fruits, grains, and vegetables (Davis, Shields, 2000; Pelletier, 2005). Crop improvement is a potential benefit of genetically enhanced or modified foods. As scientists identify genes responsible for individual food traits, those genes can be added to specific plants or crops to enhance foods. The FDA, USDA, and Environmental Protection Agency (EPA), as well as local and state government agencies, are working to ensure genetically engineered food safety. These food crops must meet the same FDA standards as other food crops.

Regulation of food biotechnology is changing. Practitioners are encouraged to stay current on the products available as well as regulation of the products. Credible, scientifically sound websites include the FDA Center for Food Safety and Applied Nutrition (http://vm.cfsan.fda.gov/~lrd/biotechm.html), the International Food Policy Research Institute (http://www.cgiar.org/ifpri/index1.htm), and the National Agricultural Biotechnology Council (http://www.cals.cornell.edu/extension/nabc/).

Nutritional Genomics: The New Frontier (Jackson, 2004)

Nutritional genetics, also known as nutrigenetics, is the area of research focused on the effects of individual gene variations on individual nutritional needs. To simplify communications around the connection between these two areas of research, they are often combined under the heading of *nutritional genomics*. This field has far-reaching potential in the future prevention of diet-related diseases; as more genetic information about individuals becomes available, there will be parallel progress in understanding how certain food components influence metabolic pathways, and subsequent long-term disease risk. From this information should develop improved therapeutic outcomes for treating existing disease and preventing disease. Nutritional genomics research is focusing upon identifying gene–diet interactions, determining the underlying mechanisms, and validating the tools developed. The following concepts provide the basis for nutritional genomic research (DeBusk, Fogarty, Ordovas, Kornman, 2005):

- Under certain circumstances and in some individuals, diet can be a serious risk factor for a number of diseases.
- Common dietary chemicals can act on the human genome (directly or indirectly) to alter gene expression or structure.
- The degree to which diet influences the balance between healthy and disease states may depend upon a person's genetic makeup.
- Some diet-modulated genes are likely to play a role in the onset, incidence, progression, and/or severity of chronic diseases.
- Dietary intervention based on knowledge of nutritional requirement, nutritional status, and genotype (e.g., personalized nutrition) can be used to prevent, mitigate, or cure chronic diseases.

The conditions that will benefit from nutritional genomic research and applications are chronic disorders like cardiovascular disease, cancers, diabetes, obesity, osteoporosis, and neurological and inflammatory disorders. In response to this research, genetic tests associated with nutritional solutions are already being sold in the marketplace. It is likely that the nutritional supplement and functional food industry will respond robustly with new products. Also, many of the nutrigenomics products now and in the future are being sold directly to the consumer. Health care providers need to be vigilant in researching the strength of the evidence before embracing such products, and be prepared to provide guidance to consumers or patients to help them navigate the marketplace because many of them will explore the options irrespective of the initial advice they may receive from a health care provider. An excellent review article (Kauwell, 2005) lists the various resources available on the Web and offers an excellent

overview of genetics concepts and their intersection with nutrition.

Here are some guidelines to consider when evaluating products and programs:

- Ensure the product can be supported with at least two confirmatory studies that demonstrate genetic associations with health risk and nutritional requirements and are published in peer-reviewed journals.
- Ensure the commercial company producing and distributing the tests and associated nutritional products has a sufficient commitment to the privacy of an individual's genetic information.
- Evaluate the nature of the recommended nutritional solutions or products to ensure they are practical and recommendations are made within the context of a healthy diet.
- If the company is providing nutritional supplements, find out how it can ensure consistency in quality and effectiveness of its products.

CONCLUSION

A variety of sound guidelines are available to help foster healthy eating habits. These guidelines range from detailed information on human nutrition requirements for various nutrients (DRIs) to suggestions for making wise food choices (MyPyramid).

New and exciting research on possible health-promoting effects of vitamins, antioxidants, phytochemicals, and enhanced foods make these products highly enticing to consumers. They appeal to the desire for longevity and good health. Unfortunately, promoters often capitalize on these consumer desires by promoting and selling products long before their benefits have been proven. Indeed, in many cases, it is only after consumers have used these products that their harmful effects appear. Sometimes it is too late.

Consumers should be guided:

- To get antioxidants and phytochemicals from foods rather than supplements (except for vitamin E and possibly vitamin C).
- Not to take individual phytochemicals. Evidence of beneficial effects is scant, and doses and safety are unknown.

- To know that functional foods are not the answer to health. Some are an improvement over the original product; however, many are not.
- To evaluate the source of the information. Is it from a credible source? Is the claim justified by science? Is it based on many studies or just one?
- That the best approach is a varied diet of whole foods, rich in fruits, vegetables, whole grains, legumes, and low-fat dairy products.

The conscientious clinician needs to point out to patients that the most prudent nutritional security is a diet that adheres to MyPyramid and is generous in fruits and vegetables, with a focus on natural, less-processed food choices, as well as awareness of one's own unique nutritional needs in relation to food preferences and lifestyle (for example, iron needs for women, and high-quality protein sources for vegetarians). The use of a daily multivitamin supplement is also a good idea. On the other hand, self-supplementing on compounds with unproven effects can be expensive and useless at best, and may cause serious harm (see Chapter 10). Always use reliable resources for research updates.

SUMMARY AND IMPLICATIONS FOR DENTISTRY

The dental health professional should consider it his or her role to conduct diet or nutrition risk assessment relative to general and oral health, to provide diet education relative to oral disease management, and to refer patients to RDs for medical nutrition therapy. In addition, every oral health professional needs to understand the principles underlying basic diet adequacy and to be able to provide diet education relevant to oral and overall health. The dietary guidelines and MyPyramid provide a mechanism for such guidance. Familiarity with current concepts such as functional foods and food biotechnology will enable health professionals to address patient questions and provide meaningful guidance. The dental team should develop professional relationships with local RDs to facilitate referrals of patients who need further nutrition care (see Chapters 22, and 23 for information on diet screening and assessment and nutrition resources).

QUESTIONS PATIENTS MIGHT ASK

Q. Aren't the RDAs fairly useless because of the focus on the minimum human requirements rather than what people actually need to be healthy?

A. No, this is a common misconception. The RDAs are actually the best judgment of actual requirements for health. Most are based upon the average requirement for health (not minimum) plus a margin of safety to allow for individual variation. The RDAs are revised often, precisely because our knowledge about the types and amounts of nutrients needed to be healthy increases rapidly.

Q. Because my life is so hectic, isn't it best just to take vitamin supplements and not worry about the food choices on a daily basis?

A. No, this is *not* a good idea! Supplements do not provide all of the substances needed for health. Supplements do not provide carbohydrates, proteins, fats, fiber, or phytochemicals. Many of the studies on diet and health show associations between various *foods* and health. It is not always clear what constituents of the food have the beneficial effects. Supplements are meant as just that— supplements to a good foundation diet, not substitutes for a good diet.

REFERENCES

American Cancer Society: *ACS Nutritional Guidelines.* 1999. Retrieved October 12, 2005, from http://cancer.org/docroot/NWS/content/NWS_5_1x_ACS_Nutrition_Guidelines.asp

American Dietetic Association: Nutrition and you: Trends 2000. Retrieved January 2000 from http://www.eatright.org/pr/2000/010300e.html

American Dietetic Association: Position of the American Dietetic Association: Functional foods. *J Am Diet Assoc.* 2004; 104(5): 814–26.

American Heart Association: Dietary guidelines for healthy american adults. Retrieved from http://www. americanheart.org

Anderson P, Milner J (eds): Highlights of ILSI Functional Foods Meeting: Reports from the Special Conference on

Functional Foods for Health Promotion: Making Sense of the Science. *Nutr Today* 2004; 39(3):122–127.

Backgrounder: Functional foods. In *Food Insight Media Guide*. Washington, DC: International Food Information Council Foundation, 1998.

Blot WJ, Li JY, Taylor PR, Guo W, Dawsey S, Wang GQ, et al.: *Natl Cancer Inst* 1993; 85(18):1483–92.

Cao G, Booth SL, Sadowski JA, Prior RL: Increases in human plasma antioxidant capacity after consumption of controlled diets high in fruit and vegetables. *Am J Clin Nutr* 1998; 68:1081–87.

Cao G, Russell RM, Lischner S, Prior RL: Serum antioxidant capacity is increased by consumption of strawberries, spinach, red wine or vitamin C in elderly women. *J Nutr* 1998; 128:2383–90.

Clydesdale FM: ILSI North America Food Component Reports. *Crit Rev Food Sci Nutr* 1999; 33(3):203–316.

Craig, WJ: Phytochemicals: Guardians of our health. *J Am Diet Assoc* 1997; 97(10):S199–S204.

Davis S, Shields J: Food biotechnology: Can you answer these consumer questions? *Educators Resource* 2000; 35:8–9.

DeBusk M, Fogarty, Ordovas, M, Kornman, K: Nutritional genomics in practice: Where do you begin? *J Am Diet Assoc* 2005; 105(4):589–98.

U.S. Department of Health and Human Services, Food and Drug Administration: 21 CFR Part 101 [Docket No. 98N-0044] RIN 0910-AB97. *Regulations on Statements Made for Dietary Supplements Concerning the Effect of the Product on the Structure or Function of the Body.* AGENCY: Food and Drug Administration, HHS.ACTION: Final rule.

Goodman GE, Thornquist MD, Balmes J, Cullen MR, Meyskens FL Jr, Goodman, et al.: The beta-carotene and retinol efficacy trial: Incidence of lung cancer and cardiovascular disease mortality during 6-year follow-up after stopping beta-carotene and retinol supplements. *J Natl Cancer Inst* 2004; 96(23):1729–31.

Halliwell B: Why and how should we measure oxidative DNA damage in nutritional studies? How far have we come? [Review] *Am J Clin Nutr* 2000, 72(5):1082–87.

Halliwell B: Antioxidant defence mechanisms: From the beginning to the end (of the beginning). [Review] *Free Radical Res* 1999–2000; 31(4):261–72.

Halliwell B: Effect of diet on cancer development: Is oxidative DNA damage a biomarker? [Review] *Free Radical Biol & Med* 2002; 32(10):968–74.

Institute of Medicine, National Academy of Sciences: *Dietary Reference Intakes for Calcium, Phosphorus, Magnesium, Vitamin D, and Fluoride.* Washington, DC: National Academies Press, 1997.

Institute of Medicine, National Academy of Sciences: *Dietary Reference Intakes for Energy, Carbohydrate, Fiber, Fat,* *Fatty Acids, Cholesterol, Protein, and Amino Acids (Macronutrients).* Washington, DC: National Academies Press, 2005.

Institute of Medicine, National Academy of Sciences: *Dietary Reference Intakes for Thiamin, Riboflavin, Niacin, Vitamin B_6, Folate, Vitamin B_{12}, Pantothenic Acid, Biotin, and Choline.* Washington, DC: National Academies Press, 1998.

Institute of Medicine, National Academy of Sciences: *Dietary Reference Intakes for Vitamin C, Vitamin E, Selenium, and Carotenoids.* Washington, DC: National Academies Press, 2000.

Institute of Medicine, National Academy of Sciences: *Dietary Reference Intakes for Water, Potassium, Sodium, Chloride, and Sulfate.* Washington, DC: National Academies Press, 2004.

International Food Information Council: Functional foods. May 2004. Retrieved from http://www..ific.org/nutrition/functional/index.cfm

Jackson, K: Pioneering the frontier of nutrigenomics. *Todays Dietitian.* 2004:34–37.

Kauwell, GP: Emerging concepts in nutrigenomics: A preview of what is to come. *Nutr Clin Pract* 2005; 20: 75–87.

Lin B-H, Frazão E, Guthrie J: Food and Drug Administration, *Away-from-Home Foods Increasingly Important to the Quality of the American Diet.* Community Nutrition Institute. CNI report February 19, 1999. 4–5.

National Research Council, Subcommittee on the 10th edition of the RDAs, Food and Nutrition Board, Commission on Life Sciences: *Recommended Dietary Allowances,* 10th ed. Washington, DC: National Academy Press, 1989.

Pelletier, DL: Science, law, and politics in the Food and Drug Administration's genetically engineered foods policy: FDA's 1992 Policy Statement. *Nutr Rev* 2005; 63(5):171–181.

Pennington, JA, Spungen, Douglass J: *Bowes & Church's Food Values of Portions Commonly Used*, 18th ed. Baltimore: Williams Wilkins, 2004.

Rock C: Dietary Reference Intakes, antioxidants, and beta carotene. *J Am Diet Assoc* 1998; 98(12):1410–11.

Standing Committee on the Scientific Evaluation of Dietary Reference Intakes and Its Panel on Dietary Antioxidants and Related Compounds: *Dietary Reference Intakes: Proposed Definition and Plan for Review of Dietary Antioxidants and Related Compounds.* Washington, DC: National Academies Press, 1998.

University of Minnesota Nutrient database, http://www.ncc.umn.edu/ABOUTNCC.htm

U.S. Department of Health and Human Services and U.S. Department of Agriculture: *Dietary Guidelines for Americans 2005*, 6th edition. Washington, DC: U.S. Government Printing Office, 2005.

USDA Nutrient database, http://www.nal.usda.gov/fnic/foodcomp/

USDA MyPyramid, http://www.MyPyramid.gov

U.S. Food and Drug Administration, http:///www.FDA.gov

Virtamo J, Pietinen P, Huttunen JK, Korhonen P, Malila N, Virtanen MJ, et al.: ATBC Study Group. Incidence of cancer and mortality following alpha-tocopherol and beta-carotene supplementation: A postintervention follow-up. *JAMA* 2003; 290(4):476–85.

Yates AA, Schlicker SA, Suitor CW: Dietary Reference Intakes: The new basis for recommendations for calcium and related nutrients, B vitamins and choline. *J Am Diet Assoc* 1998; 98(6):699–706.

Chapter **3**

Energy Balance and Weight Control

Jennifer Weston and Johanna T. Dwyer,
with the assistance of Jennifer Eveland

OBJECTIVES

The student will be able to:
- Describe the factors affecting energy balance and how to determine energy needs.
- Understand the components of body weight and how body fat and its distribution are measured.
- Discuss the characteristics of various weight-loss methods, both healthful and unhealthful.
- Understand the consequences of both underweight and overweight on oral and on general health.

INTRODUCTION

Attaining and maintaining optimal weight is a challenge for many people. After remaining relatively stable from 1960 to 1980 in the United States, the prevalence of obesity essentially doubled from 15% in 1980 to 30% in 2000 (Flegal, 2002). Currently, 65% of the U.S. population is either overweight or obese. About 34% of the population is overweight as defined by having a body mass index (BMI) between 25 to 29, and about 31% are defined as obese, having a BMI of 30. Table 3–1 shows the BMI charts. Today, obesity is even more common in minority populations (Flegal, 2002). Approximately 1% of the adult population is moving into the obese category every year, and many more are becoming overweight (Ogden, Flegal, Carroll, Johnson, 2002).

In 2000, poor diet (including obesity) and physical inactivity were found to be the second leading causes of preventable deaths in the United States. These factors accounted for 400,000 U.S. deaths (more than 16% of all deaths) (Ali, 2004). Obesity accounts for $100 billion in health care expenses per year; about 5.5 to 7.8% of all U.S. health care costs; lost productivity due to days lost from work; and increased disability (Kortt, 1998; Wolf, 1998).

Underweight can have serious side effects as well, especially among the elderly, the ill, and those on highly restrictive diets. Both underweight and obesity (particularly severe obesity) are associated with increased mortality when compared to those in a healthy weight range. There were over 111,000 excess deaths from obesity and 34,000 excess deaths due to underweight in 2004 (Flegal, 2005). Most of the obesity-related deaths were due to diseases made worse by excess weight. At least some of the deaths connected to underweight were due to underlying health problems that caused weight loss. This chapter reviews the factors that influence energy balance, describes how to determine energy needs, reviews the factors that contribute

TABLE 3–1 Body Mass Index Chart

BMI	19	20	21	22	23	24	25	26	27	28	29	30	31	32	33	34	35	36
	Normal						*Overweight*					*Obese*						
Height (inches)							*Body Weight (pounds)*											
58	91	96	100	105	110	115	119	124	129	134	138	143	148	153	158	162	167	172
59	94	99	104	109	114	119	124	128	133	138	143	148	153	158	163	168	173	178
60	97	102	107	112	118	123	128	133	138	143	148	153	158	163	168	174	179	184
61	100	106	111	116	122	127	132	137	143	148	153	158	164	169	174	180	185	190
62	104	109	115	120	126	131	136	142	147	153	158	164	169	175	180	186	191	196
63	107	113	118	124	130	135	141	146	152	158	163	169	175	180	186	191	197	203
64	110	116	122	128	134	140	145	151	157	163	169	174	180	186	192	197	204	209
65	114	120	126	132	138	144	150	156	162	168	174	180	186	192	198	204	210	216
66	118	124	130	136	142	148	155	161	167	173	179	186	192	198	204	210	216	223
67	121	127	134	140	146	153	159	166	172	178	185	191	198	204	211	217	223	230
68	125	131	138	144	151	158	164	171	177	184	190	197	203	210	216	223	230	236
69	128	135	142	149	155	162	169	176	182	189	196	203	209	216	223	230	236	243
70	132	139	146	153	160	167	174	181	188	195	202	209	216	222	229	236	243	250
71	136	143	150	157	165	172	179	186	193	200	208	215	222	229	236	243	250	257
72	140	147	154	162	169	177	184	191	199	206	213	221	228	235	242	250	258	265
73	144	151	159	166	174	182	189	197	204	212	219	227	235	242	250	257	265	272
74	148	155	163	171	179	186	194	202	210	218	225	233	241	249	256	264	272	280
75	152	160	168	176	184	192	200	208	216	224	232	240	248	256	264	272	279	287
76	156	164	172	180	189	197	205	213	221	230	238	246	254	263	271	279	287	295

Source: Adapted from National Heart, Lung, and Blood Institute, 1998.

to body weight, and discusses the dynamics of appropriate and inappropriate weight management.

ENERGY METABOLISM

Energy needs, energy output, and the energy potential from foods are measured in kilocalories (1000 calories), usually abbreviated simply as *calories*. A *calorie* is the energy needed to raise the temperature of 1 kilogram of water at a specified temperature by 1 degree Celsius (or 1.8 degrees Fahrenheit). Foods provide the energy needed for the body.

Energy Sources

Energy needs are met by consuming the energy-yielding nutrients: carbohydrates, proteins, and fats, as well as by alcoholic beverages. Carbohydrates (sugar and starch) and protein each provide 4 cal/gram, alcohol provides 7 cal/gram, and fat yields 9 cal/gram when metabolized

(after adjusting for absorption and other factors). Water, dietary fiber, vitamins, and minerals do not provide any food energy (IOM, 2005).

The calories provided by a given food are determined by the food's composition. A food composition table such as the USDA Nutrient Database for Standard Reference (http://nal.usda.gov/fnic/foodcomp/Data/SR17/sr17.html) is useful to determine the caloric contribution of a food. Total calories may also be calculated from the food's nutrient components if they are known. For example, if an 8 oz. glass of whole milk is comprised of 12 g carbohydrate, 8 g protein, 8 g fat, and 216 g water, it will provide 152 calories:

$$216 \text{ g water} \times 0 \text{ kcal/g} = 0 \text{ calories}$$
$$12 \text{ g carbohydrate} \times 4 \text{ cal/g} = 48 \text{ calories}$$
$$8 \text{ g protein} \times 4 \text{ kcal/g} = 32 \text{ calories}$$
$$+ 8 \text{ g fat} \times 9 \text{ kcal/g} = \pm 72 \text{ calories}$$
$$244 \text{ g TOTAL} = \textbf{152 calories}$$

								Extreme Obesity										
37	38	39	40	41	42	43	44	45	46	47	48	49	50	51	52	53	54	
								Body Weight (pounds)										
177	181	186	191	196	201	205	210	215	220	224	229	234	239	244	248	253	258
183	188	193	198	203	208	212	217	222	227	232	237	242	247	252	257	262	267
189	194	199	204	209	215	220	225	230	235	240	245	250	255	261	266	271	276
195	201	206	211	217	222	227	232	238	243	248	254	259	264	269	275	280	285
202	207	213	218	224	229	235	240	246	251	256	262	267	273	278	284	289	295
208	214	220	225	231	237	242	248	254	259	265	270	278	282	287	293	299	304
215	221	227	232	238	244	250	256	262	267	273	279	285	291	296	302	308	314
222	228	234	240	246	252	258	264	270	276	282	288	294	300	306	312	318	324
229	235	241	247	253	260	266	272	278	284	291	297	303	309	315	322	328	334
236	242	249	255	261	268	274	280	287	293	299	306	312	319	325	331	338	344
243	249	256	262	269	276	282	289	295	302	308	315	322	328	335	341	348	354
250	257	263	270	277	284	291	297	304	311	318	324	331	338	345	351	358	365
257	264	271	278	285	292	299	306	313	320	327	334	341	348	355	362	369	376
265	272	279	286	293	301	308	315	322	329	338	343	351	358	365	372	379	386
272	279	287	294	302	309	316	324	331	338	346	353	361	368	375	383	390	397
280	288	295	302	310	318	325	333	340	348	355	363	371	378	386	393	401	408
287	295	303	311	319	326	334	342	350	358	365	373	381	389	396	404	412	420
295	303	311	319	327	335	343	351	359	367	375	383	391	399	407	415	423	431
304	312	320	328	336	344	353	361	369	377	385	394	402	410	418	426	435	443

Energy Balance

When energy intake and energy needs (as measured by energy output) are in balance over a long period (i.e., weeks or months—not days) body weight stays constant and the body is said to be in a state of *energy balance* (Frary, Johnson, 2004). See Table 3–2 for an explanation of energy balance.

Weight gains or losses are states of *energy imbalance*. The body is in *positive energy balance* when extra energy consumed is stored as fat or glycogen (the body's storage form of carbohydrate) or used to meet growth needs. A person is in *negative energy balance* when energy needs exceed energy supplies (regardless of the reason). Causes of negative energy balance may include disease (which may decrease energy intake and raise energy output due to fever), excessive physical activity (which increases energy output over intake), malabsorption, and decreased caloric intake (due to fasting, weight-loss diet, eating disorder, or disease-induced anorexia) (Alpert, 1990). Negative energy balance causes weight loss, which may include losses of various proportions of lean tissue, fat, and water. For example, temporary weight loss unrelated to energy balance occurs when body water losses are excessive, as they are in dehydration, excessive sweating, or even high-protein low-carbohydrate diets. Total fasting for days or weeks causes excessive losses of lean tissue, water, and fat. The body's lean cells are largely water. Water comprises 50–60% of most normal adults' total body weight (Pitts, 1959, 1974). Healthful reducing diets result in losses that are predominantly fat, while maintaining nutritional status in other respects.

Factors Contributing to Energy Requirements

Three basic factors that usually contribute the most to an individual's total energy needs are:

- Resting energy expenditure (REE) (sometimes referred to as resting metabolic rate [RMR] or basal metabolic rate [BMR])
- Energy expended in physical activity and arousal (EEPAA)
- Thermic effect of food (TEF)

In adults, the REE and the EEPAA account for the vast majority of the energy requirements. The TEF accounts for very little of total energy requirements (Food and Agriculture Organization of the United Nations [FAO], 2004).

Resting Energy Expenditure (REE)

REE is the major component of energy output, and accounts for about 60–75% of daily energy expenditure. REE is the energy expended when lying in bed awake (without moving or eating) for 24 hours. It is the energy used by the body when at rest to maintain essential life functions such as respiration, circulation, organic compound synthesis, ion exchange across cell membranes, central nervous system function, excretion of waste, and so on. These functions usually produce enough heat to maintain body temperature at normal levels in typical environments. Organs that have large metabolic demands, such as the liver, gut, brain, kidney, and heart, have the highest energy requirements per gram of tissue. In a lean adult, the activity of organs accounts for approximately 75% of resting energy expenditure, even though the organs constitute only 10% of total body weight. Adipose tissue (fat) consumes less than 5% of resting metabolic rate although it usually accounts for 20% or more of body weight (North American Association for the Study of Obesity [NAASO], 2004). Resting skeletal muscle consumes only 20% of resting metabolic rate, but represents about 40% of total body

---

TABLE 3–2 The Balance of Energy

Energy Balance: [Calorie Intake = Calorie Output] → Weight Stability
Most people should be in relative energy balance over periods of weeks, months, etc.

Energy Imbalance
Positive Energy Balance: [Calorie Intake > Calorie Output] → Weight Increases
Circumstances when individuals are in positive energy balance include growth, pregnancy, lactation, when building muscle mass, fat deposition, when rebuilding glycogen stores.
Negative Energy Balance: [Calorie Intake < Calorie Output] → Weight Decreases
Circumstances when individuals are in negative energy balance include intentional weight loss, hypocaloric dieting, starvation, undernutrition, fasting, wasting diseases (cancer, AIDS), excessive exercise, malabsorption, excessive vomiting or diarrhea, restrictive eating disorders.

weight. Skeletal muscles use even more energy during activity and after activity when they are repleting their glycogen stores.

Body heat production can be measured to determine REE directly by means such as direct calorimetry chambers or indirectly using metabolic carts to measure the amount of oxygen consumed and carbon dioxide expelled at rest. However, in clinical situations, a more practical approach is to estimate REE using developed formulas.

A variety of factors can affect REE. Fevers and some wasting diseases (such as some cancers and AIDS) cause increased energy output or losses of energy-providing nutrients resulting in increased REE. Fever disrupts mechanisms in the hypothalamus of the brain that regulate temperature and increases REE by about 7% Fahrenheit (F) (or 13% Celsius [C]) for each degree increase in body temperature above normal (98.6 degrees F or 37 degrees C). REE increases during normal growth periods such as during childhood and adolescence when lean muscle mass is increasing. Resting energy expenditure tends to decrease as adults age, due to the decline in the amount of lean tissue. Females, older adults, and malnourished individuals have a lower REE than males, younger adults, and healthy people. Starvation and, to a lesser extent, hypocaloric diets (a diet lower in calories than one's requirements) result in decreased lean body mass and associated decreased REE. Some diseases such as hypothyroidism also result in decreased REE, but these conditions are relatively rare. Table 3–3 lists factors that may affect REE.

Energy Expenditure for Physical Activity and Arousal (EEPAA)

Physical activity is a major and largely controllable component of energy expenditure and therefore it is important for determining total energy needs. Energy expenditure in physical activity is the most variable component of the REE (Schoeller, 2001). Physical activity is defined as *any* body movement produced by muscles that results in increased energy expenditure (USDHHS, 1996). In contrast, exercise is considered to be more vigorous as well as planned, structured, and repetitive bodily movement done to promote or maintain physical fitness.

Energy expenditure during physical activity is based chiefly on body movement, duration and type of physical activity, body weight, and to a lesser extent, on efficiency of movement. For example, a heavy,

TABLE 3–3 Factors Affecting Resting Energy Expenditure (REE)

Higher REE	Lower REE
Younger age	Older age
Children, adolescents	During sleep
Taller, thinner people (more surface area)	Shorter, rounder people (less surface area)
Fever	Fasting/starvation
Pregnancy	Malnutrition
Hyperthyroidism	Hypothyroidism
Higher lean body mass	Lower lean body mass
Stress	Higher % body fat
Men	Women
Certain medications (e.g., levothyroxine)	Certain medications
Smoking (nicotine)	
Caffeine	
Hot and cold environmental temperatures	
Illness (Cancer, AIDS, respiratory problems, hypertension, heart failure)	

Sources:
National Academy of Sciences, 2002
Poehlman, Horton, 1999
Whitney, Cataldo, Rolfes, 2002
Williams, 1997

physically untrained and uncoordinated male walking 100 yards expends more energy than his leaner, fit, and coordinated friend who walks the same distance at the same rate. Physical activity not only increases energy expenditure, but the REE can be elevated for up to 24 hours after the activity has ended (IOM, 2005). Estimations of increased postactivity energy expenditure vary depending on the duration and intensity of exercise, and is always much less than the amount of energy expended during the exercise itself (Bahr, 1987; Poehlman, 1991; Van Baak, 1998, 1999).

Approximately 50% of America's youth aged 12–21 are not regularly physically active (USDHHS, 1996); more than 60% of American adults are not physically active on a regular basis; and 25% of the adult population is not active at all. The proportion of the U.S. population reporting no leisure-time physical activity is higher among women than men, higher among African Americans and Hispanics than whites, higher among older adults than younger adults, and higher among the less affluent than the more affluent. Participation in all types of physical activity declines strikingly as age or grade in school increases.

The surgeon general's report on physical activity and health concluded all people benefit from regular physical activity. Including a moderate amount of physical activity (e.g., 30 minutes of brisk walking, 15 minutes of running, or 45 minutes of playing volleyball) on most days of the week has significant health benefits (USDHHS, 1996). The American College of Sports Medicine (ACSM) recommends participating in an aerobic activity for at least 30 minutes, 5 days each week if weight loss is a major goal (ACSM Guidelines). The 2005 *Dietary Guidelines for Americans* recommend that "adults engage in approximately 60 minutes of moderate to vigorous intensity activity on most days of the week to help manage body weight and prevent gradual, unhealthy body weight gain in adulthood. To sustain weight loss in adulthood, at least 60 to 90 minutes of daily moderate-intensity physical activity are recommended." The health benefits of physical activity include the following (*Dietary Guidelines for Americans 2005*):

* Increases physical fitness
* Helps build and maintain healthy bones, muscles, and joints
* Builds endurance and muscular strength
* Helps manage weight
* Reduces the risk of certain chronic diseases, including high blood pressure, stroke, coronary artery disease, Type 2 diabetes, colon cancer, and osteoporosis
* Promotes psychological well-being and self-esteem
* May aid in managing mild to moderate depression and anxiety.

Thermic Effect of Food (TEF)

The thermic effect of food (TEF), also known as food-induced thermogenesis, specific dynamic action, or the specific effect of food, is the energy the body uses for eating, digesting, absorbing, transporting, metabolizing, and storing the energy derived from food. TEF accounts for 7–13% of the daily energy consumed and is directly proportional to the size of the meal ingested (Schutz, Bessard, Jequier, 1984). The larger the meal (e.g., the more calories eaten), the more energy it takes to metabolize, store, and process it. TEF values vary for each macronutrient: 0 to 3% for fat; 5 to 10% for carbohydrate; 20 to 30% for protein (Acheson, 1993); and 10 to 30% for alcohol (Westerterp, Wilson, Rollard, 1999). People eat mixed meals with many different macronutrients, and differences between meals in TEF are usually slight. A typical mixed meal composed of 30% calories from fat, 55% calories from carbohydrate, and 15% of calories from protein results in a TEF of only 6–11% of the total caloric intake.

Thermogenesis may also be induced by nicotine, caffeine, exercise, and altered circumstances (such as recovery from trauma, stress, starvation, or exposure to extreme cold or heat). Shivering, also called cold-induced adaptive thermogenesis, occurs when skeletal muscles move involuntarily and produce heat in response to cold temperatures. The extent to which this occurs depends on the insulation available from body fat and from protective clothing. Usually these other thermogenic effects are very small and can be disregarded.

Other Factors Affecting Total Energy Requirements

Growth Energy is required for growth and development throughout the life span and requirements increase during specific life stages. The most rapid growth is in utero during pregnancy, followed by early infancy, late infancy, childhood, and adolescence, and therefore energy needs are greater during these times. In general, energy needs increase throughout childhood, peak in adolescence, and then level off or even diminish as the adolescent becomes an adult (except during pregnancy and lactation, when energy needs increase to levels greater than those needed for adolescence).

The metabolic and physiologic changes that occur during pregnancy that cause maternal weight gain include the growth and development of the fetus and placenta, increased maternal fat stores, increased maternal blood volume, and changes in breasts and other tissues. Energy is expended in building these tissues and in growth. The heavier weight of the pregnant woman also increases the energy she expends with physical activity (Hark, Morrison, 2003). Lactation requires energy for milk production as well. Pregnancy and lactation are discussed in depth in Chapter 17).

Illness, Injury, or Stress Critically injured or ill patients are hypermetabolic (that is, they have very high energy outputs) and also exhibit accelerated catabolism (tissue breakdown), which leads rapidly to malnutrition if left untreated. Energy needs tend to be higher for thermal injuries, severe trauma, central nervous system

(CNS) insult, sepsis, and certain conditions such as wasting diseases like cancer, chronic obstructive pulmonary disease, alcohol abuse, and coronary heart disease because they are associated with additional stress, hormonal changes, and protein catabolism.

How to Determine Energy Needs

Clinically, energy requirements are estimated using various detailed equations based on sex, age, stage of life (e.g., pregnancy), and physical activity level (PAL) as indicated by a physical activity factor or coefficient *(PA)*. The PA is incorporated into the equation to determine total energy needs. The sedentary category is consistent with basic energy needs for daily living. Table 3–4 shows an example of a total energy requirement calculation.

Because individuals who are ill, stressed, or have experienced trauma may have higher energy needs than healthy individuals, *"stress factors"* are used to calculate the additional amount of calories needed to meet hospitalized patients' increased caloric needs (Barak, Wall-Alonso, Sitrin, 2002; Roubenoff, Roubenoff,

TABLE 3–4   Estimating Total Energy Requirements for Adults

Men 19 years and older (normal weight)
$662 - 9.53 \times \text{Age (y)} + PA \times [15.91 \times \text{Weight (kg)} + 539.6 \times \text{Height (m)}]$

Women 19 years and older (normal weight)
$354 - 6.91 \times \text{Age (y)} + PA \times [9.36 \times \text{Weight (kg)} + 726 \times \text{Height (m)}]$

Overweight and obese men 19 years and older
$1086 - 10.1 \times \text{Age (y)} + PA \times [13.7 \times \text{Weight (kg)} + 416 \times \text{Height (m)}]$

Overweight and obese women 19 years and older
$448 - 7.95 \times \text{Age (y)} + PA \times [11.4 \times \text{Weight (kg)} + 619 \times \text{Height (m)}]$

Normal and overweight or obese men 19 years and older
$864 - 9.72 \times \text{Age (y)} + PA \times [14.2 \times \text{Weight (kg)} + 503 \times \text{Height (m)}]$

Normal and overweight or obese women 19 years and older
$387 - 7.31 \times \text{Age (y)} + PA \times [10.9 \times \text{Weight (kg)} + 660.7 \times \text{Height (m)}]$

Note: PA = physical activity level; 1 kg = 2.2 lb; 1 m = 39.37 in.
Source: Adapted from the Institute of Medicine 2002. Retrieved June 30, 2005, from, http://www.nap.edu. Adapted with permission from Carol Frary and Rachel Johnson.

Physical Activity Level (PAL) and Physical Activity Coefficients (PA)

Physical Activity Level	*Physical Activity Coefficient*
Sedentary	1.0–1.39
Low active	1.4–1.59
Active	1.6–1.89
Very active	1.9–2.5

Source: Adapted from the Institute of Medicine, 2002. Retrieved June 30, 2005, from http://www.nap.edu.

Example: Obese Adult Male Aged 45
$PA = 1.2$ (sedentary)
$\text{TEE} = 864 - 9.72 \times \text{Age (y)} + PA \times [14.2 \times \text{Weight (kg)} + 503 \times \text{Height (m)}]$
$\text{TEE} = 864 - 9.72 \times 45y + 1.2 \times [(14.2 \times 113.6kg) + (503 \times 1.828m)]$
$\text{TEE} = (864 - 437.4) + 1.2 (1613 + 504.8)$
$\text{TEE} = 426.6 + 2541$
$\text{TEE} = 2968$ calories

1990). In these cases, the individual's TEE is multiplied by the stress factor to get total caloric requirements. Stress factors may range from 1.0 to 2.05, depending on the severity of the insult to the patient (Slone, 2004).

WEIGHT AND BODY COMPOSITION AS MEASURES OF HEALTH

Body weight alone is not a good indicator of health status. Body composition is more important than weight in determining health status. For example, some lean, very fit and muscular football players were rejected from the draft during WWII because they were "overweight." However, these men were later drafted because they were not "overfat." In the U.S. Army today, before individuals are declared obese, several more valid measures of body composition are used.

The Body Mass Index (BMI)

Body mass index (BMI) is an indicator of relative weight status that has been found to correlate with body fat and is used to categorize obesity on a population level. However, it does not distinguish between lean, fat, and bone tissue, and thus is not a highly precise estimate of body fatness. BMI is also a rough indicator of the increased risk for some weight-related chronic

degenerative diseases such as high blood pressure and hyperlipidemia (Melanson, Dwyer, 2002). BMI is a single number, useful in expressing the relationship between body weight and height. It can be determined using a formula [BMI = weight (kg)/height (m^2) or (weight (lb)/height (in^2)) × 703], or by using Table 3–1.

Normal BMI is 18.5–24.9. Those who are above or below this healthy range should consult their physician for help. A BMI of 25.0–29.9 is classified as overweight and is associated with increased risk of hypertension and gallstones as well as other risks (National Heart, Lung, and Blood Institute [NHLBI], 1998). A BMI of 30 or greater is considered obese and is associated with an increased risk of these many chronic degenerative diseases as well as other conditions, such as sleep apnea. A BMI of 40 or more is considered morbidly obese. As obesity increases, so does the likelihood of risk of actual chronic degenerative disease, orthopedic difficulties, and psychological problems. Table 3–5 shows body weight classification by BMI, body fat percentage, and health-related risks.

Body Fat Distribution

Body fat distribution is important because it provides additional information about the potential health risks at any given level of BMI. There are two main fat distribution patterns. A central fat distribution pattern (sometimes

TABLE 3–5 Body Weight Classification by BMI and Body Fat Percentage and Health-Related Risks

BMI Category	Classification	Body Fat (%)		Risk of Diabetes (Type 2), High Blood Pressure, or Heart Disease Relative to Having a Healthful Weight and Waist Size	
		Men	Women	Waist Circumference (35 in. or less in women; 40 in. or less in men)	Waist Circumference > 35 in. in women; < 40 in. in men)
<18.5	Underweight				
18.5–24.9	Normal	13–21	23–31		
25.0–<29.9	Overweight	21–25	31–37	Increased	High
30.0–34.9	Obese Class I	25–31	37–42	High	Very high
35.0–39.9	Obese Class II	>31	>42	Very high	Very high
≥40	Obese Class III (extreme obesity)			Extremely high	Extremely high

Sources: Adapted from National Institutes of Health; NHLBI, 1998; IOM, 2005, pp. 5–15.

referred to as apple-shaped or android) occurs when the majority of both the subcutaneous fat (fat underneath the skin) and visceral fat (intra-abdominal fat, surrounding the internal organs) is in the abdominal region. A peripheral fat distribution pattern (sometimes referred to as pear-shaped or gynoid) occurs when the majority of the subcutaneous fat is in the hip and thigh regions. See Figure 3–1 for an illustration of these fat distribution types. Even though it is more common for females to have a gynoid

fat distribution pattern and males to have an android fat distribution pattern, either one may occur in both sexes. Central obesity is associated with greater health risk for cardiovascular disease, breast cancer, and some other cancers than a peripheral fat deposition pattern (Melanson, Dwyer, 2002) due to the larger amount of visceral fat and apparently to its role in metabolism. It is important for individuals to be aware of their fat distribution pattern.

Waist circumference is the most useful measure for determining a rough indication of body fat distribution. The measurement is taken with a measuring tape at the smallest area below the rib cage above the level of the umbilicus (belly button). Waist circumferences of 40 inches (in.) (102 centimeters [cm]) in men and 35 in. (88 cm) in women is indicative of central obesity, which is associated with increased risk of Type 2 diabetes, high blood pressure, and heart disease (NHLBI, 1998). Those with a high waist circumference should see their doctors.

Waist-to-hip ratio (WHR) is sometimes used for assessing body composition. The WHR is calculated by dividing the waist circumference by the hip circumference. Males with WHR greater than 1.0 and females with WHR greater than 0.8 are considered to be at risk for chronic diseases. However, this method requires measures of both waist and hip and because it is a ratio that is difficult to interpret. Therefore, the waist circumference is preferable for estimating abdominal fat.

More Precise Measures of Body Composition

More precise body composition measurements used to obtain estimates of body fatness include (Melanson, Dwyer, 2002):

- bioelectrical impedance analysis (BIA)—fat and lean body mass
- dual energy X-ray absorptiometry (DEXA)—fat mass, lean body mass, and bone
- hydrodensiometry (underwater weighting)—fat and lean body mass
- plethysmography (air displacement Bod Pod)— fat and lean body mass

HEALTHY VERSUS UNHEALTHY WEIGHT

A healthy weight is a range of weights for height within the range known to be associated with lowest mortality from insurance company statistics. The healthy weight

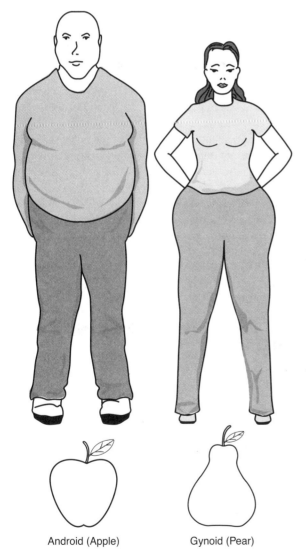

Android (Apple)   Gynoid (Pear)

FIGURE 3–1   Apple (android) and pear (gynoid) fat distribution pattern illustrations.

range is a BMI between 18.5 and 25.0; no more than one BMI unit within this range should be gained during adulthood because an increased BMI tends to signal the buildup of fat tissue (Melanson, Dwyer, 2002). For one to be at a healthy weight, there should be an absence of central body obesity; no medical conditions that increase the risk of overweight; and no wasting illnesses causing weight loss.

Underweight

Underweight is defined as having a BMI of less than or equal to 18.5. According to the Centers for Disease Control and Prevention and the National Center for Health Statistics (1999–2001) about 2% of U.S. adults are underweight; over 3% of women and only 1% of men are underweight. Young adults (aged 18–24) and older adults (above age 75) are about twice as likely as adults in other age groups to be underweight (Schoenborn, Adams, Barnes, Vickerie, Schiller, 2004).

Food intake and consequently weight can decrease as a result of wasting diseases such as cancer, infectious diseases accompanied by fevers, severe illnesses, and malabsorption, but also due to depression, restrictive eating disorders, and some medications. Whenever a patient reports unintended weight loss, he or she should be referred to a physician. A low BMI resulting from unexplained weight loss should *always* be followed up as it may signify the presence of acute mental or physical disease. The risk of underweight is considerable in old age because thin, frail elders lack fat reserves to draw on if they become acutely ill, and thus may waste (lose lean tissue) as a result. Excessive weight loss may cause dentures to become ill-fitting, making it difficult to maintain regular food intake. Those who are underweight are less able to deal with malnutrition and their immune systems may be impaired, increasing risk and severity of infectious diseases. The very underweight also have fewer reserves to recover from injuries.

Underweight pregnant women are more likely to give birth to low-birth-weight infants who have greater health risks than heavier infants. Too little body fat can also adversely affect metabolism and health. For survival, men require at least 3% body fat and women require at least 12% body fat (Williams, 1997). Infertility may become a problem with seriously underweight young women who suffer from physical or psychological conditions that cause weight loss. On its own, undernutrition causes decreased blood estrogen

and loss of weight and fat tissue. Low body fat drives estrogen levels still lower because there is less conversion of androgen to estrogen in the absence of fat tissue. These low estrogen levels in turn cause decreased bone buildup, which, if untreated, may lead to osteoporosis. Osteoporosis and bone loss are therefore also associated with weight loss and extreme underweight as in conditions such as anorexia nervosa. Underweight individuals who suffer from cancer are at greater risk of death, perhaps because they have few reserves.

Eating disorders are also major contributors to weight loss and underweight and are discussed in detail in Chapter 19. Those with bulimia nervosa who vomit frequently have increased gastric acid contact with the teeth, resulting in dental enamel demineralization.

Overweight and Obesity

Overweight is defined as having a BMI of greater than or equal to 25, but less than 30. *Obesity* is defined as having a BMI greater than or equal to 30. Being overweight or obese increases the risk of many diseases and conditions, including hypertension; dyslipidemia (for example, high total blood cholesterol or high levels of triglycerides); Type 2 diabetes; coronary heart disease; stroke; gallbladder disease; osteoarthritis; sleep apnea and respiratory problems; and some cancers (endometrial, breast, and colon) (Bray, 2000; Kushner, Blatner, 2005). Obesity is also associated with increased disability, decreased health-related quality of life, increased health care use, and increased mortality (Doll, Petersen, Stewart-Brown, 2000).

Child and Adolescent Overweight and Obesity

The prevalence of overweight among children has risen from 5% in 1960 to 15% in 2000 (Flegal, 2002). In 2004, approximately nine million children over six years of age were overweight (IOM, 2004). Overweight and obesity are defined differently for children than for adults. Weight and height values should be plotted on a growth chart issued by the Centers for Disease Control and Prevention (CDC)(http://www.cdc.gov/nchs/about/major/nhanes/growthcharts/clinical_charts.htm). These growth charts allow a comparison of the child to other children of the same age and sex. A child with a BMI between the 85th and 95th percentile is considered "at risk for overweight." Children are considered overweight or "at risk for obesity" when their BMI exceeds the 95th percentile. Overweight children have increased risks of high blood pressure, Type 2 diabetes mellitus, sleep apnea, high cholesterol, and psychological problems such as poor body image and depression (Dietz, 1998; Faith, 2004). Overweight children are also more likely to become overweight adults with poor health for longer periods than children who are not overweight (Allison, Fontaine, Manson, Stevens, Van Itallie, 1999). Therefore prevention of obesity is very important (Swinburn, Seidell, James, 2004)

Healthcare professionals routinely track BMI, offer relevant evidence-based counseling and guidance, serve as role models, and provide leadership in their communities for obesity prevention efforts. Health professionals' training programs and professional organizations (including those in dentistry) should require that students learn about overweight prevention so that health professionals have the awareness and skills to tackle weight issues (IOM, 2004). Expert guidelines recommend limiting child television viewing to no more than one to two hours per day (Calamaro, Faith, 2005). Table 3–6 details environmental risk factors for obesity in children.

Causes of Obesity

Although obesity is recognized as a chronic disease, it is still stigmatized and perceived by many as being caused by lack of self-control and bad habits (Puhl, Brownell, 2003). In fact, obesity is the result of a complicated interaction between genes and the environment. The major causes of obesity are increased food intake and lack of physical activity (Keim, Blanton, Kretsch, 2004).

Physiology and Genetics

The mechanisms regulating food intake and body weight are complex. They include both central (central nervous system) controls through the neuroendocrine system, peripheral controls through gut hormones, and other factors. Fat tissue produces hormones important in controlling body weight as well. These include two hormones produced solely in fat cells (adipocytes): adiponectin, which is reduced in obese people, and leptin, which is increased in obese individuals. High blood insulin levels (hyperinsulinemia) are also common among obese persons and so are levels of insulin-like growth factor (IGF1). It is thought that changes in these hormones in obese persons may be involved with links

to chronic degenerative diseases such as some of the hormone-dependent cancers and diabetes.

Between 30 and 40% of the variance of weight between individuals is likely to be genetic (Bouchard, Perusse, Rice, Rao, 2004; Cummings, Schwartz, 2003). For the majority of those who are obese, it has been suggested that there are those with a strong genetic predisposition to obesity and those with a slight genetic susceptibility to obesity (Loos, Bouchard, 2003).

A relatively small proportion of obesity in the population can be explained by mutations in single genes involved in the regulation of energy balance. The very rare Prader-Willi syndrome is an example. The majority of obesity cases, however, have a larger environmental component.

Environmental Factors

Food choices, physical activity levels, and the "built environment" can all contribute to obesity. The built environment refers to elevators, lack of sidewalks or bike paths, and other factors in the physical environment that favor inactivity and predispose people to sedentary habits. The social environment helps promote excessive caloric intake and discourages physical activity, often leading to weight gain (European Food Information Council [EUFIC], 2005; Gillis, 2003; Gore, Foster, DiLillo, Kirk, Smith West, 2003).

Many of these factors in our environment today may persuade individuals to make inappropriate food choices leading to weight gain (Grimm, Harnack, Story, 2004; Halford, Brown, Pontin, Dovey, 2004). Theoretically, eating 200 calories more every day than one's daily energy needs could lead to a weight gain of a few pounds each year. One recent national study found that average calorie intakes were 2700 calories/day, an increase of 530 calories, or 25%, between 1970 and 2000 (Flaherty, 2004). The majority of these extra calories came from refined grain products, calorically sweetened soft drinks, and alcohol (USDA, 2002). The powerful impact of the environment on food choice has encouraged several campaigns on the part of consumer advocates and nutritionists to encourage eating establishments to make lower calorie and more nutritious options available. Some progress has been made. For example, McDonald's discontinued the "super size" option for its fries and drinks (Associated Press [AP], 2004), and it has increased its menu offerings to include more vegetable and fruit options. Schools have reassessed their food services and the availability and

TABLE 3–6 Environmental Risk Factors That May Contribute to Childhood Overweight and Obesity

Risk Factor	Manifestations/Statistics in United States	Implications on Energy Balance and Diet Quality
Decreased physical activity in both daily life and exercise	– Few children live close enough to walk to school – There is often a lack of sidewalks, which forces children to face danger by walking in the street – Reduced physical education class time and frequency due to budget cuts (Luepker, 1999; Yackel, 2003) – Reduced recess time in schools	– Concerns with the safety of children often lead parents to fear allowing children to walk or play outside, and result in sedentary indoor activities (Peters, 2004) leading to decreased energy expenditure
Increased sedentary lifestyle	– Children in the U.S. spend an average of at least 2 hours each day watching television or playing video games, compared to other activities (Larson, 1999) – 99% of adolescents have a TV in their home and 65% of adolescents have TVs in their bedrooms (Roberts, 1999)	– TV viewing may decrease REE (Dietz, 1994) and it may correlate with increased body fat (Dietz, 1985) and body mass (Gortmaker, 1996) (Dietz, 1985)(Berkey, 2000) – Sedentary behavior provides a setting for increased snacking and exposure to food in commercials (Faith, 2001) – The odds of being overweight were 4.6 times greater for youth watching more than five hours of television per day compared with those watching 0 to 2 hours (Gortmaker et al., 1996) – Increased TV viewing results in decreases in fruit and vegetable consumption and increases nonnutritive food consumption (Boynton-Jarrett, 2003) – TV viewing may displace time spent doing higher-energy expending activities and may increase energy consumption – Increased TV viewing often results in more snacking and less meal eating and results in more calories consumed overall (Gortmaker, 1996) (Gore, 2003)
Increased exposure to food advertising	– Children see 40,000 commercials per year on television alone (Kunkel, 2001) – The majority of foods marketed to children are those low in nutritional value and high in "empty calories, fat and/or sugar" (French, 2001; Story, 2004)	– Children who watch television significantly increase their food consumption after watching food advertisements (Halford, 2004) – Children's perceived need for sweets increases after watching TV advertisements (Lewis, 1998) – Weekday TV viewing has been positively associated with eating at fast-food restaurants among adolescents (French, 2001)

Factor	Description	Evidence
Family influence	– Parents with poor nutritional habits that include dietary excess who lead sedentary lifestyles role model these behaviors for their children – Parental obesity – Fewer family meals and more snacking – More meals eaten away from home	– Snacking more often leads to consumption of less nutritious foods – Increased potential for consuming more calories when eating outside the home – Children are more likely to be obese if they have obese parents
Eating environment in schools	– Increasing amounts of fast food served in schools – Increased number of vending machines in schools, which usually offer a variety of energy-dense candies and chips loaded with fat (Kubik et al., 2003), and soft drinks – Soda companies negotiate lucrative contracts with many school systems (called pouring rights), which provide the schools with needed financial and in-kind resources in return for allowing free usage of sodas throughout the day – Decreased time given to meals at lunch	– Use of vending machines tends to displace intake of more nutritious foods (Ballew, 2000) – For every vending machine present in schools, fruit consumption decreases by 11% (Kubik, 2003) – Shortened meals may lead to increased snacking
Increased availability and usage of sweetened beverages (soft drinks, juice drinks) without moderating intakes of other foods	– A 12 fl oz soft drink contains approximately 160 kcal and 40 g sugar (contributes no nutritional value to the diet) – Added sugars account for 20% of children's daily calories (<10% recommended) (Guthrie, 2000) – Soft drinks may be replacing more nutritious beverages such as milk among children and adolescents. – Soft drink consumption has increased by almost 500% in the past 50 years (Ludwig, 2001)	– Soft drink consumption has been associated with increased calorie intake, increased body weight, and juvenile obesity (Gillis, 2003) – Children who often use soft drinks take in 10% more calories and are more likely to be overweight than children who rarely drink them (Ludwig, 2001) (Gillis, 2003) (Swinburn, 2004) (Guthrie, 2000) – When added sugars in the diet exceed 25% of total calories, micronutrient intake may be inadequate (DRI, 2002)
Increased availability and consumption of fast food/poor food choices	– Food portions from fast-food restaurants tend to be large – Fast-food restaurants typically use value pricing for larger sizes, encouraging the purchase and consumption of excess calories.	– Overly large portion sizes contribute to obesity (Young, 2002) (Goldberg, 2004) – Children consume too much fat, saturated fat, and sodium and not enough fruits, vegetables, or calcium (USDA FaNS, 2001a) (USDA FaNS, 2001b) – More than 2/3 of US children consume more than 30% of their calories from fat (<30% recommended) (USDA FaNS, 2001a) (USDA FaNS, 2001b)

content of soda machines (Kubik, Hannan, Perry, Story, 2003).

WEIGHT MANAGEMENT

Weight management involves weight loss (or gain) to optimal weight, and weight maintenance to maintain weight at a healthy level. Weight issues are emotionally and physiologically complicated. Because attaining and maintaining a healthy weight is often a lifelong battle, prevention is better than attempts at a cure. Patients should concentrate on achieving or maintaining a healthy weight longterm with appropriate lifestyle changes. These include developing healthier eating behaviors and activity patterns to avoid weight gains, instead of putting their faith in short-term weight-loss "miracles." Moderate weight loss (no more than 1 to 2 pounds (lb) per week unless under a physician's direction) increases the chances of maintaining long-term weight at healthy levels. Even modest (5–10%) weight reduction in obese persons results in clinical improvements of several health-related parameters, even if the individual remains clinically obese (Melanson, Dwyer, 2002). Smoking increases health risks at any given BMI, so smokers have an additional reason to lose weight as well as to give up smoking. Heath care professionals should emphasize the importance of even small weight losses to patients. Patients often have unrealistic goals for weight loss. Such losses are rarely possible, but more modest goals are likely to be achieved.

Characteristics of Sound Weight Management

The following characteristics represent a sound, health-promoting weight management plan (Dwyer, Melanson, 2002):

* a nutritionally adequate, balanced, and varied diet
* a hypocaloric diet
* adaptability to individual health needs
* increased physical activity
* behavioral modification
* psychological and social support
* reasonable cost

A sound long-term eating plan should follow the recommendations set forth by the USDA's MyPyramid (http://www.mypyramid.gov) (USDA, 2005). Another

important part of successful lost weight maintenance is the support from family, friends, and professionals to help motivate the dieter and instill confidence.

Negative energy balance (energy output > input) is necessary for weight loss. Physical activity alone without control over energy intake is unlikely to be sufficient enough to cause weight loss. An adult with a BMI between 25 and 35 should aim to reduce his or her usual intake by 300 to 500 calories per day. This usually leads to a loss of roughly a pound a week, since 3500 calories equals approximately 1 lb of body fat. An adult with a BMI of greater than 35 can safely eliminate 500 to 1000 calories from his or her usual intake (which is even higher) for a 1 to 2 lb weight loss per week. This typically can be accomplished with reducing diets of about 1200 calories per day; the amount of weight loss will vary depending on how many calories the individual was previously consuming. A good eating plan for maintaining weight at healthy levels provides balance, variety, and moderate consumption of all food groups in the USDA MyPyramid (http://www.mypyramid.gov).

Activity

In addition to limiting energy intake, increasing total energy expenditure by increased physical activity is important (Donnelly et al., 2004). Very vigorous exercise may also increase muscle mass and consequently increase resting metabolism slightly on a temporary basis, at least until muscle glycogen stores are restored (USDHHS, 1996).

Diet Guidelines

As a general rule of thumb, a minimum of 65–70 g of protein is needed daily. While on a very low-calorie diet (VLCD), 1.5 g of high-quality protein per kilogram of desirable body weight per day is recommended. If the dieter suffers from certain diseases or is physically stressed, protein needs may be higher because nitrogen losses may be increased in these states. On 900–1200 kcal/day (low-calorie diets [LCDs], daily protein intake should be at least 1 gram per kilogram (g/kg) ideal body weight. Reducing diets above 1200 kcal/day should provide at least the Recommended Dietary Allowance (RDA) for protein (0.8 g/kg ideal body weight). Protein levels should remain at this level after weight loss has stopped and weight maintenance has begun (Dwyer, Melanson, 2002; Laquatra, 2004).

Carbohydrates should account for at least 100 g in the diet to spare protein. Currently the amount of carbohydrates in weight-loss diets varies greatly. Some "low carbohydrate" diets are less than 100 g, whereas low-fat regimes may be very high in carbohydrates (> 200 g). In weight maintenance diets it is usually recommended that carbohydrates provide 55–60% of calories and even more for athletes.

Fat should provide no more than 30% and no less than 20% of daily calories. Small amounts (3–6 g) of essential fatty acids should be included to prevent essential fatty acid deficiency (Dwyer, Melanson, 2002). Some fat is also needed to absorb and transport fat-soluble vitamins (A, D, E, and K).

The fatigue some dieters associate with hypocaloric diets is often due in part to dehydration, especially if they have also increased their physical activity and exercise regimes dramatically (Dwyer, Melanson, 2002). Body water losses of as little as 2% have been associated with decreased physical and mental performance, and impaired thermoregulation (Kleiner, 1999). Thus, a minimum of eight glasses of water or noncaloric and nondehydrating fluids (64 oz/day) is important for good health. A tip for patients who wish to lose weight is to drink a glass of water with every craving, wait at least 5 to 10 minutes, and then decide if hunger is truly present.

Table 3–7 Provides the *Dietary Guidelines for Americans 2005* recommendations for weight management and physical activity.

TABLE 3–7   *Dietary Guidelines for Americans 2005*: Key Recommendations for Weight Management and Physical Activity

Weight Management
To maintain body weight in a healthy range, balance calories from foods and beverages with calories expanded.
To prevent gradual weight gain over time, make small decreases in food and beverage calories and increase physical activity.

To Those Who Need to Lose Weight
Aim for a slow, steady weight loss by decreasing calorie intake while maintaining an adequate nutrient intake and increasing physical activity.

Overweight Children
Reduce the rate of body weight gain while allowing growth and development. Consult a health care provider before placing a child on a weight-reduction diet.

Overweight Adults and Overweight Children with Chronic Diseases or on Medication
Consult a health care provider about weight-loss strategies prior to starting a weight-reduction program to ensure appropriate management of other health conditions.

Physical Activity
Engage in regular physical activity and reduce sedentary activities to promote health, psychological well-being, and a healthy body weight.

To reduce the risk of chronic disease in adulthood: Engage in at least 30 minutes of moderate-intensity physical activity, above usual activity, at work or home on most days of the week.
For most people, greater health benefits can be obtained by engaging in physical activity of more vigorous intensity or longer duration.
To help manage body weight and prevent gradual, unhealthy body weight gain in adulthood: Engage in approximately 60 minutes of moderate- to vigorous-intensity activity on most days of the week while not exceeding caloric intake requirements.
To sustain weight loss in adulthood: Participate in at least 60 to 90 minutes of daily moderate-intensity physical activity while not exceeding caloric intake requirements.

Children and Adolescents
Engage in at least 60 minutes of physical activity on most, preferably all, days of the week.

Older Adults
Participate in regular physical activity to reduce functional declines associated with aging and to achieve the other benefits of physical activity identified for all adults.

Source: USDHHS and USDA, 2005.

Characteristics of Unsound Weight Management

Total fasts and weight control diets of less than 600–900 calories (VLCDs) are rarely advisable except when administered under medical supervision. These diets are difficult to adhere to and are often inadequate in micronutrients and macronutrients. To prevent shortfalls of micronutrients, a multivitamin and mineral supplement is recommended if the daily energy intake is less than 1200 calories (Dwyer, Allison, Coates, 2005). If energy intakes are severely restricted, the body slows down in multiple ways: Voluntary physical activities may decrease; lean tissue decreases, which leads to a lower REE; the cost of moving the body lessens; and consequently total energy output is reduced. These changes partially nullify the caloric deficit (Dwyer, Melanson, 2002). For those who are dieting on their own, more moderate low-calorie regimes are advisable. Patients should always be directed to a registered dietitian (RD) for weight-loss management and supervision.

Beverages containing caffeine or alcohol should not be encouraged because they increase diuresis.

Eating disorders are also common problems of primarily young adult women, and result from misguided attempts to lose weight. Eating disorders are discussed in detail in Chapter 18.

Weight-Loss Diet Options

About 45 million Americans diet each year. This "feeds" about $46 billion (*Tufts University Health and Nutrition Letter*, 2005) into the burgeoning weight-loss industry. About $1 to $2 billion of that is spent on weight-loss programs alone (AP, 2005). Weight-loss attempts have been reported by 28% of men and 44% of women in the United States (Serdula et al., 1999). A recent study found that 45% of adolescent girls and 21% of adolescent boys reported currently trying to lose weight (Neumark-Sztainer, Croll, et al. 2002; Neumark-Sztainer et al., 2002).

Many people who are obese also have other health problems that require diet therapy. It is important that they work with a doctor and RD to choose reducing diets that also accommodate these problems.

Commercial Weight-Loss Programs

People differ in the kinds of weight-loss program that suits them best. Some find it easier to have a very structured eating plan with proportioned liquid or solid meals, whereas others can tolerate more flexibility. As long as the program is a sound one, individual choice should be encouraged.

Weight-loss programs vary from inexpensive and readily affordable to elaborate and costly. There is no direct correlation between the cost and the effectiveness of a weight-loss program.

Diet Books

Today's most popular diet books vary greatly in diet recommendations, and all promise significant weight loss. However, there is very little evidence that over the long run any of the various currently popular combinations of macronutrients in unusual amounts (low carbohydrate, low fat, high protein, etc.) cause greater amounts of fat loss at the same caloric intake than reducing diets that are more balanced in their nutrient composition (Foster et al., 2004). Table 3–8 provides an evaluation and comparison of some popular diet books.

Low-carbohydrate, high-protein, high-fat diets have become increasingly popular, and many best-selling diet books have promoted this approach (*Consumer Reports*, 2002). The low-carbohydrate advocates claim that high carbohydrate consumption causes insulin overproduction, and blame this for obesity. However, obesity itself causes insulin overproduction. Low-carbohydrate diets typically restrict carbohydrate intake to less than 90 g per day (Schoeller, Buchholz, 2005). Glucose (a simple carbohydrate) is an essential energy source for the brain, red blood cells, and the renal medulla; the daily requirement is ~180 g/day (Mann, 2001). Because the body is no longer receiving enough carbohydrate through dietary means on a low-carbohydrate diet, the body begins to use its carbohydrate stores (~1000 g glycogen) for fuel (Mann, 2001). Glucose is stored as glycogen with some water—as these stores are used up, water is lost as well. In addition, the body may use its own protein stores to make glucose; carbohydrate can be produced in the body by gluconeogenesis (protein breakdown to maintain blood sugar) if sufficient protein is available. At least 50–100 g of dietary carbohydrate is needed to sustain central nervous system activity. Less than this amount may lead to excessive protein breakdown and raises protein requirements (Melanson, Dwyer, 2002). For every gram of protein broken down, 3 g of water are released, leading to further water losses, contributing to the overall rapid weight loss during the initial phase of a low-carbohydrate diet (Van Itallie, 1980). This initial rapid weight loss may be encouraging

TABLE 3-8 Evaluation of Popular Diet Books

Book Title	Nutritional Issues and Concerns
Zone Diet	– Lower in carbohydrates – Higher in protein – Lacking in vitamins and minerals – Nutrient deficiencies – May cause coronary heart disease or kidney damage
Sugar Busters*	– Lower in carbohydrates, fiber, vitamins, minerals, and phytochemicals – Nutrient deficiencies – Fatigue, weakness, irritability – Possible long-term effects: kidney and liver damage, heart disease
The "New" Atkins Diet Revolution: Induction (Phase 1)	– Very low in carbohydrates – Very high in protein and fat (especially saturated fat) – Deficient in vitamins and minerals, especially calcium (multivitamin, mineral, and essential fatty acid supplements recommended), fiber, and phytochemicals – Too much fat and saturated fat – Too few fruits, vegetables, grains, dairy, and legumes – Initial loss is mostly water weight – Tends to have high dropout rates – Requires rigid adherence and strict carbohydrate counting – Meant to be followed for 2 weeks (but says people may be on it for 6 months) – Does not teach lifelong weight-loss practices – High fat intake, rapid weight fluctuations, and ketosis may adversely affect the heart – May cause kidney damage – "Safe for short-term use except for people with decreased kidney function" – "Not appropriate for pregnant women and nursing mothers"
The "New" Atkins Diet Revolution: Ongoing Weight Loss (Phase 2)	– Promotes strict carbohydrate counting, which may be difficult to maintain – Ketosis may still occur – May lead to dehydration, electrolyte imbalances, and kidney damage – Not recommended for those with decreased kidney function
Dean Ornish "Eat More, Weigh Less" Life Choice Program	– Higher in carbohydrates – Low in fat, especially essential fatty acids (linoleic and alphalinolenic acids), monounsaturated and polyunsaturated fats. – Highly restrictive diet that eliminates many foods considered healthy (oils, avocados, nuts, seeds, fish, etc.) – Tends to have high dropout rates – Very low fat intake may lead to endocrine problems (amenorrhea in women), essential fatty acid deficiencies, and reduced absorption of the fat-soluble vitamins (A, D, E, K) – Extremely high fiber/bulk diet, which will lead to constipation/hard stools if large quantities of water are not consumed to keep intestinal contents soft
Dr. Phil's Ultimate Weight Solution, Stages 1 and 2	– Low in calories – A diet this low in calories will most likely not meet the RDAs for vitamins and minerals – Low in carbohydrates – Regime requires a lot of supervision – Provides (overly) simple advice for complex emotional, eating, and family issues – Diet recommendations are universal, regardless of sex, age, height, or weight – Weight loss likely due to low-calorie diet (~1200 kcal/day)

(continued)

TABLE 3-8 Evaluation of Popular Diet Books (Continued)

	– Low calorie level may cause fatigue, dizziness, weakness, or fainting
	– Recommends reducing caloric intake to below most individuals' REE while also engaging in an exercise program
The South Beach Diet, Phase 1	– Low in fiber (~9 g on average)
	– Very low in carbohydrates
	– High in saturated fat
	– High in fat
	– Very low in carbohydrates
	– Vitamin and mineral deficiencies
	– Promotes potentially dangerous accelerated weight loss
	– Initial loss is mostly water, which may lead to dehydration and electrolyte imbalances
	– Highly restrictive and difficult to maintain
	– Completely eliminates healthy foods (fruits, some vegetables, etc.)
	– "No mandatory exercise"
The South Beach Diet, Phase 2	– High in fat (although low in saturated fat)
	– Low in carbohydrates
	– Recommends avoiding healthy foods such as bananas, watermelon, potatoes, and carrots
	– Considers some healthy foods as "bad" and recommends avoiding them
	– "No mandatory exercise"

*Includes other similar diets based on the glycemic index that are high in protein and low in carbohydrates, including *The Carbohydrate Addict's Diet, Protein Power*, and *The Glucose Revolution*.

Sources:
Agatston, 2003
American Dietetic Association, 2004
Atkins, 1998
Atkins, 2004
Consumer Reports, 2005
Dwyer, Melanson, 2002
Eades, Eades, 1999
Leighton Steward, Bethea, Balart, Andrews, 1999
Melanson, Dwyer, 2002
McGraw, 2004
Miller Foster-Powell, Burani, 2001
Ornish, 1993
Sears, 1995

for some dieters and aid in dietary compliance; however, the loss is mostly water (~1.9 kg in the first 10 days) (Yang, 1976).

The body then adapts to use fat as a greater percentage of its fuel. When fats are used excessively as fuels, they are converted to ketones (acidic by-products of fat metabolism). Ketosis, or the presence of abnormally high levels of ketones in the blood, may then occur. Normally the blood ketone levels are low, but in starvation, untreated diabetes, and when the diet is very high in fats and low in carbohydrates, the levels rise. Symptoms of ketosis include general tiredness, abrupt or gradually increasing weakness, dizziness, headaches, confusion, abdominal pain, irritability, nausea and

vomiting, sleep problems, and bad breath (Blackburn Phillips, Morreale, 2001). Appetite is often reduced during ketosis, further encouraging the dieter to comply with the diet and consume fewer calories.

Studies have shown that after one year, those following low-carbohydrate regimes have not achieved more weight loss or kept it off longer than those on other regimes. If the dieter suddenly increases carbohydrate intake after a low-calorie, low-carbohydrate regimen, it often leads to very rapid weight gain, due to water retained as glycogen stores are built back up, and return of appetite (Melanson, Dwyer, 2002). Side effects and complications of very low-carbohydrate diets include dehydration, electrolyte losses, muscle weakness, nausea, fatigue, and vitamin and mineral (especially calcium) deficiencies.

Diet Foods and Products

Currently there are thousands of reduced-fat, fat-free, and low-calorie processed foods and beverages available on the market (Melanson, Dwyer, 2002). Many of these products contain carbohydrate and/or fat substitutes. (See Chapter 4 for further information on sugar substitutes, and Chapter 6 for further information on fat substitutes.) Despite the availability of reduced-fat and reduced-calorie products, obesity rates continue to rise. Indeed, even these products can cause weight gain when overall diets are higher in calories than the body needs.

Oral Nutritional Supplements and Meal Replacements

Oral nutritional supplements were first created for clinical use to provide elderly and ill patients with a micronutrient-rich, calorically dense beverage. Today, these products (e.g., Boost, Ensure, and Glucerna) are also marketed to healthy adults to supplement their daily food intake. These supplements are not necessarily low in calories, providing about 230–400 calories per 8 oz can (http://www.ross.com/productHandbook/adultNut.asp). Other oral nutritional supplements such as Slim-Fast are targeted specifically to those trying to lose weight.

Other types of weight-loss products and plans consist of various combinations of specific products and calorie-controlled meal plans (*Consumer Reports*, 2005; Slim-Fast website). These beverages, bars, and snacks might be a good option as meal replacements for the dieter who has difficulty in making food choices and tends to overeat. However, they are not appropriate as a sole food for long-term dieting and could be hazardous if followed incorrectly without any medical supervision (Dwyer, Melanson, 2002). All of the meal replacement products are designed to be eaten with additions of conventional foods that supply dietary fiber, other nutrients, additional calories, and fluids (Dwyer, Melanson, 2002).

Commercial and Self-Help Weight-Loss Programs

Each year, millions of Americans enroll in commercial and self-help weight-loss programs (Tsai, Wadden, 2005). Generally, commercial weight-loss programs provide people with social support and a structured plan

for losing weight with others who have similar problems. These programs are categorized as follows: non-medical (WeightWatchers, Jenny Craig); medically supervised (Optifast); and self-help (Take Off Pounds Sensibly, Overeaters Anonymous). None of these programs are required to submit data on safety or efficacy to the government. Therefore, it is important for a physician to be involved for evaluating patient suitability. However, the Federal Trade Commission (FTC) may intervene when it suspects that manufacturers are making false or misleading claims. Those wishing to engage in such programs should evaluate each one carefully to see which one will fit their lifestyle and needs best. Table 3–9 compares the costs and characteristics of some major commercial weight-loss programs in the United States.

Dietary Supplements for Weight Loss

Dietary supplements may be used in weight reduction to provide nutrients inadequate in calorie-restricted diets, or for alleged benefits in stimulating or enhancing weight loss via reducing appetite or increasing REE (Dwyer et al., 2005). Nutrient-providing dietary supplements are indicated when diets do not adhere to the RDA levels for micronutrients or protein. There is little evidence at present, however, that any dietary supplements now on the market stimulate weight loss. Ephedra (or *Ma huang*) and ephedrine-containing supplements, either with or without caffeine, were widely used for stimulating weight loss from the mid-1990s through 2004 (Dwyer et al., 2005). Several studies showed that ephedra increased short-term weight loss; however, it posed serious health risks to some, including arrhythmias, heart attack, and stroke (Agency for Healthcare Research and Quality, 2003; Shekelle et al., 2003; Thomas, 2005). Therefore, the FDA banned ephedra-containing supplements in 2004 on the grounds that they present "a significant or unreasonable risk of illness or injury when used according to its labeling or under ordinary conditions of use" (Food and Drug Administration [FDA], 2004).

Medications for Weight Loss

In the 1990s the FDA banned two appetite suppressants (Redux and Fenfluramine) from pharmacy shelves after reports of primary pulmonary hypertension, heart valve abnormalities, and death were associated with their use (Moyers, 2005). There was also a risk of significant

TABLE 3–9 Characteristics of Major Weight-Loss Programs

Program	Characteristics
WeightWatchers	– Requirements to join: • Must be at least 5 pounds above the minimum weight for your height (BMI = 20) and age • Must not have an active diagnosis of bulimia nervosa • Must not be pregnant or breastfeeding – Staffed by successful lifetime members (successful program completers) – Recommends a low-calorie, low-fat, high-fiber exchange diet, where clients prepare their own meals – Choose either Flexible POINTS (Flex plan) or No Counting Plan (Core plan) – Plans do not exclude any food group – Plan does not recommend consuming extreme quantities of macronutrients – Physical activity encouraged by distributing "Get Moving" booklet
Jenny Craig	– Staffed by company-trained counselors – Asserts that clients should learn to manage their weight "one simple change at a time" – Low-calorie diet of prepackaged Jenny Craig meals only – Weekly contact with client's personal consultant – Offers telephone counseling 24 hours a day, 7 days a week, as needed – Requires clients to purchase the company's prepackaged meals – Physical activity encouraged through audiotapes for walking – Behavior modification provided through a manual on weight-loss strategies
LA Weight Loss	– Staffed by company-trained counselors – Recommends a low-calorie diet where clients prepare their own meals – Physical activity encouraged through an optional walking videotape – Behavior modification is included in individual counseling sessions three times per week
OPTIFAST (Novartis Nutrition)	– Designed to treat individuals with a BMI ≥ 30 or a BMI of 25.0 to 29.9 who have other medical problems caused by their weight – Staff qualifications: Licensed physician and other health care providers – When used as directed, the 800–1500 kcal/day plans each provide complete, balanced nutrition including at least 100% of the recommended daily intake for protein and all essential vitamins and minerals – Physical activity modules, behavior modification, stress management, and social support included in weekly mandatory lifestyle classes – Consists of a three-phase program: 12–18 weeks of rapid weight loss, a 3-to-8-week transition phase, and long-term maintenance – Medical monitoring mandatory for first two phases – Group sessions offered – Some telephone support available
Take Off Pounds Sensibly (TOPS)	– Nonprofit, noncommercial weight-loss support group – Led by laypersons who have struggled with weight or eating problems (group leader elected by local chapter) – Weekly meetings include private weigh-ins and a group meeting – Program provides members with positive reinforcement and motivation to adhere to food (low-calorie diet exchange plan) and exercise plans (to be made with health care provider) – Philosophy is that desire to change comes from within an individual and the most effective way to sustain change is to provide a supporting environment – Website allows members to interact in chat rooms
Overeaters Anonymous (OA)	– Nonprofit, noncommercial weight-loss support group – Led by laypersons (volunteer chapter leaders)

– Weekly meetings are held in neutral environments such as churches, temples, and meeting halls
– Believes that obesity results from compulsive eating, which, in turn, is considered the consequence of sadness, loneliness, and other untoward emotions
– Participants frequently report they are addicted to food
– Encourages members to develop a "food plan" with a health care professional and a sponsor (another member in the program)
– Members are encouraged to "call in" their food plans to their sponsors
– Seeks to guide participants to physical, emotional, and spiritual recovery
– Behavior modification provided with a 12-step approach, similar to that of Alcoholics Anonymous (AA)
– Physical activity plan advised to be made with a health care provider

Sources:
Dwyer, Melanson, 2002
Tsai, Wadden, 2005
WeightWatchers, 1999
Take Off Pounds Sensibly (TOPS) website
Take It Off and Keep It Off, 1989
Consumer Reports, 2005
Overeaters Anonymous website
OPTIFAST website
Consumer Reports, 2004

bleeding during periodontal surgery, root canal treatment, or tooth extractions with these products; dry mouth was also a problem.

Pharmacologic intervention is a sound option for adults who are obese (BMI > 30), or who have a BMI > 27 that is associated with an obesity-related condition, such as sleep apnea, Type 2 diabetes, dyslipidemia, or hypertension. Today, there are several FDA-approved antiobesity prescription medications on the market. *None of these medications should be used with children, pregnant or lactating women, or those who are ill* (Pronsky, Redfern, Crowe, Epstein, 2004), and all should be used in association with diet and physical activity.

Table 3–10 summarizes these weight-loss medications.

Surgical Approaches to Weight Loss

Surgical therapy may be recommended for some adults who have tried and failed to lose weight and are suffering from complications of severe obesity (BMI = 40 or BMI = 35) with comorbid conditions. This is often called bariatric surgery. The most common type of bariatric surgery is gastric bypass. It is expensive and is often not covered by health insurance, but for some patients it may be the only option left (Buchwald, 2005;

Kelly et al., 2005; Miller, 2004). In the past, jaw wiring (maxillomandibular fixation) was also used as a weight-loss procedure, but it is rarely performed today.

Long-Term Weight Maintenance

Losing weight is difficult but it is even more difficult to maintain weight at optimal levels. People who have lost weight often have difficulty maintaining lower, healthier weight because their calorie requirements are lower. It is critical that those who have lost weight maintain the loss by eating carefully according to the *Dietary Guidelines* and MyPyramid, and engaging in physical activity and exercise at least 60–90 minutes daily.

IMPLICATIONS OF WEIGHT ON ORAL HEALTH

Weight loss can have several implications in oral health. Weight loss can cause dentures to no longer fit properly. Nutritionally unsound diets can affect oral soft tissue integrity, undermining healing and response to dental treatment. Over longer periods, changes in bone health caused by calorie-restricted diets may contribute to tooth loss.

TABLE 3-10 Approved Antiobesity Medications by the Food and Drug Administration

Drug	Brand Name(s)	Proposed Mechanism	Common Side Effects
Sibutramine hydrochloride*	Meridia	Combined serotonin–norepinepherine reuptake inhibitor	Increased heart rate and blood pressure, constipation, xerostomia, insomnia, nausea, abdominal pain
Orlistat*	Xenical	Reversible gastrointestinal lipase inhibitor (causes malabsorption of dietary fat)	Oily stools, flatus with discharge, fecal urgency, increased levels of urinary oxalate (rare)
Phentermine HCl	Phentride, Terenine, Adipex, Fastin, Obenix, Oby-Cap, Oby-Trim, Zantryl	Anorectic; stimulates norepinepherine and possibly dopamine release	Increased heart rate and blood pressure, xerostomia, agitation, insomnia, nausea, diarrhea, constipation, hives
Phentermine resin	Ionamin	See Phentermine	See Phentermine
Diethylpropion	Tenuate	See Phentermine	Arrhythmia, tachycardia, elevation of blood pressure, dyskinesia, blurred vision, dizziness, insomnia, anxiety, depression, diarrhea, xerostomia, unpleasant taste, nausea, constipation, hives
Phendimetrazine tartrate	Obezine, Bontril, Adipost	See Phentermine	Restlessness, insomnia, agitation, increased heart rate and blood pressure, xerostomia, nausea, abdominal pain, constipation, diarrhea, polyuria
Benzphetamine	Didrex	See Phentermine	Increased heart rate and blood pressure, constipation, xerostomia, insomnia, hives, psychotic episodes at recommended doses, depression following withdrawal

*Approved for long-term use.

Source: Reprinted from Moyers S: Medications as adjunct therapy for weight loss: Approved and off-label agents in use, *J Am Diet Assoc,* 2005; 105(6): 948–959. Copyright © 2005, with permission from the American Dietetic Association.

Gastric bypass surgery may result in changes in eating patterns toward small semisolid or liquid meals of cariogenic foods, thus increasing caries risks. If patients are also taking weight-loss drugs that cause dry mouth, risks may be very high for caries.

SUMMARY AND IMPLICATIONS FOR DENTISTRY

Adults often see their dental professional more frequently than they do their physician. Therefore, it is important for dental team members to refer patients who have weight-related problems to a physician or registered dietitian for appropriate care.

Dental team members **SHOULD** encourage patients to:

* Know their BMI, if their fat distribution pattern is risky, and if they are obese, underweight, or at risk of these conditions.
* Exercise 60 minutes per day if normal weight or 60–90 minutes per day if overweight or after weight loss and encourage and praise overweight or obese patients if they become more physically active.

* Engage in safe weight-loss methods under a physician's and dietitian's guidance.
* Eat well-balanced meals and increase physical activity following the *Dietary Guidelines* for Americans and MyPyramid (http://www.mypyramid.gov).
* Implement appropriate diet and oral hygiene measures to lessen risks of caries secondary to xerostomia and low saliva levels, especially among patients who have had head and neck surgery.

Dental team members should **NOT**:

* Sell or recommend weight-loss diets. Rather, encourage healthful eating habits and physical activity to improve overall health and well-being. Refer patients who need to lose or gain weight to their physicians.
* Advise patients to take dietary supplements for weight loss because they are of questionable safety and efficacy. However, encourage the use of vitamin and mineral supplements (and electrolytes on very low-calorie diets) during weight loss.
* Suggest over-the-counter weight-loss medications to patients. If patients are adamant about taking a diet drug, refer them to their primary care physician. If a patient is currently taking dietary supplements or weight-loss medications, make sure he or she is under medical supervision.

QUESTIONS PATIENTS MIGHT ASK

Q. Is it better for your weight to eat three large meals a day or small, frequent meals?

A. Generally, it is better to eat balanced but smaller, frequent meals throughout the day. The body's metabolism is better supported when the body is fed in a regular, consistent way. Erratic eating patterns with more than four hours between meals and snacks may cause the body to fight back against what it perceives as deprivation and uncertainty. It may cause the metabolic rate to drop, and it may signal the body to preferentially store calories as fat instead of spending them freely.

Q. I'm hungry all the time, even if I've just eaten. Is something wrong with my metabolism?

A. Chances are that nothing is wrong with your metabolism. If you are frequently tired you may want to go to your physician to get your thyroid levels checked. Listen to your body. Follow your hunger cues and try to determine if you are truly hungry (or just bored, tired, thirsty, or upset). Some physiological signs of hunger (in the order that they tend to occur) are: rumbling, or empty stomach sensation; decreased energy, particularly during physical activity; decreased ability to focus; irritability; headache; feeling weak or shaky; and nausea and cold sweats (Brown University Health Services, 2005). It takes at least 20 minutes for your brain to register that your stomach is full and you should stop eating. Try to eat at a slower pace to give your body time to secrete the appropriate hormones for digestion and satiety. After you eat, wait a half an hour and reassess your hunger. In addition, think about the composition of the meal you just consumed. Was it composed of primarily processed carbohydrates? Did you have any fiber (whole grains, vegetables, fruits)? Fiber keeps us feeling fuller for longer. Did you eat enough protein and fat? Protein and fat are more satiating and take longer to digest than carbohydrates. Do you drink enough with meals? Drinking at least 8 fluid ounces (fl oz) of liquid (preferably water) with your meal may promote an earlier sensation of satiety.

Q. If I skip breakfast, will I lose weight faster because I'll be eating fewer calories throughout the day?

A. Not necessarily. Breakfast is considered an important meal because it breaks the overnight fasting period (which is typically 8 hours), replenishes your supply of glucose, and provides other essential nutrients to keep your energy levels up throughout the day. Several studies have shown that those who skip breakfast may consume more calories during the other meals of the day or consume more snacks.

Q. I'm a middle-aged woman who's tried many different diets and even fasting to try to lose weight since I was a teenager. I am a yo-yo dieter: My weight has gone up and down 50 lb in the past 25 years. I can't seem to keep the weight off. I'm too busy and tired to exercise. Why is this happening?

A. Metabolic changes occur during rapid weight loss and weight gain (yo-yo dieting). Rapid weight loss tends to consist of lean mass. Decreasing lean mass decreases REE, thus decreasing overall daily energy expenditure. When one resumes the increased caloric intake (goes off the diet), the weight gained is mostly fat, which is not metabolically active and does not raise the REE. Your metabolism has most likely slowed due to the constant caloric restriction, loss of lean mass, lack of exercise, and fat regain. Exercise would help burn more calories, increase your energy, and rebuild the lost lean mass, which will help increase REE. Eating small, frequent, balanced meals with enough protein should also help improve your energy levels.

CASE STUDY

At her previous dental checkup, Ms. Brody was 125 lb, a generally healthy, thin, white 27-year-old-PhD student. When she arrived for her 6-month dental visit, the dental examination revealed no recurrent caries, but generalized gingival recession and pocket depths of 4–5 millimeters(mm) on posterior maxillary and mandibular first and second molars. She said she brushes and flosses after every meal, when she wakes in the morning, and before she goes to bed, and uses a firm bristle toothbrush.

She appears to have lost a significant amount of weight since you've seen her last. She is 5 feet 5 inches tall and is now 100 lb. She reports that her appetite has significantly decreased "due to stress" and she's been having diarrhea a few times a day not long after she eats. She reveals that she has lost weight over the past 6 six months and that she's "tired all the time" and "weak." Ms. Brody says that she is not dieting to lose weight. Her daily activities include writing papers and teaching classes at a university. She does not exercise regularly, but she leisurely walks to the grocery store 1 mile away twice a week.

She informs you that two months ago her psychiatrist had prescribed Prozac (fluoxetine) to help with anxiety and depression. Ms. Brody is a vegetarian and lactose intolerant. She avoids milk, but eats some cheeses while taking dairy pills (lactase enzyme). She reports "grazing" on small portions of food throughout the day because she is never "really hungry." You have determined that she is consuming an average of about 1300 calories and 25 g of protein per day. She chews about a pack of sugar-free gum per day.

Questions:

1. Calculate her current BMI and her BMI 6 months ago. How would you classify Ms. Brody's weight 6 months ago? How would you classify her weight now?
2. What is Ms. Brody's healthy weight range?
3. Is she at risk for any diseases or disorders?
4. What are her most significant nutrition issues?
5. What may be contributing to her weight loss? Given the rapid rate of weight loss, what kinds of tissue were most likely lost?
6. What nutrition and oral health recommendations would you make for Ms. Brody?

REFERENCES

Agatston, A: *The South Beach Diet*. New York: Random House, 2003.

Agency for Healthcare Research and Quality: *Ephedra and Ephedrine for Weight Loss and Athletic Performance Enhancement: Clinical Efficacy and Side Effects*. Evidence Report/Technology Assessment Number 76: AHRQ Publication No. 03-E022. February 2003. Retrieved July 6, 2005, from http://www.ahrq.gov/clinic/epcindex.htm#complementary.

Allison DB, Fontaine KR, Manson JE, Stevens J, Van Itallie TB: Annual deaths attributable to obesity in the United States *JAMA* 1999; 282:1530–38.

Alpert S: Growth, thermogenesis, and hyperphagia. *Am J Clin Nutr* 1990; 52:784–92.

American College of Sports Medicine: *ACSM Guidelines for Healthy Aerobic Activity*. Retrieved June 20, 2005, from http://www.acsm.org/pdf/Guidelines.pdf.

American Dietetic Association: Nutrition fact sheet: Popular diets reviewed. 2004. Retrieved from htpp://www.eatright.org.

Associated Press: Diet plan success tough to weigh. January 3, 2005. Retrieved July 15, 2005, from http://www.cbsnews.com/stories/2005/01/03/health/main664519.shtml.

Associated Press: McSupersizes to be phased out. March 3, 2004. Retrieved June 15, 2005, from http://www.cnn.com/2004/US/03/02/mcdonalds.supersize.ap.

Atkins RC: *Dr. Atkins' New Diet Revolution*, Rev. ed. New York: Avon Books, 1998.

Atkins RC: *The Atkins Essentials*. New York: HarperCollins, 2004.

Bahr R, Ingnis I, Vaage O, Sejersted OM, Newsholme EA: Effect of duration of exercise on post exercise O_2 consumption. *J Appl Physiol* 1987; 62:485–90.

Barak N, Wall-Alonso E, Sitrin MD: Evaluation of stress factors and body weight adjustments currently used to estimate energy expenditure in hospitalized patients. *Parenteral and Enteral Nutr* 2002; 26(4):231–37.

Blackburn GL, Phillips JCC, Morreale S: Physician's guide to popular low-carbohydrate weight-loss diets. *Cleveland Clin J Med* 2001 68(9): 761.

Bouchard C, Perusse L, Rice T, Rao DC: Genetics of human obesity. In Bray G, Bouchard C (eds): *Handbook of Obesity*. New York: Marcel Dekker, 2004.

Bray GA: Overweight, mortality, and morbidity. In Bouchard C (ed): *Physical Activity and Obesity*. Champaign, IL: Human Kinetics, 2000:31–53.

Buchwald H: Bariatric surgery for morbid obesity: Health implications for patients, health professionals, and third-party payers. *J Am Coll Surg* 2005; 200(4): 593–604.

Calamaro CJ, Faith MS: Preventing childhood overweight. *Nutr Today* 2005; 39(5):194–99.

Consumer Reports: The truth about dieting. June 2002:26–32.

Consumer Reports: Rating the diets from Atkins to Zone. June 2005.

Cummings DE, Schwartz MW: Genetics and pathophysiology of human obesity. *Annu Rev Med* 2003;54:453–71.

Dietz WH: Health consequences of obesity in youth: Childhood predictors of adult disease. *Pediatrics* 1998;101:518–25.

Dietz WH, Bandini LG, Morelli JA, Peers KF, Ching PL: Effect of sedentary activities on resting metabolic rate. *Am J Clin Nutr* 1994; 59:556–59.

Dietz WH Jr, Gortmaker SL: Do we fatten our children at the television set? Obesity and television viewing in children and adolescents. *Pediatrics* 1985; 75:807–12.

Doll H, Petersen SE, Stewart-Brown SL: Obesity and physical and emotional well-being: Associations between body mass index, chronic illness and the physical and mental components of the SF-36 questionnaire. *Obes Res* 2000; 8:160–70.

Donnelly JE, Smith B, Jacobsen DJ, Kirk E, Dubose K, Hyob M, et al.: The role of exercise for weight loss and maintenance. *Clin Gastroenterol* 2004; 18(6): 1009–29.

Dwyer JT, Allison DB, Coates PM: Dietary supplements in weight reduction. *J Am Diet Assoc* 2005; 105:S80-S86.

Dwyer JT, Melanson KJ: Dietary treatment of obesity. Endotext.com. (2002). Retrieved April 15, 2005, from http://www.endotext.com/obesity/obesity18/obesity18.htm.

Eades MR, Eades MD: *Protein Power*. New York: Bantam Books, 1999.

European Food Information Council: Determinants of food choice. *EUFIC Review* N17, April 2005. Retrieved July 13, 2005, from http://www.eufic.org/images/Eufic%20review_17_final.pdf.

Faith MS, Calamaro CJ, Dolan MS, Pietrobelli A: Mood disorders and obesity. *Curr Opin Psychiatry* 2004; 17:9–13.

Fat chance? Making sense of the new research on weight and mortality. *Tufts University Health and Nutr Lett* 2005; 23(5).

Flaherty J: Who made America fat? *Tufts Nutr* Fall 2004; 6(1): 19.

Flegal KM, Carroll MD, Ogden CL, Johnson CL: Prevalence and trends in obesity among U.S. adults, 1999–2000. *JAMA* 2002; 228:1723–27.

Flegal KM, Graubord BI, Williamson DF, Gail MH: Excess deaths associated with underweight, overweight and obesity. *JAMA* 2005; 293:1861–67.

Food and Agriculture Organization of the United Nations: Chapter 2: Principles and definitions. In *Human Energy Requirements: Report of a Joint FAO/WHO/UNU Expert Consultation*. 2004. Retrieved July 9, 2005, from http://www.fao.org/documents/show_cdr.asp?url_file=/docrep/007/y5686e/y5686e04.htm.

Food and Drug Administration: FDA issues regulation prohibiting sale of dietary supplements containing ephedrine alkaloids and reiterates its advice that consumers stop using these products. February 6, 2004. Retrieved July 6, 2005, from http://www.cfsan.fda.gov/~lrd/fpephed6.html.

Foster GD, Wyatt HR, Hill JO, McGuckin BG, Brill C, Mohammed BS, et al.: A randomized trial of a low-carbohydrate diets for obesity. *N Engl J Med* 2003; 348: 2082–90.

Frary CD, Johnson RK: Chapter 2: Energy. In Mahan LK, Escott-Stump S (eds): *Krause's Food, Nutrition and Diet Therapy*, 11th ed. Philadelphia: WB Saunders, 2004.

Gillis LJ: Food away from home, sugar-sweetened drink consumption and juvenile obesity. *J Am Coll Nutr* 2003; 22:539–45.

Gore SA, Foster JA, DiLillo VG, Kirk K, Smith West D: Television viewing and snacking. *Eat Behav.* 2003; 4(4):399–405.

Gortmaker SL, Must A, Sobol AM, Peterson K, Colditz GA, Dietz WH: Television viewing as a cause of increasing obesity among children in the United States, 1986–1990. *Arch Pediatr Adolesc Med* 1996; 150:356–62.

Grimm GC, Harnack L, Story M: Factors associated with soft drink consumption in school-aged children. *J Am Diet Assoc* 2004; 104:1244–49.

Halford JC, Brown V, Pontin EE, Dovey TM: Effect of television advertisements for foods on food consumption in children. *Appetite* 2004; 42(2):221–25.

Hark L, Morrison G: *Medical Nutrition and Disease*, 3rd ed. Malden, MA: Blackwell, 2003.

Institute of Medicine, National Academy of Sciences: *Dietary References Intakes of Energy, Carbohydrate, Fiber, Fat, Fatty Acids, Cholesterol, Protein, and Amino Acids (Macronutrients)*.2005. Retrieved July 10, 2005, from http://www.nap.edu/openbook/030908373/html/93.html.

Institute of Medicine, National Academy of Sciences: Preventing childhood obesity: Health in the balance. Report Brief. September 2004. Retrieved July 6, 2005, from http://www.iom.edu.

Keim NL, Blanton CA, Kretsch MJ: America's obesity epidemic: Measuring physical activity to promote an active lifestyle. *J Am Diet Assoc* 2004; 104(9).

Kelly J, Tarnoff M, Shikora S, Thayer B, Jones DB, Amour Forse R, et al.: Best practice recommendations for surgical care in weight loss surgery. *Obesity Res* 2005; 13(2): 227–33.

Kleiner S: Water: An essential but overlooked nutrient. *J Am Diet Assoc* 1999; 99:200–206.

Kortt M, Langley P, Cox E: A review of cost-of-illness studies on obesity. *Clin Ther* 1998; 20:772–79.

Kubik MY, Hannan PH, Perry CI, Story M: The association of the school food environment with dietary behaviors of young adolescents. *Am J Pub Health* 2003; 93:1168–73.

Kushner RF, Blatner DJ: Risk assessment of the overweight and obese patient. *J Am Diet Assoc* 2005; 105:S53–S62.

Laquatra: Chapter 24: Nutrition for weight management. In Mahan LK, Escott-Stump S (eds): *Krause's Food, Nutrition and Diet Therapy*, 11th ed. Philadelphia: WB Saunders, 2004.

Leighton Steward H, Bethea MC, Balart LA, Andrews SS: *Sugar Busters!* New York: Ballantine Books, 1999.

Loos RJF, Bouchard C: Obesity—is it a genetic disorder? *J Intern Med* 2003; 254:401–425.

Mann J: Chapter 6: Carbohydrates. In Bowman BA, Russell RM: *Present Knowledge in Nutrition*, 8th ed. Washington, DC: ILSI Press, 2001.

McGraw P: *The Ultimate Weight Solution Cookbook*. New York: Free Press, 2004.

Melanson K, Dwyer JT: Popular diets for treatment of overweight and obesity. In Wadden TA, Stunkard AJ (eds): *Handbook of Obesity Treatment*. New York: Guilford Press, 2002:249–82.

Miller K: Obesity: Surgical options. *Best Pract Res Clin Gastroentero 2004;* 18(6): 1147–65.

Miller JB, Foster-Powell K, Burani J: *The Glucose Revolution Life Plan*. New York: Marlowe & Company, 2001.

Mokdad AH, Marks JS, Stroup DF, Gerberding JL: Actual causes of death in the United States. *JAMA* 2000; 291:1238–45.

Morley, JE, Thomas, DR, Wilson, MMG: Appetite and orexigenic drugs. *Ann of Long Term Care Supplement II* Oct., 2001: 1–12.

Moyers S: Medications as adjunct therapy for weight loss: Approved and off-label agents in use. *J Am Diet Assoc* 2005; 105(6).

National Heart, Lung, and Blood Institute: Obesity Education Initiative Expert Panel on the Identification, Evaluation, and Treatment of Overweight and Obesity in Adults. *Clinical Guidelines on the Identification, Evaluation, and Treatment of Overweight and Obesity in Adults*. Bethesda, MD: Author, 1998.

Neumark-Sztainer D, Croll J, Story M, Hannan PJ, French S, Perry C: Ethnic/racial differences in weight-related concerns and behaviors among adolescent girls and boys: Findings from Project EAT. *J Psychosom Res* 2002; 53:963–74.

Neumark-Sztainer D, Story M, Hannan PJ, Perry CL, Irving LM: Weight-related concerns and behaviors among overweight and non-overweight adolescents: Implications for preventing weight-related disorders. *Arch Pediatr Adolesc Med* 2002; 156:171–78.

North American Association for the Study of Obesity: Childhood overweight. 2005. Retrieved July 22, 2005; from http://www.naaso.org/information/childhood_over-weight.asp.

North American Association for the Study of Obesity: Principles of energy metabolism slide talk. (2004). Retrieved June 25, 2005; from http://www.obesityonline.org/slides/index.cfm.

Ogden CL, Flegal KM, Carroll IMD, Johnson CL: Prevalence and trends in overweight among U.S. children and adolescents, 1999–2000. *JAMA* 2002; 288:1728–32.

OPTIFAST website, http://www.optifast.com/index.jsp.

Ornish D: *Eat More, Weigh Less: Dr. Dean Ornish's Life Choice Program for Losing Weight Safely While Eating Abundantly*. New York: HarperCollins, 1993.

Overeaters Anonymous website, http://www.oa.org/index.htm

Peters JC: Social change and obesity prevention: Where do we begin? *Nutr Today* 2004; 39(3):112–17.

Pitts RF: Ionic composition of body fluids. In *The Physiological Basis of Diuretic Therapy*. Springfield, IL: Charles C Thomas, 1959.

Pitts RF: *Physiology of the Kidney and Body Fluids*, 3rd ed. Chicago: Year Book Medical Publishers, 1974:11–35.

Poehlman ET, Horton ES: Chapter 5: Energy needs and assessment and requirements in humans. In Shils ME,

Olsen JA, Shike M, Ross AC (eds): *Modern Nutrition in Health and Disease*, 9th ed. Philadelphia: Lippincott Williams & Wilkins, 1999:95–104.

Poehlman ET, Melby CL, Goran MI: The impact of exercise and diet restriction on daily energy expenditure. *Sports Med* 1991; 11:78–101.

Pronsky ZM, Redfern, Crowe, Epstein: *Food Medication Interactions*, 13th ed. Birchrunville, PA: Food Medication Interactions, 2004.

Puhl RM, Brownell KD: Psychosocial origins of obesity stigma: Toward changing a powerful and pervasive bias. *Obes Rev* 2003; 4:213–27.

Roubenoff RA, Roubenoff R: Nutritional support of the acutely and chronically ill patient. In Taylor R (ed): *Difficult Medical Management*. Philadelphia: WB Saunders, 1990.

Schoeller DA: The importance of clinical research: The role of thermogenesis in human obesity. *Am J Clin Nutr* 2001; 73:511–516.

Schoeller DA, Buchholz, AC: Energetics of obesity and weight control: Does diet composition matter? *J Am Diet Assoc* 2005; 105:S24 S28.

Schoenborn CA, Adams PF, Barnes PM, Vickerie JL, Schiller JS: Health behaviors of adults: United States, 1999–2001. National Center for Health Statistics. *Vital Health Stat* 10(219): 2004.

Schutz Y, Bessard T, Jequier E: Diet-induced thermogenesis measured over a whole day in obese and non-obese women. *Am J Clin Nutr* 1984; 40:542–52.

Sears, B: *Enter the Zone: The Dietary Road Map to Lose Weight & More*. New York: HarperCollins, 1995.

Serdula MK, Mokdad AH, Williamson DF, Galuska DA, Mendlein JM, Heath GW: Prevalence of attempting weight loss and strategies for controlling weight. *JAMA* 1999; 282:1353–58.

Shekelle PG, Hardy ML, Morton SC, Maglione M, Mojica WA, Suttorp, MJ, et al.: Efficacy and safety of ephedra and ephedrine for weight loss and athletic performance: A meta-analysis. *JAMA* 2003; 289:1537–45.

Slim-Fast website, http://www.slim-fast.com

Slone DC: Nutritional requirements in the critically ill patient. *Crit Care Clin* 2004; 20:135–57.

Swinburn BA, Seidell JC, James WP: Diet, nutrition, and the prevention of excess weight gain and obesity. *Public Health Nutr* 2004; 7:123–46.

Take It Off and Keep It Off: Based on the Successful Methods of Overeaters Anonymous. Chicago: Contemporary Books, 1989.

Take Off Pounds Sensibly (TOPS) website, http://www.tops.org/.

Thomas PR: Dietary supplements for weight loss? *Nutr Today* 2005; 40(1).

Tsai A, Wadden TA: Systematic review: An evaluation of major commercial weight loss programs in the United States. *Ann Intern Med* 2005; 142:56–66.

USDA Agriculture Fact Book 2001–2002. Chapter 2: Profiling food consumption in America. 2002. Retrieved June 25, 2005, from http://www.usda.gov/factbook/index.html.

U.S. Department of Health and Human Services and the U.S. Department of Agriculture: Chapter 4: Physical activity. In *Dietary Guidelines for Americans 2005*. 2005. Retrieved from http://www.health.gov/dietaryguidelines/dga2005/document/html/chapter 4.htm.

U.S. Department of Health and Human Services, Centers for Disease Control and Prevention: *Physical activity and health: A report of the Surgeon General (1996)*. Retrieved June 20, 2005, from http://www.cdc.gov/nccdphp/sgr/summary.htm.

Van Baak MA: Physical activity and energy balance. *Public Health Nutr* 1999; 2(3a):335–339.

Van Baak MA, Saris WHM: Exercise and obesity. In Kopelman PG, Stock MJ (eds): *Clinical Obesity*. London: Blackwell Science, 1998.

Van Itallie T: Diets for weight reduction: Mechanisms of action and physiological effects. In Bray G (ed): *Obesity: Comparative Methods of Weight Control*. London: John Libbey, 1980.

Weight Watchers, http://www.weightwatchers.com

Westerterp KR, Wilson SA, Rolland V: Diet induced thermogenesis measured over 24 h in a respiration chamber: Effect of diet composition. *Int J Obes Relat Metab Disord* 1999; 23(3):287–92.

Whitney EN, Cataldo CB, Rolfes SR: Chapter 8: Energy balance and body composition. Table: Factors that affect BMR p. 247. In *Understanding Normal and Clinical Nutrition*, 6th ed. Belmont, CA: Wadsworth Group/Thompson Learning, 2002.

Williams SR: Chapter 7: Energy balance and weight management. In *Nutrition and Diet Therapy*, 8th ed. St. Louis: Mosby, 1997.

Wolf AM, Colditz GA: Current estimates of the economic cost of obesity in the United States. *Obesity Res* 1998; 6:97–106.

Yang MU, Van Itallie TB: Composition of weight lost during short-term weight reduction. Metabolic responses of obese subjects to starvation and low-calorie ketogenic and nonketogenic diets. *J Clin Invest* 1976; 58:722–30.

Chapter **4**

Carbohydrates, Diabetes, and Associated Health Conditions

Stacy A. Weill and Linda Boyd

OBJECTIVES

The student will be able to:

- Describe the chemical composition of carbohydrates.
- Classify the carbohydrates and provide food sources of each.
- Detail carbohydrate digestion, absorption, and transport in the body.
- Discuss carbohydrate metabolism in the body.
- Detail the recommended dietary guidelines for carbohydrate intake.
- Discuss the etiology, types, symptoms, and management strategies for diabetes mellitus.
- Describe the characteristics of the common alternative sweeteners.

INTRODUCTION

In today's society, *carbohydrates* are often misunderstood. The diet book industry has helped convince the public that carbohydrates (including sugars) are responsible for obesity (they aren't) and a host of other ills. This is unfortunate because carbohydrates are important components of a healthy diet and serve many important functions in the body. When people think of carbohydrates, they often think simplistically of bread and pasta. Although they may equate sucrose with the word *sugar*, in fact there are several different sugars that are found commonly in grains, fruits, vegetables, and milk.

The term *carbohydrate* denotes a class of nutrients that ranges from the simple sugars like glucose to the complex carbohydrates like starch and the indigestible fibers. Digestible carbohydrates are considered the major source of fuel in humans. They are widely distributed in food and are inexpensive sources of energy. The brain requires glucose alone as an energy source.

CARBOHYDRATE FUNCTIONS

Carbohydrates serve a variety of essential functions in the body (Weigley, Muller, Robinson, 1997):

- The primary function is to provide a source of energy to facilitate body metabolism and control body temperature.
- Carbohydrates are essential for brain and nervous tissue function.
- Carbohydrates (and fats) "spare protein." In other words, when there is sufficient carbohydrate and fat in the diet to meet energy needs, protein is spared to be used for its primary role of tissue synthesis, and is not metabolized for energy. However, when there is insufficient carbohydrate or fat in the diet, protein is diverted to be used primarily for energy and is not available for tissue regeneration.
- Carbohydrates are required for proper fat metabolism. When there is too little carbohydrate, products of fatty acid metabolism called ketones accumulate in the blood and can be harmful.
- Carbohydrates are needed for structural compounds in the body such as chondroitin sulfate, needed for development of cartilage, bone, and nervous tissue. They also help form the "ground

substance," which is the foundation for collagen formation.
- Carbohydrates combine with nitrogen to form nonessential amino acids.

CARBOHYDRATE CHEMISTRY

Carbohydrates are formed in plants through the process of photosynthesis. Green plants use water from the soil, energy from the sun, and carbon dioxide from the air to synthesize carbohydrates. Thus carbohydrates are made of hydrogen, oxygen, and carbon. When used for energy in the body, each gram of carbohydrate yields 4 kilocalories (kcal).

Ethanol is an alcohol that is made by fermentation of food carbohydrates. Ethanol is metabolized somewhat like a fat in the body, and yields 7 kcal/g.

CLASSIFICATION

Carbohydrates may be classified from simple sugars (monosaccharides, disaccharides) to complex polysaccharides (starch, fiber) (Table 4–1). The most important monosaccharide is glucose. Disaccharides are formed by linking two monosaccharides together to form maltose, lactose, and sucrose. Complex carbohydrates or polysaccharides, such as starch and fiber, are longer chain glucose molecules. Approximately half of dietary carbohydrates are polysaccharides (Figures 4–1 and 4–2).

Most of the sugars end with the suffix *–ose;* their respective digestive enzymes end with the suffix *–ase.* An example would be the disaccharide sucrose and its digestive enzyme sucr*ase*, or the starch amylose and its digestive enzyme amyl*ase.*

Monosaccharides

The simplest carbohydrates are the monosaccharides glucose, fructose, and galactose. Glucose is the final breakdown product of carbohydrates in the body and is the major energy source for the body. Glucose and the other monosaccharides are known as simple sugars. The three monosaccharides—glucose, galactose, and fructose—are all six-carbon hexoses. Glucose is the most abundant simple sugar in nature and the most nutritionally important. Monosaccharides are essentially the only form of carbohydrate that can

TABLE 4–1   Classification and Food Sources of Carbohydrates

Complex Carbohydrates: *Starch*	Breads, rolls: whole grain, white, enriched, pita, pumpernickel, bagels, English muffins, quick breads, muffins, biscuits, cakes, waffles
	Breakfast cereals: cooked and ready to eat
	Grits
	Crackers: rye crisp, saltines
	Snacks: pretzels
	Pastas: macaroni, spaghetti
	Rice
	Legumes: soybeans, dried beans (kidney, navy, pinto), dried peas (black-eyed, split, chickpea, lentils)
	White and sweet potatoes, corn, taro, plantain, breadfruit
	Whole, unprocessed grains, vegetables, fruits, legumes
Dietary Fiber	Whole grain breads, cereals,
	Unpeeled vegetables
	Whole fruits
	Whole cooked peas, beans
Simple Carbohydrates: *Disaccharides:*	**Sucrose:** cane, beet, maple sugar, fruits, and vegetables
	Maltose: malting of cereal grain by starch hydrolysis, beer, cereals
	Lactose: milk only
Monosaccharides	**Glucose:** (dextrose, grape sugar, corn sugar) fruits, vegetables, corn syrup, honey
	Fructose: (levulose, fruit sugar) fruits, vegetables, corn syrup, honey
	Galactose: occurs only from lactose hydrolysis
Added Sweeteners	Simple carbohydrates such as cane sugar, corn sugar, corn syrup, high-fructose corn syrup, maltodextrin, dextrose, fructose
	Soft drinks, table sugar, bakery items, jams, jellies, gelatin desserts, popsicles, preserved cereals, cakes, cookies, donuts, pies, salad dressings, catsup, frozen meals
	Some vitamins and medications

be absorbed directly by the body. The body can convert galactose and fructose into glucose. The majority of glucose is stored in the liver and muscle as glycogen. Some is circulating in the blood to maintain serum glucose levels. The amount of glucose normally stored as glycogen provides approximately 14 to 24 hours of stored energy.

Glucose (also known as dextrose) can be found naturally in many fruits and in some vegetables. Specific food sources include grapes, oranges, corn, and carrots.

Galactose is found in milk as part of the molecule lactose. It can also be found in some legumes. Fructose (also known as levulose) is the sweetest of the monosaccharides, and can be found in honey and many fruits (Table 4–2 shows the relative sweetness of sugars).

Disaccharides

The major disaccharides are sucrose, maltose, and lactose. Of the disaccharides, sucrose currently furnishes approximately one-third of the total carbohydrate in the average Western diet. Sucrose is composed of one glucose and one fructose molecule, and is found abundantly in fruits and vegetables. Table sugar is sucrose derived from sugar cane and sugar beets. Molasses is an intermediary product in sugar refinement. Brown sugar is manufactured by spraying molasses onto refined sucrose. Sucrose enhances the flavor and desirability of many foods. It is also the most predominant food preservative used in the world today.

Maltose is composed of two glucose units and is formed from the hydrolysis of starch. Most common sources are beer, malt beverages and cereals, and malt liquor.

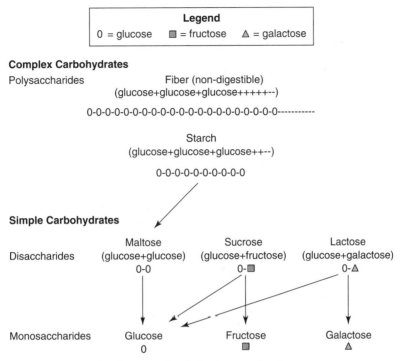

FIGURE 4-1 Classification of carbohydrates in food.

Lactose is composed of one molecule of glucose and one molecule of galactose. Lactose, also known as milk sugar, is unique to mammals. It is not naturally present in plant products. Lactose is found in milk and related dairy products, which are major dietary sources of nutrients needed for calcification of bones and teeth.

Polysaccharides

Polysaccharides are composed of many glucose molecules linked together in different configurations (from approximately 400 to hundreds of thousands of glucose molecules). The food polysaccharides include starches,

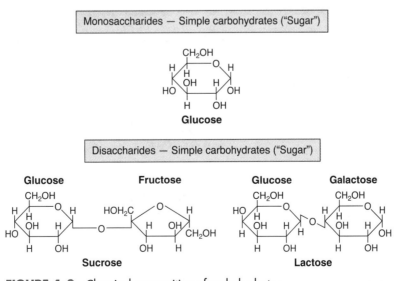

FIGURE 4-2 Chemical composition of carbohydrates.

TABLE 4–2 Relative Sweetness of Sugars in Comparison to Sucrose

Carbohydrate	Percent
Fructose	150–175
High-fructose corn syrup (HFCS)	150
Sucrose	**100**
Glucose	70
Dextrin	30
Lactose	15
Starch	not sweet

Source: From *Robinson's Basic Nutrition and Diet Therapy,* 8/E by Weigley/Mueller/Robinson, © 1997. Reprinted with permission.

glycogen, and the dietary fibers. The manner in which the glucose units are joined together determines polysaccharide digestibility. Mucopolysaccharides such as chondroitin sulfate are not food carbohydrates but are structural carbohydrates found in the body.

Starch and Glycogen

The two major forms of starch include amylose and amylopectin. Both amylose and amylopectin are digestible. Glycogen, the animal storage form of glucose, is similar to amylopectin. Starch is found in grain and grain foods, legumes, potatoes, and unripe fruits.

Fiber

Dietary fiber is mostly indigestible and is not used for energy by the human body; however, fiber has other important roles in the body (Table 4–3). Fiber promotes gastrointestinal function and motility, and may help in the prevention or management of several health conditions. Fibers can be further described by their classification as insoluble and soluble fiber.

Insoluble Fiber Insoluble fiber is what was formerly called "roughage." Insoluble fibers include cellulose, hemicellulose, and lignin, and provide the structure for plant cell walls. Insoluble fibers are found in whole grain breads and cereals; vegetables such as lettuce, asparagus, artichokes, popcorn, root vegetables, legumes, and peas; apples; and bran.

Insoluble fibers do not dissolve, but they do hold water. This allows them to help speed up transit time through the gastrointestinal tract by providing bulk to the stool and increasing peristaltic movement in the gastrointestinal tract. This function is important in the prevention of disease states such as diverticulitis, hemorrhoids, and constipation. Because of its ability to act like a sponge, insoluble fiber may also help control cholesterol levels by preventing cholesterol from returning through the enterohepatic pathway (liver recycling of bile salts and cholesterol). Insoluble fiber may also play a part in controlling the absorption of glucose, thus providing help in controlling blood glucose levels in people with diabetes.

TABLE 4–3 Food Fiber

Types of Fiber	Major Food Sources	Potential Health Effects	Possible Mechanisms
Insoluble			
Cellulose	Wheat bran	• May help prevent:	• Increases bulk
Hemicellulose	Cereals, vegetables; navy, kidney, lima, pinto beans; Fruit and vegetable skins	constipation diverticulosis and diverticulitis hemorrhoids	• Speeds stool through bowel (laxative) • Minimizes bowel contact with carcinogens
Lignin	Vegetables	• May help reduce cancer risk	
Soluble			
Gums and Mucilages	Barley Legumes: navy, pinto, lima beans Oat bran	• Aids in satiety • Stabilizes blood sugar • Helps lower blood cholesterol • Improves mineral nutriture	• Delays stomach emptying (slowing glucose release into the bloodstream) • Binds with bile acids preventing absorption
Pectin	Fruit		• Aids mineral absorption (except calcium)

The ability to be highly absorptive may also be a detriment, as fiber is not selective in its absorption and may also delay or prevent the absorption of essential vitamins and minerals. Particularly high amounts of fiber can cause diarrhea. High amounts of fiber without adequate water can cause constipation. Thus, it is important to drink plenty of water with a high-fiber diet.

Soluble Fiber Soluble fiber differs from insoluble fiber in that it dissolves and forms gels around substances to hinder their absorption. Soluble fiber is found primarily in gums, pectins, and mucilages. Food sources of soluble fiber include most fruits, oats, barley, and some legumes. In general, soluble fiber delays gastric emptying and increases gastrointestinal transit time. Soluble fiber also plays an important role in food production. It is used as a stabilizer, as in the case of guar, or to stop ice crystals from forming, as in the case of carageenan. Soluble fiber also has some of the same health benefits as insoluble fiber and may decrease glucose absorption and help lower blood cholesterol.

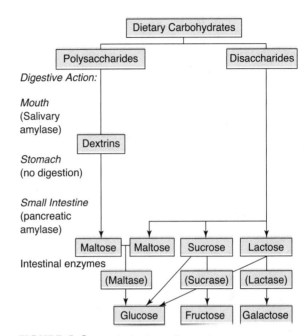

FIGURE 4–3 Carbohydrate digestion.

CARBOHYDRATE DIGESTION, ABSORPTION, TRANSPORT, AND STORAGE

The initial stage of carbohydrate digestion is both mechanical and chemical (Figure 4–3). Mechanical digestion begins in the mouth with the chewing and grinding of food. Healthy dentition is important to this process. Many forms of carbohydrate, especially those consumed raw, and many fruits and vegetables require adequate chewing to prepare them for further digestion in the stomach and small intestine.

Chemical digestion also begins in the mouth when the enzyme amylase (ptyalin), in saliva, hydrolyzes the alpha −1,4 bonds of the starch molecule. Saliva also facilitates the progression of food from the mouth to the pharynx and esophagus, through its moistening ability.

When carbohydrates enter the stomach, they are processed with more mechanical movements as the stomach mixes and churns the food to prepare it for entry into the small intestine.

Carbohydrate breakdown is completed in the small intestine with the aid of specific enzymes on the brush border (villi) of the small intestine (e.g., the

disaccharidases sucrase, maltase, and lactase) that complete disaccharide digestion. The remaining monosaccharides are absorbed across the intestinal lumen and transported to the liver. Glucose and galactose are absorbed by active transport, and fructose is absorbed by diffusion. In the liver, galactose and fructose are converted to glucose. The glucose is released into the blood and carried to the cells to be used for energy as needed.

Excess glucose may also be stored as glycogen in the liver or muscle cells. The process of converting glucose into glycogen for storage is known as glycogenesis. The body has the capacity to store approximately 14 hours of glucose in the form of glycogen.

Within 1 to 4 hours after carbohydrate ingestion, digestion is complete. Only the indigestible fibers and a small portion of any ingested starch may remain.

CARBOHYDRATE METABOLISM

The disposition of carbohydrates throughout the human body is determined by energy demands (Levin, 1999). The liver and kidney control glucose metabolism through tightly controlled hormone regulation. After carbohydrates enter cells, they are metabolized to carbon dioxide, hydrogen, and water through complex aerobic and anaerobic processes outlined in Figure 4–4.

Glucose molecules may proceed through glycolysis or be diverted into the hexose monophosphaste shunt (HMS). The HMS is responsible for producing the five-carbon sugar ribose, used in RNA and DNA synthesis. The glucose molecule completes a very precise transition where each step is enzyme mediated. The six-carbon glucose molecule is split into two three-carbon molecules (glyceraldehyde 3-phosphate). They progress through a series of conversions into pyruvate. Each step is capable of producing energy. Further conversion of pyruvate and entrance into the tricarboxylic acid (TCA) cycle is dependent on the presence of oxygen. Without the presence of oxygen, or an anaerobic environment, the pyruvate molecule may ultimately become lactate. In cells that lack mitochondria, such as the erythrocyte (red blood cell), glycolysis is the only provider of adenosine triphosphate (ATP) energy. In the presence of oxygen, or an aerobic environment, the complete phosphorylation of pyruvate occurs and the molecule may then progress into the TCA cycle (Krebs cycle or citric acid cycle).

The pyruvate molecule enters the TCA cycle as acetyl coenzyme A (CoA) and progresses through a series of conversions into oxaloacetate. During

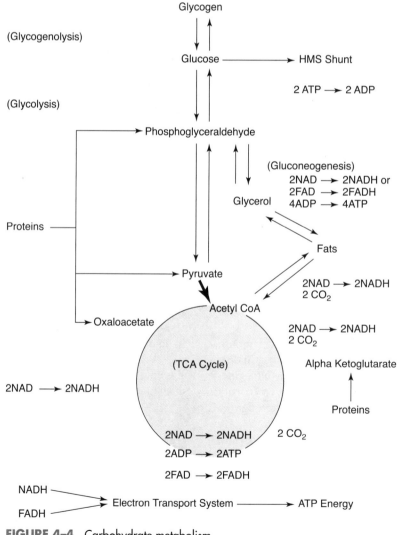

FIGURE 4–4 Carbohydrate metabolism.

this transformation energy is produced. The electron transport system provides the final steps of oxidative phosphorylation. The electrons transported by the electron carriers, nicotinamide adenine dinucleotide (NAD) and flavin adenine dinucleotide (FAD), progress through a series of reactions, with the final result being the production of ATP energy. At the end of the electron transport system, oxygen accepts the electron and becomes water.

The other macronutrient fuels, lipid and protein, feed into the metabolic system at various different points. However, without the presence of glucose, the system malfunctions. The importance of adequate carbohydrate ingestion is essential to burn fat as well as protein for fuel.

In conclusion, through the ingestion of food, human beings are able to produce enough energy to maintain all bodily functions, with the only by-products being carbon dioxide and water.

CARBOHYDRATES AND BLOOD GLUCOSE REGULATION

Blood glucose regulation is crucial to the normal functioning of the human body; the body has elaborate homeostatic mechanisms to maintain stable blood glucose levels (Figure 4–5). Normal fasting blood glucose concentration ranges from 60 to 120 milligrams per deciliter (mg/dL) in a healthy individual. After a meal, the blood glucose level may rise to approximately 140 mg/dL. When blood glucose levels are too low, the pancreas releases the hormone glucagon, which stimulates the liver to breakdown stored glycogen into glucose.

During times of stress the hormone epinephrine may have a similar metabolic effect as glucagon. Additionally, other hormones such as the corticosteroids, which are most important postsurgically or during sepsis, can have similar effects. The breakdown

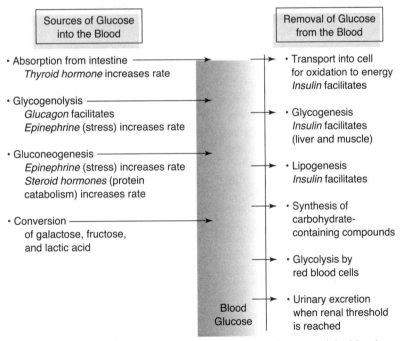

FIGURE 4–5   Blood sugar maintenance. Normally after a meal the blood sugar rises to about 140 mg/dL. After a night's fast the blood sugar level is about 60 to 100 mg/dL. The blood sugar level increases by the release of glucose from glycogen, the synthesis of glucose from glycerol and from some amino acids, and of course through absorption of sugars from the intestinal tract. The blood glucose level fails as the liver removes some of it for the synthesis of glycogen, the conversion of glucose to fats, and the synthesis of other compounds.

of glycogen into glucose is most commonly known as glycogenolysis.

Conversely, when blood glucose levels are too high, the pancreas releases the hormone insulin, which helps transport glucose into the cells for use as energy or in the case of excess intake, for storage as glucagon or fat. Unregulated blood glucose levels may result in hypoglycemia (low blood sugar) or hyperglycemia (high blood sugar). Both situations may have dire consequences on the normal functioning of the human body as evidenced in diabetes mellitus. Diabetes mellitus is discussed in more detail in Chapter 11.

CARBOHYDRATE REQUIREMENTS AND FOOD SOURCES

The new Dietary Reference Intakes for carbohydrates suggest that carbohydrates should supply between 45 and 65% of daily calories (IOM, 2005). Both children and adults should consume at lease 130 grams (g) of digestible carbohydrate daily. This is based on the minimum amount of carbohydrates needed to produce sufficient glucose for brain funtion. Most people consume far more. Complex carbohydrates (starches) should provide the greater part of carbohydrate intake. Of the 45 to 65% total daily recommendations for carbohydrates, approximately 14 g per 1000 calories should be from fiber (soluble and insoluble). The average diet today contains only 8 to 12 g of fiber per day compared to the 20–35 g recommended. The best food sources of fiber are whole grains, fruits, and vegetables. A whole grain is the entire edible part of any grain. Whole grain products have more fiber than refined because they contain the bran and germ, which contain most of the fiber. The whole grain has three components (Figure 4–6):

- the bran or outer layer: high in B-complex vitamins, minerals, and fiber
- the endosperm or inner part of the grain: mostly carbohydrate and protein; endosperm is the source of white flour
- the germ: the sprouting part of the grain, which contains vitamin E, B, trace minerals, and a little protein and fat

Added sugars should not exceed 25% of total calories to ensure sufficient intake of essential

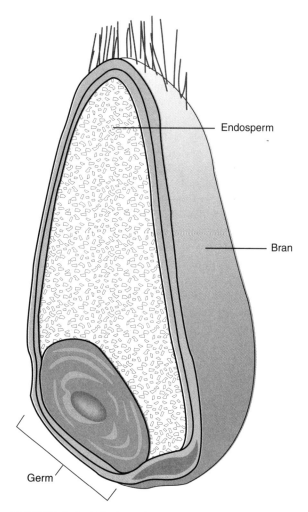

FIGURE 4–6 Whole grain.

micro-nutrients (IOM, 2005). These are part of the "discretionary calories" category and should not exceed the allowance given for each specific calorie level. More information on each level and its associated added sugars recommendation can be found at http://www.health.gov/dietary guidelines.

Despite recommendations, the largest percentage of total dietary carbohydrate consumed is often simple sugars instead of complex carbohydrates. This may contribute to increased incidence of dental caries. Excessive carbohydrates may contribute to chronic diseases as well if they are low in fiber and high in fat.

The U. S. Department of Agriculture (USDA) updated its food guide pyramid in 2005. The update—

called MyPyramid—was done to reflect the new *Dietary Guidelines* including balancing food intake with physical activity. The pyramid was essentially tipped on its side to show the importance of including foods from all the food groups. The width of the bands show the proportion of the foods one should eat from each food group. The groups containing carbohydrates (e.g., the grains, vegetables, fruit, milk, and even the meat group, which contains legumes) reflect the *Dietary Guidelines* suggestion that 45–65% of daily caloric intake come from carbohydrates. The bands of each group are much wider at the base in an effort to remind people to eat foods from each group with lower amounts of added fats and sugars. Stairs appear at the side of the pyramid to remind the reader that exercise is also an important part of overall diet and fitness. In addition, instead of using the former "one pyramid fits all" technique the USDA created 12 different pyramids that reflect the differences in caloric needs and activity levels. The changes were made in an effort to address the criticism that the original pyramid confused people and encouraged them to eat excessive amounts of certain foods including carbohydrates regardless of their classification, thus contributing to the obesity epidemic now facing many parts of the world.

All plant sources contain carbohydrates. With the exception of milk, animal products contain little carbohydrate (only glycogen in liver). Table 4–1 shows food sources of carbohydrates.

EFFECTS OF TOO LITTLE CARBOHYDRATE

Carbohydrate deficiency is rare because carbohydrates are found abundantly and are inexpensive. One sign of deficient carbohydrate intake in some people is hypoglycemia, or low blood sugar. In the absence of sufficient carbohydrate, lipid catabolism occurs, increasing ketones (acid by-products of fat metabolism) in the blood and urine. Despite many claims in the popular press, this condition is rare. When it is accurately diagnosed, the proper dietary approach is to eat several small meals a day containing a mix of complex carbohydrates (high in fiber), proteins, and fat; to avoid eating sugary foods by themselves; to limit caffeine; and to have fruit or juice if symptoms occur. Too little dietary fiber increases risk of constipation, diverticulosis, and hemorrhoids.

EFFECTS OF TOO MUCH CARBOHYDRATE

There are no specific direct effects of excessive carbohydrate consumption. However, too much carbohydrate translates into too many calories, which may contribute to weight gain. Too many "empty calorie" sweets and sweetened beverages can replace more nutritious foods and can contribute to decreased micronutrient (vitamins and minerals) intake. Many sweet foods also contain high amounts of fat, which has twice as many calories as carbohydrates. Also, frequent consumption of carbohydrate-containing foods increases the risk of dental caries.

CURRENT CARBOHYDRATE-RELATED ISSUES AND CONCERNS

Diabetes Mellitus

Diabetes mellitus encompases a group of disorders characterized by high levels of serum (blood) glucose (hyperglycemia) resulting from insulin resistance by the body cells, impaired insulin secretion by the pancreas, and/or increased hepatic glucose production (Edelman, 1998). Nearly 18.2 million (6.3% of the population) Americans have diabetes, and approximately 5.2 million of those cases are undiagnosed (Centers for Disease Control and Prevention, [CDC], 2003).

There are several classifications of diabetes including prediabetes, Type 1, Type 2, gestational diabetes, and others associated with genetic syndromes, drugs, illness, and so on (CDC, 2003) (Table 4–4). The most common types of diabetes mellitus is Type 2.

It takes an average of 4 to 7 years for Type 2 diabetes to be diagnosed. As a result, 21% of newly diagnosed cases have signs of retinopathy and 14% of cases have signs of peripheral vascular disease (PVD) (American Diabetes Association, 2004). Over $132 billion were spent on health care costs for the care of people with Type 2 diabetes in 2002 (American Diabetes Association, 2003). This health care cost estimate includes both direct medical costs and indirect costs such as disability, work loss, and premature mortality.

Prediabetes

Prediabetes is a relatively new classification that was formerly called impaired glucose tolerance (IGT). Approximately 41 million people in the United States (21.1% of the population), ages 40 to 74 years, have

TABLE 4–4 Types of Diabetes

Type	Characteristics
Type 1 (formerly called insulin-dependent or juvenile-onset diabetes mellitus)	• 5–10% of diabetes cases • Most diagnosed by age 20 • Likely to display characteristic symptoms: polyuria, polydipsia, polyphagia • Usually thin or normal weight • Lack of insulin from beta cells, normal insulin receptors • Risk factors thought to be genetic, environmental, or autoimmune • Usually requires insulin therapy
Type 2 (formerly called non-insulin-dependent or adult-onset diabetes mellitus)	• 90–95% of diabetes cases • Risk increases with age (usually over 40), but onset is decreasing with increasing obesity in younger persons • Often not symptomatic • Associated with obesity • Defects in insulin receptors rather than insulin secretion • Risk factors include obesity, age, genetic, environmental • May or may not require insulin or oral agents
Gestational Diabetes (formerly pregnancy diabetes)	• Present in 2–5% of pregnancies • Usually resolves after pregnancy • Risk factor for Type 2 diabetes • Screening is standard in 24th to 28th week of pregnancy • Risk factors: family history, ethnicity, obesity • Health risk to mother and fetus
Other Types of Diabetes Mellitus	• Only 1–2% of diabetes cases • Result from genetic syndromes, drugs, surgery, infections, other illnesses

prediabetes (CDC, 2003b). These people are more likely to develop diabetes and may already be experiencing some adverse health effects. People with prediabetes are at a 50% higher risk of cardiovascular disease compared to people with normal blood glucose (Hanley, 2002). Lifestyle changes such as regular exercise, a healthy diet, and modest weight loss may delay or prevent the onset of Type 2 diabetes for those with prediabetes. In the STOP-NIDDM Trial, lifestyle modifications in people at risk for diabetes reduced the development of diabetes by 58% (Bourn, Mann, McSkimming, Waldron, Wishart, 1994).

Type 1 Diabetes Mellitus

Type 1 diabetes is also called insulin-dependent diabetes mellitus (IDDM) or juvenile-onset diabetes. IDDM accounts for 5–10% of all diagnosed cases of diabetes and affects approximately 210,000 in the United States (CDC, 2003b). Most Type 1 diabetics are diagnosed by age 20, with peak incidence between ages 10 and 14 (American Diabetes Association, 1993). Type 1 diabetes results from inadequate insulin secretion by the beta islet cells of the pancreas. This may be due to autoimmune mechanisms as antibodies to pancreatic islet cells are found in 85–90% of people at initial diagnosis of Type 1 diabetes (Franz, 1996). As a result, glucose cannot be taken up by cells and rises in the blood above normal levels (hyperglycemia). Excess is excreted in the urine, and body cells become "starved" for energy. As the excess glucose builds up in the blood, the body tries to excrete it through frequent urination.

Type 1 diabetics are likely to exhibit the classic symptoms of diabetes often referred to as the 3 Ps: polydipsia (excessive thirst), polyphagia (excessive appetite), polyuria (excessive urination), as well as weight loss, dehydration, and electrolyte disturbances.

As the carbohydrate-deprived body breaks down fats for energy, waste products (ketones) rise in the blood. If blood ketone levels rise too high, life-threatening ketoacidosis can develop (Franz, 1996). Management of Type 1 diabetes usually requires frequent self-blood glucose monitoring and daily insulin injections, as well as diet control and exercise.

Type 2 Diabetes Mellitus

Type 2 diabetes mellitus was previously referred to as non-insulin-dependent diabetes mellitus (NIDDM) or adult-onset diabetes. However, because Type 2 diabetics may also require insulin, the earlier designations were dropped. Prevalence of Type 2 diabetes increases with age and affects nearly 16.8% of the U.S. population between 65 and 74 years of age (CDC, 2003). Type 2 diabetes accounts for 90–95% of all diagnosed diabetes cases, and the incidence is increasing in the United States and throughout the world in part due to the increasing incidence of obesity (Edelman, 1998). In the past it was uncommon for children to develop Type 2 diabetes mellitus, but due to the increase in obesity, the incidence of Type 2 diabetes mellitus is also appearing in at least 4% of obese children in the United States (Zachary, 2004). Risk factors for Type 2 diabetes include older age, obesity, genetic component, environmental determinants, previous diagnosis of prediabetes, hypertension, high triglyceride levels, history of vascular disease, physical inactivity, race or ethnicity, polycystic ovary syndrome, history of gestational diabetes, or delivery of a baby weighing 9 pounds or more (American Diabetes Association, 2005).

People with Type 2 diabetes may have defects in secretion of insulin by the pancreas (as in the Type 1 diabetic), increased hepatic glucose production, and/or defects in the action of insulin at the cellular level (insulin resistance). Typically the body does produce some insulin, but cells do not recognize it and thus do not allow cellular glucose uptake. Insulin must bind to receptors on the cells in order for the glucose to enter the cell. In Type 2 diabetes mellitus, there is a defect in this system. These patients may suffer complications such as vision disorders (retinopathy), diminished sense of feeling in the extremities (neuropathy), increased susceptibility to infection, and general decline in organ function. The high rates of morbidity and mortality are due primarily to cardiovascular and cerebral vascular diseases (Edelman, 1998). People in the early stages of diabetes may experience few symptoms, making diagnosis difficult.

Gestational Diabetes Mellitus

Gestational diabetes mellitus (GDM) develops in 2–5% of all pregnancies, typically in the second or third trimester (CDC, 1997). This type of diabetes usually resolves after the birth, but nearly 63% of women who have had gestational diabetes will develop Type 2 diabetes in the future (CDC, 2003). Risk factors include ethnicity, family history, and obesity.

Infants born to mothers with poorly controlled GDM have an increased incidence of macrosomia (large babies), neonatal hypoglycemia, birth trauma, and possibly subsequent childhood and adolescent obesity (Adams Li, Nelson, Ogburn, Danilenko-Dixon, 1998). Fetal morbidity may also be increased with GDM, so early diagnosis is crucial to achieve glycemic control (Franz, 1996). A majority of women with GDM will require insulin through the term of their pregnancy.

Diagnosis of Diabetes Mellitus

A confirmed fasting blood glucose level of greater than 126 mg/dl on three occasions indicates a diagnosis of diabetes (CDC, 1997). Blood glucose levels consistently over 126 mg/dl result in an dramatic increase in the prevalence of diabetic complications before the clinical diagnosis of diabetes. Prediabetes is diagnosed by confirmed fasting blood glucose between 100 and 125 mg/dl (American Diabetes Association, 2005). The goal for fasting blood glucose levels is less than 100 mg/dl (American Diabetes Association, 2005). The glucose tolerance test may be used to diagnose gestational diabetes. In the glucose tolerance test a person's blood glucose is measured after fasting at least eight hours and then two hours after drinking a glucose-rich beverage.

Recognizing Diabetes Signs and Symptoms: Hypoglycemia and Hyperglycemia

Hypoglycemia is diagnosed when blood glucose is less than 70 mg/dl, although this may vary from person to person. The strongest predictor of a hypoglycemic event is the number of previous hypoglycemic events, so as part of the medical history, patients whould be asked their history of hypoglycemic episodes (Diabetes Control and Complications Trial Research Group, 1997). Hypoglycemia may occur when the patient has taken diabetes medication but has delayed eating. Symptoms of hypoglycemia may include mental confusion, blurred vision, weakness, agitation, shakiness, sweating, and anger. When the patient shows signs of hypoglycemia, treatment with a rapidly absorbed source of sugar, such as orange juice or soda, will quickly return blood sugar levels to normal. Patients should be encouraged to maintain good control, because the frequent use of simple carbohydrates to alleviate hypoglycemic episodes may contribute to increased caries risk and weight gain.

Patients with diabetes who require insulin or oral medications should have dental appointments early in the day, following breakfast. Sources of rapidly absorbed sugars like orange juice should be readily accessible in the dental office. In addition, it is advisable to include a glucose monitor in an emergency kit, and be diligent in minimizing patient anxiety and eliminating pain to reduce the risk of rapid changes in blood glucose levels (Vernillo, 2003).

Hyperglycemia can occur when an individual has delayed taking the appropriate hypoglycemic medication and glucose has increased abnormally in the blood. The patient may exhibit the same symptoms seen in hypoglycemia.

Diabetes Management

The goal of diabetes treatment is to maintain blood glucose levels as near to normal as possible at all times. Management must involve diet, exercise, and possible hypoglycemic medications. Diabetes management requires a multidisciplinary effort and patient cooperation (Edelman, 1998). Good diabetes control will reduce complications such as retinopathy, nephropathy, neuropathy, and cardiovascular disease (Tamborlane, Ahern, 1997).

Dietary Management of Diabetes Mellitus
Dietary therapy provided by a registered dietitian for diabetes mellitus is similar to recommendations for a healthy, low-fat diet. The total amount of carbohydrate consumed and its distribution evenly throughout the day are the most important aspects of glycemic control (Franz et al., 1994). Diabetics no longer have to totally avoid foods with sugar (Franz et al., 1994). Moderate calorie restriction and increased physical activity are recommended for those diabetes patients needing to lose weight (Franz et al., 1994). Even modest weight loss can improve glycemic control.

Dietary principles for persons with diabetes mellitus include the following:

- Follow the *Dietary Guidelines for Americans* and the food guide pyramid: 20% of calories or less from protein, 50% of calories or more from carbohydrates, and 30% of calories from fat (less than 10% of calories from saturated fat, 10–15% of calories from monounsaturated fats).
- Sucrose and sucrose-containing foods should be consumed only as part of an overall healthy diet.
- Eat small, frequent meals and snacks.
- Achieve and maintain a healthy weight.
- Maintain regular physical activity after consulting with a physician.
- Limit alcohol if diabetes is not well controlled.

People taking insulin must be regular about the timing of meals and administration of insulin to attain optimum glycemic control, as skipping meals after insulin administration may result in hypoglycemic episodes. For many people with diabetes, it is recommended that they eat more frequent small meals to help maintain the blood glucose at more even levels. The daily food intake may be divided into as many as six small meals and snacks. Carbohydrate counting has become a well-accepted method of ensuring appropriate carbohydrate distribution throughout the day, and is taught in most diabetes treatment programs.

Oral Implications of Diabetes Mellitus The control of diabetes is imperative for overall health and quality of life as well as for the health of the oral soft tissues. Periodontal disease is a common complication of diabetes mellitus (Loe, 1993); poorly controlled Type 2 diabetic patients have a higher prevalence and severity of periodontal disease than nondiabetics (Saxe et al., 1989; Soskolne, 1998). Patients with poorly controlled diabetes are at higher risk for alveolar bone loss, and the severity of periodontal disease is greater than in those with good control (Taylor et al., 1998). Patients with uncontrolled hyperglycemia also have poor responses to periodontal therapy.

Conversely, the presence of periodontal disease may impact metabolic control of diabetes (Soskolne, 1998). Studies have found that controlling periodontal inflammation results in a decreased in the HbA_{1c} and lower insulin doses (Grossi et al., 1997; Herriges et al., 2005; Seppala, Seppala, Ainamo, 1993). Consultation with the physician may be required to determine the status of diabetic control before proceeding with invasive periodontal therapy.

Patients whose blood glucose levels are not well controlled may experience episodes of hypoglycemia, which they resolve with frequent use of hard candies or the like. This habit can increase risk for dental caries, especially when xerostomia is also present.

Persons with diabetes are often required to have snacks between meals to stabilize serum glucose levels. These snacks may consist of retentive carbohydrates, such as crackers, which may increase caries risk. In such cases, the dental professional may need to consult with the registered dietitian working with the patient to determine if less cariogenic snacks can be suggested. Equally important, the dental professional needs to stress the importance of careful brushing and flossing after each eating period, and should consider home fluoride therapy for the patient to aid in remineralization of early carious lesions and prevention of caries.

Lactose Intolerance

Lactose intolerance is caused by a deficiency of the enzyme lactase, which hydrolyzes lactose in the small intestine. This is not the same as a milk allergy, in which people are allergic to the protein in milk. Symptoms of lactose intolerance include bloating, gas, diarrhea, and gastrointestinal distress, which occur soon after the consumption of dairy products (the primary lactose-containing foods) (Carroccio, Montalto, Cavera, Notarbatolo, 1998).

More than half of the world's adult population has some degree of lactose intolerance. It is more common in certain ethnic population groups including blacks, Hispanics, and Asians. Lactose intolerance may develop gradually over time, getting progressively worse as the person ages. Because lactose-containing milk products are primary calcium sources in Western diets, lactose intolerance can be detrimental to calcium status and ultimately to bone health.

Although a lack of the enzyme lactase is the cause of this gastrointestinal disturbance, most people who are lactose intolerant are able to ingest some lactose, especially when provided in small doses. Thus, lactose tolerance may be improved with smaller, more frequent portions of lactose-containing foods.

Patients with lactose intolerance should be counseled on alternative ways to obtain adequate amounts of the calcium, phosphorus, and vitamin D normally found in dairy products. Due to the prevalence of lactose intolerance, there are now many lactose-reduced food products available such as low-lactose or lactose-free milk. Over-the-counter lactase replacement tablets are available to be taken just before eating. Table 4–5 lists diet suggestions for those with lactose intolerance. Depending on the extent of the problem, lactose-intolerant patients may need to be referred to competent dietary professionals for further assistance.

Dental Caries

All of the monosaccharides and disaccharides can be used as a food source for plaque bacteria and thus are cariogenic. Sucrose is considered the most cariogenic of sugars because:

- it can be stored by cariogenic bacteria for later use (the other sugars cannot).
- it is consumed in greater quantities and in greater frequency than the other sugars.
- the other sugars are found primarily in more nutrient-rich foods, whereas table sugar is an added sweetener that provides only calories.

Despite this distinction, the length of time that any sugars are present in the mouth is the most important factor in tooth demineralization. The texture and consistency of the sugar present also play a role in the process.

Although starches are considered low in cariogenic potential, salivary amylase can hydrolyze starch in the oral cavity to more cariogenic sugars. This can happen especially when poor oral hygiene habits allow starches to remain in the mouth for prolonged periods. Also, many

TABLE 4–5 Suggestions for People with Lactose Intolerance

Try small amounts of milk in soups, beverages, casseroles, etc.
Avoid large amounts of milk at any one time
Use hard cheeses (much lactose is lost in processing)
Use yogurt with active cultures and buttermilk
Use tofu that has been processed with calcium carbonate
Use lactose-reduced milk or calcium-fortified soy milk
Try Lactaid or Dairy Ease (lactase replacement) tablets just before eating
Try calcium-fortified orange juice
Take calcium supplements as needed
Read labels

of the most cariogenic foods are starch–sugar combinations such as cakes and cookies. In these cases, the starch contributes to the retentiveness of the food to increase its cariogenic potential.

The sugar alcohols are either not fermented or are only poorly and very slowly fermented by the oral flora. Additionally, most of the sugar alcohols fail to drop plaque pH levels low enough to cause enamel demineralization. Chapter 13 details the role of carbohydrates in dental caries.

MISCONCEPTIONS ABOUT CARBOHYDRATES

Causes Diabetes Mellitus?

Diabetes is a metabolic condition that impairs the body's ability to use carbohydrates. It is not *caused* by excessive carbohydrate intake. Neither Type 1 nor Type 2 is caused by overconsumption of sugar (Anderson, 1999). Carbohydrate consumption may be indirectly related to Type 2 diabetes mellitus if excessive carbohydrates contribute to the obesity that triggers this type of diabetes mellitus.

Triggers Hyperactivity?

Many parents believe that sugary foods cause their children to be hyperactive. However, all studies that attempted to determine if there was a relationship between attention deficit hyperactivity disorder (ADHD) and sugar consumption in children have been inconclusive (Kanarek, 1994; Krummel, Seligson, Guthrie, 1996; Wolraich, 1998). A meta-analysis in 1995 analyzed 16 different studies on the effects of sugar on the behavior or cognitive performance of children and found that sugar intake had no effect on either (Wolraich, Wilson, White, 1995). It is likely that situations where sugary foods are served, such as parties, cause children to be excited and overactive. However, this does not implicate the sweets directly in the level of activity.

Triggers Hypoglycemia?

Hypoglycemia, or low blood sugar, is a condition in which the blood sugar drops to below 40 mg/dL between meals (normal is between 60 and 110 mg/dL). The result can be sweating, rapid heartbeat, trembling, and hunger. In people with diabetes, hypoglycemia can occur when people take too much insulin, exercise too much, or eat too little. In most other cases this low blood sugar is linked to other serious medical problems like liver disease or pancreatic tumor. Reactive hypoglycemia is a rare condition in which the pancreas secretes too much insulin after a large meal. Symptoms occur 6–8 hours after eating. None of these conditions is caused by too much sugar in the diet. Health clinics that diagnose "sugar-induced hypoglycemia" and offer treatment with costly remedies are to be avoided (Duyff, 2002, pp.118–119).

Makes You Fat?

Too many calories from any source—carbohydrates, proteins, fats, alcohol—makes you fat. Excess calories from fat turn to body fat before extra calories from carbohydrates do. Glucose is converted to body fat only if you consume more than is needed. Indeed, people with weight problems do not necessarily consume more carbohydrates than normal-weight people (Duyff, 2002, p. 119).

ALTERNATIVE SWEETENERS

Alternative sweeteners include substances other than the carbohydrate classes of monosaccharides and disaccharides (Table 4–6). These substances may be naturally occurring or synthetic and may also be classified as caloric or noncaloric.

Sugar alcohols are derived from carbohydrate and include xylitol, mannitol, sorbitol, and lactitol. Sugar alcohols do provide calories similar to other carbohydrates (2.3–4.0 kcal/g), but they are often used in such small quantities that the calories may be considered insignificant. On the other hand, some products may contain 25g or more of sugar alcohols, contributing 100 kcal. In large doses, these sugar alcohols have the potential to cause gastrointestinal disturbances. Sugar alcohols lend importance to dentistry in that they are also essentially noncariogenic.

Common alternative sweeteners include saccharin, aspartame, and acesulfame K. New additions to this category of sweeteners including Sucralose, Alitame, and Sweetener 2000. Sucralose has recently received FDA approval for use in the United States. A sweetener available in health food stores as a dietary supplement but not approved by the FDA as food additive is Stevia.

Saccharin, a derivative of petroleum, is used in various food products in the United States. Saccharin is

TABLE 4–6   Common Sugar Substitutes

Name	Brand Name	Chemical Name/Formula	Sweetness Compared to Sucrose (by Weight)	Energy Provided (Calories/Gram)	Safety and Regulatory Issues / History	Acceptable Daily Intake (ADI)* [mg/kg Body Weight]
Saccharin (Sodium Saccharin or Calcium Saccharin)	Sweet N' Low, Sweet Twin	$C_7H_4NNaO_3S \cdot 2H_2O$ (sodium saccharin)	300 ×	0	1977: The Food and Drug Administration (FDA) proposed a ban because rats developed bladder cancer after large doses of saccharin. 1980: Congress reversed ban 1991: FDA withdrew saccharin ban and required warning labels after several studies suggested risks were lower than previously anticipated 2000: Congress repealed law requiring warning labels on saccharin-containing products.	5
Aspartame	Equal, NutraSweet, NaturaTaste, SweetMate, Sugar Twin	methyl ester of the dipeptide of the amino acids l-aspartic acid and l-phenylalanine	160–200 ×	4 (the amount typically used to sweeten foods is so small that aspartame usually adds no calories per serving)	1981: Approved by the FDA May be harmful to those with Phenylketonuria (PKU), who cannot metabolize the amino acid phenylalanine The label of any food containing aspartame must bear the following statement: "PHENYLKETO-NURICS: CONTAINS PHENYLALANINE."	50
Acesulfame potassium (Acesulfame K or Ace K)	Sunett, Sweet One	Potassium salt of 6-methyl-1,2,3-oxathiazine-4(3H)-one 2,2-dioxide	100–200 ×	0	1988: Approved by the FDA	15
Sucralose	Splenda	1,6-dichloro-1,6-dioxy-β-D-fructo-	500–700 ×	0; typically packaged with	1998: Approved by the FDA	9

(continued)

TABLE 4–6 Common Sugar Substitutes (Continued)

Name	Brand Name	Chemical Name/Formula	Sweetness Compared to Sucrose (by Weight)	Energy Provided (Calories/Gram)	Safety and Regulatory Issues / History	Acceptable Daily Intake (ADI)* [mg/kg Body Weight]
		furanosyl 4-chloro-4-deoxy-α-D-galactopyranoside		maltodextrin (4 kcal/g) for bulking and stability purposes		
Sugar Alcohols (Sorbitol, Xylitol, Lacitols, Mannitol, Maltitol, Erythritol)	No brand names	Polyols	0.4–1.0 ×	~ 2.4–4.0	May cause bloating, gas and/or laxative effect in large doses (> 20 g) Generally Recognized As Safe (GRAS)	No ADI established
Stevia (Stevia rebaudiana Bertoni)	No brand names	Stevia rebaudiana is a shrub composed of glycosides named steviosides and rebaudiosides that yield its sweet taste	250–300 ×	0	1991: deemed an "unsafe food additive" by FDA 1995: Stevia is permittedas a dietary supplement	No ADI (dietary supplement)

*ADI is defined as the amount of sweetener that can be safely consumed on a daily basis over a person's lifetime without any adverse effects.
Source: Adapted by Jennifer Weston from:
International Food Information Council (IFIC) Resource Kit on Low Calorie Sweeteners.
Stillings Trends in foods—nutrition-conscious consumers affect the food industry. *Nutr Today.* September–October 1994.
Wikipedia. Sugar substitutes. Retrieved from http://en.wikipedia.org/wiki/Sugar_substitute

used primarily in soft drinks and tabletop sweeteners. It is also used in cosmetics and some pharmaceuticals. Because saccharin crosses the placenta, it is not recommended for use by pregnant women.

Aspartame containins two amino acids, phenylalanine and aspartic acid, and is roughly 200 times sweeter than sucrose. It is unstable when used at prolonged high temperatures and therefore not suitable for cooking. It is found in a wide variety of products including soft drinks and other beverages, tabletop sweeteners, milk beverages, frozen desserts, candies, and baked goods. Aspartame should not be used by individuals with the condition phenylketonuria (an inborn error of phenylalanine metabolism), and is not recommended for use by individuals with epilepsy.

Acesulfame potassium or acesulfame K is approximately 200 times sweeter. It is often blended with other low-calorie sweeteners to improve taste. Acesulfame K is currently found in soft drinks, dry beverage mixes, instant coffee and tea, dairy products, and candies. The sweetner is not metabolized by the body and is excreted unchanged by the kidneys.

Sucralose is the newest nonnutritive, intense sweetener to be approved by the FDA. It is formed from sucrose and results in a water-soluble, crystalline powder that is approximately 600 times sweeter than sucrose. It is used in all the same products as the other alternative sweeteners. Like acesulfame K it can be used in baked goods because of its stability at high temperatures.

The FDA-approved alternative sweeteners used in the United States—including saccharin, aspartame, acesulfame K, and sucralose—have all been found safe for human consumption at recommended levels of use.

Stevia is a shrub found primarily in South America whose leaves have been used for centuries by people in Paraguay and Brazil to sweeten their beverages. Stevia contains stevioside, a glycoside that is 250–300 times sweeter than sugar, depending on the concentrations of the solution. Despite its wide spread use in other countries for quite some time, the FDA continues to have concerns about the safety of the herb and has not approved it as a food additive. In September of 1995 the FDA lifted a 4-year import ban of stevia, approving its use as a dietary supplement or as a dietary ingredient of a supplement, but not as a food additive or ingredient. The ruling allowed the sale of stevia as long as the bottle or package clearly labels it as a dietary supplement.

Recommendations for children are given in relation to their body weight and amounts are generally less than one packet of artificial sweetener per day. Special consideration should be given to the fact that children need calories for growth and development. Artificial sweeteners probably should not be fed at all to infants or children less than 2 years old. Because noncarbohydrate sweeteners cannot serve as food sources for oral bacteria, they can be considered noncariogenic.

SUMMARY AND IMPLICATIONS FOR DENTISTRY

Carbohydrates are important nutrients. They range in size in foods from simple sugars to complex polysaccharides. They may be indigestible, as in fiber, or digestible, as in starches and sugars.

Liberal use of complex carbohydrates (fibers and whole grain starches) has been associated with beneficial health effects such as reduced risk of caners and heart disease and improved glucose levels. There are many misconceptions about potential harmful effects of sugars on health. The major risks from excess sugars are dental caries and excess calories.

Patients should be encouraged to:

- obtain the majority of carbohydrates from foods such as grains, fruits, and vegetables, rather than from lower nutrient sweets.
- increase intake of high-fiber foods such as bran, raw fruits and vegetables, and whole grains.
- reduce caries risk, limit sugary foods (candy, cake, cookies, soda) to mealtimes rather than between meals.

QUESTIONS PATIENTS MIGHT ASK

Q. Are sugar-free foods also calorie free?

A. Not necessarily. If the food contains fat, protein, or alcohol (all energy sources), it could provide significant calories.

Q. Can a person eat too much fiber?

A. Certainly. In children, a high-fiber diet may fill them up and blunt their appetite for other nutritious foods. Excess fiber can also interfere with absorption of vitamins and minerals. For adults, an excess of 35 g of fiber a day over time can lead to gas, diarrhea, cramps, and bloating.

CASE STUDY #1

A recent immigrant from Mexico complains that her child frequently suffers from intestinal problems including diarrhea, flatulence (excess gas), and intestinal cramps. At first, you suspect problems with safe food handling or a parasitic infection. After ruling these out through a medical consult, you have decided to send the mother to a dietitian to learn how to place the child on a dairy-free diet.

Questions:
1. What problem does this child probably have?
2. Why would you suspect this problem in an immigrant from Mexico?
3. What special dietary considerations should be emphasized to promote adequate growth and dental health?

CASE STUDY #2

A new patient comes to your office for a routine dental visit. After completing the medical history you observe that the patient has slightly elevated blood pressure. The patient has reported a family history of heart disease and moderately elevated cholesterol levels. Additionally, this patient states that he is often under stress and has difficulty finding time to complete daily tasks. The patient complains of recent gastrointestinal problems such as constipation and reports an episode of diverticulitis in the past 2 years. After a thorough dental examination you discover a moderate amount of existing restorations and new decay. The patient also exhibits slight to moderate periodontal problems. You decide to collect a diet history. The patient's physician has recommended a high-fiber diet. In response to the physician's recommendations, the patient indicates that he has started to eat more white bread and refried beans.

Questions:
1. What issues would you discuss as possible reasons for this patient's health problems?
2. How would you explain to this patient the benefits of a high-fiber diet?
3. What are some practical recommendations for increasing the intake of complex carbohydrates in the diet?

REFERENCES

Adams KM, Li H, Nelson RL, Ogburn PL Jr., Danilenko-Dixon DR: Sequelae of unrecognized gestational diabetes. *Am J Obstet Gynecol* 1998; 178(6):1321–32.

American Diabetes Association: Clinical practice recommendations: 1999 Standards of Medical Care for Patients with diabetes mellitus. *Diabetes Care* 1999; 17:1514–22.

American Diabetes Association: Economic costs of diabetes in the U.S. in 2002. *Diabetes Care* 2003; 26:917–32.

American Diabetes Association: Retinopathy in diabetes [Position Statement]. *Diabetes Care* 2004; 27 (Suppl 1):S84–S87.

American Diabetes Association: Standards of medical care in diabetes [Position Statement]. *Diabetes Care* 2005; 28(Suppl 1): S4–36.

American Diabetes Association: *Vital Statistics.* Alexandria, VA: Author, 1993.

Anderson J: Nutritional management of diabetes mellitus. In Shils M, Olsen J, Shike M, Ross AC (eds): *Modern Nutrition in Health and Disease*, 9th ed. Media, PA: Williams & Wilkins, 1999.

Berkoff N: *Nutrition for the Culinary Arts.* Upper Saddle River, NJ: Prentice Hall, 2005.

Bourn DM, Mann JI, McSkimming BJ, Waldron MA, Wishart JD: Impaired glucose tolerance and NIDDM: Does a lifestyle intervention program have an effect? *Diabetes Care* 1994; 17(11):1311–19.

Carroccio A, Montalto G, Cavera G, Notarbatolo A: Lactose intolerance and self-reported milk intolerance: Relationship with lactose maldigestion and nutrient intake. Lactase Deficiency Study Group. *J Am Coll Nutr* 1998; 17(6):631–36.

Centers for Disease Control and Prevention: *National Diabetes Fact Sheet: National Estimates and General Information on Diabetes in the United States.* Atlanta: U.S. Department of Health and Human Services, Centers for Disease Control and Prevention, 2003b.

Diabetes Control and Complications Trial Research Group: Hypoglycemia in the Diabetes Control and Complications Trial. *Diabetes* 1997; 46:271–86.

Duyff RL, American Dietetic Association: *Complete Food and Nutrition Guide.* Hoboken, NJ: J Wiley, 2002.

Edelman SV: Type II diabetes mellitus. *Adv Intern Med* 1998; 43:449–99.

Edgar WM: Sugar substitutes, chewing gum and dental caries—a review. *Br Dent J* 1998; 184(1):29–32.

Franz MJ: *Nutritional Care in Diabetes Mellitus and Reactive Hypoglycemia.* Philadelphia: WB Saunders, 1996.

Franz MJ, Horton ES, Bantle JP, Beebe CA, Brunzell JD, Coulson AM, et al.: Nutrition principles for the management of diabetes and related complications. *Diabetes Care* 1994; 17(5):490–518.

Grossi SG, Skrepcinski FB, DeCaro T, Robertson DC, Ho AW, Dunford RG, et al.: Treatment of periodontal disease in diabetics reduces glycated hemogloin. *J Periodontol* 1997; 68:713–19.

Hanley, AJ, Williams K, Sterb MP, Haffner SM: Homeostasis model assessment of insulin resistane in relation to the incidence of cardiovascular disease: The San Antonio Heart Study. *Diabetes Care* 2002: 25(7):1177–84.

Herriges B, Boyd LD, R, Madden T, Laughlin G, Chiodo G, Rosenstein D: Effect of Enhanced Anti Infective Periodontal Treatment on HbA1C in Diabetic Patients. Unpublished manuscript, Oregon Health & Sciences University, 2005.

Institute of Medicine: National Academy of Sciences, *Dietary Reference Intakes for Energy, Carbohydrate, Fiber, Fat, Fatty Acids, Cholesterol, Protein, and Amino Acids (Macronutrients)*. Washington, DC: National Academies Press, 2005.

Kanarek RB: Does sucrose or aspartame cause hyperactivity in children? *Nutr Rev* 1994; 52:173–75.

Krummel DA, Seligson FH, Guthrie HA: Hyperactivity: Is candy causal? *Crit Rev Food Sci Nutr* 1996; 36:31–47.

Levin RJ: Carbohydrates. In Shils M, Olsen J, Shike M, Ross AC (eds): *Modern Nutrition in Health and Disease*, 9th ed. Media, PA: Williams & Wilkins, 1999.

Loe H: Periodontal disease: The sixth complication of diabetes mellitus. *Diabetes Care* 1993; 16(1):329–34.

Saxe SR, Anderson JW, O'Neill MK, Kryscio RJ, et al: Bleeding and gingival indices in diabetic vs. non-diabetic patients. *J Dent Res* 1989; 68:382.

Seppala B, Seppala M, Ainamo J: A longitudinal study on insulin-dependent diabetes mellitus and periodontal disease. *J Clin Periodontol* 1993; 20:161–65.

Soskolne WA: Epidemiological and clinical aspects of periodontal disease in diabetics. *Ann Periodontol* 1998; 3:3–12.

Tamborlane WV, Ahern J: Implications and results of the Diabetes Control and Complications Trial. *Pedatr Clin North Am* 1997; 44(2):285–300.

Taylor GW, Burt BA, Becker MP, Genco RJ, Shlossman M: Glycemic control and alveolar bone loss progression in type 2 diabetes. *Ann Periodontol* 1998; 3(1):30–9.

Van Loveren C: Sugar alcohols: What is the evidence for caries-preventive and caries-therapeutic effects? *Caries Res* 2004; 38(3):286–93.

Vernillo AT: Dental considerations for the treatment of patients with diabetes mellitus. *J Am Dental Assoc* 2003; 134:24S–33S.

Weigley ES, Mueller D, Robinson C (eds): Carbohydrates. In *Robinson's Basic Nutrition and Diet Therapy*. Upper Saddle River, NJ: Prentice Hall, 1997.

Wolraich M: Attention deficit hyperactivity disorder. *Prof Care Mother Child* 1998; 8:35–37.

Wolraich ML, Wilson DB, White JW: The effect of sugar on behavior or cognition in children. A metaanalysis. *JAMA* 1995; 274(2):1617–21.

Zachary T, Bloomgarden MD: Type 2 diabetes in the young: The evolving epidemic. *Diabetes Care* 2004; 27(4):998–1010.

Chapter **5**

Protein for Systemic and Oral Health: Meeting Needs in a Multicultural World

George M. Lessard

OBJECTIVES

The student will be able to:

- List the general functions of proteins in the body.
- Describe the chemistry and structural differences among proteins.
- Discuss the digestion, absorption, and metabolism of proteins.
- Describe the metabolism of protein in the body including its role in tissue formation.
- Give the RDA for protein and list the major food sources.
- Define protein balance, complete versus incomplete proteins, and protein quality.
- Discuss the risks of too much and too little protein.
- Describe the concept of protein complementarity.
- Discuss the benefits and possible risks of plant-based diets.

INTRODUCTION: ROLE OF PROTEINS IN THE BODY

Proteins play crucial roles in almost all processes and structures of the body. Protein mediates most of the actions of life. It is necessary for growth and for the continued maintenance of systemic and oral health. The term *protein*, meaning "of the first rank," should appropriately be applied to this important class of molecule.

Proteins are critical to all life processes. Every structure and activity of the human body is, at least in part, dependent upon protein. In order to carry out the body's activities, up to 50,000 different proteins must be made. Every one of these protein molecules is synthesized using the same 20 component amino acids. The proteins differ from each other in the number, order, and types of amino acids they contain.

Some proteins have a primary structural role. Muscles contain about half of the body's protein. Other proteins have a primary role of binding and thus controlling access to other molecule. Enzymes are proteins that serve as chemical catalysts, speeding up chemical reactions. Proteins also act as signaling molecules, organizing and harmonizing many biological processes that are carried out by the catalytic actions of proteins. Proteins provide protection and are combined with other molecules in conjugates.

The cells of the body are constantly being broken down and new cells are formed to replace them. Thus protein is required throughout life and especially during growth periods such as pregnancy, infancy, and childhood. Table 5–1 shows the roles of protein in the body.

THE CHEMISTRY OF PROTEINS

Proteins are made up of amino acids. The term *amino acid* is derived from the presence of both an amino group (NH_2) and an acid group (COOH) attached to the central carbon of the molecule. Proteins differ from each other as a result of the types of amino acids they contain and the sequencing of these amino acids. Each amino acid is built on a similar overall plan containing the same four elements of carbon (C), hydrogen (H), oxygen (O), and nitrogen (N). In some cases a fifth element is present, sulfur (S). However, the amino acids differ from each other in their side group or side

TABLE 5–1 Roles of Protein in the Body

Class	Example and Function
Structural	Collagen: matrix protein of skin, bones, and teeth Crystallin: structural protein of eye lens
Transport and binding	Hemoglobin: oxygen transport Ferritin: iron storage
Enzymes (names end in –ase)	Salivary amylase: catalyzes the breakdown of starch to sugar in the mouth Pepsin: digests protein in the stomach
Regulation	Insulin: a hormone that regulates uptake and storage of glucose Calmodulin: involved in regulation of calcium-mediated processes
Protection	IgA: antibodies found in saliva that neutralize foreign substance Histatins: salivary antibacterial proteins
pH regulation	Sialin: salivary pH buffering protein
Protein conjugates	Glycoproteins: salivary mucins Lipoproteins: low-density lipoproteins (LDL), chylomicrons Nucleoproteins: chromatin, nucleosomes

chains (R). Figure 5–1 shows the structure of an amino acid. Figure 5–2 shows the structure of side groups.

Many amino acids are structurally asymmetric and thus have two possible forms (D and L) that are mirror images of each other. Most organisms, however, make and use only one of these forms, the L form, directly in making protein. The L-amino acids serve as protein building blocks for all living organisms.

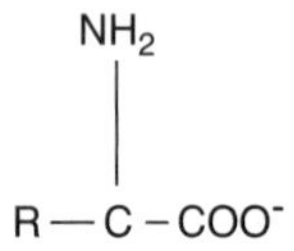

FIGURE 5–1 An amino acid.

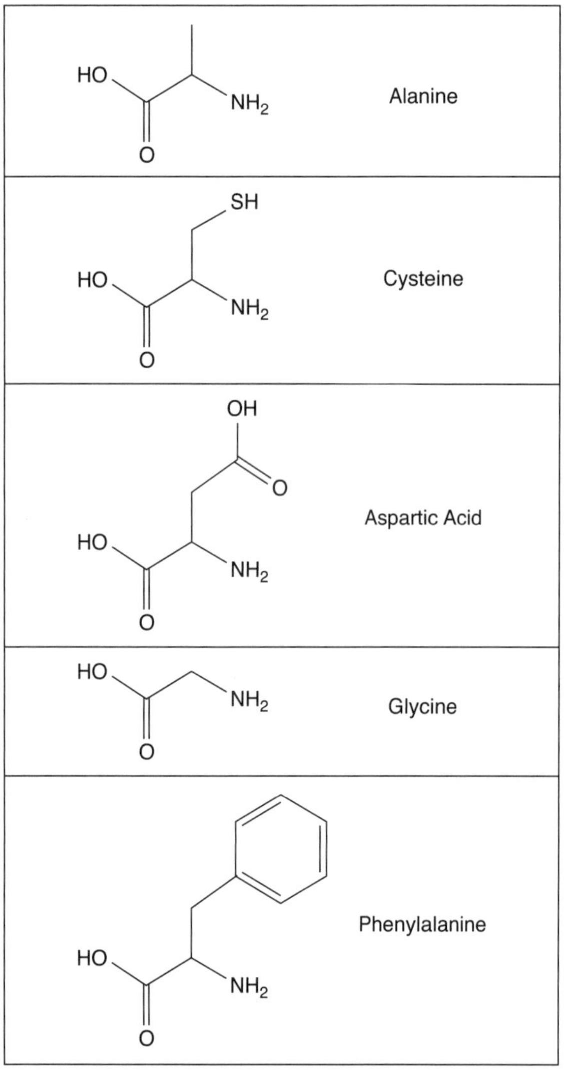

Dispensable Amino Acids

Human beings can make more than half of the specific amino acids they need. These are termed dispensable amino acids. Dispensable amino acids may be made from carbohydrates or other metabolic intermediates and are made in adequate amounts to meet the needs of the body.

Fully or Conditionally Indispensable Amino Acids

Nine of the 20 amino acids cannot be synthesized in adequate amounts by the body to meet its needs. These are called the indispensable amino acids. Because our bodies can't make them at all or cannot make them at a rate appropriate to need, they must be derived from foods.

Under special circumstances certain amino acids may become indispensable. This is what occurs when inadequate intake or the inability to metabolize phenylalanine (as in the inherited disease, phenylketonuria) limits the amount of tyrosine (a product of phenylalanine metabolism) formed. Under these circumstances, tyrosine becomes a conditionally indispensable amino acid (see Table 5–2 and Figure 5–3) (IOM, 2005).

TABLE 5–2 Indispensable and dispensable or Conditionally Indispensable Amino Acids

Indispensable	Dispensable or Conditionally Indispensable
Histidine	Alanine
Isoleucine	Argenine
Leucine	Aspartic acid
Lysine	Cysteine
Methionine	Cystine
Phenylalanine	Glutamic acid
Threonine	Glycine
Tryptophane	Serine
Valine	Tyrosine
	Proline

FIGURE 5–2 Examples of side group.

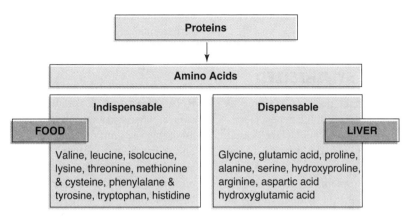

FIGURE 5–3   Indispensable versus dispensable amino acids.

When two amino acids are joined, water is eliminated and a peptide bond is formed. Two amino acids joined by a peptide bond is known as a *dipeptide*. When a third amino acid is added, a *tripeptide* is formed, the three amino acids being connected by two peptide bonds. More amino acids added to the growing molecule will convert it to an *oligopeptide* (small peptide), and finally, when many amino acids are joined together by many peptide bonds, a *polypeptide* or *protein* has been synthesized (Figure 5–4).

Each protein is unique, differing from every other protein. The structure of proteins can generally be categorized as either fibrous (elongated) or globular (rounded) structures. This is determined first by the number and order of amino acids.

Simple proteins like insulin or collagen contain only amino acids. Conjugated proteins contain other components in addition to amino acids. Myoglobin and hemoglobin include iron-containing heme groups, so are called heme proteins. Salivary proteins contain sugars and sugar acids such as sialic acid (from saliva)

that make them better able to bind water. The sugars attached to the protein confer their names, *glycoproteins* or *mucins*. Gustin, a zinc-binding protein associated with taste bud function, is a *metalloprotein*.

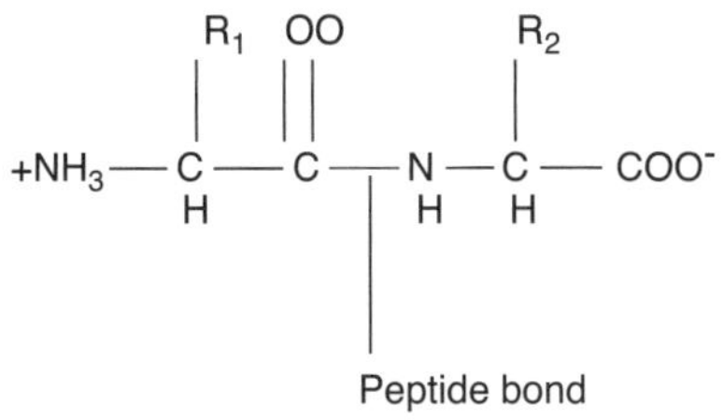

Proteins exert their function because the sequence of amino acids, the *primary structure* determines their shape. Changing the shape of a protein is termed *denaturation*. Heat, salt, and solvents can denature proteins. Cooking of eggs denatures the egg white protein, albumin, to yield a white opaque denatured protein (cooked egg white). Denatured proteins are biologically inactive, which explains why heat can be used in sterilization.

The primary structure folds spontaneously into helical (α-helix), sheetlike (β-structure) bends (β-turns) or other structural motifs that arise because of the kinds and sequence of amino acids in the protein. Together these conformational motifs are called *secondary structure*.

Because of interactions between amino acid side chains the secondary structures self-assemble, folding into rounded shapes, forming globular proteins. These side-chain interactions yield what is referred to as the *tertiary structure*. Myoglobin is a globular oxygen-binding protein that gives muscle much of its red color. It has a complex tertiary structure. A multi-subunit protein has one more level of structure than does a simple globular protein like myoglobin. The association of subunits is defined as *quaternary structure*. Hemoglobin, the red

FIGURE 5–4   A dipeptide.

Peptide bond

oxygen-transporting protein found in red blood cells, is a multi-subunit protein.

HOW PROTEINS ARE SYNTHESIZED

The information needed to make proteins is stored in the genetic information of each cell in the genes. Genes are segments of deoxyribonucleic acid (DNA) that encode the sequence of amino acids that make up the protein. The DNA in the chromosome contains all the genes needed to make all the proteins for not only that cell, but for the entire body of that individual, for his or her entire life.

Assembling the Information: Transcription

In order to utilize the genetic information, copies must be made and transported to the site at which protein is to be synthesized (Figures 5–5a and 5–5b). Thus, a gene is transcribed into a copy made of ribonucleic acid (RNA). The process is called *transcription*, the product is called a *messenger RNA (mRNA)*. Each protein is made from a unique mRNA.

Transcription is selective; messenger RNAs are made only as needed and generally under tight control. Regulation of transcription involves generalized hormonal as well as local control, responding to systemic as well as local demands. Thus, the rate of protein synthesis is determined in part by the rate at which transcription takes place.

Making the Protein: Translation

The instructions for making a protein, its messenger RNA, move out of the nucleus and attach to *ribosomes*, where proteins are synthesized. The ribosomes assemble the amino acids necessary to make a protein and knit them together using peptide bonds. The amino acids cannot be directly attached to each other, but first need to be attached to adaptor molecules called *transfer RNA (tRNA)*. Amino acids attached to tRNA are recognized by the ribosome in the order programmed by the messenger RNA, each amino acid-tRNA corresponding to one coding unit (codon) of the messenger RNA. Thus multiple tRNAs, each specifically binding one amino acid serve as the source of amino acids for protein synthesis. *Translation*, the making of protein, depends on an mRNA and amino acid tRNAs in conjunction with the ribosome. Because each protein differs in the number, kind, and sequence of amino acids, the shape and function of each protein is unique and specific to its role in the cell.

Following translation, modifications take place to the structure of proteins. Metals may be bound, heme groups may be inserted, sugars may be attached to the surface, and amino acids may be hydroxylated or oxidized. All these changes take place after synthesis

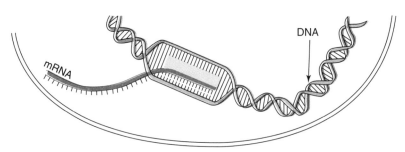

1. The DNA serves as a template to make strands of messenger RNA (mRNA). Each mRNA strand copies exactly the instructions for making some protein the cell needs.
2. The mRNA leaves the nucleus through the nuclear membrane. DNA remains inside the nucleus.
3. The mRNA attaches itself to the protein-making machinery of the cell.

FIGURE 5–5a DNA and RNA: genes and messenger RNA.

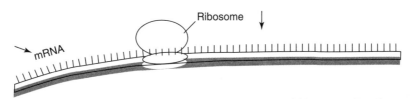

4. Another form of RNA, transfer RNA (tRNA), collects amino acids from the cell fluid. Each tRNA carries its amino acids to the mRNA, which dictates the sequence in which the amino acids will be attached to form the protein strands. Thus the mRNA ensures the amino acids are lined up in the correct sequence.

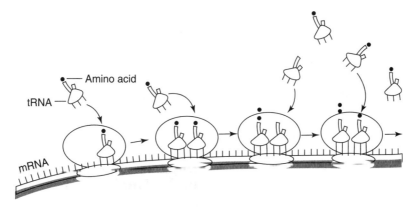

5. As the amino acids are lined up in the right sequence, and the ribosome moves along the mRNA, an enzyme bonds one amino acid after another to the growing protein strand. The tRNA are freed to return for more amino acids. When all the amino acids have been attached, the completed protein is released.

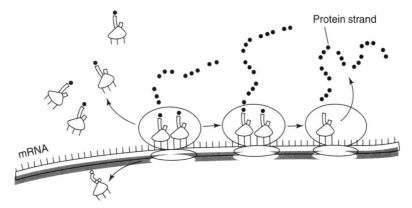

6. Finally the mRNA is degraded. It takes many words to describe these events, but in the cell, 40 to 100 amino acids can be added to a growing protein strand in only a second.

FIGURE 5–5b Translation: ribosomal protein synthesis.

and are called *post-translational modifications*. Many salivary and mucosally synthesized proteins are modified by addition of sugars to become glycoproteins and mucins.

Mutations and Sequence Errors

The amino acid sequence of proteins is determined by the sequence of bases in the DNA. A single alteration in a gene can lead to an incorrect substitution sequence of the protein, and the protein may be altered. For example, a sequencing error leads to the disease, Sickle-Cell Anemia.

PROTEIN DIGESTION AND ABSORPTION

Proteins are found in almost all foods. When protein is eaten as part of the diet, it is not absorbed directly, but must first be broken down into its component amino acids (Figure 5–6). This is a three-stage process.

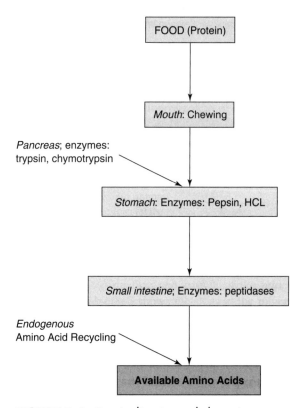

FIGURE 5–6 Protein digestion and absorption.

Digestion begins in the mouth with the moistening effect of saliva and the shredding, tearing, and grinding done by the teeth. Moistening the food creates a bolus, which can more easily mix with acid and enzymes in the stomach.

Digestion in the Stomach

The food bolus passes down the esophagus and enters the stomach where hydrochloric acid, secreted by cells in the stomach lining, denatures the protein and provides an environment conducive to digestion. Other cells in the stomach lining produce an inactive enzyme, pepsinogen. The acidic environment converts the pepsinogen to the active *protease* (protein-cleaving enzyme), pepsin. The pepsin breaks the polypeptide chain at numerous sites, yielding intermediate-length polypeptides, small polypeptides, and some amino acids.

Digestion and Absorption in the Small Intestine

Further breakdown of the polypeptides takes place in the small intestine. It involves cleavage by proteases produced by both the pancreas and villi of the small intestine itself. The variety of proteases (aminopeptidase, carboxypeptidase, enteropeptidase, chymotrypsin, trypsin, and others) is needed to cleave peptide bonds associated with the full range of protein encountered. The end result of this complex digestive process is a mixture of amino acids and short peptides, which are absorbed by the small intestine and distributed through the portal system. Under most conditions, proteins are not absorbed directly into the bloodstream. If this absorption occurs in infants or in certain disease states, allergies may develop to food proteins.

AMINO ACID METABOLISM

Once a protein is degraded to amino acids, those molecules may be reused or recycled for other purposes. The liver is the site of amino acid synthesis. Most amino acids are utilized in the formation of protein. A small percentage of amino acids are broken down to provide energy or to create other molecules.

The first step in amino acid metabolism is the removal of the amino groups from the amino acids. Enzymes called *aminotransferases* or *transaminases* use vitamin B_6 to exchange nitrogen between amino acids. Other enzymes may remove nitrogen from amino acids. The ammonia derived in this way from amino acids is used by the liver to form urea, which is excreted in the urine. Because of its importance, nitrogen metabolism is very carefully regulated in the body (Newby, Price, 1998).

All indispensable, as well as most dispensable amino acids are derived from the diet. Thus, protein is an important nutrient, both in terms of its quality and its quantity. In developed nations, most children and adults receive far more protein than is needed for optimum growth or maintenance. However, even in the United States, among people who are chronically ill, institutionalized, and elderly, there is a risk of protein malnutrition. In other parts of the world, protein-calorie malnutrition may be a serious concern, especially for children.

PROTEIN REGULATION IN THE BODY

Because protein is so important in the body, protein intake, maintenance, metabolism, and losses are carefully regulated (Figure 5–7). As the body grows, some proteins outlive their usefulness, and are oxidized or damaged. Intracellular proteases break down these proteins, degrading them to amino acids. This process, called protein turnover, is a normal bodily function; approximately 250 g of protein are turned over each day. With adequate dietary sources of protein, turnover is generally balanced with tissue synthesis in mature adults to give no net gain (anabolism) or loss

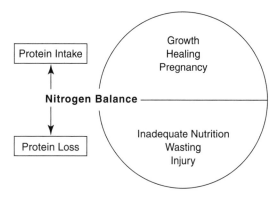

FIGURE 5–8   Nitrogen balance.

(catabolism) of protein. This condition is termed *nitrogen balance* (Figure 5–8). In circumstances of protein-calorie malnutrition—in major illness, stress, or in certain wasting diseases—more protein is lost than is synthesized. Where there is a net loss of body protein the individual is in *negative nitrogen balance*. A healthy growing child is making new protein far in excess of protein breakdown, and thus is said to be in *positive nitrogen balance*.

THE QUALITY OF PROTEINS IN FOOD

Protein quality is defined as the ability of a protein to support growth. Food proteins differ in overall quality. If a food protein has a ratio of amino acids that does not match the needs for human growth, and this is the sole

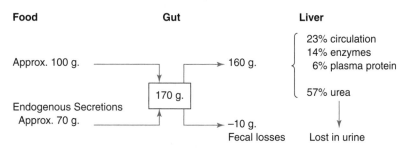

(approx. 50 g. from sloughed mucosal cells
approx. 17 g. from intestinal juices)

The free amino acid pool turns over constantly due to flux from dietary sources and recycled amino acids from tissue protein breakdown.

FIGURE 5–7   Body use of protein.

source of protein in the diet, growth will be impaired. The body can make the dispensable amino acids, so it is not critical that those be present in any specified amount. However, if a food protein contains a limiting amount of at least one indispensable amino acid needed for growth, all growth can be impaired. Such a protein is called an *incomplete* protein. For example, the proteins of cereal grains have a limiting amount of the amino acid lysine. Certain bean proteins are limited in methionine content. So if a person's sole protein sources contained only incomplete proteins, growth would be impaired.

A *complete protein* sustains optimal growth because all indispensable amino acids are present in proper proportions. Almost all proteins derived from animal sources (meat, fish, milk, and eggs), as well as soy protein, are complete and could serve as a single source of protein for growth and maintenance for health (gelatin, an incomplete protein, is an exception).

Most people eat a variety of proteins from plants and animals. Although a plant protein may have a relative limitation of one amino acid, eating more than one source of plant proteins generally will provide sufficient amounts of all amino acids. This concept, called *protein complementation*, applies not only during a single meal but also extends over a longer time. In part this is due to the role of intestinal proteins that serve as amino acid reservoirs to make up for transient amino acid limitations. For individuals who choose to eat only plant-derived foods, complementation can be important. Complementation is observed in many ethnic cuisines around the world. Lysine-poor tortillas and methionine-poor beans complement each other. A wide combination of protein sources in the diet helps ensure adequate protein quality (Table 5–3).

Food proteins are rated for protein quality. In most cases quality is measured with respect to a reference protein. Such a protein has an appropriate amino acid ratio and is digestible. For many years egg

TABLE 5–4   High- versus Low-Quality Proteins

Protein	PDCAAS Score
Egg albumin	1.00
Soy	0.99
Beef	0.92
Pinto beans	0.63
Whole wheat	0.44

protein was considered the reference protein and was given a value of 100. Recently a *protein digestibility-corrected amino acid score* (*PDCAAS*) has become the standard for determining protein quality. The Food and Agriculture Organization (FAO) and World Health Organization (WHO) standard compares the amino acid score of a food protein with the reference standard. This PDCAAS score serves as the basis for the daily values for protein shown on food labels (see Table 5–4).

PROTEIN REQUIREMENTS AND FOOD SOURCES

The greater the body mass, the more protein is turned over and the more protein is needed to maintain homeostasis. For healthy adults, the protein RDA is 0.8 g/kg body weight. For infants and children and for pregnant females the value is slightly higher, reflecting the increased rates of growth for these individuals. The protein RDA for 50 kg (110 lb) adult woman eating a mixed diet would be 46 g, for a 70 kg (160 lb) man, 56 g. Higher quality proteins may allow a slight reduction in protein intake. Approximately 15% of calories are typically obtained from protein. For an individual taking in 1800 kcal/day, this would translate to 240 kcal from protein, the equivalent of approximately 60 g of

TABLE 5–3   Complete versus Incomplete Proteins

Complete Protein	Deficient in	Incomplete Protein	Deficient in
Egg albumin	No amino acid	Pinto beans	Methionine
Soy	No amino acid	Whole wheat	Lysine

protein per day. Although this value correlates well with the RDA for individuals eating a normal diet, it may not apply to individuals on low-calorie or high-calorie diets. The amount of protein needed relates to body mass, growth, and protein replacement, and thus must be evaluated differently depending upon the individual.

In developed countries such as the United States, average protein intakes may exceed the RDA by two to three times, far more than can be appropriately used by the body for growth. A single ounce of meat provides 7 g of protein. Thus, an 8 oz steak provides 56 g of protein, the entire dietary recommendation for a day for an adult man. Other foods, often not thought of as protein-rich, may alone provide sufficient protein to meet dietary needs. A serving of vegetables provides approximately 2 g of protein, a glass of milk, 8 g. In developed countries it is not difficult for an individual, whether on an omnivorous or plant-based diet, to meet the protein RDA (Table 5–5).

Effects of Excessive Protein Consumption

For most healthy adults in the United States and Canada, the problem of protein nutrition is generally one of excess rather than deficiency. When a high-protein diet supplies more protein than can be used by the body it must be broken down to amino acids. These, in turn, will be metabolized further to yield energy and release excess nitrogen. The nitrogen thus released must be cleared from the blood through the action of the liver and kidneys, creating an added load on these organs. Although there is no upper limit on protein consumption, there do not appear to be any benefits to protein overconsumption (Metges, Barth, 2000). Because the high protein intake seen in developing countries often comes from eating large amounts of meat, and because meats contains a high content of saturated fats and cholesterol, eating such diets increases the risk for heart disease and stroke. Most truly high-protein diets lack adequate fruit and vegetable intake, which limits intake of other important nutrients.

High-protein diets may have effects on calcium metabolism. As protein increases in the diet, calcium excretion increases, which may be related to calcium uptake or bone loss (Kerstetter, O'Brien, Insogna, 2003). Especially common among postmenopausal women, although not limited to this group, osteoporosis is a serious concern and is discussed in Chapter 11 (Ginty, 2003). Because osteoporosis can affect alveolar bone density, excessive protein intake can have oral sequelae as well.

There has been a great deal of interest in protein supplementation, especially among body builders and health enthusiasts. Nothing in the literature suggests that healthy, well-fed individuals benefit from protein supplements. Other informational sources promote amino acid supplementation as a means of achieving optimal health. Unfortunately, amino acid supplements do not improve health. In fact, in a number of cases, they have been implicated in premature death. Adequate protein intake, as part of a well-chosen, balanced diet, provides the best means of promoting growth and muscle development.

EFFECTS OF PROTEIN DEFICIENCY

For sensitive populations, protein deficiencies can still occur. Among children of low socioeconomic rank who are not provided good diets and persons who are chronically ill, hospitalized, and elderly, whether living alone or in an institution, protein deficiency can be a serious problem. In other parts of the world protein-energy malnutrition may be a serious and threatening condition, especially for the young. For oral health even a single event of protein-energy deficiency in the first year of life leads to delayed deciduous tooth eruption, delayed loss of primary teeth, and greater caries experience in both primary and permanent teeth (Alvarez, 1995). Protein-energy malnutrition has also been implicated in reduced cytokine effects, and the suppression of the acute phase response, both critical in the response to periodontal pathogens and resistance to periodontal disease (Enwonwu, 1995)

Protein-Energy Malnutrition

Inadequate caloric and protein intake may lead to a severe condition known as protein-energy malnutrition (PEM). Two forms of PEM have been identified: marasmus and kwashiorkor. They are differentiated on the basis of clinical observations and are related to the time frame of the PEM. Although most examples of PEM are seen in children, others at risk (people who are homeless or elderly, substance abusers, patients in

TABLE 5–5   Dietary Reference Intakes for Protein

Nutrient	Function	Life Stage Group	RDA/AI* g/d[a]	AMDR[b]	Selected Food Sources	Adverse Effects of Excessive Consumption
Protein and amino acids	Serves as the major structural component of all cells in the body, and functions as enzymes in membranes, as transport carriers, and as some hormones. During digestion and absorption dietary proteins are broken down to amino acids, which become the building blocks of these structural and functional compounds. Nine of the amino acids must be provided in the diet; these are termed indispensable amino acids. The body can make the other amino acids needed to synthesize specific structures from other amino acids.	Infants			Proteins from animal sources, such as meat, poultry, fish, eggs, milk, cheese, and yogurt, provide all nine indispensable amino acids in adequate amounts, and for this reason are considered "complete proteins." Proteins from plants, legumes, grains, nuts, seeds, and vegetables tend to be deficient in one or more of the indispensable amino acids and are called "incomplete proteins." Vegan diets adequate in total protein content can be "complete" by combining sources of incomplete proteins that lack different indispensable amino acids.	While no defined intake level at which potential adverse effects of protein was identified, the upper end of AMDR is based on complementing the AMDR for carbohydrate and fat for the various age groups. The lower end of the AMDR is set at approximately the RDA.
		0–6 mo	9.1*	ND[c]		
		7–12 mo	11.0	ND		
		Children				
		1–3 y	**13**	**5–20**		
		4–8 y	**19**	**10–30**		
		Males				
		9–13 y	**34**	**10–30**		
		14–18 y	**52**	**10–30**		
		19–30 y	**56**	**10–35**		
		31–50 y	**56**	**10–35**		
		50–70 y	**56**	**10–35**		
		>70 y	**56**	**10–35**		
		Females				
		9–13 y	**34**	**10–30**		
		14–18 y	**46**	**10–30**		
		19–30 y	**46**	**10–35**		
		31–50 y	**46**	**10–35**		
		50–70 y	**46**	**10–35**		
		>70 y	**46**	**10–35**		
		Pregnancy				
		≤18 y	71	**10–35**		
		19–30 y	71	**10–35**		
		31–50 y	71	**10–35**		
		Lactation				
		≤18 y	71	**10–35**		
		19–30 y	71	**10–35**		
		31–50 y	71	**10–35**		

Note: The table is adapted from the DRI reports, see http://www.nap.edu. It represents Recommended Dietary Allowances (RDAs) in **bold type**. Adequate intakes (AIs) in ordinary type followed by an asterisk (*). RDAs and AIs may both be used as goals for individual intake. RDAs are set to meet the needs of almost all (97 to 98 percent) individuals in a group. For healthy breastfed infants, the AI is the mean intake. The AI for other life stage and gender groups is believed to cover the needs of all individuals in the group, but lack of data prevents being able to specify with confidence the percentage of individuals covered by this intake.
[a]Based on 1.5 g/kg/day for infants, 1.1 g/kg/day for 1–3 y, 0.95 g/kg/day for 4–13 y, 0.85 g/kg/day for 14–18 y, 0.8 g/kg/day for adults, and 1.1 g/kg/day for pregnant (using pregnancy weight) and lactating women.
[b]Acceptable Macronutrient Distribution Range (AMDR).
* The range of intake for a particular energy source that is associated with reduced risk of chronic disease while providing intakes of essential nutrients. If an individual consumed in excess of the AMDR, there is a potential of increasing the risk of chronic diseases and insufficient intake of essential nutrients.
[c]ND = Not determinable due to lack of data of adverse effects in this age group and concern with regard to lack of ability to handle excess amounts. Source of intake should be from food only to prevent high levels of intake.
Source: Reprinted with permission from *Dietary Reference Intakes for Energy, Carbohydrate, Fiber, Fat, Fatty Acids, Cholesterol, Protein, and Amino Acids (Macronutrients).* Copyright © 2005 by the National Academy of Sciences. Courtesy of the National Academy Press, Washington, D.C.

improperly managed institutions) individuals may also suffer from inadequate food and protein intake and suffer the same outcomes.

Marasmus is the *chronic* form of PEM, resulting from long term protein-energy deficits. Marasmus is most often seen in children who have had insufficient food over a long time (Figure 5–9). It is most common among children from 6 to 18 months, and represents not only inadequate caloric intake but also inadequate protein, indispensable fatty acids, vitamins, and minerals. Children experiencing marasmus may not be receiving adequate mother's milk and often may subsist on liquid diets, deficient in the nutrients required for growth and even for minimal sustenance. The malnutrition leads to muscle (including heart muscle) weakening, impairment of brain and nervous system development, and ultimately to a reduction in cognitive ability. The child with marasmus often appears to be old and shriveled.

Kwashiorkor is the *acute* form of PEM, which develops from a sudden and recent food deprivation. It is most common in children between the ages of 18 and 24 months. The term derives from a Ghanaian term, which reflects the effects of weaning of a first child at the time the second child is born. Kwashiorkor develops when the child is weaned to a low-nutrient diet from the complete nutrition provided by breast milk. The condition rapidly develops from a deficiency of indispensable amino acids for the growing child. It may also develop as a result of an infection or weakened condition that changes the nutritional needs of the child. The child's fluid balance, maintained through blood protein levels, is disturbed. Edema develops in the face and abdomen. Because the amino acid tyrosine is lacking, the hair pigment melanin is not made. Hair color and texture changes. The skin cannot replace damaged cells; scaly, patchy skin textures develop and sores develop that may not heal. The lack of iron-binding proteins leads to higher levels of unbound iron, which promotes bacterial growth. Hemoglobin and other blood proteins are not synthesized so that the child becomes weak and anemic. Antibodies are proteins produced by the body to protect against infection. In kwashiorkor, immune response is often suppressed and immunoglobulins may even be broken down to provide needed amino acids. The combination of infection, fever, and electrolyte imbalances may lead to heart failure and sudden death. Fluid and electrolyte imbalances may trigger dysentery, an intestinal infection with subsequent diarrhea. Treatment of the condition often requires rehydration and electrolyte therapy (Figure 5–10).

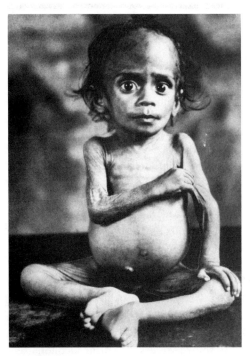

FIGURE 5–9 Child with marasmus.
Source: World Health Organization.

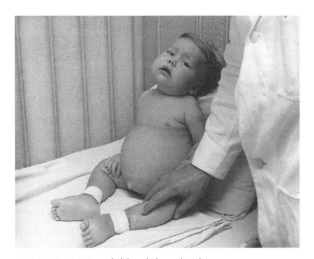

FIGURE 5–10 Child with kwashiorkor.
Source: F.A.O. Food and Agriculture Organization of the United Nations.

In summary, marasmus and kwashiorkor are different stages in the same process. Marasmus is the body's adaptation to starvation. Kwashiorkor is the condition arising from a failure of that adaptation to meet the body's demands. This may explain the concurrent existence of both diseases in the same community, and may help to understand the combined characteristics (marasmus and kwashiorkor) seen in the condition of some individuals.

TREND TOWARD PLANT-BASED DIETS (SABATE, RATZIN-TURNER, BROWN, 2001)

Traditional human diets have met the protein requirements of those who consumed them. As the number of different cultural backgrounds in North America increases, defining a Canadian or American diet becomes more and more difficult. *The Recommendations for Diet and Health (Diet and Health)*, the *Food Choice Pyramid*, and other food guides assist consumers in making good food choices (Vegetarian Diets, 1997). All recommend food selections to minimize fat and increase fruit and vegetable consumption, and base the human diet on complex carbohydrates. As cultural diversity and recommendations change, the time has come to reconsider which protein sources best meet protein requirements.

The traditional American diet (meat and potatoes diet) still predominates in many areas of the country. Most protein is derived from red meat, poultry, and fish. In reaction to the nutrient-poor diets experienced by their ancestors and having the knowledge that protein was indispensable for growth, most individuals equated a high-meat diet with a good diet.

Starting in the 19th century and developing rapidly during the latter half of the 20th century, a number of North Americans shifted their diets into one variant or another of what has been commonly called a *vegetarian diet*. The term *vegetarian* has become so broadly understood that it is confusing (Willett, 1999). Table 5–6 lists common reasons why people become vegetarians. Table 5–7 shows types of vegetarians. Vegetarians are individuals who eat foods derived directly from plants. At the one extreme, the *vegan* eats nothing but plant products, eliminating any animal products including dairy products or eggs. Most "vegetarians" are *lactovegetarians* or *lacto-ovovegetarians*, eating plant products but also including dairy products

TABLE 5–6   Rationales for Following Vegetarian Diets

A healthier diet
Avoidance of additives, chemicals
Return to more natural foods
Respect for animal life
Religious: diet as a means of achieving a balanced, righteous life
"Alternative" medicine or "self-healing" using foods as preventatives or cures

TABLE 5–7   Types of Vegetarians

Semivegetarian	Avoids red meat; eats fish and poultry, eggs and dairy in addition to plant products
Lacto-ovovegetarian	Supplements plant foods with eggs and dairy products
Lactovegetarian	Supplements plant foods with dairy products only
Pure vegetarian (vegan)	Eats only vegetables and fruit
Fruitarian	Eats only fruits

and possibly eggs in their diets. Further along the continuum, many Americans are fast becoming *semivegetarians*, individuals who eat primarily plant-derived foods but who occasionally add red meat, poultry, or fish as a way of increasing variety and adding flavor to their diets.

Many individuals have chosen to identify their diets as *plant-based diets* rather than label themselves *vegetarians*. Plant-based diets better meet the various recommendations and food guides than do the traditional North American diets. Many of the cultural cuisines brought to the United States by new immigrants, in fact, can be classified as plant-based diets.

Benefits of Plant-Based Diets

It is difficult to isolate the dietary benefits of vegetarian diets (Table 5–8). Most vegetarians have a lifestyle that differentiates them from other individuals. Some tend not to smoke, excessively drink alcohol, use illicit drugs, or engage in other risk-engendering activities (Fraser, 2003). More vegetarians are physically active than the population as a whole. Nevertheless, certain

TABLE 5-8   Benefits versus Possible Concerns of Vegetarian Diets

Benefits	*Concerns*
Ease of meeting nutritional guidelines (lacto-ovovegetarians)	Caloric adequacy for pregnant females and children (primarily vegans)
Decreased risk for death from colon cancer, coronary heart disease (CHD) (all vegetarians)	Mineral (iron, zinc, calcium) adequacy (primarily vegans)
Decreased incidence of obesity (all vegetarians)	Vitamin B_{12}, D adequacy (vegans only)
Decreased incidence of hypertension (all vegetarians)	Need for advanced nutritional knowledge (vegans only)
Lower risk for developing diabetes (all vegetarians)	

Source: Rajaram, Sabate, 2000; Sabate, 2003; Sanders, 1999.

factors appear to be directly related to diet (Leitzmann, 2005). Vegetarians generally maintain a healthier body weight (especially vegans who do not eat any animal products, but derive all their nutrients from high-fiber, high-carbohydrate foods). They maintain a healthier blood pressure (most likely related to body weight and the intake of fiber, fruits, and vegetables). Fewer vegetarians suffer from coronary heart and arterial diseases, probably due in part to the reduction in saturated fat and cholesterol consumption (Key, Appleby, 2001). Vegetarians moving to a meat-rich diet show harmful changes in blood lipids; omnivores who move to a vegetarian diet show improvement in the same measures. Individuals who have a semivegetarian diet have blood lipid profiles that are intermediate between the two extremes (Fraser, 2003). Vegetarians have less of certain types of cancer, especially colon cancer (Mills, 2001). High-fat, high-protein, low-fiber diets appear to promote development of these cancers in some people.

In 1999, the FDA approved a new health claim for food labels related to soy protein. This health claim is based on evidence that including soy protein in a low-saturated-fat-and-cholesterol diet may reduce the risk of coronary heart disease by lowering blood cholesterol levels (USDHHS, FDA, 1999).

In general, plant-based diets can be designed to meet nutritional recommendations with ease. The naturally occurring high-fiber, low-fat, vitamin-, mineral-, and antioxidant-rich plant-based foods have beneficial effects for many of the common chronic health conditions that affect Americans (Nestle, 1999).

Precautions for Those Following Vegetarian Diets

Poor diet planning can lead to problems with any diet. High-fat lactovegetarian diets containing cheeses, sour cream, and other fats and oils can lead to many of the same harmful outcomes as experienced by persons eating a high-fat meat diet. Because nutrient needs increase under conditions of pregnancy, lactation, infancy, childhood, and illness, people following restricted vegetarian diets (vegan) must give special care to making good food choices at these times (Hackett, Nathan, Burgess, 1998).

Plant-based foods generally are not as energy-dense as are animal-derived foods. It takes a larger amount of food to meet energy needs. This may be advantageous for adults but can be harmful for small children. The child may feel full before he or she has eaten enough to meet nutritional needs. Only through careful planning—including cereals, beans, nuts, and other energy-rich foods in the diet—can the child meet protein requirements. Vegan children are often below norms for growth and size and may have difficulty meeting vitamin and mineral requirements without supplementation. A child eating dairy products and eggs generally does not experience any of these problems as long as good nutritional principles are followed.

Diet Planning for Vegetarians

If diets are planned to provide adequate energy for growth and health, protein needs are not difficult to meet. For the vegan, because only plant proteins are consumed, it may be necessary to take in more than the expected amount of protein to counteract the slightly lower amino acid scores for most plant proteins. Complementation can help overcome this problem. For the lactovegetarian and lacto-ovovegetarian, protein intake is seldom a problem. The vegetarian food pyramid identifies a number of good protein sources including milk, eggs, legumes, and soy protein products that, when chosen wisely, exceed recommendations (Haddad, Sabate, Whitten, 1999).

Iron, zinc, and calcium intake should be monitored for adequacy. For those who eat milk and eggs, the same cautions should be observed as are followed by those who eat meat. For vegans, calcium can be supplied in adequate amounts by consuming tofu, green vegetables, and some nuts, but adequacy must be carefully monitored (Weaver, Proulx, Heaney, 1999).

For vegetarians who eat milk and eggs, vitamins D and B_{12} are seldom a problem. For these individuals, vitamin D can be obtained by exposure to sunlight and through vitamin D fortified milk. For the vegan, vitamin D supplements may be necessary. Vitamin B_{12} is often identified as the nutrient most at risk for the vegan. However, eating cereals or other foods supplemented with vitamin B_{12}, or taking B_{12} supplements, will provide adequate B_{12} intake (Stabler, Allen, 2004). Figures 5–11 and 5–12 show vegetarian food guides for

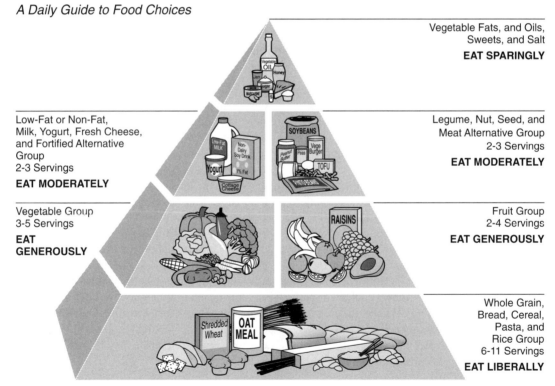

The Vegetarian Food Pyramid *(US)*
A Daily Guide to Food Choices

Vegetable Fats, and Oils, Sweets, and Salt
EAT SPARINGLY

Low-Fat or Non-Fat, Milk, Yogurt, Fresh Cheese, and Fortified Alternative Group
2-3 Servings
EAT MODERATELY

Legume, Nut, Seed, and Meat Alternative Group
2-3 Servings
EAT MODERATELY

Vegetable Group
3-5 Servings
EAT GENEROUSLY

Fruit Group
2-4 Servings
EAT GENEROUSLY

Whole Grain, Bread, Cereal, Pasta, and Rice Group
6-11 Servings
EAT LIBERALLY

FIGURE 5–11 The Vegetarian Food Pyramid (US).
Sources: Melina V, Davis B, Harrison V: *Becoming Vegetarian*. Summertown, TN: Book Publishing Company, 1995; Davis B, Melina V: *Becoming Vegan*. Summertown, TN: Book Publishing Company, 2000; Melina V, Forest J: *Cooking Vegetarian*. New York: Wiley, 1998.

(Canada)
Vegetarian Food Guide Rainbow

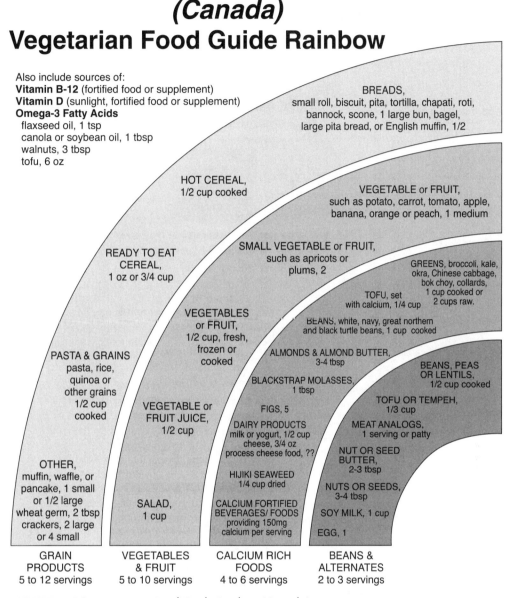

Also include sources of:
Vitamin B-12 (fortified food or supplement)
Vitamin D (sunlight, fortified food or supplement)
Omega-3 Fatty Acids
 flaxseed oil, 1 tsp
 canola or soybean oil, 1 tbsp
 walnuts, 3 tbsp
 tofu, 6 oz

BREADS,
small roll, biscuit, pita, tortilla, chapati, roti,
bannock, scone, 1 large bun, bagel,
large pita bread, or English muffin, 1/2

HOT CEREAL,
1/2 cup cooked

VEGETABLE or FRUIT,
such as potato, carrot, tomato, apple,
banana, orange or peach, 1 medium

READY TO EAT
CEREAL,
1 oz or 3/4 cup

SMALL VEGETABLE or FRUIT,
such as apricots or
plums, 2

GREENS, broccoli, kale,
okra, Chinese cabbage,
bok choy, collards,
1 cup cooked or
2 cups raw.

TOFU, set
with calcium, 1/4 cup

VEGETABLES
or FRUIT,
1/2 cup, fresh,
frozen or
cooked

BEANS, white, navy, great northern
and black turtle beans, 1 cup cooked

PASTA & GRAINS
pasta, rice,
quinoa or
other grains
1/2 cup
cooked

ALMONDS & ALMOND BUTTER,
3-4 tbsp

BEANS, PEAS
OR LENTILS,
1/2 cup cooked

BLACKSTRAP MOLASSES,
1 tbsp

TOFU OR TEMPEH,
1/3 cup

FIGS, 5

VEGETABLE or
FRUIT JUICE,
1/2 cup

MEAT ANALOGS,
1 serving or patty

DAIRY PRODUCTS
milk or yogurt, 1/2 cup
cheese, 3/4 oz
process cheese food, ??

NUT OR SEED
BUTTER,
2-3 tbsp

OTHER,
muffin, waffle, or
pancake, 1 small
or 1/2 large
wheat germ, 2 tbsp
crackers, 2 large
or 4 small

HIJIKI SEAWEED
1/4 cup dried

NUTS OR SEEDS,
3-4 tbsp

SALAD,
1 cup

CALCIUM FORTIFIED
BEVERAGES/ FOODS
providing 150mg
calcium per serving

SOY MILK, 1 cup

EGG, 1

| GRAIN PRODUCTS 5 to 12 servings | VEGETABLES & FRUIT 5 to 10 servings | CALCIUM RICH FOODS 4 to 6 servings | BEANS & ALTERNATES 2 to 3 servings |

FIGURE 5–12 Vegetarian Food Guide Rainbow (Canada).
Sources: Melina V, Davis B, Harrison V: *Becoming Vegetarian.* Summertown, TN: Book Publishing Company, 1995;
Davis B, Melina V: *Becoming Vegan.* Summertown, TN: Book Publishing Company, 2000; Melina V, Forest J: *Cooking
Vegetarian.* New York: Wiley, 1998.

Vegan Food Guide Pyramid *(US)*

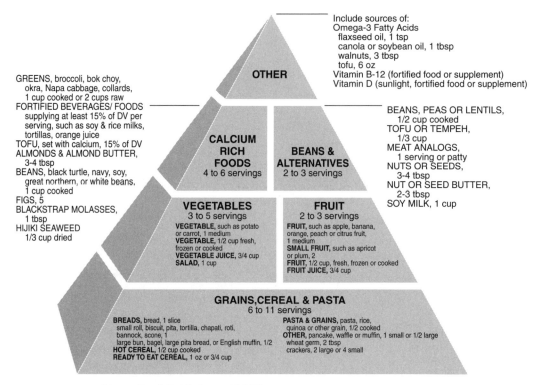

FIGURE 5–13   Vegan Food Guide Pyramid (US).
Sources: Melina V, Davis B, Harrison V: *Becoming Vegetarian*. Summertown, TN: Book Publishing Company, 1995; Davis B, Melina V: *Becoming Vegan*. Summertown, TN: Book Publishing Company, 2000; Melina V, Forest J: *Cooking Vegetarian*. New York: Wiley, 1998.

the United States and Canada. Figures 5–13 and 5–14 show vegan food guides for the United States and Canada.

SUMMARY AND IMPLICATIONS FOR DENTISTRY

Protein is of prime importance for the development of all body tissues and structures. Many different types of diets can meet protein needs. Protein deficiency can affect the growth and development of oral tissues and structures and can increase susceptibility to general and oral infections. Protein in excess can reduce calcium retention and subsequent bone health. Many people are changing to a plant-based diet for a variety of reasons. These types of diets can have many health benefits if implemented wisely. Plant-based diets can

be of high quality or can pose health risks, depending on their protein composition. In our changing cultural milieu, and in light of what is now known about proteins and the body's requirements, a person can embrace many different means of achieving optimal protein nutrition.

QUESTIONS PATIENTS MIGHT ASK

Q. How do I go about following a healthy vegetarian diet?
A. There are many good books available detailing how to make wise vegetarian food choices. In general a sound vegetarian diet is based upon the food guide pyramid, using alternative protein sources in place of animal protein sources. Because most of the vegetable proteins do not have a complete complement of indispensable amino acids, it is important to

(Canada)
Vegetarian Food Guide Rainbow

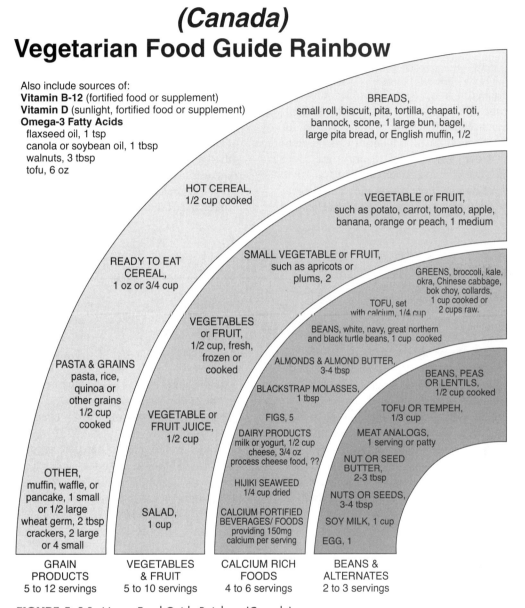

Also include sources of:
Vitamin B-12 (fortified food or supplement)
Vitamin D (sunlight, fortified food or supplement)
Omega-3 Fatty Acids
  flaxseed oil, 1 tsp
  canola or soybean oil, 1 tbsp
  walnuts, 3 tbsp
  tofu, 6 oz

BREADS,
small roll, biscuit, pita, tortilla, chapati, roti,
bannock, scone, 1 large bun, bagel,
large pita bread, or English muffin, 1/2

HOT CEREAL,
1/2 cup cooked

VEGETABLE or FRUIT,
such as potato, carrot, tomato, apple,
banana, orange or peach, 1 medium

READY TO EAT
CEREAL,
1 oz or 3/4 cup

SMALL VEGETABLE or FRUIT,
such as apricots or
plums, 2

GREENS, broccoli, kale,
okra, Chinese cabbage,
bok choy, collards,
1 cup cooked or
2 cups raw.

TOFU, set
with calcium, 1/4 cup

VEGETABLES
or FRUIT,
1/2 cup, fresh,
frozen or
cooked

BEANS, white, navy, great northern
and black turtle beans, 1 cup cooked

PASTA & GRAINS
pasta, rice,
quinoa or
other grains
1/2 cup
cooked

ALMONDS & ALMOND BUTTER,
3-4 tbsp

BEANS, PEAS
OR LENTILS,
1/2 cup cooked

BLACKSTRAP MOLASSES,
1 tbsp

TOFU OR TEMPEH,
1/3 cup

VEGETABLE or
FRUIT JUICE,
1/2 cup

FIGS, 5

DAIRY PRODUCTS
milk or yogurt, 1/2 cup
cheese, 3/4 oz
process cheese food, ??

MEAT ANALOGS,
1 serving or patty

NUT OR SEED
BUTTER,
2-3 tbsp

OTHER,
muffin, waffle, or
pancake, 1 small
or 1/2 large
wheat germ, 2 tbsp
crackers, 2 large
or 4 small

HIJIKI SEAWEED
1/4 cup dried

NUTS OR SEEDS,
3-4 tbsp

SALAD,
1 cup

CALCIUM FORTIFIED
BEVERAGES/ FOODS
providing 150mg
calcium per serving

SOY MILK, 1 cup

EGG, 1

GRAIN
PRODUCTS
5 to 12 servings

VEGETABLES
& FRUIT
5 to 10 servings

CALCIUM RICH
FOODS
4 to 6 servings

BEANS &
ALTERNATES
2 to 3 servings

FIGURE 5–14 Vegan Food Guide Rainbow (Canada).

Sources: Melina V, Davis B, Harrison V: *Becoming Vegetarian.* Summertown, TN: Book Publishing Company, 1995;
Davis B, Melina V: *Becoming Vegan.* Summertown, TN: Book Publishing Company, 2000; Melina V, Forest J: *Cooking Vegetarian.* New York: Wiley, 1998.

choose high-quality vegetable proteins whenever possible. The more restrictive you plan to be, the more important it is to choose protein sources wisely. You may also need a one-a-day type of multivitamin and mineral supplement.

Q. Don't I need extra protein to build muscle for my athletic activities? I take a protein drink for that reason.

A. It is a misconception that extra protein is needed for muscle building. A small amount of extra protein may be needed, but calories (energy) are more important. The average American and Canadian often eat a lot more protein than they really need. The extra just turns into extra calories while putting stress on the kidneys to excrete the nitrogenous waste. So with a nutritious diet that meets the food pyramid guidelines, extra protein drinks add primarily extra cost.

Q. Isn't it true that strict vegan diets are nutritionally deficient?

A. Not necessarily. Strict vegans have to be more careful than less restrictive vegetarians to ensure that their diet meets nutritional requirements. However, this can be done with careful food choices and often the use of supplements. Nobody should become a vegan casually, without careful study and attention to reliable resources.

CASE STUDY

Joanne Gilmartin is a 21-year-old patient, seen in your office for a routine visit. She informs you that she has been following a strict vegan diet for the past year and plans on continuing to do so. She has recently been married and is looking forward to starting a family. Her diet consists mainly of bread, rice, cereal, and fruits and vegetables, with little concern for protein sources. She reports that she has lost 10 pounds since initiation of the vegan diet and says she feels great. She is planning on bringing up her future children as vegans as well, as she believes that this is the most healthy eating approach. She is currently 5 feet 3 inches tall and weighs 121 pounds.

Questions

1. What are the risks associated with Joanne's eating pattern?
2. Are all vegetarians at risk for protein deficiency?
3. How could Joanne get adequate protein in her diet while remaining vegan?
4. Do you have any oral health concerns about Joanne?
5. What would you tell Joanne regarding her plans to bring up her future children vegan?

REFERENCES

Alvarez JO: Nutrition, tooth development, and dental caries. *Am J Clin Nutr* 1995; 61:410S–16S.

Enwonwu CO: Interface of malnutrition and periodontal disease. *Am J Clin Nutr* 1995; 61:430S–36S.

Fraser GE: Risk factors for cardiovascular disease and cancer among vegetarians. In *Diet, Life Expectancy, and Chronic Disease*. New York: Oxford University Press, 2003:203–239.

Ginty F: Dietary protein and bone health. *Proc Nutr Soc* 2003; 62:867–76.

Hackett A, Nathan I, Burgess L: Is a vegetarian diet adequate for children? *Nutr Health* 1998; 12(3):189–95.

Haddad EH, Sabate J, Whitten CG: Vegetarian food guide pyramid: A conceptual framework. *Am J Clin Nutr* 1999; 70(3 Suppl):615S–34S.

Institute of Medicine, National Academy of Sciences: *Dietary Reference Intakes for Energy, Carbohydrate, Fiber, Fat, Fatty Acids, Cholesterol, Protein, and Amino Acids (Macronutrients)*. Washington, DC: National Academies Press, 2005.

Kerstetter JE, O'Brein KO, Insogna KL: Low protein intake: The impact on calcium and bone homeostasis. *J Nutr* 2003; 133:855S–61S.

Key TJ, Appleby PN: Vegetarianism, coronary risk factors, and coronary heart disease. In Sabate J (ed): *Vegetarian Nutrition*. Boca Raton, FL: CRC Press, 2001:33–54.

Leitzmann C: Vegetarian diets: What are the advantages? *Forum Nutr* 2005; 57:147–56.

Metges CC, Barth CA: Metabolic consequences of a high dietary-protein intake in adulthood: Assessment of the available evidence. *J Nutr* 2000; 130:886–89.

Mills PK: Diet and cancer risk. In Sabate J (ed): *Vegetarian Nutrition.* Boca Raton, FL: CRC Press, 2001:55–90.

Nestle M: Animal v. plant foods in human diets and health: Is the historical record unequivocal? *Proc Nutr Soc* 1999; 58:211–18.

Newby FD, Price SR: Determinants of protein turnover in health and disease. *Miner Electrolyte Metab* 1998; 24:6–12.

Rajaram S, Sabate J: Health benefits of a vegetarian diet. *Nutrition* 2000; 16531–3.

Sabate J: The contribution of vegetarian diets to health and disease: A paradigm shift. In Proceedings of the Fourth International Congress on Vegetarian Nutrition. *Am J Clin Nutr* 2003; 78(Suppl):502S–7S.

Sabate J, Ratzin-Turner RA, Brown JE: Vegetarian diets: Description and trends. In Sabate J (ed): *Vegetarian Nutrition.* Boca Raton, FL: CRC Press, 2001:3–17.

Sanders TA: The nutritional adequacy of plant based diets. *Proc Nutr Soc* 1999; 58:265–69.

Stabler SP, Allen RH: Vitamin B_{12} deficiency as a worldwide problem. *Annu Rey Nutr* 2004; 24:299–326.

U.S. Department of Health and Human Services, Food and Drug Administration: Food labeling: Health claims; soy protein and coronary heart disease. *Federal Register* 1999; 64(206):57699–57733. Retrieved from http://wais.access .gpo.gov

Vegetarian diets: Position of the American Dietetic Association. *J Am Diet Assoc* 1997; 97:1317–21.

Weaver CM, Proulx WR, Heaney R: Choices for achieving adequate dietary calcium with a vegetarian diet. *Am J Clin Nutr* 1999; 70(3 Suppl):543S–48S.

Willett WC: Convergence of philosophy and science: The Third International Congress on Vegetarian Nutrition. *Am J Clin Nutr* 1999; 70(3 Suppl):434S–38S.

Chapter **6**

Lipids in Health and Disease

Linda Boyd and Carole A. Palmer

OBJECTIVES

The student will be able to:
- Describe the functions of lipids.
- Identify the classes of lipids.
- Describe fat digestion, absorption, and transport.
- Recognize the difference between the terms *serum cholesterol* and *dietary cholesterol*.
- Discuss the relationships between dietary fat and cardiovascular disease.
- Give an overview of the effects of lipids on serum cholesterol levels.
- Make general recommendations to patients on fat intake.
- Understand the possible oral implications of dietary fats.

INTRODUCTION

Lipids (fats) are a group of organic compounds that include triglycerides (fats and oils), phospholipids, and related compounds called sterols (including 7-dehydro-cholesterol—a precursor for vitamin D—and cholesterol). Like carbohydrates, lipids are composed of carbon, hydrogen, and oxygen. They may also contain other constituents such as phosphorus, nitrogen, carbohydrates, and proteins. Some lipids must be provided in the diet, whereas others can be synthesized in the body. Lipids are more calorically dense than either carbohydrate or protein. Each gram of fat provides 9 kcal of energy (compared with 4 kcal of energy produced per gram of carbohydrate or protein). Lipids are insoluble in water, but soluble in organic solvents. They are transported by or readily dispersed in fats and oils (Brody, 1999).

Lipids are widely distributed in food and in the body. Certain fatty acids and vitamins that must be dissolved in fat are essential in the diet because the body cannot manufacture them. Lipids are also of current interest due to their implications in cardiovascular disease and prevention.

FUNCTIONS OF FAT IN THE BODY

Lipids serve many functions in the body. They:

- provide the body with essential fatty acids.
- serve as a major source of energy (after carbohydrate), and reduce the body's need to break down protein for energy.
- serve as a reserve of stored energy (adipose tissue).
- facilitate fat-soluble vitamin absorption.
- cushion vital body organs.
- help maintain body insulation and temperature.
- provide a sense of fullness and satiety owing to their slow digestion.
- enhance the palatability of foods by absorbing and retaining flavors.
- provide moisture, texture, and tenderness to food.
- emulsify, stabilize foams, aerate batters, transfer heat, and carry pigments (Mattes, 1998).

TYPES OF CIRCULATING FATS

A variety of types of fats circulate throughout body tissues to provide the myriad important functions listed above.

Simple Lipids

Dietary fats and oils are often called simple lipids (Figure 6–1). Fats are usually solid at room temperature. Oils tend to be liquid. Simple lipids contain only fatty acids and glycerol. Glycerol is a 3-carbon alcohol with a structure similar to glucose.

Triglycerides

Triglycerides make up approximately 95–98% of fat found in foods and in body tissues (Krummel, 1997; Linder, 1991). Fat in this form is the most efficient way to store calories in the body until they are needed for energy. A majority of the triglycerides in the body are stored in adipose tissue. The adipose tissue gives the body an almost unlimited storage capacity for energy reserves.

Triglycerides have three fatty acids linked to a glycerol molecule. The fatty acids attached to the glycerol determine the type of fatty acid molecule. Fatty acids consist of a chain of carbon atoms with hydrogens attached and an acid group (-COOH) at the end. About 90% of fatty acids have an even number of carbon atoms (NRC, 1989). A fatty acid varies by the length of the carbon chain and the degree of saturation. The length of the fatty acid molecule and the degree of saturation influence how the fat is used in the body. The classifications according to the length of the carbon chain are:

- short-chained (less than 6 carbons)
- medium-chained (6 to 10 carbons)
- long-chained (12 or more carbons)

Short- and medium-chain fatty acids tend to be oxidized immediately, rather than deposited as triglycerides or phospholipids (Brody, 1999). The degrees of fatty acid saturation are:

- saturated (no double bonds; all are saturated with oxygen)
- monounsaturated (contains a single double bond)
- polyunsaturated (contains more than one double bond)

Saturated Fatty Acids

Fatty acids become saturated when they have all the hydrogen atoms they can carry. The process by which double bonds become saturated with hydrogen is

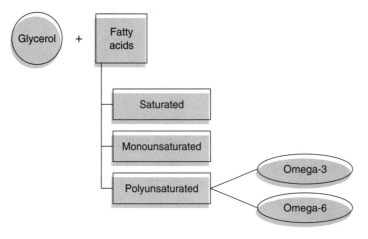

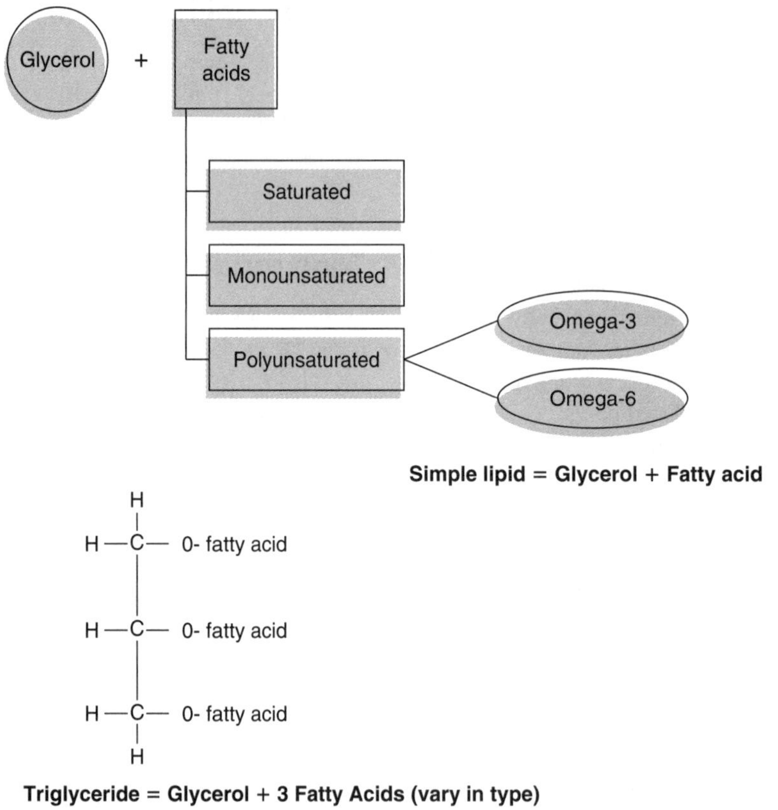

Simple lipid = Glycerol + Fatty acid

$$
\begin{array}{c}
\text{H} \\
| \\
\text{H} - \text{C} - \text{O- fatty acid} \\
| \\
\text{H} - \text{C} - \text{O- fatty acid} \\
| \\
\text{H} - \text{C} - \text{O- fatty acid} \\
| \\
\text{H}
\end{array}
$$

Triglyceride = Glycerol + 3 Fatty Acids (vary in type)

FIGURE 6–1   Model of basic lipid structures.

termed *hydrogenation*. Hydrogenation is also used to turn polyunsaturated liquid fats such as oils into more spreadable products. When this occurs, the new product is no longer polyunsaturated (Figure 6–2).

Saturated fatty acids are found primarily in animal products (beef, chicken, pork, dairy products) and certain vegetable oils (palm, palm kernel, cottonseed, and coconut oil) (Krummel, 1997). The major saturated fat found in foods is palmitic acid (16 carbons) and stearic acid (18 carbons) (NRC, 1989). Generally the more saturated the fat, the more solid the food will be at room temperature (e.g., butter or lard). The exception is vegetable oils, which remain liquid.

Saturated fatty acids have been implicated in raising total serum cholesterol and low-density lipoprotein (LDL) cholesterol levels in the blood. These are both risk factors for cardiovascular disease (Dreon et al., 1998). Palmitic, myristic, and lauric acids have the greatest cholesterol-raising effect of the saturated fatty acids (Committee on Diet and Health, 1989). A report from the Nurses' Health Study suggests that by replacing 5% of energy from saturated fat with energy from unsaturated fats the risk of coronary heart disease will be reduced by 42% (Hu et al., 1997). Stearic acid is unique among saturated fatty acids in that it appears to have a neutral effect on serum cholesterol (Kris-Etherton, Shaomei, 1997).

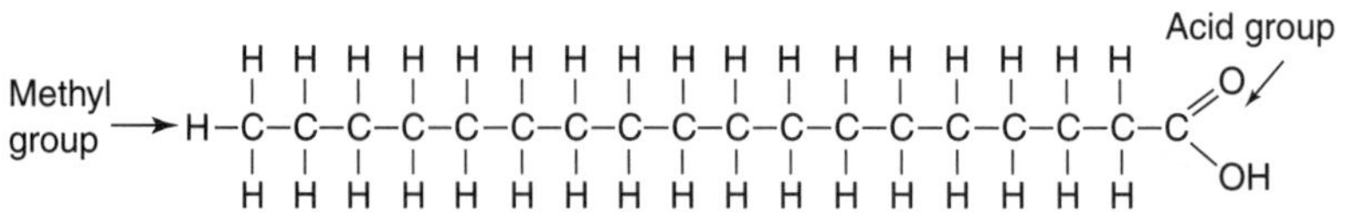

Acid group

Methyl group →

$$
\text{H} - \text{C} - \text{C} - \text{C} - \text{C} - \text{C} - \text{C} - \text{C} - \text{C} - \text{C} - \text{C} - \text{C} - \text{C} - \text{C} - \text{C} - \text{C} - \text{C} - \text{C} - \text{C} \overset{\displaystyle O}{\underset{\displaystyle OH}{=}}
$$

FIGURE 6–2   Saturated fatty acids: all double bonds saturated with hydrogen (example: stearic acid).

Monounsaturated Fatty Acids

Monounsaturated fatty acids (MUFAs) have one double bond in their carbon chains (Figure 6–3). MUFAs are found primarily in plant foods. The most common MUFA found in foods is oleic acid. Good sources of oleic acid include olive oil, canola oil, peanuts and peanut oil, pecans, almonds, and avocados. MUFAs have little effect on overall total serum cholesterol levels, but they do reduce plasma triglycerides (2–25%) and very-low-density lipoproteins (VLDLs) (Garg, 1998), both of which are risk factors for cardiovascular disease. MUFAs also increase high-density lipoproteins (HDLs) by up to 6–22% (Kris-Etherton, Shaomei, 1997). HDLs are also called "good cholesterol" because high HDL levels tend to have a protective effect against heart disease (Colyar, 2002).

Polyunsaturated Fatty Acids (Essential Fatty Acids)

Polyunsaturated fatty acids (PUFAs) have two or more double bonds in their carbon chains (Figure 6–4). PUFAs are divided into two classes: omega-3 fatty acids and omega-6 fatty acids. The human body cannot make these fatty acids so they are considered *essential fatty acids* and must be obtained from food sources. PUFAs have been reported to significantly lower total cholesterol as well as lower LDL cholesterol, but they do not increase HDL cholesterol (Kris-Etherton, Shaomei, 1997). People with a higher consumption of foods high in PUFAs, such as oil-based salad dressing, may have a reduced risk of fatal cardiovascular events (Hu et al., 1999). However, on the whole, reducing saturated fat is twice as effective in lowering serum cholesterol levels as increasing PUFAs (Kris-Etherton, Shaomei, 1997).

Omega-3 (n-3) Fatty Acids Omega-3 (n-3) fatty acids belong to the alpha-linolenic acid (ALNA) family. Until recently linolenic acid was considered the only omega-3 fatty acid important in human nutrition, but recent research suggests the significance of eicosapentaenoic acid (EPA) and docosahexanenoic acid

(DHA) as well. EPA and DHA can be synthesized from linolenic acid, but this is a slow process and generally food sources are needed to attain adequate levels. Omega-3 fatty acids are involved in the development and function of the retina and cerebral cortex. DHA is the most abundant omega-3 fatty acid found in the membranes of photoreceptors of the retina and membranes of the brain (Innis, 2003). Adequate levels are particularly important in fetal life and infancy when nervous tissue development is occurring at a rapid rate.

Alpha-linolenic acid has antiarrhythmic effects, and may be protective against fatal ischemic heart disease (Bemelmans et al., 2000; Hu et al., 1999). The American Heart Association Scientific Statement released in 2002 reviewed the evidence from randomized controlled studies about the beneficial effects of omega-3 fatty acids on cardiovascular disease. The recommendation is to include two servings of fatty fish per week along with vegetable oils and nuts high in ALNA to reduce the progression of arteriosclerosis and incidence of cardiac events (Kris-Etherton, Harris, Appel, 2002). A dietary approach to increasing omega-3 fatty acid intake is preferable over the use of fish oil supplements because the availability of contaminant-free supplements may be an issue (Kris-Etherton et al., 2002).

Omega-3 fatty acids also appear to have a significant effect on the number and functional activities of immune cells. For those with autoimmune disease and possibly the hyperinflammatory trait that may be associated with cardiovascular disease or periodontal disease, there may be some benefit to a diet high in omega-3 fatty acids.

Omega-3 fatty acids can be found in cold-water marine fish (salmon and mackerel) and in some plant oils (soybean and canola oils) and leafy vegetables. The AI (Adequate Intake) for omega-3 fatty acids is 1.1 to 1.6 g per day (IOM, 2005).

Omega-6 Fatty Acids The omega-6 (n = 6) fatty acid family includes linoleic acid. Omega-6 fatty acids are necessary primarily for growth, reproduction, and

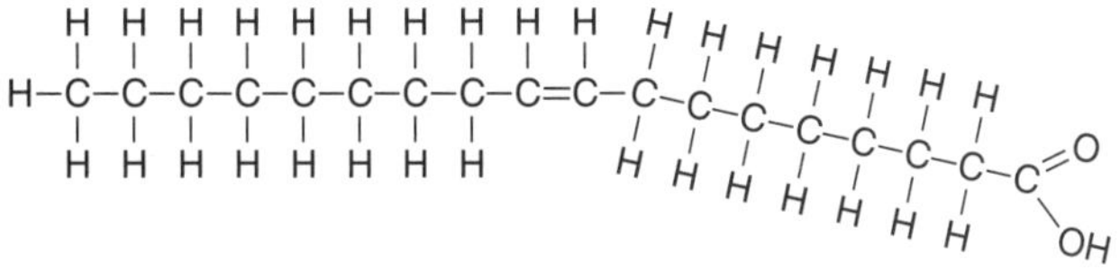

FIGURE 6–3 Monounsaturated fatty acids: one double bond (example: oleic acid).

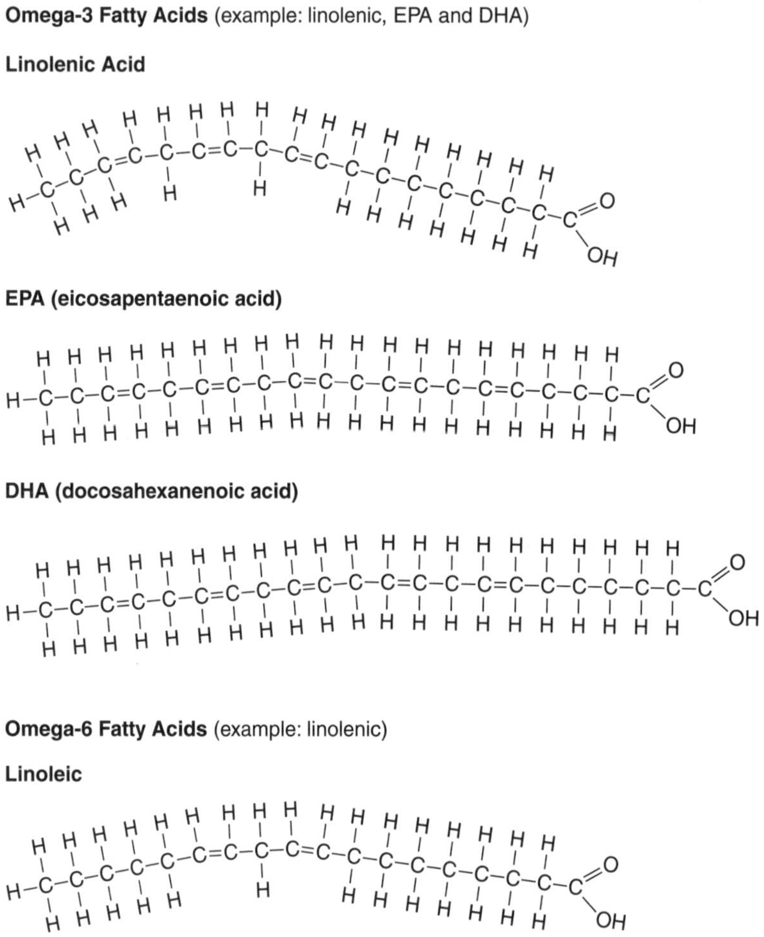

Omega-3 Fatty Acids (example: linolenic, EPA and DHA)

Linolenic Acid

EPA (eicosapentaenoic acid)

DHA (docosahexanenoic acid)

Omega-6 Fatty Acids (example: linolenic)

Linoleic

FIGURE 6-4 Polyunsaturated (essential) fatty acids: two or more double bonds (two classes: omega-3 and omega-6).

maintenance of skin integrity. The AI for omega-6 fatty acids is 12 to 17 g per day (IOM, 2005).

Trans Fatty Acids

Trans fatty acids are unsaturated fatty acids with at least one double bond. Most naturally occurring unsaturated fatty acids are in the *cis*-form in which the hydrogen atoms are both on the same side of the double bond. In the *trans*-form, the hydrogen atoms are on opposite sides of the double bond. The trans-isomer occurs in food processing when hydrogen is added to unsaturated fats in the hydrogenation process.

High intakes of trans fatty acids result in elevated total and LDL cholesterol and lower HDL cholesterol

levels (IOM, 2005; Lichtenstein, 1997). Although saturated fat intake is still a greater risk factor for cardiovascular disease than trans fatty acid intake, a reduction in the intake of both is recommended. Trans fatty acids constitute a minor component of the diet and are of lower importance than avoiding obesity, total fat, and saturated fat.

About 20–25% of trans fatty acids are naturally occurring in meats and dairy products (Allison et al., 1999). The remaining 75–80% of trans fatty acids in the American diet are from sources such as stick margarine, shortening, commercial frying fats, high-fat baked goods, and salty snacks. Changing from stick margarine to soybean oil and semiliquid margarine results in an

Comparison of Dietary Fats

DIETARY FAT

Falty acid content normalized to 100 percent

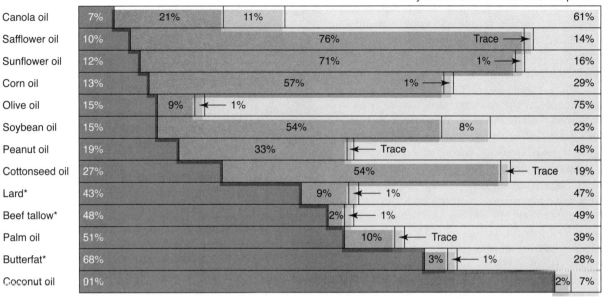

DIETARY FAT	Saturated Fat	Monounsaturated Fat	Linoleic Acid	Alpha-linolenic Acid
Canola oil	7%	21%	11%	61%
Safflower oil	10%		76%	Trace	14%
Sunflower oil	12%		71%	1%	16%
Corn oil	13%		57%	1%	29%
Olive oil	15%	9%	1%	75%
Soybean oil	15%		54%	8%	23%
Peanut oil	19%	33%	Trace	48%
Cottonseed oil	27%	54%	Trace	19%
Lard*	43%	9%	1%	47%
Beef tallow*	48%	2%	1%	49%
Palm oil	51%	10%	Trace	39%
Butterfat*	68%	3%	1%	28%
Coconut oil	91%			2%	7%

*Cholesterol Content (1mg/Tbsp): Lard 12; Beef tallow 14; Butterfat 33, No cholesterol in any vegetable-based oil.

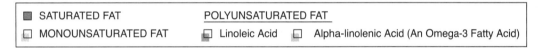

■ SATURATED FAT	POLYUNSATURATED FAT	
☐ MONOUNSATURATED FAT	☐ Linoleic Acid	☐ Alpha-linolenic Acid (An Omega-3 Fatty Acid)

FIGURE 6–5   Distribution of the types of fats in common high-fat foods.
Source: POS Pilot Plant Corporation Saskatoon, Saskatchewan, Canada, June 1994.

11–12% reduction in LDL cholesterol (Lichtenstein, Ausman, Jalbert, Schaefer, 1999). Reducing consumption of fried prepared food, hard margarine, and commercially baked goods and snacks such as cookies and crackers will also lower trans fatty acid intake. If hydrogenated fat is the first ingredient listed on the label, the product will be high in trans fatty acids. In general, the softer the margarine or cooking fat, the less saturated fat and trans fat the product contains. Beginning on January 1, 2006, the FDA required that food labels declare the amounts of trans fatty acids contained in foods and dietary supplements (USDHHS, FDA, 2005).

Very few foods are composed of only one type of fat. Most are a combination of a variety of fats. In general, however, foods are characterized by the fatty acids present in the highest quantity in the foods. So canola oil and olive oil are considered high in monounsaturated

fat, and coconut oil is high in saturated fat. Figure 6–5 shows the fat distribution in a variety of common food oils.

COMPOUND LIPIDS: LECITHIN AND OTHER PHOSPHOLIPIDS

Compound lipids differ from trigylcerides in that there are only two fatty acids attached to the glycerol backbone. The third position on the glycerol backbone is replaced by a phosphorus- and nitrogen-containing molecule. This structure gives phospholipids an affinity for water-soluble and fat-soluble molecules, which enhances their transport functions as part of interior and exterior cell membranes. About 40% of the cell membrane is made up of phospholipids. Phospholipids can be synthesized in the body or obtained from the diet. The phospholipid lecithin (phosphotidylcholine) is a major constituent of cell membranes and contains not only a phosphorus molecule but also a choline segment. Lecithin plays a role in the transport of fatty acids and cholesterol (Krummel, 1997). Lecithin is not considered an essential nutrient because adequate amounts can be produced endogenously to meet the body's needs. Lecithin is found in egg yolk, soybeans, peanuts, spinach, and wheat germ. Lecithin is also used in commercial food preparation as an emulsifier. Lecithin supplementation is not recommended due to a lack of research on the efficacy of lecithin supplements (IOM, 1998). Large intakes of lecithin can result in gastrointestinal distress, sweating, salivation, and anorexia.

Sphingomyelin is found as a component in the myelin sheath around nerve tissue and in the brain. Sphingosine-based lipids also are components of the membranes of all cells and are involved in the regulation of cell growth, cell-to-cell adhesion, and signal transmission from an outside stimulus to the interior of the cell (Brody, 1999). These phospholipids are not required in the diet. Cephalins (necessary for blood clotting) and lipontols are other phospholipids that are found in high concentrations in nerve tissue.

DERIVED LIPIDS

Derived lipids are fatlike compounds that originate from other lipids. Examples are sterols, bile acids, sex hormones, and the eicosanoids such as prostaglandins, leukotrines, and thromboxanes.

Sterols

Sterols are a group of compounds that have a complex chemical ring structure. The rings contain carbon, hydrogen, and oxygen with a variety of side rings. Sterols are important precursors for many essential substances including bile acids, vitamin D, steroid hormones (estrogens and androgens), and glucocorticoids.

Cholesterol

Cholesterol is a sterol that has many essential functions in the body. It is:

- an essential structural component of all cell membranes.
- instrumental in providing stabilization to the membrane structure.

- a precursor for the sex hormones.
- a precursor for aldosterone (involved in the control of blood pressure).
- a precursor for bile acids (important in helping regulate serum cholesterol levels).

High concentrations of cholesterol are also found in the adrenal glands, where glucocorticoid hormones are synthesized, and in the liver, where it is synthesized and stored.

The body can manufacture all the cholesterol that is needed primarily in the liver and intestines, so a dietary source of cholesterol is *not* required. The intestines synthesize most of the endogenous cholesterol in humans, and the liver uses most of the cholesterol it synthesizes for bile acid production (Brody, 1999). Generally about one-third of cholesterol comes from dietary sources and the rest comes from endogenous synthesis.

In the skin, sunlight converts 7-dehydrocholesterol to vitamin D_3. In plants, ergosterol is converted to ergocalciferol (vitamin D_2). Both vitamin D_2 and vitamin D_3 are then converted in the body to vitamin D by hydroxylation reactions in the liver and kidney.

Cholesterol synthesized by the body should *not* be confused with serum cholesterol or dietary cholesterol. Dietary cholesterol, which is *not* required by the body, is found *only* in foods of animal origin. Sources include meat, organ meats, eggs, whole milk, cheese, and animal fats. Plants do not contain cholesterol, but they do synthesize similar compounds called ergosterol. Table 6–1 shows food sources of cholesterol.

About 60–80% of dietary cholesterol is absorbed, but only 5% of plant sterols are absorbed (Brody, 1999). The average total dietary intake of cholesterol based on the NHANES IV data is approximately 307 mg/day for men and 225 mg/day for women (CDC, NCHS, 2003). However, serum cholesterol levels are affected very little by changes in the intake of dietary cholesterol for several reasons:

- Dietary cholesterol intake is small compared with endogenous synthesis.
- A reduction in dietary intake may trigger an increase in the rate of synthesis.
- Increases in dietary cholesterol may not result in corresponding increased absorption (Brody, 1999).

TABLE 6–1   Food Sources of Cholesterol

• **NONE**

Egg white; all plant foods

• **Trace amounts**

Nonfat milk; cheese made from skim milk; low-fat and nonfat yogurt

• **Moderate amounts (<100 mg/standard serving)**

Whole milk, whole-milk cheese, cream, ice cream, butter, meat, poultry, fish, clams, crab, oysters, scallops, salmon

• **High amounts (>150 mg/standard serving)**

Egg yolk, liver, sweetbreads, brains, kidney, heart, fish roe, shrimp

Source: Adapted from *Robinson's Basic Nutrition and Diet Therapy,* 8/E by Weigley/Mueller/Robinson, © 1997. Reprinted with permission.

FAT DIGESTION, ABSORPTION, AND TRANSPORT

Digestion

Dietary fat breakdown occurs primarily in the duodenum and jejunum of the small intestine (Linder, 1991). Bile acids emulsify the fat and, along with the peristalsis of the intestine, disperse the fat into tiny droplets. These tiny droplets increase the surface area allowing the pancreatic lipases access to the lipid. Once the lipids are partially digested, they form micelles that consist of long-chain fatty acids, bile acids, and monoacylglycerols, which diffuse to the mucosal surface for absorption (Figure 6–6).

Absorption

Usually, about 95% of dietary fat and 10–15% of dietary cholesterol is absorbed. Absorption of fatty acids, phosphate, monoacylglycerols, and free cholesterol generally occurs by passive diffusion from the small intestine. The glycerol and medium-chain fatty acids, which are water soluble, are absorbed directly into the bloodstream. Once these fats are absorbed, they are packaged with small amounts of protein and then secreted as chylomicrons (a type of lipoprotein).

Transport

Chylomicrons enter the lymphatic system and then the bloodstream. Chylomicrons are large, consisting of 60% triglyceride, and give the plasma a milky appearance after a high-fat meal. Normally chlyomicrons are only fully cleared from the blood in 8 to 10 hours after a meal.

In addition to chylomicrons, several other classes of lipoproteins are assembled in the small intestine or the liver to transport lipids. Those assembled in the intestine are made up of lipids contained in the diet. The lipoproteins have similar structures: a lipid core containing triglyceride and cholesterol and a surface of phospholipid and protein. The proportions and functions of the various lipids and proteins vary with the type of lipoprotein.

Lipoproteins   Very-low-density lipoproteins (VLDLs) are mainly made up of triglycerides, small amounts of cholesterol, and some protein. Clinically, a measurement of serum triglyceride levels is a measurement of the triglyceride in VLDL and remnants of chylomicrons. The liver synthesizes most of the VLDLs. A majority of the fatty acids in VLDLs enter adipose tissue for storage.

Once in the bloodstream, adipose and/or muscle tissue remove triglycerides and protein, converting VLDL to low-density lipoprotein (LDL). LDL is the primary means of transport for cholesterol in the blood, so LDL levels correlate highly with total serum cholesterol levels. The release of cholesterol from LDL acts as a feedback control to suppress endogenous cholesterol biosynthesis (Brody, 1999). LDL is considered to be highly atherogenic, as it can be oxidized and taken up by endothelial cells, leading to the early stages of vessel damage in atherosclerosis. Reduction of LDL levels is the primary target of management of hyperlipidemia.

High-density lipoproteins (HDLs) contain high amounts of protein compared with the other lipoproteins. HDL helps remove excess cholesterol from the tissues and to the liver or other tissues in need of cholesterol. Thus high levels of HDL provide a protective effect against coronary heart disease.

Ultimately all cholesterol not used by the body for steroid hormones, bile acids, and vitamin D is returned to the liver. Cholesterol can be excreted from the body only via bile acids. Bile acids are formed by the hepatocytes in the liver, aid in emulsification of fat, and then enter enterohepatic circulation and are recycled from the intestine to the liver. Soluble fibers can bind with the bile acids in the intestine and lead to excretion in the feces, thereby reducing the amount of

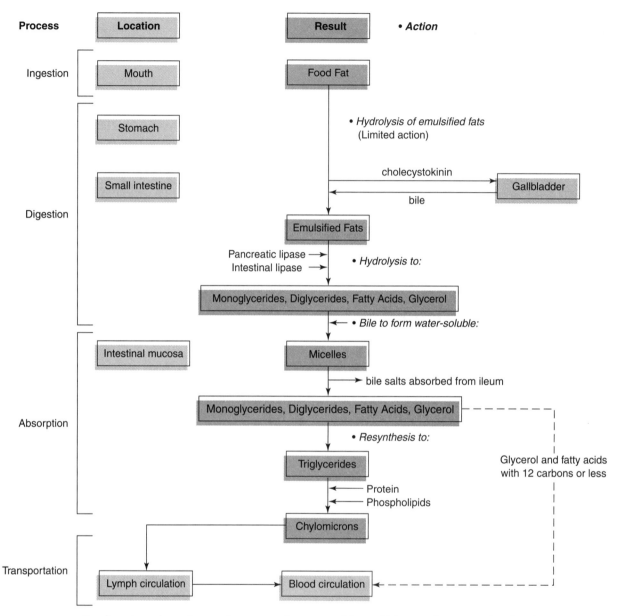

FIGURE 6-6 Fat digestion, absorption, and transport: Summary of the multiple complex steps related to the ingestion, digestion, absorption, and transportation of fats and oils.

cholesterol in the body. Soluble fibers are found in abundance in fruits, oats, and legumes.

When fat is needed for energy by the body, the triglycerides in adipose tissue are broken down by hormone-sensitive lipase. This releases glycerol and fatty acids into the bloodstream, so they are available for uptake by the cells. Glycerol can be oxidized only in liver and kidney cells. It is converted to glucose or reincorporated into triglycerides. In the liver, fatty acids are metabolized by beta-oxidation. During this process the fatty acid is broken down two carbons at a time. Beta-oxidation results in production of large amounts of adenosine triphosphate, which can then be used for energy.

DIETARY FAT RECOMMENDATIONS, CONSUMPTION, AND FOOD SOURCES

Because research over the last few decades has found significant associations between dietary fat intake and chronic diseases such as obesity, some forms of cancer, and cardiovascular disease, national dietary recommendations all suggest reducing total fat and saturated fat intakes (Table 6–2). The key to moderation is to reduce the total intake of fat and the types of fat that have been shown to increase the risk of chronic disease. Presently, there is no RDA for fat or essential fatty acids. The current recommendations are that *20 to 35%* of total calories should come from fat (IOM, 2005). The *Dietary Guidelines for Americans 2005* recommends that saturated fat not exceed 10% of calories and that cholesterol not exceed 300 mg/day (USDHHS,

TABLE 6–2 Food Choices for Lower Fat Intake

- Use nonfat or low-fat milk (skim, 1%, or 2% fat) and low-fat cheeses.
- Use egg whites or egg substitutes instead of whole eggs.
- Choose lean cuts of meat, poultry, and fish.
  - Trim off visible fat; remove skin from poultry.
  - Broil or roast instead of frying; discard drippings.
  - Refrigerate stews, soups, and nut butters after preparation and remove fat that rises to top.
- Use legumes and pastas frequently as entrees.
- Use herbs, spices, or lemon juice instead of butter or margarine to season foods.
- Use fruit or vegetable juices, like lemon, lime, and tomato.
- Use low-fat dressings or lemon juice and olive oil on salads.
- Substitute fruits for high-fat or high-trans-fat desserts like pies, pastries, cakes, cookies, or ice cream.
- Use vegetables and fruits and their juices for snacks.
- Limit high-fat cheese, dips, nuts, chips, and fatty crackers to rare occasions.
- Choose vegetable oils and margarines with poly-, mono-, or omega-3 unsaturated fatty acids.
- The first word on the ingredient list of the label should be *liquid*, because liquid oils are less saturated than those that are partially hydrogenated. Use sparingly because all oils are 100% fat.

USDA, 2005). A diet with as little as 1–2% of calories from linoleic acid will prevent fatty acid deficiency. Infant formulas should provide 3% of calories from linoleic acid. Some cholesterol is essential for infants, but older persons can synthesize all the cholesterol that is needed.

The intake of dietary fat as a percentage of total calories has decreased from a high of 43.7% in 1965 to 32–33% in 2000 (CDC, NCHS, 2003; Kennedy, Bowman, Powell, 1999). The NHANES IV estimates the average dietary intake of saturated fats in the U.S. diet is 11% (CDC, NCHS, 2003).

Some food fat is quite visible such as butter, margarine, oil, animal skins, and marbling. However, a lot of dietary fat is invisible, such as that found in milk, cheese, eggs, and processed foods. Approximately half of the fat in the American diet comes from oils, meats, and whole dairy foods. Olives and avocados are high in fat, but other fruits, vegetables, and grain products contribute little fat to the diet.

Effects of Too Little Fat

Essential fatty acids need to make up only 1–2% of total calories to prevent deficiency symptoms. The average diet contains between 5 and 10% of total calories from essential fatty acids. Those at risk for essential fatty acid deficiency include patients with fat malabsorption syndromes such as cystic fibrosis, people on very low fat diets (less than 10% of calories from fat), and premature infants. Premature infants are born before they have been able to build up their lipid stores and have greater needs because of their rapid growth. Deficiency symptoms may occur after a few weeks on a diet deficient in essential fatty acids. Symptoms include dry, scaly skin, hair loss, impaired growth, impaired wound healing, visual impairment, and possibly an impaired reproductive ability (IOM, 2005; NRC, 1989).

Effects of Too Much Fat

Gram for gram, excess fat in the diet provides twice the calories of excess carbohydrate or protein. This, in turn, contributes to an increased risk of obesity. Additionally, an intake of fat in excess of 30% of total calories increases the risk of cardiovascular disease, hypertension, diabetes, and some types of cancer. Overconsumption of saturated fat and *trans* fatty acids are an independent risk factor for cardiovascular disease because of their impact on total and LDL cholesterol concentration (IOM, 2005). Conversely, high intakes of omega-3 fatty acids reduces platelet aggregation and prolongs bleeding time, which may be beneficial in preventing heart disease (IOM, 2005).

Diet and Coronary Heart Disease (CHD)

In 2002, coronary heart disease affected 13 million (6.9%) people in the United States (AHA, 2005). Three to four million Americans may have ischemic episodes without realizing it (silent ischemia) (AHA, 2005).

Coronary heart disease results when atherosclerosis (characterized by thickening, hardening, and loss of elasticity of the artery walls) results in narrowing of arteries and restricted blood flow to all tissues. The atherosclerotic lesion is also known as plaque (Epstein, 1999). If an arterial plaque lesion ruptures, a thrombus may break off, occlude an artery, and cause sudden coronary death, acute myocardial infarction, cerebral vascular accident, or critical limb ischemia (Lowe, 1998). Figure 6–7 shows the pathogenesis of atherosclerosis.

Possible contributors to atherosclerosis include:

- the end products of the oxidation of excess blood glucose in diabetes.
- the oxidation of LDL cholesterol.
- free radicals caused by tobacco use, hypertension.
- genetic alterations.
- elevated homocysteine levels.
- infection (Epstein, 1999).

Diagnosis of CHD

Beginning at age 20, total cholesterol and high-density lipoprotein (HDL) should be measured every 5 years in people who have no history of coronary heart disease (AHA, 1995). If these values remain high on multiple occasions, then a more comprehensive lipoprotein analysis is needed to determine LDL levels. Treatment decisions are usually based on LDL levels except when CHD risk factors are present (Table 6–3).

Nonmodifiable Risk Factors for CHD

Nonmodifiable risk factors include age, gender, and heredity (National Cholesterol Education Program [NCED], 1993). Eighty-four percent of people who die from CHD are aged 65 or older (AHA, 2005). Men have a greater risk of heart attack than women. Groups at higher risk of heart disease include African Americans, Mexican Americans, American Indians, native Hawaiians, and some Asian Americans (AHA, 2005) (Table 6–4).

Modifiable Risk Factors for CHD

Modifiable risk factors include physical inactivity, tobacco use, excessive alcohol consumption, high-fat dietary intake, stress, diabetes (see Chapter 4), obesity (see Chapter 3), hypertension (see Chapter 11), hyperlipidemia, and high levels of homocysteine (Fagan,

Progression of Atherosclerosis

Normal Vessel

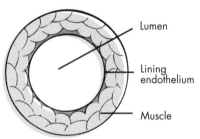

Early Injury

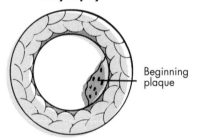

Advanced Injury

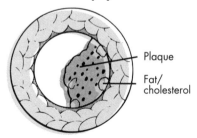

FIGURE 6–7 Progression of atherosclerosis.
Source: From *Robinson's Basic Nutrition And Diet Therapy:* 8/E by Weigley/Mueller/Robinson, © 1997. Reprinted with permission.

TABLE 6–3   Classification of Hyperlipidemia (National Cholesterol Education Program)

Classification	Total Cholesterol Level	LDL Cholesterol Level	HDL Cholesterol Level	Triglyceride Level
Desirable	<200 mg/dL	<100 mg/dL	≥60 mg/dL	<150 mg/dL
Borderline high risk	200–239 mg/dL	130–159 mg/dL	40–59 mg/dL	150–199 mg/dL
High risk	≥240 mg/dL	≥160mg/dL	40 mg/dL	200 mg/dL

From: ATP III Guidelines at a glance Quick Desk Reference http://www.nhlbi.nih.gov/guidelines/cholesterol/atglance.pdf. Accessed 05/13/06.

Deedwania, 1998; Nelson, 1998) (Table 6–4). Smoking is the major risk factor for sudden cardiac death. Tobacco users have a 70% greater level of CHD risk than nonsmokers (AHA, 2005). On average, smokers die 13–14 years earlier than nonsmokers (AHA, 2005). With smoking cessation the prevalence of cardiac events significantly decreases (Merz, Rozanski, Forrester, 1997). The risk for cardiovascular mortality due to physical inactivity is approximately 35% (Kesaniemi, 2001). Only 31% of U.S. adults engage in regular physical activity (AHA, 2005). The CHD risk for women with diabetes mellitus is up to four times higher and in men the risk is two times higher than those without diabetes (AHA, 2005).

Hyperlipidemia Hyperlipidemia, more commonly called high serum cholesterol, is a major risk factor

TABLE 6–4   Coronary Heart Disease Risk Based on Risk Factors

Characteristics of High Risk	Characteristics of Low Risk
• Male ≥45 years	• Nonsmoking
• Female ≥55 years or postmenopausal without estrogen replacement therapy	• Body mass index under 25
	• Average of ½ drink of alcoholic beverage per day
• Family history of premature coronary heart disease (definite myocardial infarction or sudden death before age 55 in father or other first-degree relative or before age 65 in mother or other female first-degree relative)	• Moderate-to-vigorous physical activity at least ½ hr per day
• Current tobacco use	• Diet high in cereal fiber, omega-3 fatty acids, and folate
• Hypertension (blood pressure > 140/90 mm Hg) or patient is receiving antihypertensive drug therapy)	
• HDL cholesterol level < 40 mg/dL (men); < 50 mg/dL (women)	
• Elevated homocysteine levels	
• Diabetes mellitus	

From: ATP III Guidelines at a Glance Quick Desk Reference. http://www.nhlbi.nih.gov/guidelines/cholesterol/atglance.pdf.

for cardiovascular disease and stroke. Hyperlipidemia results when lipid levels in the blood increase, due to either an increased rate of synthesis or a decreased rate of breakdown of lipoproteins (Thomas, 1993). This may be characterized by elevated total serum cholesterol, low-density lipoprotein (LDL), very-low-density lipoprotein (VLDL), intermediate-density lipoprotein (IDL), and/or triglyceride levels. Total serum cholesterol is composed of several kinds of lipoproteins found in the blood. A total of 60–70% of total serum cholesterol is carried on LDL, 20–30% on HDL, and 10–15% on VLDL.

LDL and VLDL are known as the "bad cholesterol" because they are implicated in the formation of athero-sclerotic plaque in the blood vessels, which leads to narrowing and stenosis. High serum levels of LDL are a major risk factor for CHD and is the primary target of cholesterol-lowering therapy (NCEP, 2002). LDL carries large amounts of cholesterol and triglycerides. High levels of LDL may occur due to inadequate numbers of LDL receptors in the liver or when the receptor sites become saturated due to too many LDL particles in the blood. HDLs are known as the "good cholesterol" because they pick up cholesterol deposited in artery walls and transport it to the liver for disposal. HDLs contain higher amounts of protein and carry less cholesterol than LDLs or VLDLs. Higher levels of HDL can provide some degree of protection from CHD.

Elevated Homocysteine Levels Homocysteine is formed in the metabolism of the dietary protein methionine (Mayer, Jacobsen, Robinson, 1996). High blood levels of homocysteine appear to be associated with damage to endothelial cells and increased platelet adhesion, which may account for its association with CHD (Mayer et al., 1996). The causes of high homocysteine levels include increasing age, male gender, decreases in renal function, disease states, drugs, and low serum levels of folate, vitamin B_6, and vitamin B_{12} (Mayer et al., 1996).

Prevention and Management of Cardiovascular Disease (CVD)

Prevention and management of CVD must be multidisciplinary. The primary goal is to reduce modifiable risk factors including:

- all types of tobacco use
- high-fat, high-saturated-fat diets leading to hyperlipidemis
- hypertension
- obesity

- inactivity
- stress
- diabetes mellitus

Management of hyperlipidemia, hypertension, and diabetes mellitus have been previously discussed and involve many of the same principles.

Dietary Management Dietary modification alone can lower blood cholesterol. The current National Cholesterol Education Program recommends a multifactorial lifestyle approach for reducing the risk for cardiovascular disease (National Cardiovascular Health Conference, 2002). This approach is referred to as therapeutic lifestyle change (TLC) and promotes use of the U.S. dietary guidelines and food guide in conjunction with the following (NCEP, 2002):

- decreased intake of saturated fat and cholesterol
- therapeutic approaches for lowering LDL (plant stanols/sterols and soluble fiber)
- weight reduction
- increased physical activity

A heart-healthy diet for all people recommends 25–35% or less of total calories from fat, less than 7% of total calories from saturated fat, and less than 200 mg/day of cholesterol (NCEP, 2002). Because it is often difficult to determine the amount of saturated fat and cholesterol consumed without detailed nutrition analysis, the dietary CAGE questions can identify common food sources of these LDL-raising nutrients. The questions are as follows (NCEP, 2002):

- **C**—Cheese: How often do you have cheese, whole milk, ice cream, cream, and/or whole-fat yogurt?
- **A**—Animal fat: How often do you have hamburger, ground meat, frankfurters, bologna, salami, sausage, fried foods, and/or fatty cuts of meat?
- **G**—Got it away from home: How often do you have high-fat meals either purchased and brought home or eaten in restaurants?
- **E**—Eat high-fat commercial products: How often do you eat candy, pastries, pies, doughnuts, and/or cookies?

The NCEP guidelines recommend up to 10% of total calories from polyunsaturated fat and up to 20% of total calories from monounsaturated fat (NCEP, 2002). Omega-3 fatty acids (found in fish, shellfish, canola, and soybean oils) are monounsaturated fats and can reduce triglycerides, have an antiinflammatory action on endothelial cells, and decrease platelet coagulation (Endres, De Caterina, Schmidt, Kristensen, 1995; Marchioli, 1999). Studies have been inconclusive as to the effects of omega-3 fatty acids on prevention and treatment of CVD, however.

Recommendations for carbohydrates are 50–60% and should be primarily complex carbohydrates including whole grains, fruits, and vegetables (NCEP, 2002). Choosing whole grains, fruits, and vegetables should facilitate reaching the goal of 20–30 g of fiber per day (NCEP, 2002). For those people with high LDL there are specific recommendations for the intake of plant sterols and soluble fiber. Soluble fibers (pectin, guar gum, psyllium, and oat bran) have been studied for their potential cholesterol-lowering effects and their intake is recommended to be 10–25 g per day (NCEP, 2002). On average an intake of 5–10 g per day of soluble fiber results in approximately a 5% reduction in LDL cholesterol levels (NCEP, 2002; USDHHS, FDA, 1998). The recommendation for plant sterols is 2 g per day and studies demonstrate a 6–15% reduction in LDL levels with this intake (NCEP, 2002). These nutrients can be found in commercial margarine.

Finally, protein should constitute approximately 15% of total calories (NCEP, 2002). Dietary protein has not been demonstrated to have a significant effect on serum LDL or other lipoproteins (Anderson, 1995). Consumption of plant proteins such as soy protein may also assist in lowering LDL cholesterol as much as 5% (Jenkins et al., 2000).

Weight reduction is recommended if patients are overweight based on the body mass index (BMI). Modest weight reduction (5–10% of body weight) lowers the total cholesterol and VLDL and LDL cholesterol levels independent of ongoing dietary modification. Thirty minutes of aerobic exercise on most days of the week is recommended to assist with weight loss and also raises HDL cholesterol levels (Ahmed et al., 1998; NCEP, 2002).

In moderation, alcohol has been shown to increase HDL levels (Ahmed, Clasen, Donnelly, 1998). The cardiovascular benefit appears to be of most benefit to men aged 45 and older and women aged 55 and older (Thun et al, 1997). However, because alcohol has the potential for addiction and abuse, its use is not recommended on a regular basis as prevention for CHD (Ahmed et al., 1998).

Very-low-fat vegetarian diets (less than 10% of total calories from fat) along with intensive lifestyle modification (aerobic exercise, stress management training, tobacco cessation, and group psychosocial support) will not only stop the progression of CVD but also result in regression of coronary atherosclerosis (Ornish et al., 1998). However, this is an extremely restrictive diet for the long term.

Oral Implications of Cardiovascular Disease

There is strong evidence of an association between periodontal disease and CHD. The formation of atheromas is an inflammatory process, and oral pathogens cause gingival and periodontal inflammation resulting in immune response. A theory exists that there may be a hyperinflammatory trait that results in a more intense inflammatory response to bacterial challenges, such as periodontal infections (Beck, Offenbacher, Williams, Gibbs, Garcia, 1998). This hyperinflammatory response may promote formation of arterial plaques (Beck et al., 1998). A 2004 meta-analysis of observational studies found that periodontal infection increases the risk of CHD by 15% compared to healthy subjects (Khader, Albashaireh, Alomari, 2004).

Summary Principles for Cardiovascular Disease Prevention

Dental practitioners can provide encouragement to maintain a healthy, moderate-sodium, low-fat diet with regular exercise. Some data suggest that people who receive health messages from multiple sources are more likely to be successful in making lifestyle changes. Good sources of literature (much of it free) include the American Heart Association, American Cancer Society, Centers for Disease Control and Prevention, and the U.S. Department of Health and Human Services.

Patients at risk for CHD should be encouraged to:

- Follow a low-fat, low-saturated fat diet.
- Choose more low-fat animal products and try more vegetable proteins such as beans, peas, and soy.
- Choose sources of omega-3 fatty acids including fish, shellfish, soybean, and canola oil.
- Eat plenty of whole grains, fresh fruits, and vegetables as sources of fiber and antioxidant nutrients.
- Attain and maintain a healthy weight.
- Be involved in regular aerobic exercise after consultation with a physician.
- Stop all forms of tobacco use.
- Prevent and manage periodontal disease with treatment by a dental professional.

FAT-FREE FOODS AND FAT REPLACERS

Fat-free and low-fat foods are being used with increasing frequency to decrease total dietary fat intake (Table 6–5). A national survey found that 76% of the U.S. population consumes low-fat, reduced-fat, or fat-free foods and beverages (American Dietetic Association, 2005). Many of these foods are not necessarily significantly lower in calories due to the addition of sugars. The increased use of reduced-fat and fat-free foods may be of concern for dental professionals because a majority of these foods such as crackers, potato chips, and cookies contain retentive carbohydrates, which are highly cariogenic (Kashket, Zhang, Van Houte, 1996; Miller, Castellanos, Shide, Peters, Rolls, 1998).

Fat replacers have also beome popular as methods of reducing dietary fat. The three common types of fat replacers are:

TABLE 6–5 Common Fat Substitutes

Name	Chemical Name/ Structure	Energy Provided (kcal/g)	Safety Issues/History
Olestra (Olean®)	Sucrose polyester (sucrose molecule with up to eight esoterically linked fatty acid tails)	0	Approved by FDA as a food additive in 1996 with a warning label stating: "This product contains Olestra. Olestra may cause abdominal cramping and loose stools. Olestra inhibits the absorption of some vitamins and other nutrients. Vitamins A, D, E, and K have been added."
			2003: Warning label requirement removed because post market surveillance results did not indicate that there were problems
			Molecules are too large to be digested/absorbed in the intestine
			Because olestra binds fat-soluble vitamins (A, D, E, K) and carotenoids and carries them with it as it is excreted, products are fortified with vitamins A, D, E, and K
			Increases the rate of removal of fat-soluble toxins such as polychlorinated biphenyls (PCBs) and dioxins from the body
Simplesse	Small, round, hydrated whey or egg protein particles (50 per teaspoon) that mimic the mouth feel of fat	1–2	GRAS (Generally Recognized As Safe)
			Cannot be used in products that are heated because whey particles break down
Oatrim	Cellulose based	0	Developed by the USDA
Salatrim	Modified soybean- and canola-oil-based fat replacer	5	Contains poorly absorbed fatty acids. Fell out of favor because of cost and difficulties in processing.

Sources: Adapted by Jennifer Weston from:
Center for Science in the Public Interest: *A brief history of Olestra.* Retrieved from http://www.cspinet.org/olestra/history.html.
Cheskin, Miday, Zorich, Filloon, 1998
Peters, Lawson, Middleton, Triebwasser, 1997
Sandler et al., 1999
Schlagheck et al., 1997
Wikipedia: *Olestra.* Retrieved from http://en.wikipedia.org/wiki/Olestra.

- fat mimetics (designed to mimic the properties of fat and usually used as a partial replacement of the fat content of a food).
- fat barriers (function by reducing absorption of fats during frying).
- fat substitutes or analogs (American Dietetic Association, 2005).

Fat substitutes contain fewer calories than fat, and can be made from protein, carbohydrate, or lipid-based compounds. Some of these fat substitutes can be used in baked goods and others degenerate and can be used only in products that are not cooked. Many of these products are made from standard ingredients such as egg whites or are already on the GRAS (Generally Recognized As Safe) list. All must undergo rigorous animal and human clinical trials to receive approval by the FDA. Table 6–5 details the common fat alternatives.

ORAL IMPLICATIONS OF FAT

Early epidemiological data have shown that Inuit people (Eskimos) with a diet high in fat intake—70–80% of total calories—have a decreased incidence of caries (Bang, Kristoffersen, 1972). The decrease in caries may also be due to the limited intake of carbohydrate in the diet of the Inuit. In later animal studies, however, fat has been associated with the inhibition of buccal and lingual (smooth surface) caries (Mundorff-Shrestha et al., 1994). Several hypotheses exist that show how the presence of fat affects the cariogenicity of the diet. A prevailing theory is that fat acts as a protective layer on the tooth surface and prevents adherence of retentive carbohydrates or enhances clearance of sugars (Bowen, 1994). Fats are used to manufacture soaps, which act as surfactants; this function may have some influence on preventing adherence of carbohydrates. Another theory is that fats have an anticariogenic effect due to the antibacterial effects of certain fatty acids (Bowen, 1994; Kabara, 1986). Optimal antimicrobial activity has been noted for fatty acids with a chain length of C12 (Kabara, Vrable, 1977). Examples of fatty acids with a chain length of C12 are lauric acid, a saturated fatty acid found in coconut and palm kernel oil, and lauroleic, an unsaturated fatty acid found in butterfat. Dental professionals need to be cautious about using this information for caries prevention because a high fat intake is implicated in several chronic diseases.

Studies utilizing omega-6 fatty acids and omega-3 fatty acids suggest these nutrients may have some beneficial effects on periodontal disease. In the studies, the use of omega-3 fatty acids in the form of 3000 mg/day capsules of fish oil resulted in decreased levels of prostaglandins and a significant reduction in gingival inflamation (Campan, Planchand, Duan, 1997; Rosenstein, Kushner, Kramer, Kazandjian, 2003). A significant reduction in pocket depth was also found with the use of omega-6 fatty acid supplements. However, these findings must be inteprepreted with caution until further clinical studies evaluate the long-term benefits and risks of pharmacologic doses of these nutrients.

However, epidemiologic data also suggest that there may be a link between obesity and periodontal disease, particularly in young adults. One study found a 2.27 times greater risk of having periodontal disease among those 18 to 34 years of age with a BMI greater than 30 kg/m (Al-Zahrani, Bissada, Borawskit, 2003; Saito, Shimazaki, Koga, Tsuzuki, Ohshima, 2001). An evaluation of NHANES III data found a greater correlation between periodontal disease and the waist-to-hip ratio (WHR measures upper body fat) (Wood, Johnson, Streckfus, 2003). These are preliminary findings, but another reason for dental professionals to be attentive to addressing an overall health dietary intake with patients.

SUMMARY AND IMPLICATIONS FOR DENTISTRY

The American Dental Association recommends following the *Dietary Guidelines for Americans* and the USDA food guide pyramid (MyPyramid) when providing nutrition guidance to dental patients. Epidemiologic and clinical research evaluating the possible association between periodontal disease and coronary heart disease also makes it imperative that any nutrition advice given to patients follow recognized national guidelines.

The following are dietary suggestions for reducing total fat and saturated fat in the diet:

- Choose plenty of whole grains, fresh fruits, and vegetables and fewer processed foods.
- Replace other fats and oils with olive or canola oil.
- Use vinegar and olive oil to replace other salad dressing at least five to six times per week.
- Read labels and choose soft margarine that does not contain trans fatty acids.
- Include several servings of fish per week.

- Choose lean cuts of meat and remove the skin from poultry.
- Use cheese in small amounts and choose low-fat or nonfat dairy products.
- Limit consumption of fried foods and commercially baked goods.
  - Recognize that reduced-fat and fat-free foods still have significant sugar content and may be retentive, which increases their cariogenicity.
  - Refer patients to their physician or a registered dietitian for more individualized meal planning, especially those with a history of cardiovascular disease.

QUESTIONS PATIENTS MIGHT ASK

Q. Because saturated fats are risk factors for heart disease, can I eat as much fat as I like as long as it is monounsaturated?

A. No, saturated fat is only one risk factor for heart disease. Obesity is another. All fats provide 9 calories per gram whether they are saturated or monounsaturated. So eating too much of any type of fat can lead to obesity. Stay within the recommended guidelines of less than 30% of calories from fat of any type to help maintain weight and prevent heart disease.

Q. I am concerned about helping my children avoid developing heart disease since we have this problem in the family. Can I start my baby on low-fat foods and skim milk as soon as she stops breastfeeding?

A. No, this is not a good idea. Children need sufficient intake of essential fatty acids to grow properly. The American Academy of Pediatrics and other respected organizations recommend that children not be given a low-fat diet until after age 2. Even then, the diet should not be extremely low in fat, but should correspond to heart-healthy guidelines of around 30% of calories from fat.

CASE STUDY

A 55-year-old woman presents for dental treatment:

Dental history: She has a history of extensive caries and has at least four to six new carious lesions at each checkup. She has mild to moderate chronic adult periodontitis that is not well controlled.

Medical history: The patient has mildly elevated cholesterol levels, but is not on any medications for it. She has a family history of high cholesterol and heart disease. Her mother had a fatal heart attack at age 65.

Nutritional status: Her physician has told her to lose weight and reduce her intake of fat and cholesterol. She has not had nutrition counseling and seems to be misinformed about fat sources. She has cut down on red meat because it is her understanding that it is the main source of fat in the diet, and eggs because they are "high" in cholesterol. Her 24-hour recall is as follows:

Breakfast
- 1 slice toast
- 1 T. butter

Lunch
- Cheese sandwich:
  - 2 slices bread
  - 1 c. coffee w/1 T. half & half
- 1 oz Raisin Bran
- ½ c. whole milk
- 1½ oz cheddar cheese
- 1 tsp. butter
- 1 T. mayonnaise
- 1 can diet soda

Afternoon Snack
- 10 reduced-fat chocolate chip cookies
- 1 c. whole milk

Dinner
- 2 oz chicken thigh & 3 oz breast, fried
- ½ c. scalloped potatoes
- 1 c. green salad w/oil & vinegar
- 1 c. whole milk

Evening Snack
- 1 c. ice cream

Questions:
1. What other factors besides dietary fat and cholesterol might be contributing to this patient's elevated cholesterol level?
2. Help the patient identify sources of saturated fat in her diet.
3. What substitutions might you recommend for high-fat, saturated-fat foods?
4. What is meant by "heart healthy" fats, and what foods are high in these fats?

REFERENCES

Ahmed SM, Clasen ME, Donnelly JF: Management of dyslipidemia in adults. *Am Fam Physician* 1998; 57(9):2192–2204.

Allison DB, Egan SK, Barraj LM, Caughman C, Infante M, Heimbach JT: Estimated intakes of *trans* fatty and other fatty acids in the US population. *J Am Diet Assoc* 1999; 99(2):166–74.

Al-Zahrani MS, Bissada NF, Borawskit EA: Obesity and periodontal disease in young, middle-aged, and older adults. *J Periodontol* 2003; 74(5): 610–15.

American Dietetic Association: Position statement of the American Dietetic Association: Fat replacers. *J Am Diet Assoc* 2005; 105(2):266–75.

American Heart Association: *Heart disease and stroke statistics—2005 update*. Dallas, TX: American Heart Association, 2005.

American Heart Association, National Heart, Lung, and Blood Institute: *Recommendations regarding public screening for measuring blood cholesterol*. NIH. Publication No. 95-3045. National Institutes of Health: Bethesda, MD, 1995.

Anderson JW: Dietary fibre, complex carbohydrate and coronary artery disease. *Can J Cardiol* 1995; 11(SupplG): 55G–62G.

ATP III Guidelines at a Glance Quick Desk Reference. http://www.nhlbi.nih.gov/guidelines/cholesterol/atglance.pdf Accessed 05-13-06.

Bang G, Kristoffersen T: Dental caries and diet in an Alaskan Eskimo population. *Scand J Dent Res* 1972; 80(5):440–44.

Beck JD, Offenbacher S, Williams R, Gibbs P, Garcia R: Periodontitis: A risk factor for coronary heart disease? *Ann Periodontol* 1998; 3:127–41.

Bemelmans WJ, Muskiet FA, Feskens EJ, de Vries JH, Broer J, May JF, et al.: Associations of alpha-linolenic acid and linoleic acid with risk factors for coronary heart disease. *Eur J Clin Nutr* 2000; 54(12):865–71.

Bowen WH: Food components and caries. *Adv Dent Res* 1994; 8(2):215–20.

Brody T: Digestion and absorption of lipids. In Brody T (ed): *Nutritional Biochemistry*. San Diego: Academic Press, 1999.

Campan P, Planchand PO, Duan D: Pilot study on n-3 polyunsaturated fatty acids in the treatment of human experimental gingivitis. *Clin Perio* 1997; 24(12):907–13.

Centers for Disease Control and National Center for Health Statistics: NHANES IV (1999–2000). *Advance Data, Vital and Health Statistics*, No. 334, April 17, 2003.

Cheskin LJ, Miday R, Zorich N, Filloon T: Gastrointestinal symptoms following consumption of olestra or regular triglyceride potato chips: A controlled comparison. *JAMA* 1998; 279(2):150–52.

Colyar MR: Lipoprotein analysis. *Adv Nurse Pract* 2002; 10:30–32.

Committee on Diet and Health, F.a.N.B: *Recommendations on Diet, Chronic Diseases, and Health*. Washington, DC: National Academy Press, 1989.

Connor WE, Neuringer M: The effects of n-3 fatty acid deficiency and repletion upon the fatty acid composition and function of the brain and retina. *Prog Clin Biol Res* 1988; 282:175–294.

Drachman DA, Glosser G, Fleming P, Longenecker G: Memory decline in the aged: Treatment with lecithin and physostigmine. *Neurology* 1982; 32(9):944–50.

Dreon DM, Fernstrom HA, Campos H, Blanche P, Williams PT, Krauss RM: Change in dietary saturated fat intake is correlated with change in mass of large low-density-lipoprotein particles in men. *Am J Clin Nutr* 1998; 67(5):828–36.

Endres S, De Caterina R, Schmidt EB, Kristensen SD: N-3 polyunsaturated fatty acids: Update 1995. *Eur J Clin Invest* 1995; 25:629–38.

Epstein FH: Atherosclerosis: An inflammatory disease. *N Engl J Med* 1999; 340(2):115–26.

Fagan TC, Deedwania PC: The cardiovascular dysmetabolic syndrome. *Am J Med* 1998; 105(A):77S–82S.

Garg A: High-monounsaturated-fat diets for patients with diabetes mellitus: A meta-analysis. *Am J Clin Nutr* 1998; 67(Suppl):577S–82S.

Hanley AJ, Williams K, Stern MP, Haffner, S: Homeostasis model assessment of insulin resistance in relation to the incidence of cardiovascular disease. *Diabetes Care* 25(7); 1177–84.

Hu FB, Stampfer MJ, Manson JE, Rimm E, Colditz GA, Rosner BA, et al.: Dietary intake of alpha-linolenic acid and risk of fatal ischemic heart disease among women. *Am J Clin Nutr* 1999; 69:890–97.

Hu FB, Stampfer MJ, Manson JE, Rimm EB, Wolk A, Colditz GA, et al.: Dietary fat intake and the risk of coronary heart disease. *N Engl J Med* 1997; 337(21):1491–99.

Innis S: Perinatal biochemistry and physiology of long-chain polyunsaturated fatty acids. *J Pediatr* 2003; 143(4):S1–S8.

Institute of Medicine, National Academy of Sciences: *Dietary Reference Intakes for Energy, Carbohydrate, Fiber, Fat, Fatty Acids, Cholesterol, Protein, and Amino Acids (Macronutrients)*. Washington, DC: National Academies Press, 2005.

Institute of Medicine, National Academy of Sciences: *Dietary Reference Intakes for Thiamin, Riboflavin, Niacin, Vitamin B_6, Folate, Vitamin B_{12}, Pantothenic Acid, Biotin, and Choline*. Washington, DC: National Academies Press, 1998.

Jenkins DJ, Kendall CW, Vidgers E, Mehling CC, Parker T, Seyler H, et al.: The effect on serum lipids and oxidized low-density lipoprotein of supplementing self-selected low fat diets with soluble fiber, soy, and vegetable protein foods. *Metabolism* 2000; 49:67–72.

Kabara JJ: Dietary lipids as anticariogenic agents. *J Environ Pathol Toxicol Oncol* 1986; 6(3–4): 87–113.

Kabara JJ, Vrable R: Antimicrobial lipids: Natural and synthetic fatty acids and monoglycerides. *Lipids* 1977; 12(9):753–59.

Kashket SJ, Zhang J, Van Houte J: Accumulation of fermentable sugars and metabolic acids in food particles that become entrapped on the dentition. *J Dent Res* 1996; 75(11):1885–91.

Kennedy ET, Bowman SA, Powell R: Dietary fat intake in the US population. *Am Coll Nutr* 1999; 18(3):207–12.

Kesaniemi A: What kind of exercise will promote health? Consensus meeting assessment about the dose-effect relationship of exercise and health. *Duodecim* 2003; 119(19):1819–22.

Khader YS, Albashaireh ZS, Alomari MA: Periodontal diseases and the risk of coronary heart and cerebrovascular diseases: A meta-analysis. *J Perio* 2004; 75:1046–53.

Krauss RM, Eckel RH, Howard B, Appel LJ, Daniels SR, Deckelbaum RJ, et al.: AHA Dietary Guidelines: Revision 2000: A Statement for Healthcare Professionals from the Nutrition Committee of the American Heart Association. *Circulation* 2000; 102:2284–99.

Kris-Etherton PM, Harris WS, Appel LJ: AHA Scientific Statement: Fish consumption, fish oil, omega-3 fatty acids, and cardiovascular disease. *Circulation* 2002; 106:2747–57.

Kris-Etherton PM, Krummel D, Russell ME, Dreon D, Mackey S, Borchers J, et al.: The effect of diet on plasma lipids, lipoproteins, and treatment of coronary heart disease in women. *J Am Diet Assoc* 1988; 88:1373–1400.

Kris-Etherton PM, Shaomei Y: Individual fatty acid effects on plasma lipids and lipoproteins: Human studies. *Am J Clin Nutr* 1997; 65(Suppl):1628S–44S.

Krummel D: Lipids. In Mahan KL, Escott-Stump S (eds): *Krause's Food, Nutrition, and Diet Therapy*. Philadelphia: WB Saunders, 1997.

Lichtenstein AH: Trans fatty acids, plasma lipid levels, and risk of developing cardiovascular disease: A statement for healthcare professionals from the American Heart Association. *Circulation* 1997; 95(11):2588–90.

Lichtenstein AH, Ausman LM, Jalbert SM, Schaefer EJ: Effects of different forms of dietary hydrogenated fats on serum lipoprotein cholesterol levels. *N Engl J Med* 1999; 340(25):1933–40.

Linder MC: Nutrition and metabolism of fats. In Linder MC (ed): *Nutritional Biochemistry and Metabolism*. New York: Elsevier Science, 1991.

Lowe GO: Etiopathogenesis of cardiovascular disease: Hemostasis, thrombosis, and vascular medicine. *Ann Periodontol* 1998; 3(1):121–26.

Marchioli R: Dietary supplementation with n-3 polyunsaturated fatty acids and vitamin E after myocardial infarction: Results of the GISSI-Prevenzione trial. *Lancet* 1999; 354:447–55.

Mattes RD: Position of the American Dietetic Association: Fat replacers. *J Am Diet Assoc* 1998; 98(4):463–68.

Mayer EL, Jacobsen DW, Robinson K: Homocysteine and coronary atherosclerosis. *J Am Coll Cardiol* 1996; 27:517–27.

Merz CN, Rozanski A, Forrester JS: The secondary prevention of coronary artery disease. *Am J Med* 1997; 102:572–81.

Miller DL, Castellanos VH, Shide DJ, Peters JC, Rolls BJ: Effect of fat-free potato chips with and without nutrition labels on fat and energy intakes. *Am J Clin Nutr* 1998; 68(2):282–90.

Mundorff-Shrestha SA, Featherstone JD, Eisenberg AD, Cowles E, Curzon ME, Espeland MA, et al.: Cariogenic potential of foods. II. Relationship of food composition, plaque microbial counts, and salivary parameters to caries in the rat model. *Caries Res* 1994; 28(2):106–15.

National Cardiovascular Health Conference 2002. http://www.nhlbi.nih.gov/resources/docs/index.htm.Accessed 05-13-06.

National Research Council: *Recommended Dietary Allowances*. Washington, DC: National Academy Press, 1989.

Nelson GJ: Dietary fat, trans fatty acids, and risk of coronary heart disease. *Nutr Rev* 1998; 56(8):250–52.

Ornish D, Scherwitz LW, Billings JH, Brown SE, Gould KL, Merritt TA, et al.: Intensive lifestyle changes for reversal of coronary heart disease. *JAMA* 1998; 280(23):2001–7.

Peters JC, Lawson KD, Middleton SJ, Triebwasser KC: Assessment of nutritional effects of olestra, a nonabsorbed fat replacement: Summary. *J Nutr* 1997; 127(Suppl):1719S–28S.

Poulter N, Chang CL, Cuff A, Poulter C, Sever P, Thom S: Lipid profiles after the daily consumption of an oat-based cereal: A controlled crossover trial. *Am J Clin Nutr* 1994; 59(1):66–69.

Rosenstein ED, Kushner LJ, Kramer N, Kazandjian G: Pilot study of dietary fatty acid supplementation in the treatment of adult periodontitis. *Prostoglandins Leukot Essent Fatty Acids* 2003; 68(3):213–18.

Saito T, Shimazaki Y, Koga T, Tsuzuki M, Ohshima A: Relationship between upper body obesity and periodontitis. *J Dent Res* 2001; 80(7):1631–36.

Sandler RS, Zorich NL, Filloon TG, Wiseman HB, Lietz DJ, Brock MH, et al.: Gastrointestinal symptoms in 3,181 volunteers ingesting snack foods containing olestra or triglycerides. *Ann Intern Med* 1999; 130:253–61.

Schlagheck TG, Riccardi KA, Zorich NL, Torri SA, Dugan LD, Peters JC: Olestra dose response on fat-soluble and water-soluble nutrients in humans. *J Nutr* 1997; 127(8Suppl):1646S–65S.

Thun MJ, Peto R, Lopez AD, Monaco JH, Henley SJ, Heath CW, Doll R: Alcohol consumption and mortality among middle-aged and elderly U.S. adults. *N Engl J Med* 1997; Dec 11; 337(24):1705–14.

U.S. Department of Health and Human Services, Food and Drug Administration: Food labeling: Health claims; soluble fiber from certain foods and coronary heart disease: Final rule. *Federal Register* 1998; 63:8103–21.

U.S. Department of Health and Human Services, Food and Drug Administration: Food labeling: Trans fatty acids in nutrition labeling, nutrient content claims and health claims. *Federal Register*, 2003; 68(133):41433–41506.

U.S. Department of Health and Human Services and U.S. Department of Agriculture: *Dietary Guidelines for Americans 2005*, 6th ed. Washington, DC: U.S. Government Printing Office, 2005.

Weigley ES, Mueller DH, Robinson, CH: *Robinson's Basic Nutrition and Diet Therapy*, 8th ed. Upper Saddle River NJ: Merrill/Prentice Hall, 1997.

Wood JL, Allison RG: Effects of consumption of choline and lecithin on neurological and cardiovascular systems. *Fed Proc* 1982; 41(14):3015–21.

Wood N, Johnson RB, Streckfus CF: Comparison of body composition and periodontal disease using nutritional assessment techniques: Third National Health and Nutrition Examination Survey (NHANES III). *J Clin Peridontol* 2003; 30(4):321–27.

Chapter 7

How the Body Uses Fluids

Carole A. Palmer

CONTENTS

OBJECTIVES

The student will be able to:

- List the functions of water.
- Discuss effects of too much or too little water on the body.
- List the risk factors for dehydration.
- Describe the importance of dehydration to oral health.
- Discuss nutritional implications of caffeine, alcohol, soft drinks, and sports drinks.

INTRODUCTION

Water is second only to oxygen in its importance to life. Although humans can last for several weeks without food, we can survive for only a few days without water.

Water is considered a macronutrient in that it is found in large quantities in the body. It comprises the body's largest constituent, comprising from 45 to 75% of total body weight. Body water is higher in men than in women and declines with age in all people. All body cells contain water. Table 7–1 shows body distribution of water. Water is comprised of hydrogen and oxygen with the formula H_2O. Body fluids are compartmentalized and separated by membranes. About two-thirds of body water is within cells (intracellular) and remains fairly constant. Fluid outside the cells (extracellular) accounts for about one-third of body water. Extracellular fluid consists of circulation (blood and lymph) and the fluid between cells or tissues (interstitial fluid).

Water is absorbed directly from the small intestine by osmosis into the circulating blood. Metabolic activities in the body use and create water. For example, water is produced when carbohydrates, fats, and proteins are metabolized. This water loss is often mistaken for true weight loss when people begin low-calorie (particularly low-carbohydrate) diets (see Chapter 3). It can be lost rapidly, and repleted just as rapidly. Water is stored primarily in the extracellular spaces. All the excretory organs, particularly the kidneys, excrete water.

FUNCTIONS OF WATER

Water is involved in most of the body's metabolic activities, and can be considered the body's universal solvent. Functions include:

TABLE 7–1 Body Water Content

Area of the Body	Water Content (Approximate Percentage)
Blood plasma	90
Muscle tissue	75–80
Adipose (fat) tissue	20
Bone	20

Source: From *Robinson's Basic Nutrition and Diet Therapy, 8/E* by Weigley/Mueller/Robinson, © 1997. Reprinted with permission.

* Facilitating digestion and absorption by serving as
  * the basis of saliva and digestive juices.
  * the solution in which nutrients are absorbed across the villi of the small intestine.
  * the transport vehicle for nutrients and other dissolved substances (e.g., oxygen) via blood and lymph.
  * the transport medium for nutrients crossing cell membranes.
* Serving as a required component of some chemical reactions.
* Serving as a product of some chemical reactions.
* Dissolving and facilitating excretion of body waste.
* Lubricating body parts such as joints.
* Maintaining body lubricants (saliva, tears, mucous).
* Regulating body temperature.

WATER REQUIREMENTS AND SOURCES

There is no specific DRI for water, but the average daily requirement is around 9 cups/day (2200 mL) for sedentary women and about 12 cups/day (2900 mL) for sedentary men (Kleiner, 1999). This is an average of about 1 mL/kcal of food consumed. Infants and children require closer to $1\frac{1}{2}$ mL/kcal. They have more water and greater surface skin area than adults do, and have higher water turnover and more limited kidney capacity due to the high solute load (dissolved particles) from the use of protein for growth. Factors that add to fluid needs include: exercise, high temperature, low humidity, high altitude, high-fiber diet, and increased fluid losses (caffeine, alcohol consumption) (Kleiner, 1999).

Most water is obtained via foods and liquids. In general, solid foods such as fruits and vegetables contribute about 1 liter or $4\frac{1}{2}$ cups/day; only a small amount is derived from cellular metabolism (about 1 cup/day), and the rest is obtained via fluid intake. It is recommended that about 5 cups of water be consumed daily. Caffeinated and alcoholic beverages increase urinary losses and can contribute even more to dehydration. An extra half-cup of water should be consumed for every cup of caffeinated or alcoholic beverage. It is also probably a good idea, especially for older people, to drink water periodically throughout the day rather than relying exclusively on thirst symptoms. Table 7–2 shows the fluid content of foods.

TABLE 7–2 Water Content of Foods

Type of Food	Water Content (Approximate Percentage)
Fruits and vegetables	70–95%
Milk	87
Cooked cereals, pasta, rice	60–85
Eggs	74
Cooked meat, poultry, fish	
Well done	40–50
Medium to rare	50–70
Cheese, hard	35–40
Bread	35
Dry cereals, crackers	3–7
Nuts, fats, sweets	0–10

Source: From *Robinson's Basic Nutrition and Diet Therapy, 8/E* by Weigley/Mueller/Robinson, © 1997. Reprinted with permission.

WATER, ELECTROLYTE, AND ACID-BASE BALANCE AND REGULATION

Several mechanisms function to maintain optimum balance of fluids in the body. These are the nervous system, which sends thirst signals to the brain; the kidneys, which conserve or excrete water; the cardiovascular system, which modulates the volume of fluid transferred; and the hormones, which also modulate retention or excretion. Normal daily water turnover (without perspiration) is about 4% of body weight in adults. The average man loses around 12 cups of water a day and consumes only 9 cups a day. The average woman loses 9 cups a day but consumes only $7\frac{1}{2}$ cups. Infants lose closer to 15% of body weight a day (or over 4 cups for a $15\frac{1}{2}$ lb infant). The majority of the water is lost from the lungs and skin. Losses from urine and stool make up the remainder. Table 7–3 shows water balance for adults.

Water is also the vehicle for dispersing electrolytes throughout the body. Electrolytes are compounds such as salts, acids, and bases. Most are minerals, but some are proteins. The functions of electrolytes are to:

- Serve as essential minerals
- Control osmotic pressure between body fluid compartments
- Maintain acid-base balance in the body

The most plentiful electrolytes are sodium, potassium, and chloride. In health, electrolyte balance is maintained in the body. In illness electrolyte imbalance often occurs. Acute infections and malnutrition both can result in severe electrolyte imbalances. Electrolyte balance is monitored as part of nutritional status assessment. Electrolyte imbalances can be fatal. A good example is death from a heart attack brought on by the electrolyte balance side effect of anorexia.

Water is also the mechanism for helping maintain acid-base balance in the body. Some body fluids are more acidic and some are more basic. The body maintains the appropriate pH (degree of acidity or alkalinity) for each fluid by homeostatic mechanisms, which include dilution, buffering, lung respiration, and kidney excretion. Normal body pH has a narrow range of 7.35–7.45, with 7.0 being neutral. Table 7–4 shows the pH of body tissues. Respiratory or metabolism abnormalities can lead to alkalosis or acidosis. Acid or alkaline foods are usually well tolerated by healthy people. However, some medications can be affected by the pH of foods and thus must be taken or not taken with these foods. Careful attention to drug instructions is essential for this reason as well as many others. For example, low-pH foods include vinegar, grapefruit, pineapple, orange and tomato juice, beer, wine, and coffee. Milk is

TABLE 7–3 Typical Water Balance for an Adult

Sources of Water		Losses of Water	
Ingested liquids	1,600 mL	Kidneys	1,500 mL
Ingested foods	700 mL	Skin	500 mL
Metabolic water	200 mL	Lungs	300 mL
		GI tract	200 mL
	Total 2,500 mL		Total 2,500 mL

Source: From *Robinson's Basic Nutrition and Diet Therapy, 8/E* by Weigley/Mueller/ Robinson, © 1997. Reprinted with permission.

TABLE 7–4   Normal pH of Various Body Fluids

Body Fluid	Normal pH Range
Saliva	6.35–6.85
Gastric juice	1.2–3.0
Pancreatic juice	7.0–8.2
Blood plasma	7.35–7.45
Overall normal body range	7.35–7.45

Note: Decreased $_p$H = more acid; increased $_p$H = more basic.
Source: From *Robinson's Basic Nutrition and Diet Therapy, 8/E* by Weigley/Mueller/Robinson, © 1997. Reprinted with permission.

almost neutral and eggs are alkaline. After foods are metabolized they may yield metabolic residues that are either acidic or base.

Signs and Symptoms of Fluid Sufficiency and Deficiency

Fluid balance is extremely important to health, yet is often overlooked in the process of health assessment. Generally, a person who is well hydrated will have skin that seems plump and well hydrated, no precipitous weight loss, and light-colored urine.

Dehydration

Dehydration can be acute or chronic, mild or severe. Acute dehydration can occur in association with intense exercise. Chronic mild dehydration may result from depressed thirst recognition, long-term poor consumption, or excess use of natural diuretics like caffeine and alcohol. Severe fluid deprivation is referred to as dehydration, and can be a serious health risk, especially in children, the elderly, and the medically compromised. Despite the body's efforts to conserve water, losses are continuous. Although thirst is the first body symptom of deficiency, 2% or more of body water may have been lost before thirst is recognized. Mild dehydration is considered to be 1% or greater loss of body weight through fluid loss. Loss of 10% of body water causes severe dehydration, and loss of 20% is fatal. Dehydration is a major cause of deaths in infants (via diarrhea) and in the elderly.

Thirst is not a reliable indicator of fluid status because many at-risk individuals may not recognize or be able to articulate thirst. This includes babies, the very ill (fever, infection, burns), and Alzheimer's sufferers, to name but a few. In the elderly, the thirst sensation is depressed, so older people may not recognize that they are dehydrated until it is too late. Other individuals, such as athletes, also have blunted thirst response during exercise and may not be sensitized to the warning signs of dehydration until they are overcome by heat stroke. Attention to hydration has become an important part of endurance athletes' training for this reason. If the level of dehydration is more than 3% of body weight loss, rehydration requires more than just use of beverages. Other osmolar intake may be needed and rehydration may require up to 24 hours.

The earliest signs of dehydration include appetite loss, headache, fatigue, flushed skin, light-headedness, dry mouth and eyes, and dark, concentrated urine with a strong odor. More advanced signs include numbness, muscle spasms, swallowing difficulty, vision difficulties, and delirium (Kleiner, 1999).

Edema

Edema, or excess fluid retention, is uncommon in healthy individuals because the kidneys easily excrete the excess water. Edema is often a sign of failure of organs such as kidneys, heart, or liver.

Water Intoxication

Although a somewhat rare condition, water intoxication can pose a significant health risk for the individual obsessed with fluid intake. It is found mainly among those with chronic mental illness (at a rate of 18%) (Hayashi, et al., 2005). It is also seen in clients with kidney disorders that reduce urine output, or patients with excessive parenteral hydration (Altieri, La Vecchia, Negril, 2003).

EFFECTS OF HYDRATION ON HEALTH AND DISEASE

Urinary Tract Stones

The prevalence of stones is higher in populations who have lower urinary volume. This is because decreased fluid leads to higher concentrations of stone-forming salts. The risk of stone formation increases with urine volumes of less than 1 liter (L) per day. Conversely, increasing fluid consumption to a level providing a urinary volume of more than 2 L/day prevents stone recurrence in the majority of patients (Borghi, Amato Briganti, Novarini, Giannini, 1996). As a rule of thumb, people at risk for stone formation should take at least a cup of fluid with each meal, between meals, before bedtime, and during the night. Fluid also needs to be increased in hotter weather and during exercise.

Cancers

There is a direct correlation between the amount of fluid consumed and the incidence of urinary tract cancers such as bladder, prostate, kidney, and testicular. The same was found with breast cancer risk. Those with lower fluid intake had higher incidence of these cancers (Stookey, Belderson, Russell, Barker, 1997; Wilkens, Kadir, Kolonel, Nomura, Hankin, 1996). There is some evidence that water itself provides greater benefit than other fluids (Michaud et al., 1999). A possible rationale is that decreased fluid intake could result in a greater concentration of carcinogens in the urine or in a lengthened contact time with the bladder mucosa due to less frequent urination. To the same extent, fluid intake decreases bowel transit time and reduces mucosal contact with carcinogens and could reduce the risk of colon cancer. Low fluid intake could also comprise cellular concentration, affect enzyme activity in metabolic regulation, and inhibit carcinogen removal. Yet, concrete association between fluid intake and cancer risk still needs further research.

Weight Control

Drinking fluids can help people feel fuller and consequently eat less. This has been shown in studies with children and adults. Replacing soft drinks with water and skim milk can help with weight control and general health, particularly in children and adolescents (Levine, 1996). (See Chapter 3 in this textbook.)

Exercise

Exercise can speed up fluid losses measurably. So, for ordinary exercise like walking, the recommendation is to have 8 oz (1 cup) of water before the walk, 4 oz every 20 minutes or so, and another cup a half-hour after the walk. Harder exercise or hotter weather means even more water should be consumed (Do You Drink Enough Water?, 1999).

Athletes often consume too few fluids, and some even induce dehydration to achieve certain weight classes. In some cases this has resulted in death. In fact, dehydration of as little as 1% decrease in body weight impairs physiologic and performance responses during exercise (Prevention CfDCa, 1998). Children show symptoms of dehydration more rapidly than adults and should be cautioned to rehydrate frequently while active, especially in hot weather.

Pregnancy and Lactation

Pregnant women need at least 1 cup of water extra per day, and breastfeeding mothers need an additional 3–4 cups.

Fluids and Oral Health of Elderly People

Decreased thirst recognition is common in elderly people, as is dehydration. Dehydration is also associated with decreased saliva because saliva is composed primarily of water. Although this is a common problem in older people, it is true at any age (Ship, Fischer, 1997). In turn, lack of saliva (xerostomia) plays a major role in oral health via its many functions in the oral cavity. These include:

- Lubricating oral tissues
- Facilitating denture retention
- Aiding in taste perception
- Preventing caries and periodontal disease via
  - Decreasing food retention
  - Buffering acids
  - Mineralizing enamel and cementum
  - Antibacterial activity

Dry mouth often leads people to try to improve moistness by using hard candies. This habit further promotes caries and does not resolve the dehydration.

In summary, the consequences of dehydration can be serious and can range from xerostomia, constipation, and fecal impaction to mental impairment, functional decline, and ultimately death (Weinberg, Minaker, 1995).

OTHER FLUIDS
Caffeine

Caffeine is a natural substance that is found in more than 60 plants. It is found in leaves, seeds, or fruits and is used to make beverages like coffee, tea, cola drinks, and chocolate. The U.S. FDA has classified caffeine as Generally Recognized as Safe, or GRAS (U.S. FDA). Nevertheless, concerns have been raised as to caffeine's safety, particularly that caffeine may contribute to adverse pregnancy outcomes, insomnia, and other problems (Eskenazi, 1999). Caffeine is a mildly addictive drug and the FDA has advised pregnant women to moderate their caffeine consumption, although they state that caffeine does not adversely affect reproduction. There is also a lack of evidence implicating caffeine in cancer, breast disease, cardiovascular disease, hypertension (high blood pressure), or stroke. Caffeine is also not a significant risk factor in osteoporosis in women who consume adequate calcium. Due to its stimulant effect, many people use caffeine to increase alertness and stay awake. People vary in their response to it. Some people feel no effect, and others may feel the effects after just one cup of coffee. In some, coffee can lead to insomnia, anxiety, and difficulty concentrating (high doses cause anxiety, insomnia, tension, nausea,

and upset stomach). Ceasing caffeine can lead to withdrawal symptoms such as headache and fatigue. Caffeine is not stored in the body and is excreted within several hours in the urine.

Moderate caffeine consumption is considered to be about three cups of coffee or about 300 mg of caffeine. The amount of caffeine varies widely among foods and brand names, and is not yet required to be on the label (Center for Science in the Public Interest, 1997). Table 7–5 shows the caffeine content of some common foods and beverages.

Alcohol

Alcoholic beverages have been researched in some detail in regard to health implications. Moderate consumption (no more than two 3 oz beverages/day) has

TABLE 7–5   Caffeine Content of Beverages and Chocolate Products

	Milligrams of Caffeine	
Item	*Typical*	*Range*
Coffee (8 oz cup)		
Brewed, drip method	85	65–120
Instant	75	60–85
Decaffeinated	3	2–4
Espresso (1 oz/cup)	40	30–50
Teas (8 oz cup)		
Brewed (major U.S. brands)	40	20–90
Brewed, imported brands	60	25–110
Instant	28	24–31
Iced (8 oz glass)	25	9–50
Some soft drinks (8 oz)	24	20–40
Cocoa beverage (8 oz)	6	3–32
Chocolate milk beverage (8 oz)	5	2–7
Milk chocolate (1 oz)	6	1–15
Dark chocolate, semisweet (1 oz)	20	5–35
Baker's chocolate (1 oz)	26	26
Chocolate-flavored syrup (1 oz)	4	4

Source: International Food Information Council Foundation: *Everything You Need to Know about Caffeine.* Washington, OC: Author.

been associated with increased HDL (good) cholesterol in older people. In patients with decreased appetite, a small alcoholic beverage before meals may help increase appetite. On the other hand, alcohol consumption is a major risk factor of oral cancer and many other cancers, particularly in association with smoking. It can also lead to alcoholism in susceptible individuals. Alcohol is a major contributor to accidents, domestic violence, elevated blood pressure, cirrhosis of the liver, and fetal alcohol syndrome. In fact, alcohol causes more harm to those under age 35 than are helped by it in later years (Scragg, 1995). Thus, the risks of alcohol consumption far outweigh the benefits, and drinking alcoholic beverages should not be encouraged except on a physician's recommendation.

Tea

Tea is the most popular beverage consumed by human society worldwide, second only to water. Tea is made from brewing the leaves of the plant *Camellia sinensis* in hot water. There are different ways of processing the leaves resulting in different types, the main three being oolong tea (most widely used in China and Taiwan), green tea (common in Asian countries and North Africa), and black tea (the main choice of Western consumers) (Trevisanato, Kim, 2000; Wu, Wei, 2003). It is important to note that herbal teas are not true tea because they are not derived from *C. sinensis*, but from other sources. Tea provides a dietary source of biologically active compounds that help prevent a side variety of diseases. It is the richest source of a class of antioxidants called flavonoids and contains many other beneficial compounds such as vitamins and minerals. In particular, tea contains 0.1 mg fluoride/cup.

More and more evidence is showing that moderate tea consumption may protect against several forms of cancer, cardiovascular disease, the formation of kidney stones, bacterial infections, and dental caries. Tea consumption may reduce the cariogenic potential of starch-containing foods; caries among children were found to be significantly reduced in children who drank a cup of tea immediately following lunch. Tea polyphenols, rather than fluoride, may be responsible for the anticariogenic effect. Tea extracts also inhibit human salivary amylase, which can affect carbohydrate digestion in the mouth.

As with anything, there are potential health concerns associated with tea. These include the caffeine content of tea, the aluminum content of tea, and the fact that tea has been shown to decrease iron absorption.

Soft Drinks (Carbonated Beverages)

Currently almost 30% of all beverages consumed in the American diet are sodas (What America's Drinking, 2006). Soda is also the "single biggest source of refined sugars in [the] American Diet" (Jacobson, 2006), and consumption has increased almost 500% in the past 50 years. The consumption of soft drinks (sweetened and artificially sweetened) has surpassed that of all other beverages including water, milk, and coffee in the United States.

Sodas are a source of empty calories in that they provide calories but no other nutritional value. Excessive consumption can lead to weight gain and take the place of more nutritious food choices. Indeed, children who often use soft drinks have 10% more calories and are more likely to be overweight than kids who rarely drink them, and have 1.6 times greater odds of becoming obese for each added can of sugar-sweetened beverage consumed per day (Giammattei, Blix, Marshak, Wollitzer, Pettitt, 2003). Teenagers drink one-half to twice as much soda as milk.

There has been some concern that heavy soda drinking may compromise bone density in children and older adults. However, these findings are somewhat controversial (Nielsen, Milne, 1998; Sun, Morton, Barrett-Conror, 1999). What remains clear, however, is that frequent sugar-containing soda use is a risk factor for dental caries. Regular and diet sodas both cause demineralization, regardless of sugar content (von Fraunhofer, Rogers, 2004). The recommendation should be moderation and not to substitute sodas for more nutritious beverages.

Sports Drinks

Sports drinks are also referred to as fluid replacement drinks or carbohydrate-electrolyte (C-E) beverages. The standard carbohydrate concentration of most C-E beverages is 4–7%. Studies have shown that these beverages do improve performance in moderate- and high-intensity exercise and that the effects of the carbohydrate and the fluid appear to be additive (Ryan, 1997). However, these beverages are also potentially cariogenic and can add unneeded calories to the diet.

SUMMARY AND IMPLICATIONS FOR DENTISTRY

* Fluids are important and often overlooked nutrients that can impact general and oral health.
* Dehydration is common in older people and can lead to xerostomia, denture slippage, and confusion.
* Caffeine and alcohol contribute to fluid losses.
* Due to concern about side effects, caffeine and alcohol should be consumed in moderation.
* Consumption of soft drinks and sports beverages can contribute to dental caries when consumed frequently.

QUESTIONS PATIENTS MIGHT ASK

Q. I always thought that caffeine was not healthy, but now people are recommending tea for health. I'm confused.

A. You are right that too much caffeine can cause problems such as inability to sleep and difficulty paying attention in school. However, it is not the caffeine that researchers are focusing on, but the many antioxidants present in teas that have been shown to have a variety of disease-preventing beneficial effects.

Q. My daughter is a runner and frequently uses beverages such as diet drinks and sports drinks. She says she needs them to keep up her fluid levels and that the drinks don't have any potential negative side effects. Is she correct?

A. Yes and no. It is true that these liquids keep her from becoming dehydrated during active exertion. The sports drinks contain electrolytes which help replace those lost through sweat. However, if she drinks the diet sodas often, the acid in them can cause tooth enamel demineralization. Water is a better choice. The sports drinks also contain carbohydrates, which add calories and can contribute to tooth decay if consumed often.

Q. My 90-year-old grandmother is a finicky eater and doesn't drink many fluids. When I caution her about this, she says that she drinks when she is thirsty and there's nothing to worry about. Is she correct?

A. No, she is not correct. As people get older, their ability to recognize thirst diminishes. This can be a serious problem because it can lead to dehydration. Dehydration, in turn, can be fatal if not prevented or reversed. You might gently suggest that she have a variety of beverages throughout the day, and to sip frequently on water or tea, for example, whether she thinks she is thirsty or not.

REFERENCES

Altieri A, La Vecchia C, Negril E: Fluid intake and risk of bladder and other cancers. *Eur J Clin Nutr* 2003; 57(2):S59.

Borghi L, Amato F, Briganti A, Novarini A, Giannini A: Urinary volume, water and recurrences in idiopathic calcium nephrolithiasis: A 5-year randomized prospective study. *Urology* 1996; 155:849–53.

Center for Science in the Public Interest: *Label Caffeine Content of Foods, Scientists Tell FDA*. Press release, 1997.

Do you drink enough water?: *Consumer Reports on Health*, November 1999, pp. 8–10.

Eskenazi B: Caffeine-filtering the facts. *N Engl J Med* 1999; 341(22):168–89.

Giammattei J, Blix G, Marshak HH, Wollitzer AO, Pettitt DJ: Television watching and soft drink consumption: Associations with obesity in 11- to 13-year-old schoolchildren. *Arch Pediatr Adolesc Med* 2003; 157(9):882–86.

Hayashi T, Ishida Y, Miyashita T, Kiyokawa H, Kimura A, Kondo T: Fatal water intoxication in a schizophrenic patient—An autopsy case. *J Clin Forensic Med* 2005; 12(3):157–59.

Jacobson, Michael F, Liquid Candy: How Soft Drinks are Harming Americans' Health. Washington, DC: Center for Science in the Public Interest 2006. http://www.cspinet.org/new/pdf/liquid_candy_final_w_new_supplement.pdf. Accessed 05/13/06.

Kleiner SM: Water: An essential but overlooked nutrient. *J Am Diet Assoc* 1999; 99(2):200–206.

Levine B: Role of liquid intake in childhood obesity and related diseases. *Curr Concepts Perspect Nutr* 1996; 8:2.

Michaud D, Spiegelman D, Clinton SK, Rimm EB, Curhan GC, Willett WC: Fluid intake and the risk of bladder cancer in men. *N Engl J Med* 1999; 340(18):1390–97.

Nielsen FH, Milne DB: Too much soda may rob bone minerals. *Proceedings of the North Dakota Academy of Science* 1998; 51:212.

Prevention CfDCa. *MMWR* 1998; 47 (RR-3):1–36.

Ryan M: Sports drinks: Research asks for reevaluation of current recommendations. *J Am Diet Assoc* 1997; 97(10): S197–S98.

Scragg RA: Quantification of alcohol-related mortality in New Zealand. *Aust NZ J Med* 1995; 25:5–11.

Ship JA, Fischer DJ: The relationship between dehydration and parotid salivary gland function in young and older healthy adults. *J Gerontol* 1997; 52(5):M310–19.

Stookey JD, Belderson PE, Russell JM, Barker ME: Correspondence re: J. Shannon et al., Relationship of food groups and water intake to colon cancer risk. *Cancer Epidemiol Biomarkers Prev* 1997; 6(8):657–58.

Sun HK, Morton DJ, Barrett-Connor EL: Carbonated beverage consumption and bone mineral density among older women: The Rancho Bernardo Study. *Am J Public Health* 1997; 87(2):276–79.

Trevisanato SI, Kim YI: Tea and health. *Nutr Rev* 2000; 58(1):1–10.

U.S. Food and Drug Administration: Foods generally recognized as safe (GRAS), http://www.cfsan.fda.gov/~dms/grasguid.html.

von Fraunhofer JA, Rogers MM: Dissolution of dental enamel in soft drinks. *Gen Dent* 2004; 52(4):308–12.

Weigley ES, Mueller DH, Robinson CH: Chapter 4: Transformation of food and fluid for body needs. In *Robinson's Basic Nutrition and Diet Therapy*, 8th ed. Upper Saddle River, NJ: Merrill/Prentice Hall, 1997:58–78.

Weinberg AD, Minaker KL: Dehydration. Evaluation and management in older adults. *JAMA* 1995; 274(19):1552–56.

What America's Drinking, http://www.ameribev.org/variety/what.asp2006.

Wilkens LR, Kadir MM, Kolonel LN, Nomura AM, Hankin JH: Risk factors for lower urinary tract cancer: The role of total fluid consumption, nitrites and nitrosamines, and selected foods. *Cancer Epidemiol Biomarkers Prev* 1996; 5(3):161–66.

Wu C, Wei Guo-Xian: Tea as a functional food for oral health. *Nutrition* 2003; 18(5):443.

Chapter **8**

The Minerals and Mineralization

Carole A. Palmer and Athena S. Papas

Source: This chapter is adapted from Weigley, Mueller, Robinson, 1997.

OBJECTIVES
The student will be able to:

- Discuss the general functions of minerals in the body.
- List the functions of each mineral, along with its major food sources.
- Describe the general manifestations of mineral deficiencies.
- Describe the oral manifestations of mineral deficiencies.
- Detail the process of mineralization of bones and teeth.
- Discuss the roles of calcium in the body including in bone physiology.
- List factors that could interfere with mineral absorption.
- Discuss the role of fluoride in tooth mineralization and the criteria for fluoride supplementation.
- Describe common effects of electrolyte imbalance.

147

INTRODUCTION: MINERALS IN GENERAL

Characteristics

The essential minerals are a group of elements that are necessary in small amounts to maintain health and function. They cannot be made endogenously and must be supplied by the diet. Table 8–1 shows the mineral distribution in the body.

Minerals are inorganic elements, meaning they do not contain carbon. It is the mineral component that remains after death or after plants or animals burn. Although this aspect of minerals has been known for thousands of years, many of the intricate functions of minerals were not known until recently. A large gray area of tentative knowledge about minerals still exists, and they are being closely studied to determine their functions in both health and disease.

Macrominerals are those needed in larger amounts (100 mg/day or more). Macrominerals include calcium, phosphorus, magnesium, sodium, potassium, and chloride. The elements sodium, potassium, magnesium, and chloride are also collectively termed *electrolytes* because they separate into electrically charged ions when dissolved in the body. Electrolytes play indispensable roles in transmitting nerve impulses, contracting muscles, keeping proper fluid levels in the body, and maintaining the proper acid-base balance of these fluids.

Microminerals are also called trace elements, and are needed in amounts of no more than a few milligrams a day. The microminerals include iron, zinc, iodine, fluoride, chromium, cobalt, manganese, molybdenum, selenium, nickel, tin, vanadium, and silicon.

Chemical Structure, Composition, and Measurement

Minerals usually exist in three states:

- Inorganic compounds (e.g., sodium chloride in cells and blood, hydrochloric acid in the stomach);
- Organic compounds (e.g., PO_4 in phospholipids in membranes; Fe; in hemoglobin; iodine, in thyroxine;
- Free ions (e.g., Cl^-, K^+, Ca^{++}).

In foods, minerals are measured in milligrams (mg) or micrograms (μg)—1 microgram = 0.000001 gram). In body fluids, mineral concentrations are expressed in milliequivalents per liter.

Minerals and vitamins (the other micronutrients) are found in all but highly refined foods. They are found in all tissues and fluids, comprising 4% of the body weight. The oldest method of measuring the total amount present in the body is by measuring the ash remaining after tissues are burned. In the human body, calcium and phosphorus comprise three-quarters of the total mineral composition.

Classification

For convenience, minerals can be divided into two groups:

- *Macrominerals* (greater than 0.005% of body weight): calcium, magnesium, phosphorus, sodium, potassium, chloride, and sulfur
- *Microminerals* (trace elements): iron, iodine, copper, manganese, zinc, cobalt, molybdenum, arsenic, nickel, selenium, chromium, silicon, tin, fluoride, vanadium

Another method of classification is according to the dietary recommendations. Traditionally, 100 mg is used as the dividing line between the macro- and the microminerals.

TABLE 8–1 Mineral Composition of the Adult Body

Mineral	Approximate Amount in Adult (70 kg body weight)
Calcium	1200 g
Phosphorus	750 g
Potassium	245 g
Sulfur	175 g
Sodium	105 g
Chloride	105 g
Magnesium	30 g
Molybdenum	9 g
Iron	4 g
Zinc	2 g
Selenium	2 g
Fluoride	1 g
Copper	150 mg
Manganese	150 mg
Iodine	30 mg
Chromium	5 mg
Cobalt	5 mg

Microminerals present in the body that might have some function are arsenic, cadmium, nickel, silicon, tin, and vanadium. Aluminum, barium, boron, bromine, gold, lead, mercury, and strontium are present in the body but have no specific known function. Lead, cadmium, and mercury are considered toxic. However, all minerals can be toxic if consumed or inhaled in large amounts for long periods.

Properties

Minerals are not affected by heat. However, food preparation can affect the mineral values of foods because minerals can be soluble in water, acids, and bases. Conversely, vegetables canned in salted water will absorb salt. The pH can make minerals either more or less soluble. For example, calcium and iron are more soluble in acids and less in bases; thus people who have achlorohydria (loss of stomach acid, common in old age) have trouble absorbing minerals, especially calcium. As with vitamins, minerals do not supply energy themselves, but are involved in all metabolic pathways of the macronutrients.

Functions

The earliest recognition of the importance of minerals was the awareness of the importance of calcium and phosphorus for bones and teeth. Over the years, the many other functions of minerals have been identified. Some general categories of mineral function include:

- *Cell structural elements:* Minerals comprise part of the structure of every cell. Calcium, phosphorus, magnesium, and fluoride provide strength and rigidity to hard structures like bones and teeth. The soft tissues, like organs and muscles, contain many minerals in their structures, including potassium, sulfur, phosphorus, and iron.
- *Regulatory functions:* Minerals are constituents of various regulatory compounds as components of vitamins, enzymes, and hormones. For example,
  - Vitamins: sulfur is a component of thiamin and biotin, and cobalt is a component of vitamin B_{12}.
  - Enzymes: selenium is a component of glutathione peroxidase (part of the body's antioxidant system), and zinc is a component of carbonic anhydrase (helps release carbon dioxide from red blood cells).
  - Hormones: iodine is a component of thyroxine.

- *Cofactors:* Minerals often function as cofactors—that is, a mineral unites with the other compound in order for that substance to function (calcium activates pancreatic lipase). In other cases, minerals act as catalysts to increase the speed of a reaction (copper speeds up the reaction to incorporate iron into the hemoglobin molecule and zinc does the same in the formation of insulin by the pancreas).
- *Nerve response regulators:* Minerals control the passage of materials in and out of cells, thereby regulating the transmission of nerve impulses and muscle contractions. For example, working together, sodium, potassium, calcium, and magnesium all regulate the various cellular pumps and cellular membrane ion channels.
- *Maintenance of water and acid-base balances:* Water balance between the inside and outside of cells depends in large part on the correct concentrations of potassium (inside) and sodium (outside). Acid-base regulation involves minerals, especially as buffer salts.

Requirements and Range of Safety

More is known about some minerals than others. A total of 15 out of 92 naturally occurring minerals are currently considered to be "essential." Sufficient scientific data exist for 8 minerals to allow a specific RDA to be set (see chapter 2). For others, a level of adequate intake (AI) is set. Some minerals present in the body do not yet have a clearly identified role. Research in these elements is ongoing. Some minerals may have no role in the human body at all, and may just happen to be in many of the many substances people consume.

Food Sources

Food sources of minerals include natural food components, contaminants, and additives. The concentration of minerals in food is determined by the food species, the soil composition, and the type of fertilizer used.

Minerals are found in all food groups, but no single food or group of foods supplies all minerals. Consuming a wide variety of wholesome foods within each group of the food guide pyramid should ensure sufficient mineral intake.

Gross mineral deficiencies or toxicities in foods are usually detected and corrected early in the food chain. Because humans are at the end of the chain, and obtain foods from a wide variety of sources, we usually are protected from these effects. If mineral deficiencies exist in soil, resulting products will not be mineral deficient, but rather will be smaller in size to adapt to the deficiency. Food processing can also affect mineral levels and availability. For example, levels of iodine and fluoride can be increased by supplementation, while refining can remove minerals.

The primary source of sodium is at the table and in food processing and preservation. Calcium is present primarily in dairy products, but is also present in a variety of fortified foods such as cereals and orange juice. Many minerals, such as calcium, magnesium, sodium, fluoride, and iron, are found in drinking water (not distilled). However, the mineral composition of water varies greatly from region to region. Only some minerals are required to be listed on package labels, so consumers cannot be sure of the kinds and amounts of all minerals found in foods.

Bioavailability

The bioavailability of minerals varies widely and can range from 90% (sodium) to less than 2% (chromium). A variety of factors determines bioavailability, including food and meal composition, processing, preparation, and body nutrient status. Some minerals are removed in processing; for example, iron and other minerals are removed from whole grains during the refining process. Iron is the only mineral added back when the refined grain product is "enriched." Whole grains contain fiber that can chelate some minerals and make them unavailable for absorption.

Factors favoring the absorption of mineral elements include:

- *Body requirement*: Growing children and pregnant women require more calcium and so absorb a higher percentage of calcium from food. People with low calcium stores will absorb more calcium than those with higher stores.
- *Chemical form*: Heme iron in animal foods is more available than is the nonheme iron found in plant foods.
- *Stomach and small intestine pH*: Calcium and iron are better absorbed in an acidic environment.
- *Presence of other nutrients*: Lactose in the intestinal tract improves the absorption of calcium; vitamin C enhances the absorption of calcium, iron, and zinc.

Factors reducing the absorption of mineral elements include:

- *Excessive intake*: High intakes of any mineral above body need may pass directly into the feces and be eliminated.
- *Mineral–mineral interaction*: High intakes of zinc (as from supplements) reduce absorption of copper; high intakes of iron reduce absorption of zinc and copper; high intakes of calcium reduce absorption of iron.
- *Chelating agents*: Substances such as oxalic and phytic acids, fiber, fat, and some medications bind minerals, thus reducing absorption.
- *Rapid digestive tract transit time*: Fiber, mineral oil, laxatives, diarrhea, and food poisoning speed up the passage of foodstuffs so there is less time for absorption.
- *Damage to the digestive tract*: Stomach and intestinal surgery, short bowel syndrome, sprue, cystic fibrosis, and intestinal parasites can cause short- and long-term mineral malabsorption.
- *Medication interactions*: Some medications may form a complex with calcium, rendering either calcium or the medication, or both, nonabsorbable.

MINERALIZATION OF BONES AND TEETH

Bones

Bone is about 60% inorganic (mineral), 25% organic (collagen), and 15% water, and has traces of proteins and mucopolysaccharides. Bone contains over a gram of calcium and phosphate as well as a variety of other minerals such as magnesium, sodium, fluoride, and other trace minerals.

Nutrients needed for healthy bone development include the minerals just listed as well as vitamins C, D, and K, and protein. Boron and manganese may also play roles in bone development (Heaney, 1999). Recent research has also shown a significant positive association between fruit and vegetable consumption and bone size. Both men and women with high intakes of fruits and vegetables had stronger bones than those with lower intakes (Tucker et al., 1999), and children with higher fruit and vegetable intakes had larger bones than those with lower intakes (Tylavsky et al., 2004).

Bone is a dynamic organ system that undergoes continuous modeling (new bone formation) and remodeling (resorption and reformation of the bone). Bone has two growth phases:

1. The formation of a protein matrix (collagen produced by osteoblasts), which can be calcified
2. Calcification (calcium phosphate is precipitated from serum)

Table 8–2 shows the process of bone mineralization. During normal growth, bone is built by osteoblast cells, broken down by osteoclasts, and subsequently rebuilt by osteoblasts in the following manner:

1. Osteoblasts secrete an amorphous, shapeless collagen protein matrix that forms the support structure of the bone, and they secrete bone mineral to provide bone strength.
2. Calcium phosphate is deposited within the spaces of the collagen fibrils (seeding or nucleation), and the amorphous mass becomes hydroxyapatite ($Ca_{10}(PO_4)_6OH_2$), the primary inorganic constituent of bone and teeth.
3. The apatite develops in ribbonlike structures within the fibrils and forms crystallites.
4. The crystallites develop into crystals. As the bone matures, the crystals displace existing water.
5. Osteoclasts are drawn to bone sites by microdamage to the bone, mechanical stress, and for other unknown reasons, and start bone resorption. Cytokines and bone-derived growth factors released by resorption attract osteoblasts. Figure 8–1 shows bone modeling and remodeling.

TABLE 8–2   Bone Mineralization

1. Osteoblast $\rightarrow$ Ca + P_4 $\rightarrow$ Amorphous mass
2. Ca + PO + Amino acid side chains $\rightarrow$ *Nucleate* $\rightarrow$ $Ca_{10}(PO_4)_6(OH)_2$ (Apatite)
3. $Ca_{10}(PO_4)_6(OH)_2$ grows in ribbons within fibrils leading to crystallites
4. Crystallites coalesce leading to crystals
5. Crystals grow and displace fluid leading to normal bone

Source: Adapted from Irving JT. In Shaw JH, Sweeney EA, Cappuccino CC, Meller SM (eds): *Textbook of Oral Biology.* Philadelphia: WB Saunders, 1978:482.

As the osteoblasts lay down new bone, bone density increases. In normal bone status, total osteoblastic activity exceeds osteoclast activity.

The highly structured crystal arrangements in calcified vertebrate tissues indicate that calcification is not a random event. Crystal development (deposition, orientation, size, shape) is controlled by several factors such as the organic matrix, the degree of phosphorylation, and the amount of ground substance (Heaney, 1999). The skeletal crystalline mass in bone is quite stable. Most crystals are extracellular and can exchange calcium and phosphorus with body fluids. This exchange is regulated by parathyroid hormone and vitamin D.

When osteoclastic activity is in excess of osteoblastic activity, bone loss and osteoporosis can result. Osteoporosis is discussed in Chapter 11. Dietary factors that can lead to excess bone losses if consumed in excess include sodium (depletes calcium), vitamin A, protein, and caffeine (Weaver, Heaney, 1999).

The mineralization of cementum and dentin is similar to that of bone.

Teeth

Enamel calcification differs from that of bone, cementum, and dentin. Mineralization and matrix formation occur together from the beginning of enamel development through its maturation. Enamel is about 95–97% mineralized, and there is only a trace of organic matrix. The apatite crystals of enamel may also be 200 times larger in volume than those of bone or dentin.

The major protein fraction in developing enamel is an aggregate of small proteins, several of which are phosphoproteins. Once the enamel is completely mineralized, only small phosphopeptides (a compound of phosphorus with two or more amino acids) remain. The rest of the protein is lost.

The calcification mechanism of enamel is not as clear as that of bone, dentin, and cementum. The most probable theory involves initial nucleation of apatite on outer layer dentin crystals followed by growth across tissue. Collagen from hard and soft tissues have similar molecular structures and composition but different fiber organization and different physical properties. The crosslinks of collagen keep the fibers organized three-dimensionally, which allows crystals to fill in between. When the collagen molecules assemble in fibrils, the regions where the crystals form become the channels

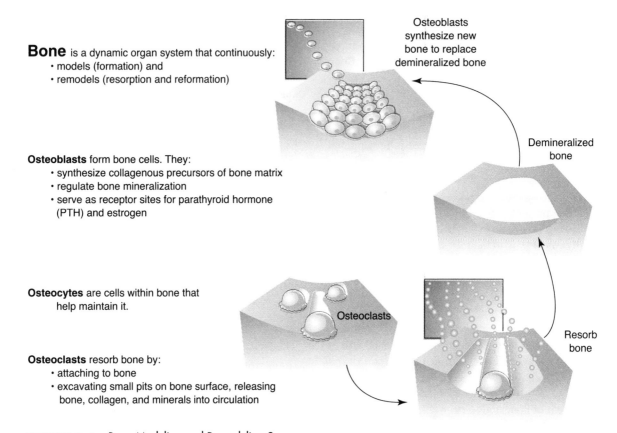

Bone is a dynamic organ system that continuously:
- models (formation) and
- remodels (resorption and reformation)

Osteoblasts form bone cells. They:
- synthesize collagenous precursors of bone matrix
- regulate bone mineralization
- serve as receptor sites for parathyroid hormone (PTH) and estrogen

Osteocytes are cells within bone that help maintain it.

Osteoclasts resorb bone by:
- attaching to bone
- excavating small pits on bone surface, releasing bone, collagen, and minerals into circulation

Osteoblasts synthesize new bone to replace demineralized bone

Demineralized bone

Osteoclasts

Resorb bone

FIGURE 8-1 Bone Modeling and Remodeling Sequence.

TABLE 8-3 Steps in Mineralization of Teeth

- Ameloblasts release calcium and phosphate.
- They form an amorphous mass.
- Calcium and phosphate are organized by the matrix.
- Nucleation occurs.
- Crystallites grow into ribbons.
- Ribbons coalesce to crystals.
- Fluid is displaced as the crystals grow.

that direct the formation and growth of the mineral crystallites. Table 8–3 shows the steps in the mineralization of teeth.

THE MINERALIZING MINERALS

The following minerals interact in the proper development and continued integrity of bones and teeth. They also serve many other important functions in the body.

Calcium

Calcium is the most abundant mineral in the body. Of the approximately 1200 g present in the adult, 99% are located in the skeleton.

Functions

Although the majority of calcium in the body is in the structure of bones and teeth, the remaining calcium has functions so essential to life that they take first priority over bone mineralization. Functions of calcium include the following:

- Regulation of ion transport across cell membranes.
- Normal muscle and nerve activity, such as heart contraction. Contraction and relaxation of the heart muscle depend on a proper ratio of calcium to sodium, potassium, and magnesium ions. Deficiency will increase the irritability of nervous

tissue and may cause tetany (sustained muscular contraction) with convulsions.

- Formation of the enzyme thrombin (together with prothrombin and thromboplastin), which acts in blood coagulation.
- A cofactor to activate enzymes such as pancreatic lipase and alkaline phosphatase.
- Activation of rennin, which causes the curdling of milk during its digestion.
- Synthesis and release of neurotransmitters (e.g., acetylcholine, serotonin, and norepinephrine), substances from nerve endings that aid in the transmission of nerve impulses.
- Chromosome movement before cell division.

Metabolism

Some calcium is absorbed in the stomach, but most is absorbed by active transport from the upper small intestine. Factors that enhance its absorption include acid pH, vitamins C and D, some amino acids, lactose, and increased body need. In blood circulation, most calcium is transported either as an ion or bound to the protein albumin.

Calcium blood levels are maintained within a narrow range and regulated by parathyroid hormone, calcitonin (a hormone produced by the thyroid), and metabolically active vitamin D (Table 8–4). For example, if blood levels begin to fall, two hormones—parathyroid hormone and the active form of vitamin D—intervene to increase calcium concentration. Opposing them is calcitonin (secreted by the thyroid gland). If calcium levels begin to rise, calcitonin is secreted and the calcium level decreases back to the normal range. The chief storage deposit of calcium is bone trabeculae in the ends of the long bones. Bones are metabolically very active tissues. Minerals can be withdrawn from the trabeculae when needed. Each day from 250 to 1,000 mg of calcium enter and leave bones. The body tends to maintain a continuous dynamic equilibrium between minerals that are stored in the bone and those found in the blood. The blood acts as a pool or reserve. The diet and bone resorption contribute to the pool, and bone and tooth formation cause the minerals to be taken from the pool. The degree of development of the bone trabeculae, where osteoid tissue is formed, and the amount of calcium deposited are directly related to the amount of calcium available from the diet. Blood within the trabeculae transports the calcium and phosphate salts to the tissues and structures that need them.

TABLE 8–4 Hormones That Regulate Calcium Metabolism

Parathyroid Hormone (PTH)
- Secretion regulated by serum calcium levels
  Low calcium →
- Bone:↑ bone resorption
- Kidneys: ↑ phosphate excretion → ↑ calcium resorption

Calcitonin
- Fine-tunes calcium metabolisms by inhibiting bone resorption
- Counters PTH

Active Form Vitamin D
(1,25 HO- Vit D)
- ↑ Calcium absorption from intestine
- ↑ Bone deposition

The body is considered to be in calcium balance when there is sufficient calcium absorbed to meet body requirements for growth and tissue regeneration. Negative calcium balance exists when insufficient calcium is consumed, and the body must mobilize calcium from bone to maintain necessary blood levels (Figure 8–2).

Excess calcium is excreted in the urine. Some calcium is found in the feces as well. Of a dietary intake of 1,000 mg of calcium, 700 to 800 mg is excreted. There is a relatively unimportant daily loss of 15 mg of calcium via perspiration. When the serum calcium level or the dietary intake is low, absorption of calcium is more efficient and thus less is excreted.

During lactation a mother loses between 150 and 300 mg of calcium daily in her milk. This is replenished by calcium either from food or from bone reserves. Normally the level of calcium in the serum is unaffected by lactation, which indicates that the body, through the homeostatic mechanism, usually functions well with respect to calcium regulation (Figure 8–3).

The body maintains tightly controlled calcium homeostatic levels in blood. To measure body stores, the bones must be radiographically analyzed. However, as much as 30–40% of bone calcium must be lost before radiographic changes are detected.

Requirements and Range of Safety

As knowledge has increased about the functions of calcium in the body, particularly its role in bone health, recommendations for calcium intake have been revised

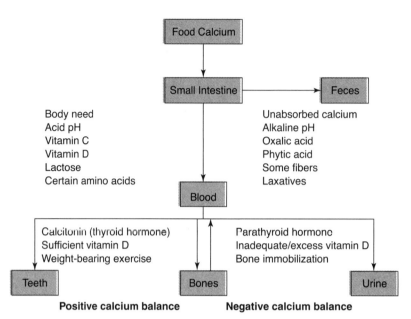

FIGURE 8-2 Factors affecting calcium balance.
Source: From *Robinson's Basic Nutrition and Diet Therapy:* 8/E by
Weigley/Mueller/Robinson, © 1997. Reprinted with permission.

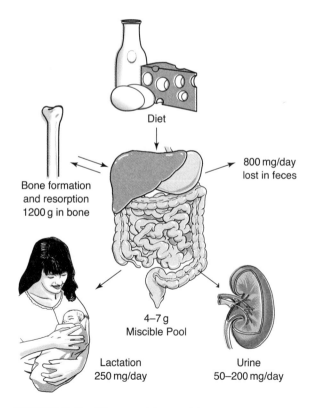

FIGURE 8-3 Dietary calcium activity.

upward and range from 1000 to 1200 mg/day for adults. Actual intakes are much lower than recommended (IOM, 1997). The upper level of safety (UL) is set at 2.5g/day.

Food Sources

Calcium is widely distributed in varying amounts in foods, with the highest concentration and bioavailability coming from milk-based dairy products. Several dark green leafy vegetables such as kale, turnip greens, mustard greens, and collards are also sources of bioavailable calcium, but unrealistically large amounts would have to be consumed daily to meet daily calcium requirements.

Other greens such as spinach, chard, and beet greens (as well as cocoa) are not good calcium sources because they contain oxalic acid, which combines with calcium to form an insoluble complex and reduces calcium absorption. Similarly, phytic acid, an organic acid found in the outer layers of whole grains, can also form a complex with some of the calcium. Legumes (peas, nuts) contain calcium, but the calcium absorption from legumes is also impaired by the phytic acid and fiber contents. Although grains are not particularly rich in calcium, they can provide substantial calcium if consumed in large quantities.

Canned fish with bones, such as herring, salmon, and sardines, are also sources of calcium if the bones are eaten. However, again, it would be impractical to consume enough of these foods to meet daily calcium requirements (Table 8–5).

Calcium Supplements

Because many people are unable to consume milk products as a result of lactose intolerance (see Chapter 4), there has been increased interest in developing alternative calcium sources. Calcium-fortified orange juice is particularly useful, as the form of calcium added to the juice (calcium citrate) is absorbed best by older individuals who suffer from lack of stomach acid. Tofu preserved in calcium is also a good alternative calcium source.

A variety of calcium supplements is available for those unable to meet calcium requirements through food. Some, such as calcium carbonate or citrate, are

TABLE 8–5 Food Sources of Calcium

200–300 mg
Milk (whole, skim, low-fat), yogurt/cup
Calcium-fortified orange juice/cup
Swiss cheese, Cheddar cheese, American cheese
    (processed)/oz
Soymilk (fortified)/cup
Tofu (with, calcium)/$\frac{1}{2}$ cup
Dried figs—5
Soynuts $\frac{1}{2}$ cup
Sardines, canned with bones/3 oz

100–200 mg/serv
Cottage cheese/$\frac{1}{2}$ cup
Collard greens, turnip greens/$\frac{1}{2}$ cup
Salmon, canned with bones/3 oz
Navy beans, baked beans, white beans (cooked)/cup
Blackstrap molasses/1 Tbsp

20–99 mg/serv
Most fruits/$\frac{1}{2}$ cup
Most vegetables/$\frac{1}{2}$ cup
Most meat, fish, peanut butter, eggs/oz
Almonds/2 Tbsp

Source: Adapted from Miller GD, Jarvis JK, McBean LD: *Handbook of Dairy Foods and Nutrition*, 2nd ed. National Dairy Council. Boca Raton, FL: CRC Press, 2000.

highly bioavailable. Natural sources such as those made from bonemeal and dolomite have calcium that is not as bioavailable. More important, they may contain harmful levels of toxic metals such as lead.

Effects of Too Little Calcium (Hypocalcemia)

Calcium deficiency becomes evident only after years of insufficient intake. People at risk for deficiency include those with insufficient calcium intake, and those with milk allergies, lactose intolerance, and malabsorptive conditions. Immobilization and lack of weight-bearing physical activity increase calcium release from bone storage; this places nonambulatory and inactive people at risk for bone loss of calcium and subsequent osteoporosis. (Osteoporosis is discussed in detail in Chapter 11 on chronic conditions) (USDHHS, 2004).

A healthy person can have a calcium intake of about 2500 mg (more than twice the RDA) without any appreciable effect on calcium excreted in the urine. About 80% of kidney stones contain calcium, chiefly as calcium oxalate.

Oral Implications of Inadequate Calcium Intake

The oral implications of inequate calcium intake, impaired absorption, and increased loss include incomplete calcification of teeth, tooth and bone malformations, increased susceptibility to dental caries, excessive periodontal bone resorption, increased tooth mobility and premature tooth loss, and increased risk of hemorrage. Recent research indicates that people in their 20s and 30s who have the least calcium intake (<500 mg/day) have the highest risk for gingival detachment (Grossi, 1998). This supports earlier research showing that postmenopausal women who lost teeth also lost bone density at a faster rate than women who did not lose teeth (Krall, Dawson-Hughes, Papas, Garcia, 1994).

Effects of Too Much Calcium (Hypercalcemia)

Conditions of calcium excess have not been observed in healthy people. When toxic signs were noted, the cause usually was related to excess vitamin D or to a disease state, such as parathyroid or kidney diseases.

Certain conditions such as idiopathic hypercalcemia (excess calcium in blood) of infancy, hypercalcinuria (excess calcium in urine), hyperparathyroidism, alkali syndrome, and kidney stones result in high levels of calcium in the blood and/or urine and ectopic calcification (calcification of the soft tissues).

Summary and Implications for Dentistry of Calcium

Calcium is essential for mineralization and a variety of other physiological functions. Insufficient calcium consumption is a major problem, especially in females. Before age 30, sufficient calcium is needed to promote peak bone mass development. Through adulthood and particularly after menopause, adequate intake is needed to help maintain bone density and counteract bone loss. Deficient consumption leads to increased risk of osteoporosis and related disorders including possible increased alveolar bone loss. For these reasons, the recommended allowances for calcium have been increased. Patients should be strongly encouraged to consume adequate calcium from a variety of sources daily. Dental professionals should provide patients with resources that will assist them in achieving adequate calcium intake.

Phosphorus

About 85% of phosphorus is located in bones and teeth. The remaining amount is found in muscles, organs, blood, and other fluids. This mineral exists either as an ion or in bound form, such as with phospholipids and phosphoproteins.

Functions

Besides its role in the formation of bones and teeth, phosphorus functions as a major buffer for the body, is a component of many enzymes, and is necessary for muscle contraction and nerve activity. Of importance, it is part of the compounds adenosine triphosphate (ATP) and adenosine diphosphate (ADP), which store and release energy according to body needs. Phosphorus is part of deoxyribonucleic acid (DNA) and ribonucleic acid (RNA).

Metabolism

Nearly all ingested phosphorus is absorbed. The presence of high levels of other cations such as magnesium, aluminum, and calcium, lessens absorption. Absorption is by both active and passive transport mechanisms, with vitamin D playing a role. On a mixed diet, absorption can range from 55 to 70%. The kidneys maintain body homeostasis by excreting more or less phosphorus, according to body needs.

Requirements and Range of Safety

The requirements are based on the amount needed to maintain serum phosphorus at the lower end of the normal range for healthy individuals at various life stages. The RDA is 700 mg/day for adults. The upper range of safety is from 3–4 g/day.

Food Sources

Phosphorus is widely found in foods and as an additive. If the diet supplies enough calcium and protein, it will tend to furnish sufficient phosphorus; dairy foods are the best sources. Plant seeds (beans, peas, cereals, nuts) and animal foods are also good sources. Additionally, many processed foods and carbonated beverages contain phosphates for nonnutrient functions such as moisture retention, smoothness, and binding. The consumption of phosphates has increased substantially over the past 20 years from both foods and additives.

Effects of Too Little Phosphorus (Hypophosphatemia)

Neither deficiency nor toxicity appears to occur in healthy people. Because the kidneys play a pivotal role in body balance, their dysfunction can lead to serious phosphorus imbalances, as can near total starvation. Excessive intake of aluminum-containing antacids can bind dietary phosphorus in the gut and produce hypophosphatemia.

Oral Implications of Phosphorus Deficiency

Phosphorus deficiency has been associated with incomplete calcification of teeth, increased caries susceptibility if present during tooth development, and increased susceptibility to periodontal disease via its effect on alveolar bone (DePaola, Tauger-Decker, Faine, 2005).

Effects of Too Much Phosphorus (Hyperphosphatemia)

The principal results of too much phosphorus include changes in the hormonal control system that regulates calcium, calcification of the kidney, possible increased porosity of the skeleton, and possible reduced calcium absorption.

Summary and Implications for Dentistry of Phosphorus

Phosphorus is an important mineral that is an essential component of all known tissues in both plants and animals. Because phosphorus is prevalent in foods, an adequate diet should provide sufficient phosphorus as well. With the increasing use of phosphates as food additives, and with increasing soda consumption, there is some concern that intakes may become excessive in the future. This is another reason to urge moderation in the use of phosphorus-containing beverages like colas.

Magnesium

The entire adult body contains about 25 g (1000 millimoles [mmol]) of magnesium, of which 50–60% is located in bones and teeth. About 40% is in muscles and organs, and the remaining (about 1%) in the extracellular fluids.

Functions

Magnesium plays a major role in bone and mineral physiology. Magnesium also

- activates more than 300 enzymes, especially those related to storing and releasing energy. (It forms complexes with ATP.)
- together with calcium, sodium, and potassium, regulates the transmission of nerve impulses and the contraction of muscles. Calcium is necessary for muscles to contract, and magnesium is necessary for them to relax.
- ensures proper DNA and RNA formation and function.
- facilitates parathyroid hormone secretion.
- ensures vitamin D conversion in the liver.
- facilitates blood clotting.

Metabolism

Magnesium absorption occurs along the entire length of the small intestine. Healthy people absorb between 40 and 60% of magnesium consumed. Body need influences absorption, which occurs by both active and passive transport. Absorption is enhanced by vitamin D and decreased by high amounts of calcium, phosphorus, and fat. Bones are magnesium's major long-term storage site. The kidney is the principal organ responsible for magnesium homeostasis. Up to 90% of filtered magnesium is reabsorbed by the kidneys in response to salt and water reabsorption and the rate of fluid flow.

High levels of dietary fiber from fruits, vegetables, and grains can decrease magnesium absorption and/or retention probably by the binding of magnesium to

phosphate groups on phytic acid. Dietary protein can also influence intestinal magnesium absorption. Absorption of magnesium is lower when protein intake is less than 30 g/day. It is somewhat difficult to determine precise body balance of magnesium. Nevertheless, the most available and commonly used test is the measurement of serum magnesium concentration.

Requirements and Range of Safety

The body is able to maintain close regulation of blood levels of magnesium. The RDAs are based primarily upon balance studies. Elderly people have relatively low dietary intakes of magnesium. This may be due to decreased appetite, decreased absorption, and increased excretion. A diet low in magnesium can place elders at risk for deficiency. The RDA for magnesium ranges from 320 to 420 mg/day for adults. The upper limit of safety is 350 mg/day of supplemental magnesium.

Food Sources

Magnesium is widely distributed in foods, but the magnesium content of foods varies. Because magnesium is a constituent of chlorophyll in plants, dark green vegetables are a particularly rich source. Whole grains and nuts are high in magnesium, whereas meats, starches, and milk are lower. Refined foods have the lowest magnesium content. "Hard" water is a reliable source as a beverage and in foods prepared with water.

About half of dietary magnesium comes from vegetables, fruits, grains, and nuts, with about one-third coming from milk, meat, and eggs.

Effects of Too Little Magnesium

Deficiency or toxicity is rare in healthy people. Deficiency can occur with prolonged vomiting, severe malabsorption, kidney disease, intestinal surgery, cirrhosis of the liver, and excessive use of over-the-counter and prescription medications that interfere with absorption or excretion (e.g., corticosteroids, diuretics). Nearly all chronic alcoholics have symptoms of magnesium depletion (Abbott, Nadler, Rude, 1994). The initial sign of magnesium deficiency is neuromuscular hyperexcitability. Latent tetany, spontaneous hand or foot spasms, and generalized seizures may also occur. Magnesium depletion is also associated with cardiac arrhythmias, atrial fibrillation, and ventricular tachycardia (Ma et al., 1995). Magnesium deficiency may also be a risk factor for postmenopausal osteoporosis and may worsen the control of diabetes.

Oral Implications of Magnesium Deficiency

Magnesium deficiency has been related to increased fragility of alveolar bone and gingival hypertrophy (DePaola et al., 2005).

Effects of Too Much Magnesium

Adverse effects of too much magnesium have been seen with excessive use of nonfood sources such as medications. The most common manifestations of excess intake are diarrhea, nausea, and cramping. Deaths from very large intake of magnesium sulfate or magnesium oxide have been reported, especially in those with renal insufficiency.

Summary and Implications for Dentistry of Magnesium

Magnesium is a mineral that works in tandem with calcium and has a variety of functions in the body. It is easily obtained if the diet contains plenty of fresh foods and whole grains. Deficiency and toxicity are uncommon and most often related to kidney disfunction. Patients should be cautioned to avoid overdoses of magnesium via supplements or drugs, as the results can be harmful.

Fluoride

Fluoride is a natural element found at varying concentrations in all drinking water as well as in soil. It is considered a beneficial nutrient and is present in trace amounts in the body. Fluoride is deposited in calcified structures of the body such as in bones and teeth. Body content of fluoride depends on intake from water and food sources.

Functions

Fluoride is important for the integrity of bones and teeth. When consumed in optimal amounts in water and food and used topically in toothpastes, rinses, and office treatments, fluoride reduces the risk and prevalence of dental caries. Fluoride also helps increase bone density (Position of the American Dietetic Association, 2000; Warren, Levy, 2003).

The relationship between fluoride and dental caries was first noted in the early part of the 20th century when it was observed that residents of certain areas of the country developed brown stains on their teeth. These stained teeth, though unsightly, were highly resistant to decay. Active research through the 1930s

culminated in the discovery that the prevalence and severity of this type of mottled enamel (dental fluorosis) were directly associated with the amount of fluoride in the water. It was later noted that fluoride consumption at "optimal" concentrations (0.7 to 1.2 parts per million [ppm]) in the water supply imparted protection against development of dental caries without staining teeth. The results of numerous long-term community trials in which fluoride has been added to water supplies at an optimal level verify the effectiveness, safety, and economy of this public health measure in reducing the prevalence of dental caries (Winston, Bhaskar, 1999). Although the early studies focused primarily on children, water fluoridation has also been found effective in preventing dental caries in adults.

More recently, the possible role of fluoride in strengthening bone and thus helping prevent fractures has inspired much new research. However, practical implications of fluoride in this process are conflicting.

Mechanisms of Fluoride Action on Teeth

Preeruptive Systemic Effects Fluoride is incorporated into the developing tooth's mineralized structure during the course of tooth development. In the presence of fluoride, the hydroxyl ion (OH) in tooth hydroxyapatite crystal $(Ca_{10}[PO_4]_6[OH]_2)$ is exchanged with the fluoride ion, forming either a mixed fluorhydroxylapatite $(Ca_{10}[PO_4]_6 FOH)$ or a fluorapatite crystalline structure $(Ca_{10}[PO_4]_6 F_2)$. The fluoride ion makes the apat crystal less soluble and thus more resistant. Prenatal fluoride is not thought to benefit developing dentition, because only minimal tooth mineralization occurs before birth (Leverett, Adair, Vaughan, Proskin, Moss, 1997). Thus, the use of systemic fluoride above amounts normally obtained through water and food is not indicated for pregnant women (NAS Subcommittee, 1990).

After birth, the infant should obtain appropriate systemic fluoride either via a fluoridated water supply or through supplementation after 6 months of age (see the section on supplementation that follows). The presence of fluoride in the dental enamel helps increase resistance to demineralization when the erupted tooth surface is exposed to organic acids. However, systemic fluoride during tooth formation is no longer believed to provide the most important benefit in preventing dental caries.

Posteruptive Systemic Effects During tooth development, fluoride is incorporated into the developing tooth's mineralized structure. Although this is no longer believed to be the most important reason for the effect of fluoride in dental caries, the presence of fluoride in the dental enamel probably increases resistance to demineralization when the tooth surface is exposed to organic acids.

Posteruptive Topical Effects The posteruptive beneficial effect of fluoride likely occurs primarily from the presence of fluoride in the fluid phase at the tooth surface. The fluoride is responsible for decreasing demineralization when the tooth is exposed to organic acids and for increasing the rate of remineralization.

After tooth eruption, fluoride is no longer involved systemically in tooth formation. However, consumed fluoride is excreted through the saliva and can contribute topically to enamel protection throughout the lifetime (Hillier et al., 2000).

Topical mechanisms are now considered the primary means by which fluoride imparts protection to teeth for children and adults (Hillier et al., 2000). Proposed mechanisms of action include the following (CDC, 2001; Featherstone, 1999):

- Increased resistance to acid demineralization
- Remineralization of incipient lesions
- Interference in the formation and functioning of dental plaque microorganisms
- Increased rate of posteruptive maturation
- Improved tooth morphology (preeruptive)

The frequency of fluoride exposure to the tooth surface is the prime factor in maintaining high fluoride concentration in the fluid phase of enamel surfaces. This helps prevent caries and enhances the remineralization of early carious lesions (Hillier et al., 2000). Topical fluoride may be particularly important in the prevention of root and coronal caries in adults and older people; it is also an effective desensitizing agent.

In addition to its direct mineralizing effect on enamel, fluoride also affects oral plaque bacteria *(Streptococcus mutans)*. The entry of fluoride into the bacterial cell interferes with acid production, thus reducing potential enamel destruction (Featherstone, 1999).

Effects on Bone Health

The skeletal content of fluoride is directly correlated with the usual fluoride intake from foods and drinking waters (depending on geographic location), and the fluoride content of the skeleton increases with age (Elbe, Deaton, Wilson, Bawden, 1992).

Fluoride is one of only a few known agents that can stimulate bone cell (osteoblast) proliferation (Farley, Wergedal, Baylink, 1983) and increase new mineral deposition (in cancellous bone, but not in cortical bone). However, early optimism that osteoporosis risk was lower in fluoridated communities has not been supported (Sowers, Clark, Jannausch, Wallace, 1991). The contribution of fluoride in drinking water, at 1 ppm (1mg/L), to skeletal fluoride content is not considered to be sufficient to prevent osteoporotic fractures, except possibly in elderly subjects with reduced renal function. An intake of fluoridated water at a level higher than 1 ppm may actually increase the risk of skeletal fractures (Hillier et al., 2000), especially over decades of exposure. The l ppm level is widely accepted as being safe and without risk of fracture (Featherstone, 1999).

Metabolism

Fluoride absorption occurs rapidly, directly from the stomach. The rate and degree of absorption depend on the solubility of the source and the amount ingested at a given time. Ingested fluoride is better absorbed from drinking water than from food. Once absorbed into the bloodstream, fluoride is either deposited into bones and developing teeth or excreted in the urine (60–70%). During tooth development, fluoride is incorporated into the developing tooth's mineralized apatite structure. This systemic effect is no longer believed to be the most important reason for the effect of fluoride in dental caries.

Requirements and Range of Safety

Requirements for fluoride are based on its uptake by bones and teeth. The RDA for fluoride is set at the level of an adequate intake (AI) and is 3 mg/day for adult women and 4 mg/day for adult men. The UL for adults is 10 mg/day.

Sources

The fluoridated community water supply is a major source of fluoride. The definition of *fluoridation* is the adjustment of the water to contain from 0.8 to 1.2 ppm of fluoride. This is the amount that has been determined to confer optimum protection against dental caries. (This is equal to 1 part of fluoride to 1 million parts water or about 1 mg per quart) (ADA, 1998). The estimated amount of fluoride consumed from fluoridated drinking water by adults ranges from 1.8 to 2.7 mg/day (Featherstone, 1999), assuming the consumption of fluoridated fluids each day. This amount may be overestimated for many females who may consume less than 1.5 L/day of water containing fluoride.

The water used in commercial and household food preparation is another source. This includes fluoridated water used to make pastas, rice, cooked cereals, soups, frozen juices, powdered beverages, ice cubes, and sodas. The fluoride content of bottled water varies and is often low (McGuire, 1989). Nevertheless, fluoride from beverages, in meal preparation, and in the reconstitution of soups and beverages can add up (Tate, Chan, 1994). For this reason, potential sources of high fluoride intake in children's diets (particularly in infants) should be identified before any fluoride supplementation is recommended (Chaudhury, Brown, Shepherd, 1990).

Home water treatment systems can also affect the fluoride content of the filtered water. Reverse osmosis systems and distillation units remove significant amounts of fluoride from water (Brown, Aaron, 1991), whereas water softeners do not seem to change fluoride levels, and water filters vary in their ability to remove fluoride from water (Robinson, Davies, Williams, 1991). Therefore, people using home water treatment systems should have their water tested by local or state public health departments or private laboratories to monitor fluoride content.

Food sources of fluoride vary greatly depending on the region's fluoride content of water and soil. Ocean fish eaten with bones (such as salmon, herring, and sardines) and tea are excellent sources (Clovis, Hargreaves, Thompson, 1988; Nutrient Data Laboratory, 2004). Bottled waters vary greatly in their fluoride content (Johnson, DeBiase, 2003). Most bottled waters contain low concentrations of fluoride, so drinking strictly bottled water may not provide sufficient fluoride to maintain optimal dental health. (See Table 8–6) Topical sources of fluoride include application in the dental office, home and school topical applications, fluoride oral rinses, and fluoride-containing dentifrices. Small amounts of fluoride from these sources may be swallowed and contribute to daily intake. This is of some concern in young children.

Fluoride Supplementation

For children who do not have fluoridated water, fluoride-containing vitamin supplements may be indicated and should be prescribed by the child's pediatrician and/or dentist. Table 8–7 provides fluoride supplementation guidelines for children. As stated previously, bonemeal and dolomite may be high in fluoride, but also may contain toxic levels of undesirable minerals like lead and arsenic.

There is little indication that the use of fluorides prenatally will confer meaningful systemic benefits to the developing fetus. Thus, there is little justification for recommending prenatal use of systemic fluoride above amounts normally obtained through water and food (NAS Subcommittee, 1990).

Although the concentration of fluoride in breast milk is very low, many mothers combine breastfeeding with formula use and may give infants drinking water between feedings. Thus, fluoride supplements are not generally recommended for breastfed infants residing in fluoridated communities.

Effects of Too Little Fluoride

No deficiency symptoms have been reported, other than the increased risk for dental caries (Report to the ad hoc Subcommittee, 1991; Riley, Lennon, Ellwood, 1999).

Effects of Too Much Fluoride

Fluoridation does not increase the incidence or mortality rate of any chronic condition, including cancer, heart disease, intracranial lesions, nephritis, cirrhosis, and Down syndrome (NRC, 1993). However, excess fluoride in developing teeth can result in fluorosis (Figure 8–4). Depending on the degree of fluorosis, the appearance of irregularly distributed patches in tooth enamel can range from chalky white to yellow, to gray, and even to brown or black. Fluorosis can occur in children when the concentration of ingested fluoride is from 2 to 8 mg/body weight. In cases of mild fluorosis, teeth are highly caries resistant in spite of the chalky white patches. This mild fluorosis, for the most part, may be detectable only during dental examinations and is not cosmetically objectionable. In recent years, with the broader availability of systemic fluoride from various sources, there has been an increase in the prevalence of mild fluorosis, which has been attributed to several factors (Horowitz, 1999; Warren, Levy, 1999):

- Early use of fluoride toothpaste
- Misused dietary fluoride supplements
- Long-term use of infant formula, particularly powder concentrates reconstituted with fluoridated water

TABLE 8–6   Fluoride in Foods and Beverages

Food or Beverage	Range of Fluoride (Content per Serving in ppm [mg/L])
Soft drinks	0.02–1.28 ppm About 77% of soft drinks had fluoride levels above 0.6 ppm (Levy, 2003).
Juices Grape juice tends to have a higher fluoride content than other juices.	0.02–2.80 ppm Over 42% had fluoride levels greater than 0.6 ppm.
Bottled waters Nonfluoride With fluoride	 0.0–2.58 ppm 0.8–4.00 ppm
Tea	1–6 ppm brewed Depends upon the amount of tea used, the fluoride in the water used, and the length of brewing (Lu, Guo, Yang).

Infant foods
Infant formulas (not reconstituted)
    Ready to feed
    Liquid concentrate
    Powder concentrate
Dry infant cereals
Ready-to-eat infant foods
Chicken products for infants are 20 times higher than infant fruit (Tomori et al.).
Soy-based formulas are higher in fluoride than milk-based formulas (Van Winkle, 1995).
	
	0.04–0.55
	0.04–0.10
	0.05–0.28
	0.05–0.52
	0.01–8.38
	0.5 mg/kg/day is the maximum amount infants above age 6 months should receive daily from all sources (Levy, 2003).

Sources: Adapted from Levy, 2003; USDA National Fluoride Database of Selected Beverages and Foods, http://www.nal.usda.gov/fnic/foodcomp/Data/Fluoride/fluoride.pdf and Tracking Fluoride in the National Food Supply, http://www.ars.usda.gov/is/pr/2004.

TABLE 8–7   Recommendation for Fluoride Supplementation 1994 Concentration of Fluoride Ion in Drinking Water

Age (Years)	<0.3	0.3–0.6	>0.6 ppm
6 mos. To 3 yrs	0.25 mg	0	0
3 to 6	0.50 mg	0.25 mg	0
6 to 16	1.0 mg	0.50 mg	0

Source: American Dental Association: *American Dental Association Supports Fluoridation.* Council on Access, Prevention, and Interprofessional Relations Report, January 1998.

- "Diffusion" (or "halo" effect) of fluoride from foods and beverages processed in fluoridated areas and consumed by people in fluoridated as well as fluoride-deficient areas

Long-term daily ingestion of 10 mg/L of fluoride in drinking water has resulted in skeletal fluorosis (*Fluoride and Oral Health*, 1994). Fluoride can be toxic if consumed in large amounts, as when small children drink topical fluoride solution from the bottle.

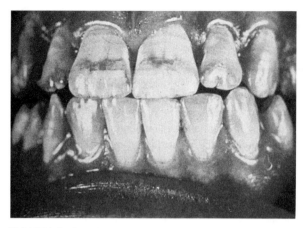

FIGURE 8–4   Fluorosis.

Summary and Implications for Dentistry of Fluoride

Fluoride is a mineral that enhances tooth and bone health when provided in optimal amounts through the life span. Fluoride increases tooth resistance to dental caries, primarily through topical effects. Fluoridation of public water supplies has been endorsed by most professional health organizations (ADA, 1998) as the most effective dental public health measure in existence. The effects of fluoride on bone are less well delineated. Fluoride is obtained primarily via fluoridated water and foods and beverages containing fluoridated water (and topical sources like dentifrices). Other food sources vary in their fluoride content depending upon the soil and water where they are grown. Highest food sources are fish, tea, and milk. The dental team should:

- see that young children obtain appropriate amounts of fluoride (Table 8–7).
- educate patients of all ages on the benefits of topical fluoride in caries prevention throughout life.
- educate patients on how to avoid excess fluoride consumption.

Summary and Implications for Dentistry of the Mineralizing Minerals

Optimal mineralization of bones and teeth is essential for lifelong health and must begin early (Table 8–8). Peak bone mass accretion occurs by age 30. Calcium is essential for mineralization and a variety of other physiological functions. Before age 30, sufficient calcium is needed to promote peak bone mass development. Through adulthood and particularly after menopause, adequate intake is needed to help maintain bone density and counteract bone loss. Insufficient calcium consumption is a major problem, especially in females. In children and teenagers, milk intake is often replaced by nonnutritious soda. Older persons may be lactose deficient and unable to tolerate milk products, which are the most concentrated natural sources of calcium.

Phosphorus is an essential component of all known tissues and is plentiful in foods. An adequate diet should provide sufficient phosphorus as well. With the increasing use of phosphates as food additives and with increasing soda consumption, there is some concern that intakes may become excessive in the future. Magnesium works in tandem with calcium and phosphorus and is also easily obtained in a diet containing plenty of fresh foods and whole grains. Patients should avoid overdoses of magnesium via supplements or drugs, as the results can be harmful.

Fluoride enhances tooth and bone health when provided in optimal amounts throughout life. Fluoride increases tooth resistance to dental caries, primarily through topical effects. Fluoridation of public water supplies has been endorsed by most professional health organizations (Position of the American Dietetic Association, 2000) as the most effective dental public health measure in existence. The effects of fluoride on bone are less well delineated. Fluoride is obtained primarily via fluoridated water and foods and beverages containing fluoridated water (and topical sources such as dentifrices). Other food sources vary in their fluoride content depending on the soil and water where they are grown. Food sources highest in fluoride are fish, tea, and milk.

Dental team members should help patients achieve optimal mineralization of teeth and bones by:

- educating them about the importance of calcium (and phosphorus and magnesium) to general and dental health.
- providing information on good mineral food sources, including alternatives to dairy products when needed.
- encouraging parents to help children increase calcium-rich beverages such as milk-based drinks in place of carbonated beverages.
- educating patients of all ages on the benefits of topical fluoride in caries prevention throughout life.

TABLE 8-8   Summary of the Mineralizing Minerals

Mineral	Metabolism and Function	Deficiency or Excess	Oral Implications	Requirements and Food Sources
Calcium	*Metabolism:* 99% in bones and teeth; 10 to 40% absorbed—aided by vitamin C, D, and lactose, hindered by oxalic acid, fiber, and basic pH *Functions:* Transport of ions; muscle contraction; blood clotting; activates enzymes; synthesis/ release of neurotransmitters	*Deficiency:* Incomplete calcification of teeth/ bones; excessive bone resorption; osteoporosis; ↑ tendency to hemorrhage; rickets; bone fragility *Excess:* Toxicity not seen	*Deficiency:* Leads to incomplete calcification of teeth; ↑ tooth mobility; premature loss of teeth	*AI:* Men and women: 1000 mg up to 50 yr, 1200 mg 51+ yr *Sources:* Milk, cheese, ice cream, fortified soymilk, fortified orange juice, green leafy vegetables (mustard and turnip greens, broccoli), sardines
Phosphorus	*Metabolism:* 80–90% in bones and teeth; vitamin D favors absorption *Functions:* Formation of bones and teeth; acid-base balance; transport of fats; enzymes for energy metabolism; protein synthesis; necessary for muscle contraction; needed for DNA/RNA	*Deficiency:* Dietary deficiency unlikely *Excess:* Potential for increased skeletal porosity	*Deficiency:* Leads to incomplete calcification of teeth—contributing to osteomalacia or osteoporosis; potential for compromised alveolar bone integrity	*RDA:* Men and women: 700 mg *Sources:* Milk, cheese, ice cream, meat, poultry, fish, whole grain cereals, nuts, legumes
Magnesium	*Metabolism:* 60% in bones and teeth; absorption ↑ by vitamin D and acid, ↓ by high amounts of calcium, phosphorus, and fat; stored in bone; kidney responsible for homeostasis *Functions:* Bone cell function; hydroxyapatite crystal formation and growth; transmits nerve impulses; muscle contraction; enzymes for energy metabolism	*Deficiency:* Dietary deficiency unlikely— occurs in alcoholism, renal failure; ↑ risk for osteoporosis and alveolar bone fragility; neuromuscular hyperexcitability; spasms; cardiac complications *Excess:* Problems usually only from excess medications containing magnesium	*Deficiency:* Leads to alveolar bone fragility; gingival hypertrophy	*RDA:* Men: 400 mg 19−30 yr, 420 mg 31+ yr; Women: 320 mg 31+ yr *Sources:* Green leafy vegetables, legumes, whole grain cereals
Fluoride	*Metabolism:* Rapid absorption directly through the stomach; better absorbed from water than food; storage in bones and teeth *Functions:* Prevents tooth decay	*Deficiency:* ↓ resistance to dental caries *Excess:* Tooth mottling; enamel hypoplasia; ↓ caries resistance interference with amelogenesis	See Deficiency and Excess	*AI:* Men: 4.0 mg; Women 3 mg *Sources:* Fluoridated water, tea, foods and beverages prepared with fluoridated water, supplements

- informing patients how to avoid excess fluoride consumption.
- warning against arbitrary mineral supplementation.

THE ELECTROLYTES

Electrolytes are substances that dissociate into charged particles (ions) when dissolved in water or other solvents, and conduct electrical currents. Sodium, potassium, and chloride are the most abundant electrolytes in the body. These three are the main ions involved in maintaining the body's osmotic pressure, and fluid and electrolyte balance (Luft, 1996b).

The body maintains fluid homeostasis by balancing water intake and output through a variety of complex mechanisms. In the body, water is present in compartments. To maintain fluid and electrolyte balance, the proper amounts and kinds of electrolytes and fluids must be maintained in the various fluid compartments. An imbalance in one is usually accompanied by an imbalance in another.

In addition to their critical role in maintaining fluid balance, short-term exchange of Na^+ and K^+ ions across cell membranes is essential for transmitting nerve impulses and signaling muscle cells to contract. Potassium also helps maintain a steady heartbeat.

The body also maintains a steady acid-base balance so that the pH of the intracellular and extracellular fluids remains almost constant. The kidneys play a gatekeeper role in fluid, electrolyte, and acid-base balance by controlling the retention and excretion of ions and fluids. This process is moderated by hormones, such as aldosterone, which promotes potassium loss and reduces sodium loss in the urine.

The body's ability to maintain fluid and electrolyte balance is critical to health. An increase in sodium concentration in the blood (plasma osmolality) triggers the thirst center in the brain. Increased water intake decreases the plasma osmolality, which deactivates the thirst response. Thirst cannot be used as a sole monitor of hydration, however, because thirst recognition may be blunted with aging. Dehydration can be fatal, especially in the very young and the very old. Fluid and electrolyte balance can be impaired after vomiting, diarrhea, heavy sweating, high fever, burns, kidney disease, and other major illnesses. The dehydration and electrolyte imbalance can result from inadequate fluid and electrolyte intake, excessive losses, or both.

Sodium

Sodium is found in every cell of the body and is the major extracellular electrolyte. Half of the total body sodium is in the extracellular fluid, 40% in bone, and about 10% in the intracellular fluid.

Functions

Sodium is the major extracellular cation. Functions of sodium include cell permeability maintenance, muscle contraction, nerve impulse transmission, and acid-base balance. Sodium facilitates nutrient absorption, such as glucose and amino acids.

Metabolism

Nearly all ingested sodium is absorbed through the small intestine via active transport with glucose. Sodium homeostasis is maintained inside the body mainly by adrenal hormone control on the amount of sodium excreted by the kidneys. When sodium intake is high, aldosterone levels decrease, causing an increase in urinary sodium excretion. The reverse reactions occur when sodium intake is below the body's needs. Hormone levels increase, resulting in decreased sodium excretion. Sodium metabolism correlates with water balance. Varying amounts of sodium are excreted through the skin (sweat) and feces.

The healthy body is able to maintain sodium balance over a wide range of dietary intakes and environmental climates. The sodium content of a 24-hour urine collection is a good indicator of the previous day's dietary intake, compared to the amount needed by the body. Blood levels are easier to collect; serum sodium concentrations are measured routinely in health care settings.

Requirements and Range of Safety

Sodium requirement depends mostly on the amount lost and that needed to maintain extracellular fluid volume. For example, fluid volume increases during times of growth, such as infancy and pregnancy. A daily intake of as little as 0.5 g of sodium can maintain sodium balance in the body. This is contrasted to the usual daily intake, which averages from 2 to 6 g/day (2,000 to 6,000 mg) or higher. The RDA for sodium is set at the level of an adequate intake (AI) and is 1.5 g/day for adult men and women. The upper level of intake (UL) is set at 2.3 g/day.

Athletes such as long-distance runners and bikers, or people doing heavy work in hot environments, have increased sodium needs due to losses in perspiration.

Such losses usually can be replaced by adding extra salt to food before and after the activity. Water intake should be increased as well (see Chapter 7). Salt tablets are not recommended. Electrolyte replacement beverages may contain up to a gram of sodium per liter. They provide no particular benefit over water in the short term because electrolytes lost during exercise are readily replaced from food. (See Chapter 11 for more details on hypertension.)

Food Sources

Since sodium enhances food flavor, much sodium consumption results from habit and taste preference. Sodium is found widely in foods naturally, but a major source of sodium is added salt (sodium chloride). Because 40% of the weight of table salt is sodium, a little more than a teaspoon will provide 2.4 g (2400 mg) of sodium. Salt not only is used in home food preparation and at the table, but also is present in many fast foods and commercially processed foods. Examples are soups, ham, bacon, luncheon meats, smoked poultry and fish, cheese, pickles, olives, catsup, relishes, gravies, and snack foods such as potato chips, pretzels, crackers, and some sodas. Sodium is present in other compounds often used in food preparation, such as monosodium glutamate, baking powder, and baking soda. About three-fourths of the sodium present in fresh foods is from the milk and meat groups. In general, foods lowest in sodium are fresh fruits and vegetables, rice, pasta, and cooked cereals. Table 8–9 lists the sodium content of foods. "Softened" water, in which calcium and magnesium are removed and sodium is substituted, often is an overlooked contributor of sodium, as is the sodium in some medications.

Effects of Too Little Sodium (Hyponatremia)

Dietary deficiencies of sodium are rare. Sodium deficiency can result from extremely heavy sweating, especially in people before they adapt to extremely hot and humid climates. Infants are especially vulnerable. Other people at risk for sodium depletion are those experiencing severe vomiting or diarrhea, or who have conditions such as adrenal gland disease or cystic fibrosis.

Effects of Too Much Sodium (Hypernatremia)

Normally, healthy people can handle high intakes of sodium. However, when the body is unable to excrete excess sodium, additional water is held in the extracellular fluid. The resulting adema or ascites is characteristic of several pathological conditions, including congestive heart failure, renal failure, excessive secretion of cortical

TABLE 8–9   Sodium Content of Foods

Food	Sodium Content (in Milligrams [mg])
Salt (1 tsp)	2132
Commercial soups (1 c)	900–2100+
Beef bouillon (1 tsp)	960
Salad dressings (bottled, 1 Tbsp)	200
Frozen dinners	500–2000
Processed meats (2–3 oz)	350–1000+
Pickle, dill, small	800
Potato chips (1 oz bag)	360
Potato, 1 cooked	6
Bread and cereal	av. 250
Milk	av. 250
Fresh fruit	0
Fresh vegetables	<50
Fresh meats	<50

hormones by tumors of the adrenal gland, and liver disease. Steroid medications used in the therapy of several conditions, such as arthritis, inflammatory diseases, and organ transplants, can also lead to sodium and water retention. About one in four Americans has some elevation of blood pressure. Nearly half of these people are salt sensitive—that is, sodium intakes considered typical for most people lead to elevation of blood pressure for them. In all of these conditions, modification of sodium intake is included as part of therapy (see Chapter 11). Recent research by the National Heart, Lung, and Blood Institute (NHLBI) indicates that even in people without hypertension, the lower the amount of sodium in the diet, the lower the blood pressure.

Summary and Implications for Dentistry of Sodium

Sodium is an essential electrolyte for maintaining fluid equilibrium in the body. Deficiency is rare, but most often associated with dehydration via exercise or elderly people who have decreased kidney function. Most people consume much more sodium than they require to meet physiologic requirements. Much of the sodium consumed is either added during cooking or at the table, or hidden in processed foods or medications. Only those who are specifically salt sensitive need to be concerned with their sodium consumption. However, because it is not apparent who is and who is not salt sensitive the guidelines for a prudent diet suggest keeping consumption to about 2 g of sodium a day. Dental professionals can help by providing resources such as Table 8–9, which shows sodium content of foods.

Potassium

Potassium is the seventh most plentiful mineral on earth (Schardt, 2004). It is the major electrolyte in the intracellular fluids; 98% of total body potassium is intracellular. Because the highest potassium concentrations are in the skeletal muscle, the total amount of body potassium is closely correlated with lean body mass.

Functions

Potassium plays an essential role in maintaining fluid balance. It also serves other crucial functions such as:

- energy metabolism
- membrane transport
- normal contractions of all muscles, including the heart
- synthesis of protein and glycogen
- maintenance of fluid pH
- transmission of nerve impulses

Metabolism

Nearly all ingested potassium is rapidly absorbed through the small intestine and colon. In healthy people, the kidneys finely regulate potassium balance and excrete excess potassium. Regulation of potassium excretion is opposite that of sodium. However, the kidneys have less control over potassium excretion than over sodium excretion. Even when a potassium deficiency exists, the kidneys continue to excrete some potassium. Some potassium is also excreted in feces. Determination of serum potassium concentrations is a routine laboratory test (Luft, 1996a).

Requirements and Range of Safety

In a healthy adult, potassium balance can be maintained easily with a balanced diet. The RDA for potassium is set at an adequate intake (AI) level of 4.7 g/day (4700 mg) for adults. However, U.S. women consume only about 2500 mg/day and men consume only about 3000 mg/day. A UL has not been set.

Food Sources

Potassium is widely distributed in food. The best sources are bananas, oranges, grapefruit, dried fruits, cantaloupe, potatoes, broccoli, carrots, celery, legumes, meat, poultry, fish, and milk. Whole grains have more potassium than refined ones. Salt substitutes usually use potassium to replace sodium. Table 8–10 lists the potassium content in common foods.

Effects of Too Little Potassium (Hypokalemia)

Normally, dietary deficiency of potassium does not occur. However, deficiency can occur with very-low-calorie diets, anorexia nervosa, alcoholism, excessive vomiting, diarrhea, tissue wasting (catabolism), or diabetic ketoacidosis. Medications such as thiazide diuretics and some antibiotics and steroids also cause potassium loss. Common deficiency symptoms include nausea, vomiting, apprehension, listlessness, muscle cramps, and weakness. The most serious side effects are cardiac arrest and respiratory failure, which can result in death. Prevention of potassium depletion is accomplished by emphasis on potassium-rich foods. Treatment is with potassium-containing medications or intravenous electrolyte replacement therapy.

Effects of Too Much Potassium (Hyperkalemia)

Potassium toxicity can result from sudden increase in dietary intake such as with improper use of salt substitutes or potassium tablets. Toxicity can also result when renal failure impairs excretion. Other causes may include severe dehydration, adrenal insufficiency, major infection, hemorrhaging into the gastrointestinal tract, or increased and rapid protein catabolism. Symptoms of toxicity include numbness of the face, tongue, and extremities; muscle weakness; and cardiac arrhythmia. Cardiac failure may ultimately occur.

TABLE 8–10 Sample Food Sources of Potassium

Food (Vegetables Cooked, Fruits Raw)	Potassium Content (in Milligrams [mg])
Potato (1)	940
Sweet potato (1)	540
Banana (1)	490
Fresh halibut or fresh tuna (3 oz)	485
Acorn squash or spinach (1/2 c)	420–450
Milk (1 cup)	370
Lentils (1/2 c)	365
Beef (3 oz)	270
Orange (1)	235
Chicken (cooked), canned tuna (3 oz)	200

Chloride

Chlorine exists nearly always as the ion chloride. It is the major anion of extracellular fluid, and provides balance with the cation, sodium. Chloride is found primarily in extracellular fluids and especially in gastrointestinal secretions and cerebrospinal fluid. Less than 15% of chloride is found in intracellular fluids. Small amounts are also found in bone, connective tissue, muscle, and nerve (Garrison, Somer, 1995, p. 156).

Functions

Chloride, along with phosphate and sulfate, is important in maintaining the acid-base balance of body fluids. Chloride is the major anion of gastric juice (hydrochloric acid—HCl). Lung function depends on the chloride ion being exchanged for another anion, bicarbonate (HCO_3) during oxygen and carbon dioxide exchange.

Metabolism

Chloride absorption occurs by passive transport, but follows along with the active transport absorption of sodium. Chloride is almost completely absorbed in the intestine. Whether chloride is present in foods or gastric juice, it is absorbed into the blood circulation in the intestines. As with sodium, the kidneys excreted excess chloride. Chloride also is excreted through the skin along with sodium in sweat, and in feces. The concentration of chloride in serum is the standard test used to determine body balance.

Requirements and Range of safety

Determining exact chloride requirements is difficult because its balance is so closely interrelated with the other electrolytes. The recommendation is set at the level of an adequate intake (AI) and is 2.3 g/day for adults. The UL is set at 3.6 g/day.

Food Sources

Most dietary chloride comes from table salt (sodium chloride) and in salt substitutes (potassium chloride). The major source of chloride is sodium chloride. Thus, any food with added salt contains chloride. It is also found in abundance in a balanced diet in foods such as eggs, fish, and meat.

Effects of Too Little or Too Much Chloride

Chloride deficiency rarely occurs, except in situations of digestive tract upsets such as vomiting, diarrhea, and gas-tric suctioning. Chloride losses usually reflect sodium losses except in the case of vomiting. Profuse sweating places people at risk, especially infants, children, and athletes. Accidental deficiency resulting from deficient infant formula results in metabolic alkalosis, potassium loss, psychomotor defects, and growth retardation.

Toxicity usually occurs only as a result of dehydration. When water is lost from the body, the concentration of chloride increases in the remaining body fluids.

Because most Americans obtain 3 to 9 g/day, too little chloride is not normally a problem. However, disease, diuretics, nasogastric suctioning, and vomiting are instances where extra chloride may be needed to correct metabolic acidosis.

Summary and Implications for Dentistry of the Electrolytes

Electrolyte balance is of great importance, and dehydration can lead to severe complications including death (Table 8–11). Dehydration can be a problem in elderly patients who may have impaired kidney function. It is thought that some of the confusion attributed to the aging process may be a result of dehydration and associated electrolyte imbalance. Dehydration can also impair denture retention.

Potassium deficiencies or toxicities are rare and usually associated with disease conditions. Diuretic medications are the most common cause of potassium loss and can be counteracted with additional intake of potassium-rich foods.

Athletes suffering from severe exertion can also become dehydrated. However, rehydration with water and a proper diet are usually sufficient and electrolyte-containing beverages should not be needed. In severe conditions such as anorexia nervosa, death can result from severe electrolyte imbalance.

Patients should moderate their intake of sodium even if they do not have a family history of hypertension. Recent research indicates that the lower the amount of sodium in the diet, the lower the blood pressure.

THE TRACE ELEMENTS

Iron

The body contains between 3 and 5 g of iron, primarily in two forms: *functional form* (hemoglobin, enzymes) and *transport and storage forms* (transferrin, ferritin,

(continued on page 174)

TABLE 8-11   Summary of the Electrolytes and Other Nonmineralizing Minerals

Mineral	Metabolism and Function	Deficiency or Excess	Oral Implications	Requirements and Food Sources (Adults Age 18+)
Sodium	*Metabolism:* Almost completely absorbed; body levels regulated by adrenal glands; excess excreted in urine, by skin *Functions:* Water balance; acid-base balance; nervous stimulation; muscle contraction; facilitates nutrient absorption	*Deficiency:* Rare, occurs with excessive perspiration; causes exhaustion *Excess:* Edema, ascites	No oral implications	*Minimum:* Men and women: 500 mg *Sources:* Table salt, baking soda and powder, milk, meat, poultry, fish, eggs
Potassium	*Metabolism:* Almost completely absorbed; body levels regulated by adrenal glands; excess excreted in urine *Functions:* Protein and glycogen synthesis; maintenance of fluid pH; transmits nerve impulse; muscle contraction	*Deficiency:* Starvation, diuretic therapy— nausea; vomiting; apprehension; listlessness; muscle cramps; weakness; ↓ peristalsis; cardiac arrest; respiratory failure *Excess:* Toxic—numbness of face, tongue, extremities; muscle weakness, cardiac arrhythmia	No oral implication	*Minimum:* Men and women: 2000 mg *Sources:* Meat, cereals, fruits, fruit juices, vegetables
Chloride Chlorine exists as ion chloride Found mostly in extracellular fluid Also in bone, connective tissue, muscle, and nerve	*Metabolism:* Absorbed along with active transport of sodium; excreted in kidneys, skin, sweat, and feces *Functions:* Regulates electrolyte balance; major anion of gastric juice; needed for lung function	*Deficiency:* Rare; associated with sodium losses; deficiency in infant formulas causes metabolic acidosis, potassium loss, psychomotor defects, growth retardation *Toxicity:* Seen with dehydration resulting in ↑ body concentration	No oral implications	*Minimum:* Men and women: 750 mg *Sources:* Primarily table salt, salt substitutes, eggs, fish, meat

TABLE 8-12 Summary of The Microminerals

Mineral	Metabolism and Function	Deficiency or Excess	Oral Implications	Requirements and Food Sources (Adults Age 18+)
Iron	*Metabolism:* 5–20% absorption—aided by acid and vitamin C; balance affected by stores, intake, losses (daily losses in urine and feces; menstrual loss); mostly in hemoglobin *Functions:* Muscle myoglobin; carries oxygen to cells; oxidizing enzymes for release of energy	*Deficiency:* Anemia (common in infants, children, young women)—shortness of breath, pallor, headache, dizziness, fatigue; ↑ heart rate; impaired psychomotor development; changes in behavior; ↓ immunity *Excess:* Toxicity possible—organ damage, skin pigmentation; cirrhosis of the liver	*Deficiency:* Leads to: angular cheilosis; pallor of lips and oral mucosa; sore, burning tongue; atrophy/ denudation of filiform papillae; glossitis; ↑ risk of candidiasis	*RDA:* Men: 8 mg; women: 18 mg *Sources:* Organ meats, meat, fish, poultry, whole grain and enriched cereals; green vegetables; dried fruits
Zinc	*Metabolism:* Gastric acid secretion important for optimal absorption; high fiber can reduce absorption *Functions:* Component of 50 metalloenzymes; normal growth and development; sexual maturation; taste and smell sensitivity; proper insulin activity; bone structure; protein synthesis; cell membrane structure; immune response; maintaining vitamin A levels; skin function; wound healing	*Deficiency:* Growth retardation; altered taste; impaired immunity; ↓ wound healing; hair loss; skin lesions; impaired reproductive ability; skeletal abnormalities *Excess:* Toxicity is rare. Large intakes lead to stomach irritation, vomiting, lack of muscle coordination, dizziness	*Deficiency:* Leads to: loss or distortion of taste and smell acuity; loss of tongue sensation; delayed wound healing; impaired keratinization of epithelial cells; epithelial thickening; atrophic oral mucosa; ↑ susceptibility to periodontal disease and candidiasis; xerostomia; ↑ susceptibility to caries if present during tooth formation	*RDA:* Men: 11 mg; women: 8 mg *Sources:* Plant and animal protein

(continued)

169

TABLE 8–12 Summary of the Microminerals (Continued)

Mineral	Metabolism and Function	Deficiency or Excess	Oral Implications	Requirements and Food Sources (Adults Age 18+)
Iodine	**Metabolism:** Absorbed throughout the digestive tract; no mechanism of conservation; chiefly in thyroid gland. **Functions:** Forms thyroxine for energy metabolism; normal physical and mental development	**Deficiency:** Endemic goiter; ↓ thyroid hormone production; hypothyroidism; ↓ metabolic rate. **Excess:** Toxicity rare	No oral implications	**RDA:** Men and women: 150 µg. **Sources:** Iodized salt, shellfish, saltwater fish
Selenium Present in all cells, especially kidney, liver and pancreas; considered an antioxidant nutrient	**Functions:** Alone or as a component of enzyme systems. Antioxidant and free radical scavenger. Major function: enzyme glutathione peroxidase. (involved in antioxidant defense system) Part of several other enzyme systems. Important for the proper functioning of the pancreas a component of sulfur amino acid metabolism, reduces mercury toxicity by binding to heavy metals, needed for normal fetal development. **Metabolism:** About 90% consumed is absorbed. No special storage spaces in the body. **Excretion:** 2/3 through urine, the rest mostly in the feces. Also via sweat and lungs with high intakes. Strong homeostasis maintained even with wide variation in intake.	**Deficiency:** Signs similar to vitamin E deficiency: muscle weakness, joint discomfort, and disorders of the heart muscle or pancreas. At risk are: vegans, especially growing vegan children, in low selenium areas. People with malabsorption syndromes can also be at risk of deficiency. **Toxicity:** Interferes with sulfur metabolism affecting several enzymes. Impairs embryonic development including bone and cartilage. Signs include: hair loss; fingernail discoloration, tenderness, and loss; and breath odor. Short-term oversupplementation caused: vomiting, hair loss, increasing fatigue, and breath odor. Severe toxicity can lead to liver disease and cardiomyopathy.	Incidence of decayed, missing, and filled teeth is higher in children living in areas where soil is high in selenium (Hakjimarkos). This relationship has also been shown in animal studies, but has not been corroborated in other human studies (Nizel, 1989, p. 211).	**RDA:** Adult men and women: 55 ug/day. UL: 400 ug/day. **Sources:** Good sources: animal protein foods such as seafood, kidney, liver, and meat; selenium content of soil determines amount available in plants. Grains are higher than fruits and vegetables

Chromium

Chromium
Adult body contains about 5 mg of chromium
Highest concentrations in muscle, fat, and skin

Function: Glucose metabolism via its role in glucose tolerance factor (GTF)
Needed for efficient uptake of insulin by cell membranes.
Synthesis of fatty acids, cholesterol, and RNA
Metabolism: Organic form appears better absorbed. Transported by transferrin and possibly albumin, globulins, and lipoproteins. No specific storage site
Excreted by the kidneys.

Deficiency: Uncommon; most at risk are people with narrow, highly refined food selections; or long-term malabsorption or those on parenteral (intravenous) nutrition.
Toxicity: Few serious side effects from excess intake from food and little data from ↑ supplement intake. Some forms of chromium are toxic, but these are not present naturally in foods or supplements.

No known oral implications

Requirements: AI- Adequate Intake is 35 mg/day for adult men and 25 mg/day for adult women.
No UL has been set at this time.
Sources: Good sources: whole grains and meats. (Refining of grains removes the chromium.) Also: yeast, cheese, mushrooms, and prunes.
Acid foods heated in stainless steel containers may absorb chromium.

Copper

Copper
Found throughout the body; largest concentration in liver, brain, heart, and kidneys

Metabolism: Acid pH enhances absorption; High zinc, calcium, magnesium, vitamin C can ↓ absorption
Competes with zinc for absorption
Main storage in liver
Functions: Collagen formation
Many enzyme systems like ceruloplasmin (involved in iron transport in blood); cytochrome oxidase (essential for release of energy from the macronutrients); superoxide dismutase (plays a role in the body's antioxidant system)
Catalyzes hemoglobin synthesis
Affects iron absorption and mobilization from tissues
Aids in phospholipid synthesis and iron utilization for hemoglobin formation
Aids in phospholipid synthesis of myelin nerve sheath

Deficiency: Uncommon in healthy people, may result from ↑ zinc or vit. C or antacids
Causes ↓ RBC formation; anemia; tissue fragility; bone demineralization; CNS disorders; diminished skin pigmentation
Toxicity: Unusual in healthy people; causes vomiting, diarrhea, increases hemachromatosis
Wilson's Disease: ↑ copper stored through body e.g., liver, brain, and eyes. Skin, hair, and eyes have a golden or greenish-golden hue.

Deficiency: leads to: ↓ trabeculae of alveolar bone; ↓ tissue vascularity; ↑ tissue fragility

RDA: Men and women: 900 ug/day
UL: 10 mg/day to protect against liver damage
Sources: Depends on amount in soil. Best sources: organ meats, liver, shell fish, meats, nuts, legumes, whole-grain cereals

(continued)

TABLE 8–12 Summary of the Microminerals (Continued)

Mineral	Metabolism and Function	Deficiency or Excess	Oral Implications	Requirements and Food Sources (Adults Age 18+)
Manganese Found in all cells, mostly in the mitochondria Of the organs, highest concentrations are in the pancreas, bone, and liver	*Functions:* Part of several enzyme systems. Enhances defenses by ↑ concentrations of antioxidant enzyme superoxide dismutase (SOD) Energy metabolism, fatty acid and cholesterol synthesis, collagen formation, urea formation, prothrombin formation, protein synthesis *Metabolism:* Poorly absorbed from the small intestine. (about 40% absorbed) ↑ calcium and phosphorus can interfere with absorption. Transported by transferrin Excreted mainly through bile and feces	*Deficiency or Toxicity:* Rarely seen in humans Toxicity seen in miners who inhaled excess. Advanced symptoms resembled Parkinson's disease or viral encephalitis: e.g., speech impairment, headaches, leg cramps, and asthenia (loss of strength)	No known oral implications	AI-Adequate Intake is 2.3 mg/day for men and 1.8 mg/day for women. UL is 11 mg/day for adults *Food Sources:* Primarily in plant foods. Soil concentration can determine food content *Best sources:* whole grains, legumes, vegetables, and fruits.
Molybdenum Adult body has small amounts Highest concentrations in the liver, adrenal glands, and kidneys Widely distributed in the environment	*Functions:* In enzyme systems, including xanthine dehydrogenase and xanthine oxidase (both involved in the formation of uric acid), and sulfite oxidase (involved in catabolism of the sulfur-containing amino acids, methionine and cysteine). Necessary (like copper) for iron metabolism in conversion of iron from ferrous to better absorbed ferric form.	*Deficiency:* Wide distribution in environment, so no deficiency seen in normal conditions Artificially induced deficiency causes nausea, vomiting, disorientation, and decreased uric acid and sulfate in the urine. A rare genetic defect in metabolism has led to mental retardation. *Toxicity:* Can increase urinary copper loss and increase blood and urine uric acid levels leading to a goutlike condition.	No known oral implications	RDA for adult men and women is 45 µg/day UL is 2000 µg/day *Food Sources:* content in plants and animals reflects soil content. *Good sources:* legumes, whole grains, meats, fish, and poultry, and nuts. Also: milk, yogurt, and cheese. Removed in refining of whole grains Low in vegetables and fruits

Mineral	Functions / Metabolism	Deficiency or Toxicity	Recommendations / Food Sources
Sulfur Present in all proteins in the body In connective tissue, skin, hair, and nails In organic sulfates and sulfides and in B-complex vitamins (thiamin and biotin), and coenzyme A	*Functions:* Cell structures as part of proteins Helps to maintain body acid base balance Important in oxidation reduction reactions. Needed for mucopolysaccharides like chondroitin sulfate and collagen ground substance Needed for sulfolipids found in liver, brain, and kidney *Metabolism:* Absorbed as a component of other nutrients or as the free ion. Excreted in the feces and urine.	*Deficiency or Toxicity:* Not seen in healthy humans. Some adverse reactions to sulfite (a food preservative containing sulfur) Sulfite presence must be stated on labels	No recommended level of intake, since diets adequate in protein supply liberal amounts of sulfur. *Food Sources:* Protein-containing foods such as dairy products, meat, fish, poultry, and legumes
Cobalt Red colored pigment	*Function:* Needed in erythropoiesis (red blood cell formation) as a component of vitamin B_{12} May be involved in the metabolism of sulfur-containing amino acids *Metabolism:* Absorbed as part of vitamin B_{12}. The majority is not absorbed and is excreted in the feces. Stored in the liver and kidney	*Deficiency:* Not shown in humans In animals deficiency produces the emaciation and wasting resulting from vitamin B_{12} deficiency *Toxicity:* Not shown in humans In animals, ↑ doses can lead to increased erythrocytes and hemoglobin as well as congestive heart failure (Garrison & Somer, 1995).	No specific requirement for cobalt separate from the requirements for vitamin B_{12}. *Food Sources:* Cobalt is found commonly in foods that are good sources of vitamin B_{12}: Examples: liver, kidney, fish, poultry, eggs, tempeh (fermented bean curd).

Metabolism: About 25–80% absorbed.
Sulfur and copper ↓ absorption
No specific storage site
Quickly excreted by the kidneys
Excreted via bile, sweat, and hair

Chronic high levels of intake can lead to impaired reproduction and growth in animals.

No known oral implications

No known oral implications

and hemosiderin). The amount of iron in the storage form reflects body demands and dietary absorption. Most of the body iron is present in blood as hemoglobin (70–80% in males). Hemoglobin consists of heme (an iron-containing compound) attached to globin (protein). A small amount of iron (about 5%) is present in muscles as myoglobin. About 1% is associated with enzyme systems, and the remaining is stored. Iron is usually bound to a protein such as hemoglobin (See Table 8–12.)

Functions

As a component of hemoglobin, iron has the crucial function of carrying oxygen from the lungs to all cells and returning with carbon dioxide. Iron is the main determinant of the cell's oxygen supply. Myoglobin serves as an oxygen reservoir in cells, especially heart and skeletal muscle. Iron also is a cofactor for many enzymes, such as those required for the release of energy from the macronutrients, conversion of beta-carotene to preformed vitamin A, and formation of collagen. In addition, iron is involved in the immune function (Dallman, 1987; Yip, Dallman, 1999).

Metabolism

Iron is absorbed via the mucosal cells of the small intestine (Peters, Raja, Simpson, Snape, 1988), transported in the blood bound to a protein (transferrin), and stored, chiefly as ferritin, in blood and other body cells

(Figure 8–5). Hemosiderin is the storage form of iron in the liver. Because iron is a component of hemoglobin, it is also found in the bone marrow and spleen. Red blood cell manufacture requires about 25 mg of iron a day. The body uses its iron economically and recycles about 95% of it. For example, after the normal life span of red blood cells (about 120 days), the cells release the iron from hemoglobin. The body then reuses the iron for the synthesis of new hemoglobin.

Iron absorption is inversely related to iron status. So when transferrin levels are low, absorption is increased and vice versa. Iron absorption also varies through the life cycle in relationship to protein needs.

Iron bioavailability from food is an important factor. The body has a great capacity to absorb greater amounts of iron from food during times of need. For example, rapidly growing children, pregnant women, and people with iron-deficiency anemia can absorb a greater proportion of iron from food compared to healthy adult men. Iron absorption, like that of calcium and some other minerals, can also be affected by food factors such as antacids, phytates, and carbonates. Factors that facilitate iron absorption include growth, pregnancy, blood loss, anemia, heme iron, vitamin C in same meal, and stomach acidity. Factors that interfere with absorption include optimal iron stores, ferric form of iron (Fe^{3+}), lack of stomach acid, tannins in tea (with meals), coffee with meals (less effect than tea),

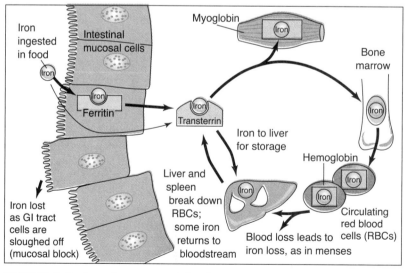

FIGURE 8–5 Iron absorption and distribution.

Source: Reprinted with permission from G. Wardlaw, *Perspectives in Nutrition.* Copyright by the McGraw-Hill Companies, Inc.

phytic acid, oxalic acid, excess calcium, phosphorus, magnesium or zinc, antacids with meals, and malabsorption disorders. For example, when ascorbic acid (vitamin C) is eaten with a nonheme iron source, the iron is converted from the +3 state to its reduced state (+2), which is much more readily absorbed. (Table 8–13 lists the factors that aid or impede iron absorption.)

The chemical form of iron (heme versus nonheme) in food is particularly important. *Heme iron* is part of the hemoglobin and myoglobin molecules, and thus occurs only in animal foods. About 40% of iron in meat, poultry, and fish is heme iron; the remaining 60% is nonheme iron. About 25% of heme iron is available for absorption.

Nonheme iron is present in both animal and plant foods. Nonheme iron constitutes more than 85% of most dietary iron. All iron in plant foods is nonheme iron. Only 5% of nonheme iron is available. Nonheme iron, such as that found in vegetables, is less well absorbed and more greatly influenced by absorption aids or impediments than heme iron.

The three main factors affecting iron balance and metabolism are iron stores, iron intake, and iron losses. Iron absorption also varies through the life cycle in relationship to needs. Rapidly growing children, pregnant women, and people with iron-deficiency anemia can absorb a greater proportion of iron from food than healthy adult men.

TABLE 8–13   Factors That Affect Iron Absorption

Increase Absorption	*Decrease Absorption*
Unmet body needs	Body needs met
Growth	Ferric iron (Fe 3^+)
Pregnancy	Nonheme iron without meat or vitamin C
Acute blood loss	Lack of stomach acid
Anemia	Tannins in tea (with meals)
Heme iron	Coffee with meals (less effect than tea)
Ferrous iron (Fe 2^+)	Phytic acid; oxalic acid
Meat in same meal	Calcium, phosphorus, magnesium, zinc
Vitamin C in same meal	Antacids with meals
Gastric acidity	Malabsorption disorders

Source: From *Robinson's Basic Nutrition and Diet Therapy:* 8/E by Weigley/Mueller/Robinson, © 1997. Reprinted with permission.

Storage amounts are different in healthy adult men and women and are referred to as the "body pool." Excretion of iron is by daily perspiration, shed gastrointestinal cells, urine, skin, hair, and nails. Usual daily losses are in the range of 1 mg. However, blood loss from any cause (menstruation, bleeding ulcers, hemorrhage) is a major cause of iron loss (NAS Subcommittee, 1990). Blood loss can cause iron losses at a rate of 10 to 40 mg/day.

The most sensitive indicators of early stage iron deficiency are serum ferritin or total iron binding capacity tests. Routine blood tests for iron deficiency anemia include hemoglobin and hematocrit tests, which detect more advanced deficiency. Normal hemoglobin levels for men are 14 to 18 g/dL and for women 12 to 16 g/dL. Normal hematocrit for males is 41–51% and for females 37–47%.

Requirements and Range of Safety

Recommended levels of dietary iron assume a 10% rate of absorption and are designed to replace daily losses, maintain stores, and avoid iron overload. They take into consideration iron bioavailability from the food supply.

The RDA for adult men is now 8 mg/day and for adult women 18 mg/day. The UL for iron was set at 45 mg/day for adults, a level above which gastric distress may occur, especially when supplements are consumed on an empty stomach. Most women average only 9 to 10 mg/day of iron, which is only half of the RDA.

Food Sources

The best food sources of iron are animal muscle foods, organ meats, legumes, whole and enriched grains, dark green vegetables, and dried fruits. Iron is the only mineral added to grains labeled "enriched." Some cereals are "fortified" with additional levels of iron. Iron-fortified foods such as grain products may play a major role in meeting iron requirements, especially in people who are vegetarians or who do not eat red meat on a regular basis.

Heme iron sources are lean muscle meats, poultry, and fish, with liver, oysters, and clams being especially high. Nonheme iron is supplied by meat, poultry, fish, legumes, and nuts; whole, enriched, or fortified grains; dried fruits; dark green leafy vegetables; and dark molasses. Dairy foods are low in iron. See Table 8–14 for the iron content of common foods.

Multivitamin supplements with iron may be indicated for those who are unable to meet iron requirements from food sources, and are prescribed routinely for pregnant women. Infant diets are supplemented with iron-fortified cereals as soon as they are weaned from breast or formula.

Effects of Too Little Iron

Iron deficiencies can result from chronic or acute blood loss; blood loss from the gastrointestinal tract (bleeding ulcers; ulcerative colitis; the blood losses that accompany parasite infestation such as hookworm); insufficient dietary intake or absorption; and increased demand such as in growth spurts, pregnancy and lactation, or combinations of these. Women are particularly susceptible to iron deficiency as a result of monthly blood loss from menstruation, which may average 28 mg of iron monthly (Garrison, Somer, 1995). Once available iron stores have been depleted, less and less hemoglobin is produced. Although body iron can be recycled, some is always lost, and eventually iron depletion and iron-deficiency anemia result. Iron deficiency can lead to iron-deficiency anemia (hypochromic mycrocytic) and reduced immune function.

Iron-Deficiency Anemia (Microcytic, Hypochromic Anemia)

Iron-deficiency anemia is the most common anemia, but anemias can be caused by many other deficiencies as well (folate, vitamin B_6, vitamin B_{12}, vitamin C, vitamin E, and copper).

TABLE 8–14 Iron Content of Common Foods

Food	Iron Content (mg)
Heme Iron = 40%;	
Nonheme Iron = 60%	
(3 oz Servings)	
Liver, beef	5.3
Oysters	5.0
Beef, ground, lean	2.1
Turkey, dark	2.0
Lamb, roast	1.7
Tuna, light	1.6
Pork, fresh, roast	0.9
Chicken, breast	0.9
Salmon, pink	0.5
Nonheme Iron = 100%	
Beans, lima, dry, cooked (1/2 c)	3.0
Beans, canned, with pork (1/2 c)	2.3
Lentils, cooked (1/2 c)	2.1
Peanut butter (2 Tbsp)	0.6
Walnut halves (1/2 oz)	0.5
Almonds, shelled (1/2 oz)	0.5
Cereals	
bran flakes (40%)	
with added iron (1 oz)	8.1
cornflakes, plain (1 oz)	1.8
oatmeal, cooked (1 c)	1.6
wheat, shredded (1 oz)	1.2
Breads	
whole wheat (1 slice)	1.0
white, enriched (1 slice)	0.7
rye, enriched (1 slice)	0.7
Nonheme Iron = 100%	
Broccoli, spear (1)	2.1
Turnip greens (1/2 c)	1.6
Spinach, cooked (1/2 c)	1.5
Peas, cooked (1/2 c)	1.3
Tomato, raw (1 med)	0.6
Potatoes, white (1 med)	0.5
Beets, cooked (1/2 c)	0.5
Beans, green (1/2 c)	0.5
Carrots, cooked (1/2 c)	0.4
Cabbage, raw (1 c)	0.4
Lettuce, iceberg (1 c)	0.3
Prunes (10)	2.4
Dates (10)	1.0
Raisins (1 oz)	0.6
Banana (1 med)	0.4
Cantaloupe (1/4)	0.3
Apple (1/2)	0.2
Orange (1 med)	0.1
Molasses	
black strap (1 Tbsp)	5.0
light (1 Tbsp)	0.9
Sugar	
brown (1 Tbsp)	0.3
white (1 Tbsp)	0.0
Cheese, cheddar (1 oz)	0.2
Milk (1 c)	0.1

Source: From *Robinson's Basic Nutrition and Diet Therapy: 8/E* by Weigley/Mueller/Robinson, © 1997. Reprinted with permission.

In iron-deficiency anemia, the red blood cells carry less hemoglobin than normal and thus have reduced ability to carry oxygen. They are also small and pale in color, so the anemia is called microcytic (small cells), hypochromic (pale color) anemia. Pallor, headache, dizziness, and fatigue are common symptoms. Severe iron-deficiency anemia can result in shortness of breath and increased heart rate as the lungs and heart attempt to compensate for reduced oxygen levels.

Anemic women tend to gain too little weight during pregnancy, are three times more likely to deliver low-birth-weight babies, and are twice as likely to deliver prematurely than women who are not anemic (Scholl, Hediger, Fischer, Shearer, 1992). Iron deficiency during critical stages of brain development in infants can cause irreversible abnormalities such as impaired short-term memory and poor test scores. Deficiency in older children is associated with hyperactivity, decreased attention span, and reduced IQ (Oski, 1993).

Lead poisoning is an important problem related to iron status. Lead interferes with the formation of hemoglobin and can result in anemia. The amount of lead absorbed is greater in people whose diets are deficient in iron, calcium, and zinc (there is competition or interference among many minerals for absorption). In lead poisoning, lead absorption is greater. A nutritionally adequate diet is essential for reducing the amount of lead absorbed. At special risk are children living in poverty where exposure to lead is highest and who are least likely to be well nourished. Children with lead poisoning exhibit poor appetites, vomiting, weight loss, hyperactivity, and learning disabilities. Severe cases can lead to convulsions and death.

Iron deficiency may be corrected with attention to the factors influencing iron absorption. By the time iron deficiency is obvious, iron supplementation usually is necessary.

Oral Signs of Iron Deficiency

Iron deficiency can result in signs such as angular cheilosis (cracks in the corners of the mouth). This oral sign is not unique to iron deficiency, however. Angular cheilosis can also result from vitamin B complex deficiency, loss of vertical dimension (proper vertical positioning of maxillary and mandibular teeth at rest), and fungal infections. Other signs of iron deficiency may include pallor of the lips and oral mucosa; sore, burning tongue; glossitis; and atrophy or denudation of filiform papillae. There may also be increased risk of candidiasis, possibly related to decreased immune function.

Effects of Too Much Iron (Hemosiderosis and Hemochromatosis)

Iron excess usually does not occur under normal circumstances because the body regulates absorption well. However, *hemosiderosis* can occur from excess intake, excess absorption, or intravenous administration of iron. Iron overload can also be a complication of any abnormal breakdown of red blood cells, such as hemolytic anemia. In this case, the transferrin becomes saturated and iron is deposited in the liver, lungs, pancreas, and other tissues. In hemosiderosis, excessive iron storage does not lead to tissue damage. It can occur when iron therapy is continued long after it is needed.

Hereditary *hemochromatosis (HHC)*, called iron overload disease, is is a genetic defect characterized by excessive absorption of iron leading to organ damage, skin pigmentation, and cirrhosis of the liver. It is the most common genetic disease in the United States, with one in eight people being silent carriers of the single HH gene mutation (CDC). People who have HHC absorb too much iron and it builds up (in toxic levels) in the liver, lungs, heart, pituitary, thyroid, joints, and other organ tissue. This toxic buildup is slow and can take years to develop, leading to diabetes, heart failure, arthritis, liver disease, impotence, depression, and other organ failure. Individuals with this disease are treated with blood transfusions. HHC is generally a disease of males in their early 30s, although it can be present in both sexes and at all ages. Concern for people with iron storage diseases was one reason why supplementation of bread with iron as a possible way to increase dietary iron (as with folic acid supplementation) is not feasible.

Additionally, in the United States every year about 2,000 children suffer iron poisoning from accidentally swallowing iron supplements formulated for adults.

Summary and Implications for Dentistry of Iron

Iron is essential for proper hemoglobin function and subsequent oxygen transport. Iron is also important for the general development of body tissues and structures including those of the oral cavity. Although research specific to dentistry is sparse, one study in rats showed that iron-deficient animals had higher caries susceptibility than iron-sufficient animals.

Iron-deficiency anemia is the most common of the anemias, and is of particular concern in women, especially in pregnancy. The daily requirement for iron is higher in women due to the need to replace monthly blood losses. Patients should be encouraged to consume a variety of iron-rich and iron-fortified foods and take a daily multivitamin if this is not possible or practical.

Zinc

Zinc is widely but unevenly distributed in plants and animals, and is the most abundant intracellular trace element (Cousins, 1999). The zinc content of the human body is 1.5 to 2.5 g, which is similar to the body content of iron (Cousins, 1999). In humans, the highest concentrations are found in the muscle (50% of total body zinc), eye, kidney, brain, liver, and male reproductive tissues. The majority of serum zinc is bound to protein.

Functions

Zinc is essential for normal growth, development, wound healing, sexual maturation, and immunity. Zinc has structural, regulatory, and catalytic functions in the body. Known structural and regulatory functions include synthesis of DNA, RNA, and proteins; normal growth, development, and sexual maturation; antioxidant activity and immunity; taste and smell sensitivity; insulin activity; bone and cell membrane structure; maintenance of normal vitamin A levels (especially for night vision); and wound healing.

As a catalyst, zinc is a component of over 50 human metalloenzymes including alcohol dehydrogenase (required for the metabolism and detoxification of alcohol and vitamin A by the liver), carbonic anhydrase (transfer of carbon dioxide from the tissues to the lungs), carboxypeptidase (splits off amino acids during protein digestion), glutamate dehydrogenase (needed for catabolism and synthesis of amino acids), alkaline phosphatase (frees phosphates for use in bone), and intestinal folate conjugase (may affect folate metabolism).

Metabolism

Zinc is absorbed actively, passively, and by carrier-facilitated transport. From 20 to 40% of the zinc is absorbed from a mixed (animal and vegetable) diet.

Adequate gastric acid secretion is important for optimal absorption. A high intake of dietary fiber (particularly phytates) can bind zinc and reduce absorption (Sandstrom, Lonnerdal, 1989). Zinc, cadmium, and copper all compete for absorption sites in the intestine. Zinc is absorbed according to body need and is transported in the blood, usually attached to the protein albumin. Zinc is found throughout the body, but has no special storage spaces. Zinc is excreted through the feces from unabsorbed zinc and from that present in digestive tract secretions. It is also lost from skin cells, sweat, and hair; a small amount is excreted in urine. Plasma zinc is considered a poor measure of zinc status because plasma levels are reduced only when the zinc pool has been depleted. Plasma zinc, leukocyte zinc, erythrocyte zinc, hair zinc, and saliva zinc are *not* considered reliable assessment tools. A functional outcome assessment such as metalloenzyme activity (commonly plasma alkaline phosphatase) is most commonly used.

Requirements and Range of Safety

Healthy adult males require about 8 mg/day of dietary zinc and females need 11 mg/day. The UL for zinc is set at 40 mg/day, based on studies showing that zinc adversely affects copper absorption at high levels of intake. The average diet provides from 10 to 15 mg/day. The majority of the zinc consumed in the United States is from animal products.

Food Sources

Zinc is widely distributed in animal foods and those plant foods that are good sources of protein. Excellent sources are oysters, organ meats, muscle meats, dark meat of poultry, eggs, legumes, peanuts, and peanut butter. Dairy foods, whole grain breads, cereals, rice, pasta, and dark green and deep yellow vegetables also make important contributions. Fruits and other vegetables are low in zinc. The zinc in animal foods such as meat is better absorbed than from plant foods. Zinc inhibitors include fiber, phytates, oxalates, ethylenediaminetetra-acetic acid (EDTA), and polyphenols (tannins). Zinc supplement lozenges have become a popular cold remedy. However, there is little good evidence that zinc lozenges can reduce the duration of common colds (Jackson, Lesho, Peterson, 2000).

Effects of Too Little Zinc

Zinc deficiency in humans was first described in the 1960s in Iran and Egypt, when young boys—who had been eating a diet in which more than half the calories were provided by unleavened whole grain bread—failed to grow and mature sexually. Although the bread was a good source of zinc, almost all of the zinc was chelated by the phytate. People at risk for zinc deficiency include anyone who is malnourished, especially rapidly growing children. There is also a hereditary disorder, acrodermatitis enteropathica, in which the inability to absorb zinc results in severe zinc deficiency.

The first response of the body to zinc deficiency is reduced growth. Other effects include impaired immunity, decreased wound healing, hair loss, skin lesions, impaired reproductive ability, and skeletal abnormalities. Immune status is closely linked to zinc status. Zinc deficiency rapidly diminishes antibody-mediated and cell-mediated immunity in humans and animals. (Zinc levels are suppressed during infections.) Even moderate zinc deficiencies can greatly alter host defense systems and lead to increased opportunistic infections and increased mortality.

Because of zinc's interrelationship with vitamin A metabolism, deficiency can contribute to night blindness. Even a borderline deficiency during pregnancy increases the risk of toxemia, premature delivery, and spontaneous abortion, and impaired fetal growth and development (Garrison, Somer, 1995).

Oral Implications of Zinc Deficiency
Patients with zinc deficiency may complain of changes in taste, such as hypogeusic (diminished taste sensitivity) and hyposmia (diminished odor sensitivity); altered tastes of saltiness, sweetness, or bitterness of foods; and lessened appetites. Through its role in immunity, it can increase susceptibility to periodontal disease, candidiasis, and dental caries (during tooth formation only). Other oral effects include delayed wound healing, defective keratinization of epithelial cells, epithelial thickening, atrophic oral mucosa, and xerostomia.

Zinc supplementation has been shown to improve immune function in several conditions including human immunodeficiency virus (HIV), childhood diarrhea, and aging (Fraker, King, Laakko, Vollmer, 2000).

Effects of Too Much Zinc
Zinc toxicity is rare. However, ingestion of large doses (more than 2 g) of zinc can result in stomach irritation, vomiting, lack of muscle coordination, and dizziness. Zinc poisoning is also possible from ingesting acid foods or beverages that have been stored in galvanized containers.

Summary and Implications for Dentistry of Zinc
Zinc is an important nutrient for wound healing and new tissue formation. Zinc deficiency can impair healing and resistance to infection and can also affect the sense of taste. Deficiency is rare, but can occur in older persons.

Iodine

Iodine exists mainly as the iodide ion. In the body, most iodine is located in the thyroid gland (about three-fourths of the iodide content of the body), with lesser amounts in skin, skeleton, and salivary and stomach and other endocrine glands. However, all cells contain tiny amounts. In the environment, iodine is unevenly distributed, with highest concentrations in ocean water and nearby coastal areas.

Functions
Iodide's major function is as a constituent of two hormones, triiodothyronine (T_3) and thyroxine (T_4). These hormones influence most organ systems of the body. For example, the hormones regulate energy metabolism, including basal metabolism, and the metabolic processing of the macronutrients. The hormones are necessary for normal physical and mental development.

Metabolism
Iodine is ingested in foods mostly as the inorganic ion (iodide) and as organic compounds (attached to amino acids). Absorption occurs rapidly and throughout the digestive tract. The ionic form is better absorbed than the organic form. Iodide is taken up by the thyroid gland from blood circulation. The kidneys promptly excrete iodide. A small amount is excreted in feces and sweat, tears, saliva, and bile. In the presence of deficiency, there is no adaptive mechanism for conserving iodine.

Proper functioning of the thyroid gland is the hallmark for optimal iodide balance. Laboratory tests to measure adequacy include measurement of iodide in urine, blood levels of T_3 and T_4 and radioactive iodide uptake by the thyroid gland.

Requirements and Range of Safety
Requirements relate to the formation of the proper amount of the thyroid hormones for healthy function and to prevent goiter. The RDAs take into account the wide distribution of iodide in regular and processed foods. Based on research into how much iodine the thyroid gland needs to regulate enzyme and metabolic

processes, an RDA of 150 µg/day was established for both men and women. To avoid overabsorption of iodine by the thyroid, adults should not consume over the UL of 1.1 mg/day (1,100 ug/day).

Food Sources of Iodine

Three major food categories contribute to iodide intake: seafood, plants grown along the seacoast, and iodized salt. The greatest natural source of iodide is seafood such as saltwater fish, shellfish, seaweed, and plants grown along the seacoast. There has been a steady decline in extra sources of iodide in the total food supply. Foods grown inland and freshwater fish are poor iodine sources. The iodine content of foods varies with the soil and water supply, fertilizers, animal feed, and food-processing methods.

The most reliable way to ensure an adequate iodide intake is to use iodized table salt. (The addition of iodine to salt was the public health intervention that helped eradicate iodine deficiency in the United States.) However, the sodium chloride used in commercially processed foods usually is not iodized.

Certain plants of the cabbage family—including cabbage, brussel sprouts, cauliflower, radishes, rutabagas, and turnips—contain natural goitrogens, which interfere with the body's use of thyroid hormones. Goitrogens are also found in raw peanuts, cassava, and some oilseeds such as rape seed. Fortunately, heating inactivates goitrogens.

Effects of Too Little Iodine (Hypothyroidism, Goiter)

Insufficient iodide leads to decreased thyroid hormone production, followed by a lowered metabolic rate. The thyroid gland enlarges in an effort to produce more hormones. The result is hypothyroidism (simple goiter). If widespread in a particular geographical area, it is called endemic goiter. Symptoms include enlargement of the thyroid gland with follicular epithelial cell hypertrophy, hyperplasia, or both. In mild deficiency, the only outward sign is slight enlargement of the thyroid gland, visible at the neckline (Figure 8–6). However, in pregnant woman, irreversible birth defects can result if the mother is unable to supply the fetus with enough iodide. Because this deficiency occurs during such a critical period of development, the baby is more severely affected than the mother. This condition is called cretinism and is characterized by low basal metabolism, dry skin, thick lips, enlarged tongue,

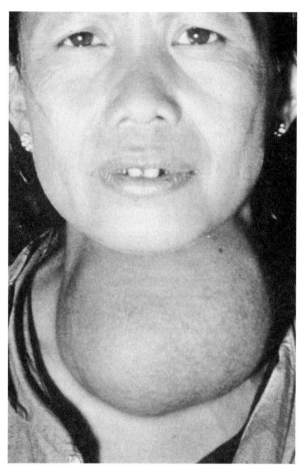

FIGURE 8–6 Goiter.

arrested skeletal and muscle development, and severe mental retardation.

Effects of Too Much Iodine (Hyperthyroidism)

Because the kidneys rapidly excrete iodide, toxicity is extremely rare. Normal concentration for protein-bound iodine in plasma and serum are 0.004 to 0.008 mg/100 mL. When concentrations exceed 20 to 35 ug/100 mL, thyrotoxicosis can occur and thyroxine synthesis can stop. However, this is reversible within weeks with decreased iodine intake.

Selenium

Selenium is a mineral present in all cells, especially in the kidney, liver, and pancreas. The selenium content of soil varies widely throughout the world, a fact that has enabled researchers to study its essential roles in human health.

Functions

Selenium functions alone or as part of enzyme systems. Its function is like that of the antioxidant and free radical scavenging ability of vitamin E. Thus, it is also considered an antioxidant nutrient. The major function appears to be its presence in the enzyme glutathione peroxidase. This is one of the enzymes involved in the body's antioxidant defense system. Selenium is part of several other enzyme systems, and is important for the proper functioning of the pancreas and the immune system. It is a component of sulfur amino acid metabolism, reduces mercury toxicity by binding to heavy metals, and is needed for normal fetal development. Selenium may also play a role in reducing the risk of colon cancer. Several studies to date have shown that people with the highest blood selenium levels had a 34% lower incidence of precancerous colon polyps than did those with lower selenium levels (Duffield-Lillico, Shureigi, Lippman, 2004).

Metabolism

Selenium is ingested in food in both the inorganic and organic forms. The organic form of selenium is more bioavailable and is absorbed mainly from the duodenum. About 90% of the selenium consumed is absorbed. No special storage spaces are evident in the body. The kidneys can excrete varying amounts of selenium. Up to about two-thirds of excreted selenium is through the urine, with the remainder mostly in the feces. However, with excessive intakes, selenium also is excreted through the sweat and lungs. Body homeostasis seems to be maintained even with wide differences in intake. The most common laboratory tests measure glutathione peroxidase levels of platelets, blood selenium levels, or urinary selenium.

Requirements and Range of Safety

It was not until 1979 that human requirements for selenium were determined, and information about selenium requirements across the life span is still limited. The RDAs are estimated from worldwide human and animal studies, and are set at 55 µg/day for adults. The UL is set at 400 µg/day.

Food Sources

In foods, selenium is found combined with sulfur-containing amino acids (methionine and cysteine). Thus, animal protein foods such as seafood, kidney, liver, and meat are the highest sources. Like iodine, the selenium content of the soil reflects the amount available in plants. So the region where individual plant foods are grown determines their selenium content. Of the plant foods, grains are higher in selenium than are vegetables and fruits.

Effects of Too Little Selenium

Signs of selenium deficiency can be similar to those of vitamin E deficiency. Examples are muscle weakness, joint discomfort, and disorders of the heart muscle or pancreas. People potentially at risk are those being fed tightly controlled nutrient solutions, and vegans (especially growing children) who eat plant foods grown in soil low in selenium. People with malabsorption syndromes can also be at risk of deficiency. In addition, low levels of selenium have been associated with compromised immune function associated with impaired antioxidant defenses.

Effects of Too Much Selenium

Selenium toxicity in animals was identified before it was recognized in humans. Cattle that grazed in areas with high amounts of selenium in the soil classically developed stiffness, blindness, hoof deformity, and hair loss. Death sometimes occurred. In humans, excess selenium can interfere with sulfur metabolism affecting several enzymes. It can also impair embryonic development, including bone and cartilage. Signs of toxicity are evident in the areas of the world where constant exposure to slightly elevated amounts of selenium exists. Abnormal observations include hair loss; fingernail discoloration, tenderness, and loss; and breath odor. Results of short-term oversupplementation resulted in vomiting, hair loss, increasing fatigue, and breath odor. Severe toxicity can lead to liver disease and cardiomyopathy.

Oral Implications of Selenium

The incidence of decayed, missing, and filled teeth is higher in children living in areas where soil is high in selenium. This relationship has also been shown in monkeys fed high-selenium water.

Chromium

Functions

Chromium is a metal that exists in both the inorganic and organic forms. The adult body contains about 5 mg of chromium, with the highest concentrations in muscle, fat, and skin. More information is known about chromium's role in animals than in human beings. Chromium is a constituent of glucose tolerance factor (GTF). This compound also contains amino acids and nicotinic acid. GTF is involved in the efficient uptake of insulin by cell membranes. Thus, chromium appears to be important for the optimal metabolism of glucose. Other possible functions of chromium are in the synthesis of fatty acids, cholesterol, and RNA.

Metabolism

The metabolic processing of chromium is under active investigation. Chromium is absorbed from the small intestine, especially the jejunum. The organic form appears better absorbed. About 0.5% of chromium is absorbed from the diet. In blood circulation, chromium is transported by transferrin and possibly albumin, globulins, and lipoproteins. No specific storage site has been located. Chromium is excreted by the kidneys.

Methods to study chromium balance in human beings are limited because chromium is so widely distributed in the environment.

Requirements and Range of Safety

Knowledge of human requirements for chromium is limited. The AI for chromium is 20–25 µg/day for women and 30–35 µg/day for men. The UL has not been set.

Food Sources

Detection of chromium content of foods and determination of chromium bioavailability are under investigation. Current information suggests chromium is present especially in whole grains and meats. (Refining of grains removes the chromium.) Other sources include yeast, cheese, mushrooms, and prunes. Commercial and home preparation of foods may be important factors. For example, stainless steel contains chromium. Acid foods heated in such containers can leach out chromium. This may explain the higher levels found in some beers and wines fermented in stainless steel vats.

Effects of Too Little or Too Much Chromium

Chromium deficiency is uncommon. People potentially at risk include those with narrow, highly refined food selections; those with long-term malabsorption; and those on parenteral (intravenous) nutrition. Some people who have insulin resistance have benefited from increased chromium. However, chromium cannot replace insulin therapy in people with insulin-dependent diabetes mellitus (IDDM).

Excessive intake of chromium from food or dietary supplements may not lead to excessive levels of chromium in the body because such tiny amounts are absorbed. More knowledge may be learned as people continue to take self-prescribed, unmonitored chromium dietary supplements. However, the chemical form of chromium in food and supplements does not appear to be toxic.

Copper

Copper is found throughout the body, with the largest concentrations in the liver, brain, heart, and kidneys. It is widely but unevenly distributed throughout the world. It was recognized to be an essential dietary element because of its role in hemoglobin formation.

Functions

Copper has many functions in the body, including an important role in collagen formation. It:

- is essential for the correct functioning of many enzyme systems: ceruloplasmin (involved in iron transport in blood); cytochrome oxidase (essential for release of energy from the macronutrients); superoxide dismutase (plays a role in the body's antioxidant system).
- catalyzes hemoglobin synthesis.
- affects iron absorption and mobilization from tissues.
- aids in phospholipid synthesis.

Metabolism

Absorption of copper appears to occur throughout the digestive tract, with most from the stomach or duodenum, where an acid pH enhances its absorption. Several factors enhance or inhibit copper absorption. For example, large amounts of zinc, calcium, magnesium, or vitamin C can decrease its absorption. Because copper competes with zinc for absorption, increased zinc can precipitate copper deficiency.

About one-third of the copper consumed is absorbed. In blood circulation, about 95% of the copper is transported as ceruloplasmin. The liver is the main storage organ; feces are the major excretion routes. Absorbed but unneeded copper is excreted into bile, which then becomes part of the feces that also contain unabsorbed copper.

Commonly used laboratory tests include superoxide dismutase (SOD) copper levels, and amounts of ceruloplasmin.

Requirements and Range of Safety

The RDA for copper is 900 µg/day for adult men and women. The UL is 10,000 µg/day.

Food Sources

The copper content of foods depends on the amount in the soil, so the amount in foods will vary. Among foods from similar geography, the highest sources are organ meats, shellfish, whole grains, legumes, nuts, mushrooms, and chocolate. Milk is a poor source. Water may be a source, especially household or institutional sources that travel through copper pipes.

Effects of Too Little Copper

Copper deficiency is unusual in healthy people. People at risk include those with malabsorption or those taking high doses of zinc, vitamin C, or antacids. Infants at risk are those born prematurely (who did not build up adequate stores) or those with persistent diarrhea. Because copper is important for normal development of nerve, blood, bone, and collagen, deficiency can result in decreased red blood cell formation and anemia. Signs can include tissue fragility, bone demineralization, central nervous system disorders, and diminished skin pigmentation. Children at risk are those fed diets composed only of milk. Menkes disease is a rare hereditary disorder, characterized by low levels of the copper-containing proteins, severe mental retardation, and sparse, steely (kinky) hair.

Effects of Too Much Copper

Copper excess is unusual in healthy people. Instances have occurred from ingesting acidic food or beverages stored in copper or brass containers; or ingesting abnormally acidic water that travels through copper tubing and valves. Symptoms include vomiting and diarrhea. High copper levels also increase hemochromatosis (iron accumulation in soft tissues). A rare hereditary disorder, Wilson's disease, is characterized by slowly increasing and potentially irreversible amounts of copper stored throughout the body, such as in the liver, brain, and eyes. The skin, hair, and eyes take on a golden or greenish-golden hue.

Manganese

Manganese is found in all body cells, mostly in the mitochondria. Of the organs, highest concentrations are in the pancreas, bone, and liver. Manganese is part of several enzyme systems. It enhances antioxidant defenses by increasing concentrations of the antioxidant enzyme superoxide dismutase (SOD).

Functions

Manganese functions as a component of many enzyme systems. However, magnesium can substitute for manganese in many enzyme systems. Other functions include energy metabolism, fatty acid and cholesterol synthesis, collagen formation, urea formation, prothrombin formation, protein synthesis, and antioxidant protection. Reliable laboratory tests for manganese have yet to be established.

Metabolism

Manganese is absorbed poorly from the small intestine. Only about 40% of consumed manganese is absorbed. Large amounts of calcium and phosphorus can interfere with absorption. Its absorption and transport in the blood is also shared with iron. For example, increased levels of iron inhibit absorption of manganese; and manganese is transported by transferrin. No particular storage location is known. Manganese is excreted mainly through the bile and feces, with little present in urine.

Requirements and Range of Safety

The RDA for manganese is set at an AI level of 310–320 mg/day for adult women and 410–420 mg/day for adult men. The UL is set at 9–11 mg/day.

Food Sources

Manganese is found primarily in plant foods. Soil concentration of manganese can determine the amount in foods. Major food sources are whole grains, legumes, vegetables, and fruits. Although tea has especially high levels, the manganese appears to be unabsorbed.

Effects of Too Little or Too Much Manganese

Neither deficiency nor toxicity from consumed manganese has been seen in humans except in extreme research conditions. Ability to maintain body balance may be due to adequate dietary sources, strong body homeostatic controls, and interchangeability of manganese and magnesium in enzyme systems. Manganese toxicity has been seen in miners who inhaled excess manganese. Symptoms in more advanced stages resembled those of Parkinson's disease or viral encephalitis and included speech impairment, headaches, leg cramps, and asthenia (loss of strength).

Molybdenum

Functions

The adult body contains small amounts (about 9 mg) of molybdenum, with the highest concentrations in the liver, adrenal glands, and kidneys. Molybdenum is widely distributed in the environment; its content in plants and animals also reflects soil content. Research has required artificial means of creating deficiencies and excesses. More information is known about molybdenum's role in plants and animals than in human beings. Molybdenum is involved in enzyme systems, including xanthine dehydrogenase and xanthine oxidase (both involved in the formation of uric acid), and sulfite oxidase (involved in catabolism of the sulfur-containing amino acids, methionine and cysteine). Because xanthine oxidase is important in converting iron from the ferrous to the better absorbed ferric form, molybdenum is necessary (like copper) for iron metabolism.

Metabolism

Molybdenum appears to be absorbed from the stomach and small intestine. About 25–80% is absorbed. Absorption is influenced by several factors. For example, sulfur and copper appear to decrease its absorption. In blood circulation, molybdenum seems to be transported in both its inorganic and organic forms. No specific storage site has been located. Molybdenum is quickly excreted by the kidneys. The body also excretes molybdenum via bile, sweat, and hair.

Requirements and Range of Safety

Knowledge about human requirements for molybdenum is also limited. The RDA is set at 45 µg/day for both adult men and women. The UL is 1700–2000 µg/day.

Food Sources

Detection of molybdenum content of foods and determination of molybdenum bioavailability are under investigation. Current information suggests molybdenum is present especially in legumes, whole grains, meats, fish, and poultry. Refining of whole grains removes the molybdenum. Other sources include nuts, milk, yogurt, and cheese. Vegetables and fruits are low in molybdenum content.

Effects of Too Little or Too Much Molybdenum

Methods to study molybdenum balance in human beings are limited. Because molybdenum is so widely distributed in the environment, neither insufficiency nor deficiency states under normal conditions have been documented. One example of an artificially induced deficiency was a patient fed parenterally, without molybdenum, for 18 months. Abnormalities included nausea, vomiting, disorientation, and decreased uric acid and sulfate in the urine. A rare genetic defect in molybdenum metabolism leads to mental retardation. Excessive intake can increase urinary copper loss and increase blood and urine uric acid levels leading to a goutlike condition.

See Table 8–12 for a summary of the microminerals including sulfur and cobalt.

Ultra-Trace Elements

The microminerals arsenic, cadmium, nickel, silicon, tin, and vanadium are present in the body in small amounts, but not enough is known about their function for them to be considered essential. This is also true of aluminum, barium, boron, bromine, gold, lead, mercury, rubidium, and strontium.

Lead, cadmium, and mercury are toxic to humans. The health effects of lead are undergoing active study. Lead is toxic to almost all body tissues. In children, environmental sources of lead such as lead paint and drinking water can cause severe cognitive disability. As people age, the lead stored in their bones can be released into the body and cause damage. Known health effects of excess lead in adults include increased risk of hypertension, decreased kidney filtration ability, declines in memory and mental abilities, and increased cataract risk through accellerated oxidative damage (Get the Lead Out, 2005). See Table 8–15 for a summary of the ultra-trace elements.

TABLE 8–15   Ultra-Trace Elements

Mineral	Metabolism and Function	Deficiency or Excess	Oral Implications	Requirements and Food Sources
Aluminum, arsenic, boron, bromine, cadmium, germanium, lead, lithium, mercury, nickel, rubidium, silicon, strontium, tin, and vanadium	Some evidence suggests a beneficial role for these in animal and human health; not enough data to define specific roles	No known deficiency; lead, cadmium, mercury, and arsenic can be toxic	No known oral implications	Requirements not established; UL set for boron at 20 mg/day, vanadium 1.8 mg/day, and nickel 1 mg/day; not enough data to set a UL for others

Source: Adapted from *Robinson's Basic Nutrition and Diet Therapy:* 8/E by Weigley/Mueller/Robinson, © 1997. Reprinted with permission.

Summary and Implications for Dentistry of the Microminerals

Iron is essential for proper hemoglobin function and subsequent oxygen transport. Iron is also important for the general development of body tissues and structures including those of the oral cavity. Although research specific to dentistry is sparse, one study in rats showed that iron-deficient animals had higher caries susceptibility than iron-sufficient animals (Sintes, Rosa, Freund, 1983). Iron-deficiency anemia is the most common of the anemias and is of particular concern in women, especially during pregnancy. Patients should be encouraged to consume a variety of iron-rich and iron-fortified foods or take a daily multivitamin if this is not possible or practical.

Zinc is an important nutrient for wound healing and new tissue formation. Zinc deficiency can impair healing and resistance to infection and can also affect the sense of taste. Older persons are at particular risk of zinc deficiency, which may contribute to decreases in the ability to taste and smell as well as to heal and resist infection. A balanced diet should provide sufficient zinc in the healthy individual.

Selenium, copper, chromium, manganese, and molybdenum are found widely in foods. Deficiencies tend to be rare. They are generally either associated with genetic abnormalities or soil deficiencies, or are artificially induced. In developed countries where the food supply is obtained from varied areas, nutrient deficiencies resulting from depleted soil are rare. Excess amounts of copper may be obtained from copper cookware. There are no direct oral implications of these nutrients, but enough is known about them to warrant determination of RDAs.

QUESTIONS PATIENTS MIGHT ASK

Q. I am a 34-year-old woman. Should I take a calcium supplement?

A. The best source of calcium is foods. If you drink 2–3 cups of milk a day and eat a variety of foods from the MyPyramid Food Guide, you will get about 800 mg of calcium. An additional cup of milk, yogurt, or some cheese will bring the intake up to the new RDAs.

Q. I am allergic to milk. What is the best calcium supplement for me?

A. Calcium carbonate is 40% calcium, so a 500 mg tablet provides 200 mg of calcium. You can select the least expensive brand. However, avoid any with bonemeal and dolomite because such natural products may be contaminated. If you are a senior citizen or have a lack of stomach acid, the best supplement for you is calcium citrate.

Q. Can too much calcium cause kidney stones?

A. A healthy person can have a calcium intake of about 2500 mg (more than twice the RDA) without any appreciable effect on calcium excreted in the urine. People who have kidney stones or who are at risk for them may excrete more calcium when they have high intakes. About 80% of kidney stones contain calcium, chiefly as calcium oxalate. Severely cutting down on calcium intake not only increases the loss of calcium from the bones but also increases the absorption of oxalate. Thus, the calcium from bone could combine with oxalate to form stones, even though calcium intake is reduced. To minimize the problem, a susceptible person should drink plenty of fluids.

CASE STUDY

Morgan, age 15 years, is not doing well in school. She is frequently absent because of headaches. When she is there, her teachers notice she is not concentrating in class. At home, her parents find her sleeping instead of doing her homework. She is irritable with her family; she never wants to do anything with them, complaining she is too tired. Even her friends have noticed she is moody and can't keep up with their high-energy activities.

At a health checkup the following screening information was obtained. Morgan is 63 in. (160 cm) tall (without shoes) and weighs 108 lb (49 kg) in light indoor clothing. Blood test results were: hemoglobin = 10 g/dL (6.2 mmol/L), hematocrit = 30%. By history, Morgan started her menses at age 12; her monthly period lasts about 1 week, with heavy flow the first 3 days. Morgan's eating habits are erratic and she is afraid of "getting fat." A typical food intake is:

Breakfast: Cold cereal with sliced banana; skim milk.
Lunch: Eats school lunch, depending on the menu. Her favorite meals are pizza, spaghetti with tomato sauce, and grilled cheese sandwiches. On other days, she just eats the foods she likes, usually the salad and applesauce or peaches. Sometimes she drinks all the milk, but usually only about half.

After school: Low-fat cookies; low-calorie soda.
Dinner: Poultry, fish, or pasta; green vegetable such as peas; salad with low-calorie dressing; low-fat cake; skim milk.
Evening snack: Pretzels; low-calorie soda.

Questions
1. What are normal levels for hemoglobin and hematocrit? What is your interpretation?
2. What are some reasons that teenage girls are especially at risk for iron-deficiency anemia? What factors apply to Morgan?
3. Why is fatigue a common symptom of anemia?
4. An iron supplement, ferrous sulfate, was prescribed for Morgan. Could a high-iron diet achieve the same results?
5. In her health class at school, Morgan learned that some foods are good sources of heme iron. What is meant by heme iron? What foods supply heme iron? What are such foods in Morgan's typical day? What other foods in her current diet are good sources of nonheme iron?
6. What nutrients enhance or interfere with iron absorption? With Morgan, plan revised meal patterns and menu structures for a typical day to improve the food combinations at meals and snacks.

REFERENCES

Abbott L, Nadler J, Rude RK: Magnesium deficiency in alcoholism: Possible contribution to osteoporosis and cardiovascular disease in alcoholics. *Alcohol Clin Exp Res* 1994; 18:1976–2082.

American Dental Association: *American Dental Association Supports Fluoridation.* Council on Access, Prevention, and Interprofessional Relations Report, January 1998.

Brown MD, Aaron G: The effect of point-of-use conditioning systems on community fluoridated water. *Pediatr Dent* 1991; 13(1):35–38.

Centers for Disease Control and Prevention: Recommendations for using fluoride to prevent and control dental caries in the United States. *MMWR* 2001; 50(RR-14):1–42.

Chaudhury NG, Brown RH, Shepherd MG: Fluoride intake of infants in New Zealand. *J Dent Res* 1990; 69(12):1828–33.

Clovis J, Hargreaves JA, Thompson GW: Fluoride intake from beverage consumption. *Comm Dent Oral Epidemiol* 1988; 16(1):11–15.

Cousins RJ: Zinc. In Shils ME, Olsen JA, Shike M, Ross AC (eds): *Modern Nutrition in Health and Disease*, 9th ed. Baltimore: Williams & Wilkins, 1999.

Dallman PR: Iron deficiency and the immune response. *Am J Clin Nutr* 1987; 46:329–34.

DePaola DM, Tauger-Decker R, Faine MP: Nutrition in relation to dental medicine. In Shils ME, Olsen JA, Shike M, Ross AC (eds): *Modern Nutrition in Health and Disease*, 10th ed. Baltimore: Williams & Wilkins, 2005.

Duffield-Lillico AJ, Shureiqi L, Lippman SM: Can selenium prevent colorectal cancer? A signpost from epidemiology. *J Nat Cancer Inst* 2004; 96(22):1645–47.

Eble D, Deaton TG, Wilson FC, Bawden JW: Fluoride concentrations in human and rat bone. *J Public Health Dent* 1992; 52:288–92.

Farley JR, Wergedal JE, Baylink DJ: Fluoride directly stimulates proliferation and alkaline phosphatase activity of bone-forming cells. *Science* 1983; 227:330–32.

Fluoride and Oral Health. Report of a WHO Expert Committee on Oral Health Status and Fluoride Use. Geneva: World Health Organization, WHO Technical Report Series # 846, 1994:11.

Featherstone JD: Prevention and reversal of dental caries: Role of low level fluoride. *Community Dent Oral Epidemiol* 1999; 27:31–40.

Fraker PJ, King LE, Laakko, T, Vollmer TL: The dynamic link between the integrity of the immune system and zinc status. *J Nutr* 2000; 130:1399S–1406S.

Garrison R, Somer E: *The Nutrition Desk Reference*, 3rd ed. New Canaan, CT: Keats, 1995.

Get the lead out: What you don't know can hurt you. *Nutrition Action Healthletter* 2005; 32(1):3–7.

Grossi S: *Low Dietary Calcium, Low Vitamin C Linked to Increased Risk of Gum Disease*. Nice, France: IADR, 1998.

Hadjimarkos DM: Effect of trace elements on dental caries. *Adv Oral Biol* 1968; 3:263.

Heaney RP: Bone biology in health and disease: A tutorial. In Shils ME, Olsen JA, Shike M, Ross AC (eds): *Modern Nutrition in Health and Disease*, 9th ed. Baltimore: Williams & Wilkins, 1999.

Hillier S, Cooper C, Kellingray S, Russell G, Hughes H, Coggon D: Fluoride in drinking water and risk of hip fracture in the UK: A case-control study. *Lancet* 2000; 355:265–69.

Horowitz HS: Proper use of fluoride products in fluoridated communities. *Lancet* 1999; 353(9163):1462.

Institute of Medicine, National Academy of Sciences; *Dietary Reference Intakes for Calcium, Phosphorus, Magnesium, Vitamin D, and Fluoride*. Washington, DC: National Academies Press, 1997.

Jackson JL, Lesho E, Peterson C: Zinc and the common cold: A meta-analysis revisited. *J Nutri* 2000; 130(Suppl): 1512S–15S.

Johnson S, DeBiase C: Concentration levels of fluoride in bottled drinking water. *J Dent Hyg* 2003; 77:161–67.

Krall E, Dawson-Hughes B, Papas A, Garcia R: Tooth loss and skeletal bone density in healthy postmenopausal women. *Osteoporosis Int* 1994; 4:104–9.

Leverett DH, Adair SM, Vaughan BW, Proskin HM, Moss ME: Randomized clinical trial of the effect of prenatal fluoride supplements in preventing dental caries. *Caries Res* 1997; 31(3):174–79.

Luft, FC: Potassium and its regulation. In Ziegler EE, Filer LJ (eds): *Present Knowledge in Nutrition*, 7th ed. Washington, DC: ILSI Press, 1996a.

Luft FC: Salt, water, and extracellular volume regulation. In Ziegler EE, Filer LJ (eds): *Present Knowledge in Nutrition*, 7th ed. Washington, DC: ILSI Press, 1996b.

Ma J, Folson AR, Melnick SL, et al.: Associations of serum and dietary magnesium with cardiovascular disease, hypertension, diabetes, insulin, and carotid arterial wall thickness: Atherosclerosis Risk in Community Study. *J Clin Epidemiol* 1989; 48:927–40.

McGuire S: Fluoride content of bottled water. *N Engl J Med* 1989; 321:836–37.

National Academy of Sciences Subcommittee on Nutritional Status and Weight Gain During Pregnancy: *Nutrition During Pregnancy*. Washington, DC: National Academy Press, 1990.

National Research Council: *Health Effects of Ingested Fluoride*. Washington, DC: National Academy Press, 1993.

Nielsen FH: Other trace elements. In Ziegler EE, Filer LJ (eds): *Present Knowledge in Nutrition*, 7th ed. Washington, DC: ILSI Press, 1996.

Nizel AE, Papas AS: *Nutrition in Clinical Dentistry*, 3rd ed. Philadelphia: WB Saunders, 1989.

Nutrient Data Laboratory, Beltsville Human Nutrition Research Center, USDA Agricultural Research Service: *USDA National Fluoride Database of Selected Beverages and Foods*. Beltsville, MD: Authors, 2004.

Oski F: Iron deficiency in infancy and childhood. *N Engl J Med* 1993; 329:190–93.

Peters TJ, Raja KB, Simpson RJ, Snape S: Mechanisms and regulation of iron absorption. *Ann NY Acad Sci* 1988; 526:141–47.

Position of the American Dietetic Association: The impact of fluoride on health. *J Am Diet Assoc* 2000; 100:1208–13.

Report to the ad hoc Subcommittee on Fluoride of the Committee to Coordinate Environmental Health and Related Programs: *Review of Fluoride Benefits and Risk*. Washington, DC: U.S. Department of Health and Human Services, 1991.

Riley JC, Lennon MA, Ellwood RP: The effect of water fluoridation and social inequalities on dental caries in 5-year-old children. *Int J Epidemiol* 1999; 28:300–305.

Robinson SN, Davies EH, Williams B: Domestic water treatment appliances and the fluoride ion. *Br Dent J* 1991; 171:91–93.

Sandstrom B, Lonnerdal B: Promoters and antagonists of zinc absorption. In Mills CF (ed): *Zinc in Human Biology*. New York: Springer-Verlag, 1989.

Schardt D. Potassium: Bones, stones, & strokes on the line. *Nutrition Action Healthletter* 2004; 31(10):8–9.

Scholl TO, Hediger ML, Fischer RL, Shearer JW: Anemia vs. iron deficiency: Increased risk of preterm delivery in a prospective study. *Am J Clin Nutr* 1992; 55:985–88.

Sintes JL, Rosa J, Freund T: Iron deficiency and dental caries: A pilot study. *Clin Prevent Dent* 1983; 5(2):3–5.

Sowers M, Clark MK, Jannausch ML, Wallace RB: A prospective study of bone mineral content and fracture in communities with differential fluoride exposure. *Am J Epidemiol* 1991; 133(7):649–60.

Tate WH, Chan JT: Fluoride concentrations in bottled and filtered waters. *Gen Dent* 1994; 42(4):362–66.

Tucker KL, Hannan MT, Chen H, Cupples LA, Wilson PW, Kiel DP: Potassium, magnesium, and fruit and vegetable intakes are associated with greater bone mineral density in elderly men and women. *Am J Clin Nutri* 1999; 69:727–36.

Tylavsky FA, Holliday K, Danish R, Womack C, Norwood J, Carbone L: Fruit and vegetable intakes are an independent predictor of bone size in early pubertal children. *Am J Clin Nutr* 2004; 79(2):311–17.

U.S. Department of Health and Human Services: *Bone Health and Osteporosis: A Report of the Surgeon General*. Rockville, MD: U.S. Department of Health and Human Services, Office of the Surgeon General, 2004.

Warren JJ, Levy SM: A review of fluoride dentifrice related to dental fluorosis. *Pediatr Dent* 1999; 21(4):265–71.

Warren, JJ, Levy SM: Current and future role of fluoride in nutrition. *Dent Clin North Am* 2003; 47(2):225–43.

Weaver CM, Heaney RP: Calcium. In Shils ME, Olsen JA, Shike M, Ross AC (eds): *Modern Nutrition in Health and Disease*, 9th ed. Baltimore: Williams & Wilkins, 1999.

Weigley ES, Mueller DH, Robinson CH: *Robinson's Basic Nutrition and Diet Therapy*, 8th ed. Upper Saddle River, NJ: Merrill/Prentice Hall, 1997.

Winston AE, Bhaskar SN: Caries prevention in the 21st century. *J Am Dent Assoc* 1999; 129(11):1579–87.

Yip R, Dallman PR: Iron. In Shils ME, Olsen JA, Shike M, Ross AC (eds): *Modern Nutrition in Health and Disease*, 9th ed. Baltimore: Williams & Wilkins, 1999.

Chapter 9

Vitamins Today

Carole A. Palmer

OBJECTIVES

The student will be able to:

- Define vitamins, and describe their functions in general.
- Differentiate between fat- and water-soluble vitamins.
- For each of the vitamins, list the major functions, general and oral effects of deficiency and excess, and food sources.

INTRODUCTION

The word *vitamin* comes from the time when these substances were erroneously thought to be protein in origin and were referred to as "vital amines." Vitamins are the most recent food substances determined to be essential nutrients. Most of the vitamins were identified in the early to middle 20th century. In the early part of the 20th century, a prime focus was on the prevention and cure of vitamin deficiency diseases such as:

- Scurvy: the scourge of sailors for centuries—result of vitamin C deficiency.
- Pellagra: a dreaded disease resulting in paralysis—result of vitamin B_3 (niacin) deficiency.
- Rickets: the cause of severely bowed legs in children—result of vitamin D deficiency.

Today, vitamin deficiency diseases have been eliminated for the most part in well-nourished societies, and current research focuses on the roles of vitamins in preventing or treating disease, enhancing overall health, and prolonging longevity.

FACTORS INFLUENCING VITAMIN STATUS

Many factors can affect ultimate vitamin status in the body:

- The vitamin content of the foods eaten is of primary importance.
- Physiological status greatly affects nutrient absorption. In general, as body stores decrease, absorption increases.
- Vitamin requirements are often increased in cases of severe illness and stress.
- Food preparation and cooking can also radically affect vitamin availability. Cooking will destroy heat-labile vitamins such as vitamin C. Prolonged storage can increase some vitamin losses through oxidation.
- There are also compounds found naturally in foods that can enhance or inhibit vitamin availability. For example:
  - Raw egg whites contain a compound that can bind biotin and prevent its absorption.
  - Enzymes in raw fish can destroy thiamine.
  - Milk is not a good source of preformed niacin, yet it is a considered a good niacin source

because it contains tryptophan, which is converted into niacin in the body.
- Niacin in corn is bound and unavailable, but it can be liberated by contact with alkali (such as when corn tortillas are prepared with an ingredient having an alkaline pH).

As a result of the interest in supplements and "fad" diets by the public, the dental team may encounter patients getting too few or too many vitamins or minerals. Severe deficiencies or toxicities may first be seen in the oral cavity, so dental team members need to be able to recognize vitamin-associated conditions and screen patients for vitamin deficiencies or toxicities. This chapter reviews the vitamin details. The screening process is detailed in Chapter 22.

CONTEMPORARY VITAMIN CONCERNS
Vitamin Deficiencies

While vitamin deficiencies are rare in healthy populations, vitamin deficiencies may be seen in individuals for a variety of reasons:

- Anyone can develop deficiencies by following vitamin deficient diets for prolonged periods.
- People with alcoholism may develop vitamin deficiencies due to poor diet and liver failure.
- Older people may develop vitamin deficiencies due to lack of appetite, poorly-fitting dentures, medications, physiological, and/or psychosocial factors (see Chapter 19).
- Anyone with physiological disorders that interfere with vitamin ingestion, digestion, absorption, or utilization may develop vitamin deficiencies.

Vitamin Overdoses and Toxicities

Vitamin safety has become more of an issue as people have increased total vitamin intake by using supplements in addition to foods. Very few food items are be consumed in amounts high enough to be harmful (an exception is polar bear liver, which contains toxic amounts of vitamin A). The known range of safety differs from vitamin to vitamin. Some have a very small range of safety, such as vitamin A or D. Others, like vitamin E, have not shown harmful effects even in quite large doses. Nevertheless, as with all foods and drugs, "too little" or "too much" can be fatal. The trick is to determine the meaning of these terms. Inadequate intake can be determined by the deficiency diseases, which can be monitored by biochemical markers. On the other hand, levels at which excesses interfere with function are more difficult to determine. In the past, it was thought that only the fat-soluble vitamins, which can be stored in body tissues, can result in toxicities. Now it is evident that very large doses of any nutrient can be harmful and even fatal. Even too much water can be fatal. Too much vitamin B_6 can cause neurological disorders.

The DRI (Dietary Reference Intake) and the UL (upper level of intake) provide good monitors of safe and unsafe levels of nutrient intake. One rule of thumb is that supplements at the level of 100% of the DRI are generally considered safe (this would be the amounts in a one-a-day type multivitamin). As intake increases above this level, so does risk. Thus higher intakes should be undertaken only under the supervision of a physician. Harmful effects of *megadoses* (very large doses, 10 times the DRI or more) continue to appear in the literature, often as a result of misguided individuals who think that "if a little is good, a lot will be even better." The topic of supplement safety is discussed in Chapter 10 on supplements.

VITAMIN FUNCTIONS, CHEMICAL STRUCTURE, AND NOMENCLATURE

Vitamins are organic substances found in most foods in small amounts and necessary for normal metabolic functioning. Each vitamin has a unique chemical structure, but all vitamins contain carbon, which classifies them as organic compounds. Many contain nitrogen. Some contain minerals such as sulfur or cobalt. Several exist in different forms, each with a different biological activity. One vitamin cannot substitute for another, nor can different vitamins be converted into another vitamin.

Humans cannot synthesize vitamins, so they must be supplied by the diet, either from food or supplements. Vitamins serve a variety of functions in the body. Some act as coenzymes in intermediary metabolism, whereas others function in oxidation/reduction (redox) reactions. It is a common misconception that vitamins are needed for energy. In fact, vitamins do not supply energy (calories) themselves, but they are needed at points along the metabolic pathways where energy is released from carbohydrates, lipids, and proteins, and, in some cases, in the conversion of one macronutrient to another.

Vitamins are consumed either preformed in their active vitamin form, or as precursors that can be converted in the body into the active vitamin (e.g., conversion of carotene to vitamin A in the liver).

Originally, vitamins were categorized into just two groups: fat-soluble (A) and water-soluble (B). Later they began to be classified according to function as well (e.g., K = Koagulation). The B-complex vitamins are also referred to as the energy-releasing vitamins because they are involved in the production of adenosine triphosphate (ATP) from the macronutrients. A subgroup of the B-complex vitamins, especially vitamins B_6, B_{12}, and folate, are involved in blood formation and are called hematopoietic vitamins. Vitamins A, C, and E are also antioxidants. The letter classification remains for most vitamins along with a number and the chemical designation (e.g., vitamin B_1 thiamine).

REVIEW OF THE FAT-SOLUBLE VITAMINS: A, D, E, K

Vitamins A, D, E, and K are called the *fat-soluble vitamins* because they dissolve in lipid and fat solvents rather than in water, are transported via the lymphatic system along with lipids, and are stored in the liver and other organs and the body's fatty tissues. They tend to be stable in foods, so losses in cooking are minimal. Absorption is reduced by the use of mineral oils and other laxatives, by bile-binding agents, and by some medications.

Vitamin A (Retinoids and Carotenoids)

Vitamin A is a group of compounds generally organized into two major classes: retinoids (preformed vitamin A found in animal foods) and carotenoids (vitamin A precursors found in certain vegetables and fruits). Retinoids exist in the body as retinal (vitamin A aldehyde), retinol (vitamin A alcohol), and retinoic acid (vitamin A acid).

Three carotenoids, alpha-carotene, beta-carotene, and beta-cryptoxanthin, are considered pro-vitamin A carotenoids because they can be converted to retinol in the body. Lycopene, lutein, and zeaxanthin are also carotenoids, but they cannot be converted into vitamin A in the body.

Functions

Vitamin A plays a major role in cell differentiation, so it is essential for reproduction, growth, bone and tooth development, synthesis and maintenance of healthy epithelia, and integrity of the immune system. Because vitamin A is essential for proper tissue epithelialization, it is important for the integrity of the oral cavity.

The most commonly recognized function of vitamin A is its role in preventing night blindness. Vitamin A is an essential component of rhodopsin, which is the eye pigment sensitive to light. When light hits rhodopsin, it splits the rhodopsin into the protein fragment (opsin) and retinal (vitamin A). In the dark, these components readily recombine if sufficient vitamin A is available. If there is deficiency of vitamin A, this regeneration is slower and the eye does not adapt as readily to the darkness (night blindness). Figure 9–1 shows the role of vitamin A in vision.

Vitamin A and the carotenoids are also potent antioxidants. They may play an important role in the prevention of many cancers, including oral cancer, as well as cataracts (Chasan-Taber et al., 1999).

Metabolism

Preformed vitamin A is more bioavailable and better absorbed than the carotenoids (Li, Tso, 2003). A small amount of the carotenoids consumed are converted to vitamin A in the intestinal wall. For every 12 µg of beta-carotene consumed from a mixed diet, 1 µg of retinol is synthesized. Consequently the efficiency of conversion

of beta-carotene to vitamin A is considered to be 12:1 on a weight basis.

About 90% of body storage of vitamin A is in the liver. Carotenoids are deposited in body fat. The majority of preformed vitamin A and the carotenoids are excreted into the bile and removed from the body via the feces. The kidney excretes some vitamin A.

When vitamin A is released from the liver to meet body needs, it is linked to specific proteins, retinol-binding protein (RBP) and transthyretin (TTR). This allows the fat-soluble vitamin A to be transported in the blood. RBP levels are maintained at a steady state in the body and prevent free retinol from circulating unchecked. This is important, as free retinol is highly toxic.

Nutrient adequacy of vitamin A is determined by assessing blood levels of either the vitamin directly or of carrier proteins. Serum carotene levels, however, reflect recent dietary intake, rather than body stores, and are not good monitors of vitamin A status.

Requirements and Range of Safety

The Recommend Dietary Allowances (RDAs) are based on a mixed diet of preformed vitamin A and carotene. In the American diet, carotene provides the majority of the vitamin A consumed, along with dietary supplements.

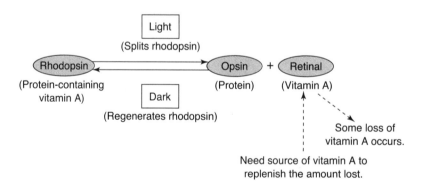

FIGURE 9–1   Role of vitamin A in vision. Rhodopsin is the eye pigment sensitive to light. When light strikes rhodopsin, it splits into its protein part (opsin) and its vitamin A part (retinal). Some vitamin A is lost in the process. In the dark, opsin and retinal rapidly recombine, provided there is an adequate supply of new vitamin A to replace the lost amount. If there is not enough vitamin A, regeneration is slow and the eyes cannot adapt to changes in light—as when a person goes from a lighted room into a dark one. The condition sometimes is called *night blindness*.
Source: From *Robinson's Basic Nutrition and Diet Therapy*: 8/E by Weigley/Mueller/Robinson, © 1997. Reprinted with permission.

There is no specific recommendation to date for the percentage of vitamin A that should come from carotenoids. The RDAs are given as retinol equivalents to adjust for a variety of food sources from a mixed diet (IOM, 2000, 2001).

> The RDA for children ranges from 300 to 600 μg/day depending upon age.
>
> The RDA for men aged 14+ is 900 μg/day.
>
> The RDA for women aged 14+ is 700 μg/day.
>
> The upper level of safety (UL) for vitamin A ranges from 600 to 3000 μg/day (0.6–3 mg/day) depending upon age.

In healthy people who get adequate vitamin A from their diets, reserves are gradually built up so that adults have sufficient stores to meet body needs for several months to more than a year. Infants and children have not yet built up such stores and are more vulnerable to the effects of dietary deficiency.

Food Sources

In U.S. and Canadian diets, the primary food sources of vitamin A are fortified grains and vegetables, followed by dairy and meat products (Tables 9–1, 9–2). About a third of the vitamin A in the U.S. food supply comes from the carotenoids in vegetables and fruits. Vitamin A is stable in ordinary processing and cooking temperatures. Frozen and canned foods may retain vitamin A for 9 months or longer. Wilted and dried vegetables and fruits and rancid fats usually lose most of their vitamin A activity to oxidation. Absorption is better from cooked foods than from raw.

The best sources of carotene are fruits and vegetables with deep yellowish orange, red, and dark green colors like pumpkin, sweet potato, carrots, spinach, canteloupe, mango, and greens (collard, kale, etc). Liberal intake of carotene-containing foods is especially important for vegetarians who rely on vegetables and fruits alone to meet their vitamin A requirements. Foods rich in carotenoids may provide some protection against certain forms of cancer, primarily because of their antioxidant properties. Public health organizations continue to recommend the consumption of fruits and vegetables rather than supplements, because it remains unknown what factors associated with fruits and vegetables are actually producing the effects.

TABLE 9–1 Food Sources of Vitamin A Precursor Carotene (as Retinal Equivalents)

- Yellow vegetables—carrot, pumpkin, sweet potato, winter squash
- Yellow fruits—apricot, cantaloupe, mango, papaya
- Green leafy vegetables—green tops of beets, turnips, mustard; chard, collards, kale, spinach, dark salad greens
- Green stem vegetables—asparagus, broccoli
- Red fruits and vegetables—tomato, red sweet bell pepper

Examples:
Peach (1 med) = 4667 RE
Raw carrot (1 med) = 2025 RE
Baked sweet potato (1 small) = 2382 RE
Cooked spinach (1/2 cup) = 875 RE
Cubed cantaloupe (1 cup) = 516.7 RE
Dried apricots (8 halves) = 202 RE
Romaine lettuce (1 cup) = 147 RE
Cooked green beans (1/2 cup) = 112 RE
Steamed broccoli (1/2 cup) = 110 RE
Cooked peas (1/2 cup) − 68 RE
Winter squash (1/2 cup) = 53 RE
Orange (1 med) = 27 RE

Preformed vitamin A is found in animal foods such as whole milk or vitamin A fortified skim milk, liver, fish, cream, butter, whole milk cheeses, fortified margarine, and egg yolk.

Supplements of vitamin A higher than RDA levels should not be taken due to the risk of toxicity. Patients should be encouraged to get their vitamin A from foods and not from supplements. Consumption should be in the range of 2–4 servings of fortified dairy

TABLE 9–2 Preformed Vitamin A Sources (High to Low)

Beef liver (3 oz) = 9011 RE
Lamb liver (3 oz) = 6366 RE
Mackerel (1 can) = 470 RE
Nonfat milk (1 cup) = 149 RE
Egg yolk (1) = 197 RE
Oyster (1) = 686 RE
Cheddar cheese (1 oz) = 86 RE
Whole milk (1 cup) = 76 RE
Butter (1 tsp) = 35 RE

products, 2–4 servings of fruits, and 3–5 servings of vegetables per day.

Effects and Oral Implications of Too Little Vitamin A

Vitamin A deficiency is rarely seen in countries where a varied diet is readily available or where vitamin A fortified foods are eaten. However, vitamin A deficiency can occur in:

- People with limited incomes or access to food
- People who eat a limited variety of foods containing vitamin A or carotene, or who severely restrict fat intake
- People with any condition of the intestinal tract that interferes with absorption, such as intestinal surgery or conditions resulting in malabsorption

In vitamin A deficiency, tissues fail to develop or regenerate properly, resulting in impaired healing (Olson 1994). As deficiency becomes more severe, symptoms such as dryness of the skin, impaired visual dark adaptation, and eye discomfort may result.

A common sign of deficiency is keratinization, or drying, scaling, and roughening of the skin, especially surrounding hair follicles (follicular hyperkeratosis). Soft, moist epithelia normally offer protection against bacteria, but as drying occurs, infections of the eyes, mouth, and respiratory and genitourinary tracts result. Xerophthalmia (dryness of the eye) develops in stages, the earliest of which is night blindness. This is followed by xerosis (drying and opaqueness) of the cornea. If treated at this point, the condition can be reversed. However, untreated xerosis progresses rapidly to the deep layers of the cornea with scarring and permanent blindness (Figure 9–2). As many as 10 million children, mostly in developing countries, become vitamin A deficient annually, and up to 500,000 go blind (Sommer, 1996). Vitamin A deficiency has also been associated with increased infectious morbidity and mortality. Children who are vitamin A deficient have a higher incidence of respiratory infections and diarrhea, and those with even mild xerophthalmia have four times the mortality rates of children who are not deficient (Ross, 1998). In countries that experience famine, vitamin A deficiency ranks second in prevalence only to protein-energy malnutrition. When the two deficiencies are present together, the prognosis is poor (Whiting, Lemke, 1999).

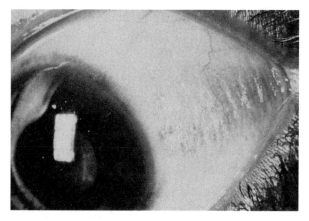

FIGURE 9–2 Xerosis (severe vitamin A deficiency).

Effects and Oral Implications of Too Much Vitamin A

Vitamin A intoxication (hypervitaminosis A) occurs primarily from oversupplementation of preformed vitamin A (such as in cod liver oil given in excess to children). High beta-carotene intake will *not* cause hypervitaminosis A. Excess carotene is extruded into the skin and fatty tissues, resulting in an orange coloration in skin and oral tissues. This coloration is particularly noticeable on the palms of the hands and may be distinguished from jaundice by the absence of changes in the sclera of the eye. Although unsightly, this skin coloration is benign and the skin color returns to normal with decreased carotene consumption.

Exposure to high doses of vitamin A (= or > 15,000 µg) for up to a few weeks, or lower but chronic doses for several months or more, can result in harmful effects. Toxicity can also result from excess intake of liver or other organ meats. Long before the toxic effects of vitamin A were known, Eskimos learned that eating polar bear liver could be fatal; a single gram of polar bear liver contains about 6000 RE of vitamin A! Those at greatest risk for toxicity are children, the elderly, and those with liver conditions (Hathcock et al., 1990). As in deficiency, toxicity can also result in impaired healing and growth. Excess vitamin A stimulates bone resorption and inhibits bone formation (Binkley, Krueger, 2000). Excess vitamin A may also be a risk factor for osteoporosis (Whiting, Lemke, 1999). Symptoms of toxicity include nausea, vomiting, abdominal pain, failure to grow in children or weight loss in adults, drying and scaling of the skin, thinning of the hair, swelling and tenderness of the long bones, joint pains, headaches, and enlargement of the liver. The condition is usually reversible when the supplement is discontinued, but full recovery may take several weeks.

In addition, in the Nurses Health Study a 48% increased risk of hip fracture in postmenopausal women was observed with intakes of vitamin A above 3000 µg (10,000 international unit [IU]) (Feskanich, Singh, Willett, Colditz, 2002).

The dental literature and individual case reports have documented cases in which failure of periodontal surgery to heal has been associated with patients' use of megadoses of vitamin A supplements (De Menezes, Costa, El-Guindy, 1984). Since vitamin A toxicity most commonly results from improper use of supplements, the FDA has limited the amount of preformed vitamin A allowed per individual pill or capsule to 5000 IU. However, it's impossible to control how many pills people choose to take!

Summary and Implications for Dentistry of Vitamin A

- Vitamin A deficiency is rare in developed countries.
- Deficiency can cause xerostomia (Anzano) and impaired healing.
- Toxicity is more common and can be fatal.
- Toxicity can cause birth defects, including abnormalities of the face, mouth, lips, and jaws. It can also interfere with epithelial tissue integrity and healing of periodontal tissues.
- Excess carotene may be manifested as orange pigmentation in skin and soft tissues, such as the soft palate and gingivae. However, this condition is generally benign and will disappear with reduced carotene consumption.

Vitamin D (Calciferol)

Vitamin D is actually a group of sterol compounds, the most important of which are vitamin D_3 (cholecalciferol), produced when 7-dehydrocholesterol in the skin is exposed to the sun's ultraviolet rays, and vitamin D_2 (ergocalciferol), produced in plants from the precursor ergosterol by ultraviolet light. Both forms of vitamin D are known by the general name calciferol, and both are converted in the body into the active form of vitamin D (IOM, 1997). This need for activation by sunlight has led vitamin D to be known as the "sunshine vitamin."

Vitamin D differs from the other fat-soluble vitamins in that it can be totally synthesized by the body, and dietary sources may or may not be required. Vitamin D activity in foods is measured in micrograms (µg), but the earlier international unit (IU) designation may be still seen on food and supplement labels.

Functions

The best known function of vitamin D is the facilitation of calcium and phosphorus absorption from the intestine and incorporation into developing bones and teeth.

Other important functions of Vitamin D are to:

- aid in the regulation of blood levels of calcium and phosphorus by influencing their resorption in the kidney (along with parathyroid hormone).
- aid in proper muscle, heart, and nerve function via regulating effects on calcium and phosphorus.
- possibly affect the cellular activity of several organs, including the skin, pancreas, and ovaries. (In this role, vitamin D functions as a hormone as it is synthesized by one organ but has its effects on other body organs.)
- play a role in decreasing the risk of breast cancer in premenopausal women in association with sunlight (Zhang, 2004).

Metabolism

Vitamin D is derived through conversion of precursors in the skin and from food sources (Figure 9–3). Ultraviolet light activates 7-dehydrocholesterol in the skin. From 50 to 80% of the vitamin D_3 produced from precursors in the skin is transported to the liver where it is transformed to 25-hydroxycholecalciferol [25(OH)D-calcidiol]. It is then transported to the kidneys where it is converted into the active form of vitamin D, 1,25-dihydroxycholecalciferol (calcitriol, or vitamin D_3 hormone). From the kidney, it is transported to the villi of the small intestine where it mediates calcium and phosphorus absorption. Food sources of vitamin D are absorbed like other lipids and transported via the lymph circulation to the liver.

Although vitamin D is found in several organs, it appears that the blood, liver, and adipose tissue are the primary storage locations. Vitamin D is excreted mainly through bile into the feces, with a small amount found in the urine.

The best measure of vitamin D status in individuals is serum 25(OH)D concentration.

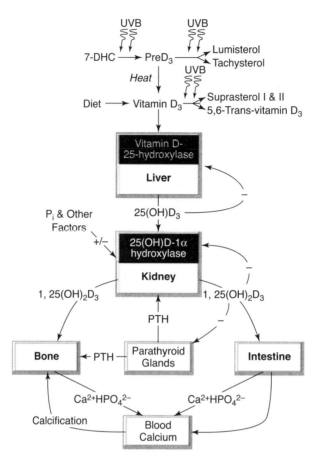

FIGURE 9-3 Photosynthesis of vitamin D_3 and the metabolism of vitamin D_3 to $25(OH)D_3$ and $1,25(OH)_2D_3$. Once formed, $1,25(OH)_2D_3$ carries out the biologic functions of vitamin D_3 on the intestine and bone. Parathyroid hormone (PTH) promotes the synthesis of $1,25(OH)_2D_3$, which, in turn, stimulates intestinal calcium transport and bone calcium mobilization, and regulates the syntesis of PTH by negative feedback.
Source: Reprinted with permission from *Dietary Reference Intake.* Copyright 2001 by the National Academy of Sciences. Courtesy of the National Academy Press, Washington, DC.

Requirements and Range of Safety

The Dietary Reference Intakes for vitamin D take into consideration availability via food sources only (as sun-mediated synthesis is too variable and difficult to assess), and are expressed as adequate intake (AI).

The AI for children, and men and women up to age 50 is 5 μg.

The AI for adults aged 51–70 is 10 μg.

The AI for seniors over age 70 is 15 μg.

The tolerable upper intake level (UL) has been set at 50 μg (2000 IU) per day.

A variety of factors can affect vitamin D requirements: These include:

• Periods of rapid growth
• Liver or kidney disorders

- Darker skinned people who produce less vitamin D
- Older people in whom slowing down of body processes may impede vitamin absorption and activation
- People who get less than a half-hour per week of sunlight (people who work at night and sleep during the day, who stay indoors, or whose clothing covers all the skin surface like veiled women or swaddled infants)
- When soot, fog, or window glass cut off ultraviolet light, thereby preventing the body from synthesizing vitamin D
- Active use of sunscreen—sunscreen SPF-8 or higher can block the sun's rays
- Use of Dilantin (phenytoin) which blocks vitamin D absorption

Food Sources

Approximately 90% of most people's vitamin D comes from sunlight, and 10% from food (especially fortified milk). Because vitamin D is stored in the body, good storage in sunny months can provide a reserve for the less sunny ones. Due to the many factors that can interfere with optimal body vitamin D synthesis, and the low natural vitamin D in foods (fatty fish and fish liver oils are the primary natural food sources) (Table 9–3), some groups (e.g., older people) may need to obtain the majority of their requirement from fortified food sources and may need supplements as well. Almost all fresh, powdered, evaporated milk, and infant formulas are fortified with 10 mg (400 IU) vitamin D per quart or its equivalent. (Human milk contains only about one-tenth this amount, but if the infant gets exposed to enough sunlight, this is sufficient.) Some breakfast cereals are also fortified with vitamin D. Most commercially manufactured cheeses, yogurts, and ice creams are not made from vitamin D fortified milk. Ingredient listings on food packages should provide information about vitamin D fortification. Vitamin D is stable in foods during storage, processing, and cooking.

Guidelines for Obtaining Sufficient Vitamin D

- **Up to age 50:** Go outside often and leave skin exposed for at least a half-hour two or three times a week (storage will last over winter). Homebound people need a supplement (rays don't pass through windows).
- **Over age 50:** Wait 10–15 minutes before applying sunscreen. Drink a quart of milk daily *or* take a supplement with 400 IU/day in the winter.

TABLE 9–3   Food Sources of Vitamin D

Salmon, sardines, herring, tuna, organ meats, vitamin D fortified milk and milk products, egg yolks, wheat germ

Examples:
Fresh salmon (3.5 oz) = 154–550 IU
Shrimp (3.5 oz) = 150 IU
Milk (1 cup) = 100 IU
Egg yolk (1 med) = 25 IU
Fresh herring (3.5 oz) = 315 IU
Beef liver (3.5 oz) = 9–42 IU
Fresh mackerel (3.5 oz) = 1150–1570 IU
Canned sardines (3.5 oz) = 1100 IU
Cheese (1 oz) = 4 IU

- **Over age 70 or diagnosed vitamin deficient:** All of the above plus take a daily multivitamin (100% DRI) *and* a 400 IU vitamin D supplement for a total of 800 IU supplemental/day.

Effects of Too Little Vitamin D

Vitamin D deficiency usually occurs in people who have insufficient exposure to sun, maintain rigidly restricted diets without vitamin D fortified foods, or have a condition that prevents the absorption of vitamin D from foods or conversion in the body (Calvo, Whiting, Barton, 2005). Vitamin D synthesis at age 80 is half that at age 20. None is produced from October through March north of 40th degree line (Philadelphia to Reno) (Hanley, Davidson, 2005). Black women living in northern latitudes have only half the vitamin D status of white women (Harris, Dawson-Hughes, 1998). Recent research has shown associations between vitamin D deficiency and muscle weakness among elderly people (Venning, 2005).

Too little vitamin D will cause severely decreased calcium and phosphorus absorption, resulting in too little calcium absorption to maintain required serum and bone levels. Calcium is then mobilized from bone to maintain steady serum levels, putting bone integrity at risk. Vitamin D deficiency is now recognized as a major cause of metabolic bone disease in the elderly. In recent studies of older hospitalized patients, more than 50% of patients studied were deficient in vitamin D (Dawson-Hughes, Harris, Krall, Dallal, 1997). The childhood form of vitamin D deficiency is rickets; the adult form is osteomalacia.

Rickets (Carpenter, 2003c; Mellanby, 1921) Rickets, the vitamin D deficiency disorder of infants and children, results in defective bone mineralization (Figure 9–4). The result is overgrown and disorganized capillaries, fibroblasts, and cartilage in areas where bone and cartilage join, resulting in soft, pliable bones that yield to pressure, enlargement of the joints, and delayed closing of the skull bones. The child may have an enlarged skull, chest deformities, poor muscle development, spinal curvature, and bowed legs. Overgrowth of cartilage at the rib–cartilage junction can result in beading of the ribs. A protruding sternum and depressions at the sides of the rib cage result in "pigeon breast." Although the fortification of milk with vitamin D (primarily) has eliminated rickets as a public health problem, there were outbreaks of rickets in the United States in the 1970s in children of strict vegetarians, who received no food sources of vitamin D (Dwyer, Dietz, Hass, Suskind, 1979).

Osteomalacia Osteomalacia, adult rickets, is rare. In osteomalacia, mineralization also fails and large areas of demineralized osteoid tissue are seen at the junctions of mineralized bone and layers of osteoblasts. Signs and symptoms include pain in the legs and lower back, and deformed bones of the spine, pelvis, and limbs, leading to spontaneous fractures. Osteomalacia has been seen after multiple pregnancies (and extremely inadequate intakes of vitamin D, calcium, and phosphorus), in people with severe malabsorption disorders (e.g., sprue, colitis, and cystic fibrosis), and in people with chronic renal disease, whose damaged kidneys are unable to convert vitamin D to its active form, and can develop bone pain and bone disease (osteodystrophy). Osteomalacia may also result from the use of some medications, depending on dosage and duration of use. For example, bile-binding agents used for their cholesterol-lowering effects, anticonvulsants, muscle relaxants, sedatives, and mineral oil can all decrease the absorption and synthesis of vitamin D. The severity of the effect depends on the dosage and duration of the medication usage.

Note: Osteoporosis differs from osteomalacia in that in osteoporosis, bone composition is normal but because more bone is mobilized than is reformed, total bone quantity is decreased. Vitamin D deficiency does not cause osteoporosis—the causes are multifactorial—but it may play a role by impairing calcium absorption (Holick, 1998). Osteoporosis is discussed in detail in Chapter 11 on chronic health conditions).

Oral Implications of Vitamin D Deficiency

Vitamin D deficiency during tooth development and calcification results in enamel and dentin hypoplasia, or incomplete development. In children with severe deficiency, the first tooth rarely erupts before 6 to 9 months of age because of delayed development. The enamel is poorly calcified and may fail to form at all in some areas. In the dentin, areas of uncalcified dentin matrix result. The earliest sign of vitamin D deficiency is a calciotraumatic line in the dentin (Nizel, Papas, 1989). Rats fed a vitamin D-deficient, low-calcium diet had greater mandibular bone resorption, more cemental resorption, and less cemental mineralization than did control animals (Golebiewska, Bielaczyc, 1997). It is also possible that the pitted enamel characteristic of rickets could increase caries risk by serving as a locus for plaque and sugar accumulation. However, despite the dental defects, an association between vitamin D deficiency and increased caries incidence has not been shown in humans. Since vitamin D deficiency is a major contributor to metabolic bone disease in elderly people, it may also be associated with alveolar bone loss. However, the research has not been done to show this to date (see Chapters 12 and 19).

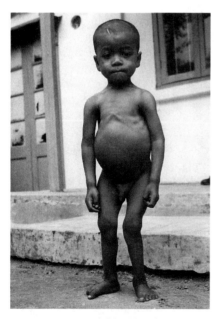

FIGURE 9–4 Child with rickets resulting from vitamin D deficiency.
Source: © World Health Organization.

Effects of Too Much Vitamin D

Hypervitaminosis D results primarily from excessive intake of supplements. It is not possible to develop hypervitaminosis from excess sun exposure alone because the body has protective feedback mechanisms to prevent this occurrence. Hypervitaminosis D is characterized by loss of appetite, increased thirst, vomiting, diarrhea, fatigue, drowsiness, and growth failure in children. Excessive supplementation of vitamin D for extended periods can result in hypercalcification of soft tissues, and ultimate death (Jacobus et al., 1992; Morita, Yamamoto, Takada, Ohnaka, Yuu, 1993; Vieth, 1999). As serum calcium levels increase, calcium salts are deposited in the soft tissues including the heart and blood vessels, lungs, and kidneys, leading to organ malfunction (Blank, Scanlon, Sinks, Lett, Kalk, 1995).

Although vitamin D at recommended levels is needed for the body to absorb calcium, too much vitamin D can also cause bone loss. According to the IOM of the National Academy of Sciences, these complications can occur with daily doses in excess of 2400 IU (600 μg).

Oral Implications of Too Much Vitamin D

Oral effects of hypervitaminosis D mimic those of deficiency and have been reported in the teeth of animals and humans (Giunta, 1998). Ameloblasts and odontoblasts are target cells for 1,25-dihydroxyvitamin d_3. An excess of vitamin D results in hypercalcemia (because of acceleration of intestinal calcium absorption) and bone resorption. This leads to disturbances in tooth matrix formation and calcification, and can result in either hypoplasia or hypocalcification, depending on the timing of the insult. Because enamel does not remodel, disturbances occurring during development remain as a permanent record.

Recently, overfortification of milk at a local dairy provided greater insight into the systemic and oral effects of vitamin D toxicity (Blank et al., 1995). A 7-year-old girl was found to have major defects in her permanent dentition. At the age of 15 months the child had been admitted to an endocrine service for failure to thrive. She had markedly elevated blood levels of calcium and had calcification of the kidneys. Oral examination revealed a healthy appearing, alert, bright female child with normal soft tissues and a normal mixed dentition. However, hypoplastic linear defects were seen on several of the erupted and partially erupted teeth. Changes noted in the deciduous central incisors were similar to those noted in the permanent central incisors. The pulp chambers of both permanent central incisors also showed significant changes.

The timing of the developmental defects of the teeth corresponded to the timing of the hypercalcemia and vitamin D intoxication. The hypoplastic lines on the crowns of the permanent central incisors and the roots of the deciduous canines corresponded to a time period of about 15 to 18 months of age. The hypocalcified line as noted radiographically corresponded to about 10 months of age, which is when the patient first received the whole milk. In addition to the dental defects noted, this child and several older individuals who had also consumed the overfortified milk were hospitalized with various degrees of kidney damage, which in some cases proved fatal (Giunta, 1998) (Figure 9–5).

Summary and Implications for Dentistry of Vitamin D

In summary, vitamin D is a particularly important vitamin for both general and oral health. Clinicians should consider the following points when they provide dietary guidance to patients:

- Sufficient vitamin D is crucial for proper mineralization of bones and teeth.
- The variations in potential body synthesis and contact with sunlight make food sources essential. The best food sources are fortified dairy products; vegetarians can purchase vegetable-based supplements.
- Older persons may need supplements as well as food sources.

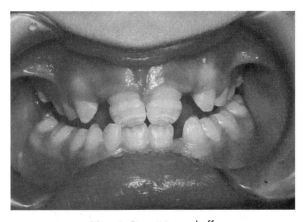

FIGURE 9–5   Vitamin D toxicity oral effects.
© John L. Giunta, DMD, MS.

- Dietary supplement use needs to be carefully monitored to prevent toxicity.
- Risk for deficiency increases with age, lack of sunlight, and poor diet.
- Risk of toxicity increases with increasing length and doses of supplements.
- Dental defects can result from deficiencies or excesses. In the developing dentition, hyper-vitaminosis D can cause both enamel hypoplasia and calcifications in soft tissues such as the pulp.

Vitamin E (Tocopherol)

Vitamin E is the general designation for several compounds that exhibit the biological activity of alpha-tocopherol. In nature, eight substances have vitamin E activity: alpha-, beta-, gamma-, and delta-tocopherol; and alpha-, beta-, gamma-, and delta-tocotrienol. Alpha-tocopherol is the most biologically active form and is the most widely distributed in foods. Measurement of vitamin E activity in foods is expressed as tocopherol equivalents (TE), based on the varying activity of the different forms of vitamin E present.

Functions

Vitamin E has many important functions in the body (Rock, Jacob, Bowen, 1996).

- It is a potent antioxidant in the body:
  - protects lipids in cell membranes from oxidation
  - prevents the hemolysis of red blood cells
  - protects vitamin A from oxidation
  - may contribute to cataract prevention along with carotenoids (Lyle, Mares-Perlman, Klein, Klein, Palta, et al., 1999)
- It acts as a scavenger to inactivate free radicals in cells. Free radicals are destructive, highly reactive atoms or molecules with one or more unpaired electrons. They are produced normally as by-products of metabolism and aging, and are also in environmental pollutants, such as smog and cigarette smoke.
- It inhibits the conversion of nitrites in pickled, smoked, and cured foods to cancer-causing nitrosamines in the stomach.
- It stimulates the immune response (Meydani et al., 1997) and helps lessen the severity of prostaglandin-mediated disorders such as inflammation and premenstrual syndrome, and circulatory disorders such as leg cramps.
- It may play a role in protecting against cardiovascular disease by preventing platelet adhesion (Rimm et al., 1993; Steiner, 1999).

Metabolism

Vitamin E is digested, absorbed, and transported similarly to the other fat-soluble vitamins. Absorption of alpha-tocopherol ranges from 20 to 80%. Absorption efficiency declines as the dosage increases (Hopkin, 2004). Vitamin E is stored in most organs, with the largest concentration found in adipose tissue. It is excreted in the bile and possibly the urine and skin.

Requirements and Range of Safety (IOM, 2000)

The requirement for vitamin E increases with increased intake of polyunsaturated fatty acids (PUFAs), due to its role as an antioxidant. The RDA of vitamin E is also measured as of alpha-tocopherol.

> The RDA for children up to age 13 ranges from 6 to 11 mg/day depending upon age.
>
> The RDA for adult men and women is 15 mg/day.
>
> The UL is 200–800 mg/day for children (depending upon age) and 1000 mg/day for adult men and women.

Food Sources

The best natural food sources of vitamin E are plant foods containing polyunsaturated fatty acids (Table 9–4). Wheat germ oil is the single richest source, whereas most fruits, vegetables, and animal foods are low in vitamin E (with the exception of egg yolk). Vitamin E is lost when whole grains are processed, so whole grains are better sources than refined flours. Fruits and vegetables combined are reported to provide more than 20% of the vitamin E in the American diet, followed by cereals, peanut butter, eggs, and nuts. Vitamin E is stable at normal cooking temperatures and in acids, but it can be destroyed by oxidation.

Effects and Oral Implications of Too Little Vitamin E

Vitamin E deficiency is extremely rare. Deficiency in humans has been seen primarily in premature infants, and people with fat malabsorption. Any person with malabsorption, such as persons with impaired pancreatic digestive function, diminished bile flow, or intestinal surgery, should be considered at risk for deficiency. Such patients usually are treated with a water-soluble vitamin E preparation.

TABLE 9-4 Food Sources of Vitamin E

Peas, lettuce, sweet potatoes, leafy vegetables, brown rice, rye, whole grain cereals, wheat germ, nuts, egg yolks, organ meats, molasses, corn oil, cold-pressed oils

Examples:
Wheat germ oil (1/4 cup) = 63.6 IU
Safflower oil (1/4 cup) = 19.5 IU
Sunflower oil (1/4 cup) = 18.3 IU
French dressing (cottonseed oil) (1/4 cup) = 13 IU
Wheat germ (1/4 cup) = 6.0 IU
Spinach (1/2 cup) = 2.2–3.3 IU
Canned peaches (1/2 peach) = 2.1–2.4 IU
Dried prunes (10 prunes) = 1.61–1.85 IU
Asparagus (5 spears) = 1.1–1.6 IU
Avocado (1/2 avocado) = 0.95–2.0 IU
Broccoli (3 stalks) = 0.8–3.4 IU
Shredded whole wheat cereal (1 cup) = 0.4–0.6 IU
Beef (3.5 oz) = 0.33–1.0 IU

Vitamin E deficiency can cause enamel defects in rats, although this has not been seen in humans. In rats, ameloblasts become disarranged, resulting in chalky white incisors (Nizel, Papas, 1989).

Effects and Oral Implications of Too Much Vitamin E

Toxicity from high intake of vitamin E has been rarely reported (Hathcock et al., 2005). This may be due to the inefficient absorption that occurs with high doses. Vitamin E intake at the level of 200 IU/day has been shown to reduce upper-respiratory infections a significant 20% in elders (Meydani et al., 1997). Megadoses of vitamin E administered intravenously, however, can lead to elevated blood lipids, interference with the vitamin K clotting mechanism, and impairment of white blood cell activity. Also increased vitamin E consumption via supplements resulted in increased gingival bleeding, particularly in those taking aspirin as well as vitamin E (Liede, Haukka, Saxen, Heinonen, 1998).

Implications for Dentistry of Vitamin E
- Vitamin E is important for immune function and as an antioxidant.
- Requirement increases with intake of polyunsaturated fatty acids.
- Excess in conjunction with aspirin intake can cause gingival bleeding.

Vitamin K (Quinone)

Vitamin K was first discovered in the 1930s and was called vitamin K after the German word "koagulation" for its role in blood coagulation. Vitamin K is found in at least three related forms: phylloquinone (vitamin K_1), commonly found in plants; menaquinone (vitamin K_2), synthesized by bacteria in the intestinal tract; and menadione (vitamin K_3), a synthetic water-soluble form.

Functions

The principal function of vitamin K is in several steps of the blood-clotting process in the liver. These include factor II (prothrombin), factor VII (proconvertin), factor IX (Christmas factor), factor X (Stuart factor), and proteins C and S. Prothrombin results from carboxylation of a precursor protein requiring vitamin K as a catalyst. Prothrombin is then converted to the enzyme thrombin in the presence of calcium and thromboplastin. Thrombin catalyzes fibrinogen into fibrin, which is the basis of a blood clot. In the absence of vitamin K or when there is a vitamin K antagonist such as coumarins (Warfarin, Dicumarol) or excess aspirin, the clotting factors will not form and blood clotting will be impaired (Figure 9–6).

Vitamin K also plays an important role in bone mineralization owing to its role in the activation of at least three proteins involved in bone formation. Vitamin K helps osteocalcin (bone protein) undergo carboxylation, which results in strengthening. If insufficient carboxyl groups attach to bone protein, the skeletal system can be weakened. Low dietary vitamin K intakes have been associated with hip fractures in elderly men and women (Booth et al., 2000). Conversely, there may be potential benefits of increased intakes of vitamin K for bone and vascular health (Vermeer et al., 2004).

Metabolism

The digestion and absorption of vitamin K require the same conditions as for the other fat-soluble vitamins. Vitamin K is stored in the liver and excreted mainly into the bile and urine. Intestinal bacteria synthesize the menaquinone form of vitamin K, but the contribution from this source to the maintenance of vitamin K status has been difficult to evaluate (Suttie, 1995). Vitamin K status is measured indirectly by tests that measure blood-clotting time.

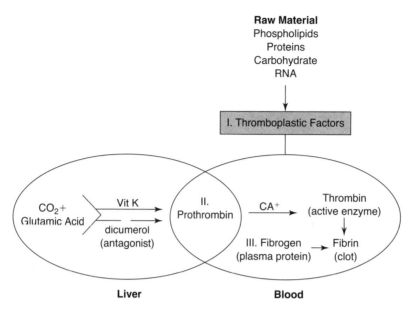

FIGURE 9–6 Blood-clotting mechanism. Without vitamin K or in the presence of a vitamin K antagonist such as coumarins (Warfarin, Dicumarol) or excessive salicylates (aspirin), prothrombin and other clotting factors cannot be formed, and the blood will not clot.

Requirements and Range of Safety (IOM, 2001; Weaver et al., 2004)

About half of the vitamin K requirement can be derived from food (plant) sources and the remainder comes from bacterial synthesis.

> The AI for children ranges from 30 to 75 μg/day, depending upon age.
>
> The AI is 90 μg/day for adult women aged 19+ and 120 μg/day for adult men aged 19+.
>
> A UL has not been set because no adverse effects have been reported for individuals consuming large amounts of vitamin K.

Food Sources

The primary dietary source of vitamin K is phylloquinone from green leafy vegetables such as broccoli, spinach, Brussels sprouts, turnip greens, lettuce, cabbage, and dried green tea leaves (Table 9–5). One serving of collards, spinach, or broccoli is equivalent to 5 times the RDA. In food, vitamin K appears stable in heat and to oxidation, but retention seems to decline when exposed to light, acid, and alkali. Vitamins A and E are antagonists of vitamin K in the body, but the exact mechanism of their interference is not known.

Patients on Warfarin therapy should have a consistent daily intake of vitamin K at the AI level (Booth, Centurelli, 1999).

Effects of Too Little Vitamin K

Newborns, those with liver disease or disrupted gastrointestinal flora, and those on antagonist medications are at greatest risk for vitamin K deficiency. Because the intestinal tract of newborns is sterile, sufficient synthesis of vitamin K may not occur until 1 week of age. Since breast milk is a poor source of vitamin K, hemorrhagic disease is a risk during the first days of life. To prevent this, a single dose of vitamin K, usually as an injection of phylloquinone (vitamin K_1), is given shortly after birth.

Severe liver disease may inhibit the synthesis of the clotting factors even when dietary vitamin K is adequate. Malabsorptions and biliary obstruction can lead to deficiency via malabsorption, as can mineral oil and bile-binding medications. Oral use of sulfa or antibiotic drugs can destroy gut bacteria and thus destroy the bacterial source of vitamin K. Some prescription and over-the-counter medications can counteract vitamin K activity (e.g., anticoagulants such as coumarins (Warfarin, Dicumarol used in treating heart disease).

TABLE 9–5 Food Sources of Vitamin K

Alfalfa, turnip greens, green vegetables, chlorophyll, cauliflower, oats, wheat, rye, soybeans, egg yolks, liver, yogurt, acidophilus, safflower oil, blackstrap molasses

Examples:
Turnip greens (2/3 cup) = 650 μg
Broccoli (2/3 cup) = 200 μg
Lettuce (2 cups) = 129 μg
Cabbage (2/3 cup) = 125 μg
Spinach (2/3 cup) = 89 μg
Beef liver (3.5 oz) = 92 μg
Cheese (3.5 oz) = 35 μg
Avocados (3.5 oz) = 20 μg
Egg yolk (1 med) = 11 μg
Peach (1/2 med) = 8 μg
Baked potato (1 med) = 6 μg

Aspirin and salicylates are also widely known for their ability to induce hypoprothrombinemia and hemorrhage.

Oral Implications of Vitamin K Deficiency

Hemorrhage could be a serious problem if an at-risk individual experiences an injury or has surgery, including oral surgery or dental prophylaxis. If possible, the use of anticoagulants should be suspended for a day or two before oral or periodontal surgery or prophylaxis.

Effects of Too Much Vitamin K

Toxicity of vitamin K has not been shown.

Summary and Implications for Dentistry of Vitamin K

* Vitamin K deficiency is rare but occurs most often in patients taking certain vitamin K antagonist medications.
* Dental team members should take a good history to determine factors that can affect vitamin K status.
* Patients on anticoagulant therapy should suspend use for 1–2 days if possible before any invasive oral soft tissue procedures are done.

SUMMARY AND IMPLICATIONS FOR DENTISTRY OF THE FAT-SOLUBLE VITAMINS

Many consumers buy and use fat-soluble vitamin supplements, unaware of potential harm. Toxicities of vitamins A and D are serious and can be fatal. Toxicity of

vitamin A causes birth defects, including abnormalities of the face, mouth, lips, and jaws. It can also interfere with epithelial tissue integrity and healing of periodontal tissues. Excess carotene may be manifested as orange pigmentation in skin and soft tissues, such as the soft palate and gingivae. However, this condition is generally benign and will disappear with reduced carotene consumption. Patients should be encouraged to get their vitamin A from foods and not from supplements (Krinsky, 2003).

Sufficient vitamin D is crucial for proper mineralization of bones and teeth. Evidence is increasing that it may be difficult to obtain sufficient vitamin D from ultraviolet light alone, so fortified food sources are essential. The best food sources are fortified dairy products; vegetarians can purchase vegetable-based supplements. The risk for deficiency increases with age, lack of sunlight, and poor diet. The risk of toxicity increases with increasing length and doses of supplements. Dental defects can result from deficiencies or excesses of vitamin D. Hypervitaminosis D can cause both enamel hypoplasia and calcifications in soft tissues such as the pulp.

Vitamin E is important for immune function and as an antioxidant. The requirement increases with intake of polyunsaturated fatty acids. There is little evidence to date for significant benefits or risks of vitamin E supplements in healthy individuals. The best sources of vitamin E are whole grains and oils.

Vitamin K deficiency is rare but occurs most often in patients taking vitamin K antagonist medications. Patients on anticoagulant therapy should suspend use for 1 to 2 days if possible before undergoing any invasive oral soft tissue procedures. Green leafy vegetables are the best sources of vitamin K. Table 9–6 provides a summary of the fat-soluble vitamins.

REVIEW OF THE WATER-SOLUBLE VITAMINS: B-COMPLEX AND C

Vitamins B-complex and C are called the *water-soluble vitamins* because they dissolve in water, are transported via active or passive transport in the portal system, and are not stored to any degree in body organs and tissues. The amount of any of the water-soluble vitamins present in the body at any time is called the "body pool." the body pool requires constant replenishment via the diet. The water-soluble vitamins can be readily oxidized by heat or light, and may leech out into cooking water, resulting in significant losses in cooking. Although toxicity like that occurring with fat-soluble vitamins is not

TABLE 9–6   Summary of Fat-Soluble Vitamins

Vitamin, Requirements, and Food Sources	Metabolism and Function	Signs and Symptoms of Deficiency or Excess	Oral Implications
Vitamin A Retinol Retinal Retinoic acid Provitamin A: Carotenes *RDA:* Adult men: 900 μg/day preformed vitamin A; women: 700 μg/day; UL: 3000 μg/day *Sources: Preformed vitamin A*: Animal foods, liver, egg yolk, butter, fortified margarine, milk, cream, cheese *Carotenoids*: Dark green leafy and deep yellow/orange/red vegetables, deep yellow and orange fruits	*Metabolism:* Preformed vitamin A more bioavailable than carotenoids; carotene converted to vitamin A in intestinal wall; bile needed for absorption; mineral oil prevents absorption; stored in liver *Functions:* Cell differentiation; bone and tooth development; healthy skin and mucous membranes; immune system integrity; vision in dim light	*Deficiency:* Night blindness; ↓ resistance to infection; xerophthalmia *Severe deficiency:* Drying and scaling of skin; eye infections; blindness *Excess:* Overdoses are toxic; skin, hair, and bone changes; abnormalities of the face, mouth, lips and jaw	*Deficiency:* Leads to inadequate differentiation of cells; impaired healing and tissue regeneration; desquamation of oral mucosa; keratosis; ↑ risk of candidiasis; gingival hypertrophy and inflammation; leukopenia; ↓ taste sensitivity; xerostomia; disturbed or arrested enamel development; irregular tubular dentin formation; ↑ caries risk *Excesses:* Mimic signs of deficiencies
Vitamin D Calciferol Precursors: • Ergosterol in plants • 7-dehydrocholesterol in skin *AI:* Men and women: 5 μg (200 IU) up to 50 yr, 10 μg (400 IU) 50–70 yr, 15 μg (600 IU) 71+ yr UL: 50 μg (2000 IU) *Sources:* Fortified milk, concentrates: calciferol & viosterol, fish-liver oils, exposure to ultraviolet rays of sun	*Metabolism:* Some storage in liver; liver synthesizes calcidiol; kidney converts calcidiol to calcitriol (active form) *Functions:* Hormone in absorption of calcium and phosphorus; mobilization and mineralization of bone	*Deficiency:* Rickets in babies → • Soft bones • Enlarged joints • Enlarged skull • Deformed chest • Spinal curvature • Bowed legs Osteomalacia in adults; osteodystrophy in renal disease *Excess:* Overdoses are toxic	*Deficiency:* Leads to abnormal bone regeneration; osteoporosis; osteomalacia; incomplete calcification of teeth and alveolar bone rickets *Excesses:* Lead to pulp calcification and enamel hypoplasia
Vitamin E Tocopherol *RDA:* Adult men and women: 15 mg α-TE *Sources:* Salad oils, shortenings, margarines, whole grains, legumes, nuts, dark green leafy vegetables	*Metabolism:* Limited stores in body—largest in adipose tissue; polyunsaturated fats increase need *Functions:* Prevents oxidation of vitamin A in intestine; protects cell membranes against oxidation; protects red blood cells	*Deficiency:* Not common, seen in infants or those with malabsorption; causes red cell hemolysis in malnourished infants *Excess:* Low toxicity	*Deficiency:* Leads to enamel defects in rats (not seen in humans to date) *Excesses:* In conjunction with aspirin, may cause gingival bleeding

Vitamin K
Quinone
AI: Adult men 120 µg/day
    adult; women: 90 µg/day
Sources: Synthesized by
    intestinal bacteria, dark
    green leafy vegetables

Metabolism: Synthesized by
    intestinal bacteria; stored
    in liver
Functions: Forms prothrombin
    for normal blood clotting;
    activation of proteins for
    bone formation

Deficiency: Prolonged clotting
    time; hemorrhage, especially
    in newborn infants; biliary
    tract disease
Excess: Toxic in large amounts

Deficiency: Leads to ↑ risk
    of candidiasis

seen, excessively high doses of several of the water-soluble vitamins have serious harmful effects in humans.

The first B-complex vitamin was a substance found in food that prevented the potential fatal condition, beriberi. It was named vitamin B in 1915. Subsequently, vitamin B was found to be eight different compounds with dissimilar properties, and they were called B-complex vitamins and named $B_1, B_2, B_3,$ and so on. Because people were accustomed to the letter classification, it has been retained for most vitamins along with the more precise chemical designation. Thus, vitamin B_1 is also called thiamine.

The B-complex vitamins are also referred to as the "energy-releasing vitamins" because they are involved in the production of ATP from the macronutrients. For example, metabolism of carbohydrates, protein, and fat require thiamine, niacin, riboflavin, pantothenic acid, and biotin A subgroup of the B-complex vitamins, especially vitamins B_6, B_{12}, and folate, are involved in blood formation and are also called "hematopoietic vitamins." Those vitamins that have antioxidant functions (A, C, E) were labeled "antioxidant vitamins."

The B-complex vitamins are found widely in foods and function closely together. All B-complex vitamins are found in yeast and liver and promote bacterial growth. The relationship among the B vitamins is such that deficiency of one impacts the others. In fact, particularly in the case of vitamins B_1 (thiamine), B_2 (riboflavin), and B_3 (niacin), deficiency of a single B-complex vitamin is rarely seen. B-complex vitamins are no longer required on food labels because deficiencies are rare and these vitamins are plentiful in food.

The B-Complex Vitamins

Vitamin B_1 (Thiamine)

Thiamine was the first of the eight B-complex vitamins to be discovered. Its deficiency disease, beriberi, was recognized as early as 2600 BC. The cause of beriberi was discovered when it was found that chickens and sailors who ate polished rice developed the severe polyneuritis characteristic of the disease, whereas those fed whole grain rice were protected (Carpenter, 2003b). The protective compound was found to be thiamine. Thiamine is unique in that it is one of the few vitamins that contains a mineral (sulfur).

Functions Like most of the B-complex vitamins, thiamine functions primarily as a component of an essential coenzyme. The particular coenzyme, thiamine pyrophosphate (TPP), is necessary for the decarboxylation of alpha-keto acids, critical to the transformation of carbohydrates (especially glucose), proteins, and fats into energy. TPP also is required as a coenzyme for the enzyme transketolase. This enzyme functions in the pathway that produces ribose, a sugar essential for the formation of DNA and RNA. Apart from its coenzyme functions, thiamine is necessary for the synthesis of acetylcholine for proper functioning of nerves. Deficiency of ACTH causes polyneuritis and memory loss. The neuritis of alcoholism is similar to the polyneuritis of thiamine deficiency.

Metabolism Thiamine is absorbed by active transport into the portal circulation. When high levels are ingested, some is absorbed by passive diffusion. There appears to be no specific storage location. The majority of thiamine is found in muscles, but some is found in the liver and other organs. Thiamine and its breakdown products are excreted in the urine.

Because thiamine is not stored, it must be frequently replenished in the diet. Thiamine has a short half-life of only 9–18 days in any tissue. Thus, there must be a constant supply available. Thiamine status is assessed indirectly by measuring red blood cell levels of the enzyme, transketolase.

Requirements and Range of Safety Requirements are based on the calorie content of the diet, especially the energy yielded from carbohydrate.

Requirements increase with increased exercise and carbohydrate intake:

> The RDA for children ranges from 0.5 to 1.2 mg/day depending upon age and gender.
>
> The RDA for adult males aged 14+ is 1.2 mg/day.
>
> The RDA for adult females aged 19+ is 1.1 mg/day.
>
> A UL has not been set for thiamine.

Food Sources Thiamine is widely distributed in small amounts in most plant and animal foods (Table 9–7). The best sources are whole and enriched grains. Thiamine is also found in dry beans and peas and vegetables, such as potatoes. Of the meats, lean pork is especially high in thiamine.

Thiamine is destroyed by heat, so thiamine can be lost during soaking or cooking of food. Thiamine can also be destroyed by alkali such as sulfur dioxide (used to dry fruits), and baking soda. So baking soda should not be used in cooking water to help preserve the green color of vegetables because it destroys the thiamine. Since thiamine is removed during the refining process, whole or enriched grains should be used. Thiamine is one of the three vitamins added to flour, breads, cereals, pasta, and rice during the "enrichment" process.

Effects of Too Little Thiamine Thiamine deficiency is rare in developed countries due to the prevalence of thiamine in food and the enrichment of refined grains. Deficiencies have been seen in malnourished homeless people, refugees from war-torn countries, some elderly people with narrow food variety, and people with decreased absorption or increased cellular utilization. Wernicke-Korsakoff syndrome is the classic thiamine deficiency seen secondary to alcohol abuse.

The classic thiamine deficiency disease is beriberi (Carpenter, 2003c). The disease is progressive in adults, but in infants, the onset can seem to be sudden, with the outcome fatal. Beriberi affects the gastrointestinal, cardiovascular, and nervous systems. Early symptoms include fatigue, irritability, depression, and loss of appetite, weight, and strength. With advanced deficiency, adult symptoms may include indigestion, constipation, headaches, unusually rapid heart rate after mild exercise, numbing of the feet, and cramping or weakness of the legs.

In patients over age 65 who had subclinical thiamine deficiency, B_1 supplementation resulted in improved sleep and energy and decreased blood pressure (Wilkinson, Hanger, Elmslie, George, Sainsbury, 1997). However, there is no scientific evidence to support supplementation with thiamine to improve energy levels or combat emotional stress in well-nourished individuals.

Oral Implications of Thiamine Deficiency Possible oral implications of deficiency include taste loss, burning tongue, and increased sensitivity of the oral mucosa. However, these symptoms are nonspecific and can result from other B-complex deficiencies as well. Thiamine deficiency alone is rare.

Effects of Too Much Thiamine Excessive oral ingestion of thiamine appears to have no adverse side effects.

Vitamin B_2 (Riboflavin)

Riboflavin was the first vitamin identified to function as a coenzyme. It is a unique yellow-green fluorescent pigment. The faint green tinge seen in skim milk is riboflavin. In foods, these color pigments are designated as "flavins."

In contrast to several other vitamins, riboflavin is stable in heat. It dissolves sparingly in water and is stable during cooking and in the presence of air and acids.

TABLE 9–7 Food Sources of Thiamine

Wheat germ (1/4 cup) = 0.47 mg
Ham (3 oz) = 0.4 mg
Cereal (RTE) = 0.38 mg (most servings)
Brewer's yeast (1 Tbsp) = 0.34 mg
Oysters (3/4 cup) = 0.25 mg
Beef liver (3 oz) = 0.23 mg
Peanuts (1/2 cup) = 0.22 mg
Green peas (1/2 cup) = 0.22 mg
Raisins (1 cup) = 0.21 mg
Collard greens (1/2 cup) = 0.14 mg
Orange (1) = 0.13 mg
Dried beans and peas (1/2 cup) = 0.13 mg
Asparagus (1 cup) = 0.12 mg
Cauliflower (1 cup) = 0.11 mg
Nonfat milk (1 cup) = 0.09 mg
Small potato (1) = 0.08 mg
Whole wheat bread (1 slice) = 0.06 mg
Brussels sprouts (1/2 cup) = 0.06 mg
Extra lean beef (3 oz) = 0.05 mg
Chicken meat (3 oz) = 0.05 mg

Note: RTE = ready to eat.

However, it is destroyed by alkali (like baking soda) and is quickly decomposed by ultraviolet rays and light. Recently there has been concern over riboflavin losses from milk kept in nonopaque containers under strong grocery store lights. As a result, more milk processors are packaging milk in paper cartons and opaque materials rather than glass bottles. In food, riboflavin is measured in milligrams.

Functions Riboflavin is known to be a constituent of several enzymes, especially riboflavin monophosphate (FMN) and flavin adenine dinucleotide (FAD). FMN and FAD function as hydrogen carriers for the oxidation reduction reactions leading to the formation of ATP. In this role, Riboflavin is involved in energy transfer reactions, which release energy from carbohydrate, protein, and fat. FMN is a component of L-amino acid oxidase, which oxidizes L-alpha amino acids and L-alpha hydroxy acids to alpha-keto acids. Flavin enzymes are also involved in the deamination of amino acids. Riboflavin is also needed for normal fatty acid and amino acid synthesis. Cellular growth cannot occur without riboflavin (Powers, 2003).

Metabolism Riboflavin exists either in the free state or in combination with other compounds, especially protein and phosphate. Riboflavin is absorbed by active transport. No site serves as a special storage depot. Riboflavin and its metabolites are excreted in the urine, which takes on a bright orange-yellow color. The activity of one of the red blood cells' enzymes, glutothione reductase, of which riboflavin is a constituent, is the laboratory test used to measure riboflavin status.

Requirements and Range of Safety Riboflavin requirements are also based upon energy consumption and need during positive protein balance. The DRIs are set at approximately 0.6 mg/1000 cal/day. Tissue reserves cannot be maintained at an intake below 1.2 mg/day.

The RDA for children ranges from 0.5 to 1.0 mg/day depending upon age and gender.

The RDA for adult men aged 14+ is 1.3 mg/day.

The RDA for adult women aged 19+ is 1.1 mg/day.

No UL of safety has been set.

Food Sources Milk, and to a lesser extent other animal products, is the best source of riboflavin (Table 9–8). Riboflavin is also found to a lesser extent

TABLE 9–8   Food Sources of Riboflavin

Beef liver (3 oz) = 3.6 mg
Low-fat milk (1 cup) = 0.52 mg
Low-fat yogurt (1 cup) = 0.39 mg
Oysters (3/4 cup) = 0.30 mg
Cereal (RTE) = 0.25–0.43 mg/serving (most RTE cereals)
Avocado (1/2) = 0.22 mg
Collard greens (1/2 cup) = 0.19 mg
Chicken meat (3 oz) = 0.16 mg
Canned salmon (3 oz) = 0.16 mg
Asparagus (1/2 cup) = 0.13 mg
Broccoli (1/2 cup) = 0.12 mg
Brussels sprouts (1/2 cup) = 0.11 mg
Spinach (1/2 cup) = 0.11 mg
Whole wheat bread (1 slice) = 0.05 mg

in plants. It is also added to refined flour during the enrichment process. Retention in foods is better than for some of the other vitamins.

Effects of Too Little Riboflavin Usually, rather than a separate condition, inadequate riboflavin status is associated with other vitamin B-complex deficiencies. Some medications, such as chloramphenicol, have been associated with riboflavin deficiency.

General signs and symptoms of deficiency include:

• growth failure
• greasy scaliness of the skin around the nose and ears
• eye fatigue, itching, burning, and watering, and extreme sensitivity to bright light
• increased capillary blood vessels in the cornea giving a "bloodshot" appearance

Oral Implications of Riboflavin Deficiency Several oral signs and symptoms are associated with insufficient intake of riboflavin including:

• cracking of the skin at the corners of the lips (angular cheilosis)
• purple-red swollen tongue (glossitis)
• inflammation of the corners of the mouth (angular stomatitis)
• edema of oral and throat mucous membranes

Effects of Too Much Riboflavin Riboflavin toxicity has not been reported, probably because riboflavin absorption appears limited.

Vitamin B₃ (Niacin)

Niacin deficiency disease, pellagra, was a problem in the United States in the early 1900s (Carpenter, 2003c), and was found to be cured by adding milk, meat, and eggs to a diet of corn, pork, hominy, and molasses. Niacin is the general term applied to the two active forms of the vitamin: nicotinamide and nicotinic acid (not related to nicotine). Niacin is a constituent of the coenzymes nicotinamide adenine dinucleoticle (NAD) and nicotinamide adenine dinucleotide phosphate (NADP). It is stable in heat, acids, light, and oxygen (air). Thus, retention of preformed niacin in foods is good, but can be lost if cooking water is discarded.

Functions Like thiamine and riboflavin, niacin functions as a coenzyme in release of energy from the macronutrients, as well as for their synthesis. It is involved in over 50 metabolic reactions. Some roles include synthesis of NAD and NADP, which function in oxidation-reduction reactions important in carbohydrate metabolism; the deamination of amino acids; and the oxidation and synthesis of fatty acids. Niacin is also essential for steroid formation, red blood cell formation, and the metabolism of several drugs. In essence, niacin is essential to the functioning of all body cells.

Metabolism Food sources of niacin are almost completely absorbed. The body is also able to transform tryptophan, an essential amino acid, into niacin. This conversion requires vitamins B_1, B_2, B_3, and B_6. Niacin status is assessed by measuring the amount of niacin metabolic by-products excreted in the urine.

Requirements and Range of Safety Determination of the requirements for niacin is complicated by the fact that the body can use tryptophan as a precursor of niacin. The RDAs take this conversion into consideration and thus are expressed as NE (niacin equivalent). Generally, 1 mg of niacin can be produced from 60 mg of tryptophan. The RDAs for niacin are based on energy intake at a level of about 6.6 mg/1000 cal.

The diet should have no less than 13 mg/day to maintain niacin balance. In the third trimester of pregnancy, women can convert tryptophan to niacin three times as rapidly as normally.

The RDA for children is from 6 to 12 mg/day depending upon age.

The RDA for adult men aged 14+ is 16 mg/day.

The RDA for adult women aged 14+ is 14 mg/day. The UL ranges from 10 to 35 mg/day depending on age.

The upper limit of safety for niacin is based upon the intake of supplements. For treatment of clinical deficiency, a safe range is considered to be from 40 to 250 mg, tapering off over time.

Food Sources Generally about half of the daily requirement is derived from tryptophan conversion. The other half is from food sources (Table 9–9). Niacin in foods is measured in milligrams of preformed niacin. Foods in typical American diets furnish about 1% tryptophan from good-quality proteins. Thus, a 60 g protein diet could supply an additional 10 NE. Meat, fish, and poultry are the chief sources of preformed niacin. Some niacin is also present in vegetables. The niacin in whole grains is bound, making much of it (up to 70%) biologically unavailable. This chemically bound niacin can be released in an alkaline environment (such as lime). Niacin is added to refined grains labeled "enriched"; such grains provide biologically available preformed niacin.

Effects of Too Little Niacin The classic niacin deficiency disease is pellagra (Carpenter, 2003c). Pellagra often is called the disease of the "4 Ds"—diarrhea, dermatitis, dementia, and death. The symptoms are progressive:

- The first signs are usually seen in the gastrointestinal tract because the cells there turn over so quickly. Diarrhea is common.
- An extremely sore and swollen tongue makes eating difficult.

TABLE 9–9 Food Sources of Niacin (as Niacin Equivalents)

Chicken (1/2) = 21.5 NE
Salmon (3 oz) = 9.6 NE
Beef (2.9 oz) = 7.1 NE
Peanut butter (2 Tbsp) = 6.2 NE
Cereal (RTE) = 5.0 mg (NE) (most RTE cereals)
Green peas (1 cup) = 4.5 NE
Potato (1 med) = 3.6 NE
Brewer's yeast (1 Tbsp) = 3.6 NE
Milk (1 cup) = 2.2 NE

- Next, skin changes appear. Dermatitis is symmetrical—that is, on both hands, both forearms, both legs. The exposed parts of the body are more affected, leading to sensitivity to the sun.
- As the disease advances, mental changes become evident, such as depression, disorientation, delirium, and dementia.
- Without treatment, the ultimate outcome is death.

Oral Implications of Niacin Deficiency Oral signs and symptoms of deficiency are much the same as with riboflavin:

- Angular cheilosis (lip fissures)
- Stomatitis (inflammation in corners of mouth)
- Tongue: sore, swollen, smooth, scarlet red color
- Secondary infection with fungi or bacteria as in acute necrotizing ulcerative gingivitis
- Inflammation of oral mucosa leading to painful eating and swallowing

Effects of Too Much Niacin Toxic effects from food sources of nicotinamide have not been seen. However, toxic effects have resulted from the use of nicotinic acid for the treatment of heart disease (levels of around 3000 mg or greater). Potential beneficial effects include decreased total cholesterol and LDLs and increased HDLs, but harmful side effects can also occur. The most immediate and obvious symptoms are uncomfortable sensations from flushing of the skin, accompanied by skin redness. More serious side effects include heartburn, gastric ulcers, and elevated blood glucose levels. Time-release niacin supplements may increase risk of liver damage and should be monitored closely by a physician. Otherwise, unless a person has a proven niacin deficiency, large doses of niacin are not indicated.

Summary and Implications for Dentistry of the B-Complex Vitamins

- Deficiencies of thiamine, riboflavin, and niacin are rare in developed countries due to the prevalence of these vitamins in foods and the enrichment of refined grains.
- Deficiency of only one of these vitamins and not the others is rare.
- Deficiency, when it does exist, is seen primarily in elderly people and alcoholics.

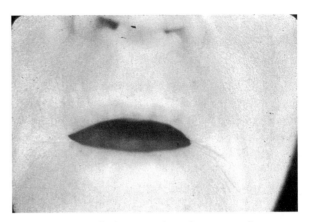

FIGURE 9–7 Cheilosis (cracks in the corner of the mouth).

- Oral signs and symptoms of deficiency are similar for all of the B-complex vitamins and include:
  - cracking of the skin at the corners of the lips (angular cheilosis) (Figure 9–7)
  - purple-red swollen tongue (glossitis)
  - inflammation of the corners of the mouth (angular stomatitis)
  - edema of oral and throat mucous membranes
  - sore, swollen, smooth, scarlet red colored tongue (glossitis)
  - secondary infection with fungi or bacteria as in acute necrotizing ulcerative gingivitis
  - inflammation of oral mucosa leading to painful eating and swallowing
- Supplements are not usually needed for those having a healthy diet.
- Supplementation of niacin for cholesterol control needs to be under the careful supervision of a physician.

The Hematopoeitic Vitamins

Vitamin B$_6$ (Pyridoxamine)

Vitamin B$_6$ consists of a group of related compounds, all with some vitamin activity: pyridoxine (mostly in plant products), pyridoxal, and pyridoxamine (mostly in animal products). Pyridoxine is the most stable. All forms can be destroyed by light, especially in neutral and alkali mediums. Measurement of vitamin B$_6$ in foods is in milligrams.

Functions Vitamin B$_6$ is unique in that most of its enzyme systems are involved in protein metabolism, rather than in the release of energy. Vitamin B_6 is a constituent of the coenzyme pyridoxal phosphate (PLP), a coenzyme needed for nitrogen metabolism. PLP is involved in protein amination, de-amination, and transamination. It is needed for normal development and function of red blood cells, and for the normal synthesis of hemoglobin. In this role, vitamin B_6 can be classified as a hematopoietic vitamin.

Vitamin B_6 also helps remove sulfur from sulfur-containing amino acids, and is necessary for the conversion of tryptophan to niacin. It is also required for the conversion of glycogen to glucose, and is involved in selenium function.

Metabolism Vitamin B_6 usually is present in a bound form in food. It is liberated during digestion, passively absorbed, and transported in blood circulation. Although the liver does store some vitamin B_6, most of it is located throughout the body, especially in the muscles. The vitamin itself, along with metabolic by-products, is excreted in the urine. To evaluate vitamin B_6 status, a number of urine tests are performed. The presence in the urine of xanthurenic acid, a product of faulty tryptophan metabolism, is one test for B_6 deficiency.

Requirements and Range of Safety The RDAs for vitamin B_6 (pyridoxine) are based upon protein intake, at a level of 0.016 mg/g protein for adults. When protein intake increases or when the body's needs for protein increase, as during pregnancy, vitamin B_6 requirements increase. The RDA for B_6 is based upon a diet of 100 g of protein.

The RDA for children ranges from 0.5 to 1.0 mg/day depending upon age.

The RDA for adult men aged 14–50 is 1.3 mg/day and for men over age 50 is 1.7 mg/day.

The RDA for adult women aged 14–50 is 1.2–1.3 mg/day and for those over age 50 is 1.5 mg/day.

The UL ranges from 30 to 100 mg/day depending upon age.

Food Sources Vitamin B_6 is found in all foods, plant and animal, with the exception of fat and sugar. Vitamin B_6 appears to be more bioavailable from animal sources (Table 9–10). However, its bioavailability and retention are best in minimally processed animal foods. Absorption is usually greater than 75% for most foods.

TABLE 9–10   Food Sources of Vitamin B_6 Pyridoxine

Banana (1 med) = 0.48 mg
Avocado (1/2 med) = 0.42 mg
Hamburger (3 oz) = 0.391 mg
Chicken (3 oz) = 0.34 mg
Fish (3 oz) = 0.289 mg
Potato (1 med) = 0.2 mg
Collard greens (1/2 cup) = 0.17 mg
Cooked spinach (1/2 cup) = 0.161 mg
Brown rice (1/2 cup) = 0.127 mg
Green peas (1/2 cup) = 0.11 mg
Walnuts (8–10 halves) = 0.109 mg
Peanut butter (2 Tbsp) = 0.096 mg
Wheat germ (1 Tbsp) = 0.055 mg

It binds with fiber and with other substances in plants. Vitamin B_6 is lost when whole grains are milled, and is not one of the three vitamins added to enriched grains. Food retention varies, as it is destroyed by heating and freezing.

Effects of Too Little Vitamin B_6 Symptoms of deficiency in adults include irritability, depression, confusion, anemia, nausea, seborrheic dermatitis, peripheral neuritis, ataxia, convulsions, and abnormal EEG. Vitamin B_6 deficiency has a serious effect on brain function because it plays an important role in the synthesis of several neurotransmitters. Vitamin B_6 deficiency has been implicated along with B_{12} and folate deficiency as a risk factor for heart attack. One mechanism is via the association of vitamin B_6 with the amino acid homocysteine. Homocysteine requires vitamins B_6, B_{12}, and folic acid for its metabolism. In the absence of one or more of these vitamins, homocysteine levels build up in the blood and can cause heart attacks. Low vitamin B_6 status has also been linked to higher levels of high-sensitivity C-reactive protein (CRP) and fibrinogen, both of which are markers for the arterial inflammation that can raise risk for coronary artery disease (Low levels of vitamin B_6, 2004). Vitamin B_6 deficiency can also have serious effects on amino acid metabolism. In the 1950s vitamin B_6 was inadvertently destroyed during sterilization of infant formula. Since infancy is a time of rapid formation of body proteins, deficiency soon became apparent. The infants fed this formula had reduced growth rates, nervous irritability, hypochromic anemia, and convulsions. They recovered promptly when adequate vitamin B_6 was provided. All commercial formulas for infants now supply sufficient vitamin B_6 to meet infants' needs.

Vitamin B_6 deficiency can impair immune function via its effects on protein synthesis and cell division. Vitamin B_6 deficiency reduces T-helper cell production and induces a decrease in lymph cell production (Malouf, 2005).

Several medications affect B_6 absorption or metabolism: Isoniozid, used for the treatment of tuberculosis, binds vitamin B_6 so that it cannot be utilized by the body. If the intake of vitamin B_6 is not increased, neurological problems may occur. Penicillamine, a medication used in the treatment of Wilson's disease, increases the loss of the vitamin in the urine. Amphetamine, chlorpromazine, reserpine, and oral contraceptives affect tissue concentrations. Renal dialysis treatments remove the vitamin. In these conditions, supplements of vitamin B_6 are recommended.

Oral Implications of Vitamin B_6 Deficiency Oral deficiency signs, as with other B-complex vitamins, include:

- Stomatitis—inflammation of oral mucous membranes
- Cheilosis—cracks in the corners of the mouth
- Glossitis—inflammation of the tongue

Effects of Too Much Vitamin B_6 The use of vitamin B_6 in doses >1 g/day over time to treat conditions such as premenstrual syndrome, asthma, and some sensory neuropathies has resulted in cases of neurotoxicity and photosensitivity (IOM, 1998).

Folate (Folic Acid, Pteroylmonoglutamic Acid)

Folate is the general term applied to several forms of the vitamin, including folic acid and pteroylmonoglutamic acid. It was discovered as an antianemic factor for treating anemia in pregnant women and was found to exist in green leaves, hence the term *folic* (foliage). Because of its role in blood formation, it is classified as a hematopoietic vitamin. Because of its role in blood formation, like vitamins B_6 and B_{12}, it is classified as a hematopoietic vitamin. Like vitamin B_{12}, the amount in foods and the body is so small that it is measured in micrograms (Carpenter, 2003d).

Functions Folate functions in coenzyme systems, particularly in amino acid metabolism, and participates in the regeneration of a number of enzymes. Folate is essential for DNA synthesis and cell division. It is needed for rapidly dividing cells, such as red blood cells and fetal cells, and in body systems where cells turn over rapidly, such as the gastrointestinal tract.

Metabolism Folate is both passively and actively absorbed, and transported in the blood circulation, usually attached to a protein. The major storage depot is the liver. Once folate is absorbed, the body appears to retain most of it. Some is excreted into the bile, but then it is reabsorbed.

Synthetic folic acid is significantly more bioavailable than food folate. Bioavailability of food folate is half that of folic acid used in supplements. Evaluation of folate status is by the laboratory measure of red blood cell concentration.

Requirements and Range of Safety Requirements of folate are related to folate's function in cell division. Requirements are particularly high during periods of rapid growth and development as in pregnancy and fetal development. The RDAs take into consideration that, on average, about half of folate in food is digested and absorbed. The RDAs are given in dietary folate equivalents (DFE) to account for both food and supplement sources, which have different bioavailability. RDAs are the same for both sexes (Bailey, 1998; IOM, 1998).

The RDA for children ranges from 150 to 300 µg/day depending upon age.

The RDA for adult men and women is 400 µg/day.

The UL ranges from 300 to 1000 µg/day depending upon age.

The UL has been set for folic acid from fortified food and supplements only, because food folate intake is not a potential problem. The UL of 1000 µg/day is based on the progression of neurological symptoms in B_{12} deficient people who are taking excess folic acid.

Food Sources Plant foods, such as vegetables, legumes, and fruits, are the best sources (Table 9–11). Many animal foods also supply folate. The bioavailability and retention in foods vary. Heating can destroy folate; milling grains removes some folate as well. Commercial and food preparation can destroy up to 95% of the folic acid content. Acids, including vitamin C with its antioxidant properties, protect folate. Thus, fresh oranges and fresh or frozen orange juice are important food sources of folate.

TABLE 9–11 Food Sources of Folate

Brewer's yeast (1 Tbsp) = 313 µg
Beef liver (3 oz) = 123 µg
Raw spinach (1 cup) = 106 µg
Cooked spinach (1/2 cup) = 82 µg
Orange juice (6 oz) = 102 µg
Romaine lettuce (1 cup) = 98 µg
Iceberg lettuce (1 cup) = 0–20 µg
Cooked beets (1/2 cup) = 66 µg
Avocado (1/2 med) = 59 µg
Cooked broccoli (1/2 cup) = 44 µg
Wheat germ (2 Tbsp) = 40 µg
Cooked red beans (1/2 cup) = 34 µg
Banana (1 med) = 33 µg
Brussels sprouts (1/2 cup) = 28 µg
Whole wheat bread (1 slice) = 16 µg
White bread (1 slice) = 10 µg

Breakfast cereals and infant formulas have been fortified with folic acid for several years. Since January 1998, all commercial breads have been fortified at the level of 1.4 µg/g (140 µg/100 g) of product. This form of folic acid is well absorbed and provides an average increase in intake of 100 µg/day. It is also recommended that women of childbearing age take a daily multivitamin supplement with 400 µg of folic acid in addition to daily food sources.

Effects of Too Little Folate People at risk for folate deficiency are those who have inadequate intakes or interference with folate metabolism. Conditions that can interfere with folate metabolism include gastrointestinal problems or drug interferences. Antacids can increase stomach and small intestine alkalinity, thus reducing folate digestion or absorption. Sulfosolozine, phenytoin, and alcohol interfere with absorption and cellular utilization. Methotrexate, a powerful antitumor medication, is a folate antagonist; this is the basis for the medication's effectiveness against rapidly dividing cancer cells (Mason, Levesque, 1996).

Anemia: Classic folic acid deficiency results in macrocytic (megaloblastic) anemia. Because this anemia can also result from vitamin B_{12} deficiency, it is important that the correct diagnosis be made. If folic acid is given to correct B_{12} deficiency, the anemia will be corrected but the neurological problems will persist and are irreversible. In one measure to prevent this from happening, over-the-counter folate supplements can contain no more than 400 µg, the RDA level for pregnant women.

Birth defects: Folic acid deficiency in pregnancy can cause babies to be born with neural tube defects (spina bifida), a severe condition affecting the formation of the nerves of the spinal cord, and resulting in infant paralysis. This is considered a major public health problem, and is particularly problematic because the effects of deficiency on the fetus occur in the first 6 weeks of pregnancy, often before women are aware that they are pregnant. An added 400 µg/day of folic acid is estimated to prevent about 47% of neural tube defects (Daly et al., 1997; Pfeiffer, Rogers, Bailey, Gregory, 1997).

Heart disease and high blood pressure: Direct association has been shown between increased risk of heart disease and low intake of folic acid via the amino acid homocysteine (Morrison, Schaubel, Desmeules, Wigle, 1996; Rosenberg, 2001). High levels of homocysteine in the blood can lead to increased risk of heart attack and stroke. Folic acid is required for normal degradation of homocysteine, and folic acid (and/or vitamin B_{12} and B_6) deficiency can result in abnormally high serum levels of homocysteine (Gauthier, Keevil, McBride, 2003; Robinson et al., 1998).

In the Nurses Health Study of more than 150,000 women, women aged 27–44 who got at least 1000 µg/day of folic acid had a 46% less risk of high blood pressure than those who got less than 200 µg/day. Older women who got 1000 µg/day had an 18% lower risk than those who had the lowest intake (Forman, Rimm, Stampher, Curham, 2005).

Cancer: Recent studies suggest that folate can play an important role in the prevention of breast cancer, especially among women consuming alcohol (Zhang, 2004).

Oral Implications of Folate Deficiency Because the oral tissues have rapid cellular turnover, a folic acid deficiency may increase gingival sensitivity to plaque irritation. In one study, significantly greater inflammation was seen in subjects with no supplementation compared with those taking 4 mg of folic acid per day. The findings suggested that supplementation may increase gingival resistance to local irritants (Vogel, Deasy, 1978). Oral signs and symptoms of deficiency, as with other B-complex vitamins, include:

- burning tongue and oral mucosa
- red, sore, swollen tongue
- angular cheilosis
- gingivitis

Effects of Too Much Folate The only known concern of excess intake of folate is in cases where there is a vitamin B_{12} deficiency. High folate intakes can mask the signs of the deficiency by curing the anemia but not the neurological effects. As a result, the neurological effects can progress and may be irreversible.

Vitamin B_{12} (Cobalamin)

Vitamin B_{12} has the most complex chemical structure of any of the vitamins and is the only one containing the mineral cobalt, which gives it a dark red color. Cyanocobalamin is the synthetic source of the vitamin. Vitamin B_{12} appears to be formed only by microorganisms and to be present only in animal foods. Plant foods may be a source only if they inadvertently contain animal particles or microorganisms. Vitamin B_{12} can be destroyed by heavy metals and by strong oxidizing and reducing agents.

Functions (Carpenter, 2003d) Vitamin B_{12} performs several vital reactions as a constituent of two major coenzymes, methylcobalamin and 5-deoxyadenosylcobalamin, Major functions of vitamin B_{12} include DNA formation, the division and maturity of red blood cells, and the activation and interconversion of amino acids. Vitamin B_{12} is involved in the synthesis of nucleoproteins via its involvement in the metabolism of purines and pyrimidines, and the manufacture of neurotransmitters and the myelin sheath of nerves. Through its involvement in neurologic activity, B_{12} may help prevent depression and other neurological disturbances, particularly in elderly people.

Metabolism Vitamin B_{12} is unique in its absorption process. For vitamin B_{12} to be absorbed, it must be combined with a glycoprotein secreted from the parietal cells of the stomach, called *intrinsic factor*. (Vitamin B_{12} in food is often termed *extrinsic factor*.) The intrinsic factor, with the aid of calcium, binds to the vitamin B_{12} and facilitates its absorption in the small intestine in an acid environment. Vitamin B_{12} is then released and absorbed into the blood circulation bound to proteins.

This prevents it from being readily excreted by the kidneys. Some is excreted into bile and eliminated in the feces; up to 75% is then reabsorbed. Unlike other water-soluble vitamins, vitamin B_{12} is stored in the body, chiefly in the liver. About one-third is in the muscle, bone, skin, lungs, kidneys, and spleen. Absorption is about 70% and is inversely related to intake at higher levels of consumption.

Even if adults completely stop eating animal foods, they have supplies estimated to last 20 to 30 years. The same does not hold true for children because they have not had enough time to develop stores.

Blood levels of vitamin B_{12} or its metabolites are examples of laboratory tests used to measure status.

Requirements and Range of Safety Requirements are based on worldwide studies of people who eat different levels of animal or plant foods. The adult RDA is the requirement for growth and development.

The RDA for children is 0.9–1.8 µg/day depending upon age.

The RDA for adult men and women is 2.4 µg/day.

There is no UL because no dangers are known with doses as high as 1000 µg/day.

Food Sources The only food sources of vitamin B_{12} are animal products (Table 9–12); plant foods are lacking in vitamin B_{12}. The best sources are organ meats, clams, oysters, yeast, and other animal products. Strict vegetarians (vegans) may get vitamin B_{12} from sea vegetables and fortified soy milk, but B_{12} is unavailable in

TABLE 9–12   Food Sources of Vitamin B_{12}

Salt-water fish, pork, organ meats, eggs, milk, and milk products

Examples:
Beef liver (3 oz) = 68 µg
Canned clams (1/2 cup) = 19.1 µg
Canned oysters (3.5 oz) = 18 µg
Tuna (2 oz) = 1.32 µg
Yogurt (1 cup) = 1.06 µg
Nonfat milk (1 cup) = 0.95 µg
Halibut (3 oz) = 0.85 µg
Egg (1 large) = 0.77 µg
Chicken (3 oz) = 0.36 µg
Cheddar cheese (1 oz) = 0.23 µg

fermented foods such as miso and tempeh. Synthetic B$_{12}$ supplements are also available. Limiting the processing and heating of animal foods can aid retention.

For adults over age 51, sources of vitamin B$_{12}$ should be primarily fortified foods or supplements, which can be absorbed in the absence of stomach acid (Yates, Schlicker, Suitor, 1998).

Effects of Too Little or Too Much Vitamin B$_{12}$
Inadequacy of vitamin B$_{12}$ can result from:

* lack of stomach acid (achlorhydria)
* lack of intrinsic factor
* interference with absorption as in intestinal surgery
* insufficient dietary sources

B$_{12}$ deficiency resulting from dietary deficiency is rare, but can occur in people following a strict vegetarian diet with no animal sources over a prolonged period. It can also occur in others who for one reason or another fail to consume sufficient vitamin B$_{12}$ sources. For example, a 14-year-old boy was diagnosed with B$_{12}$ and folate deficiency in the absence of any malabsorption. The patient's diet consisted of french fried potatoes, peanut butter and jelly sandwiches on white bread, and an occasional glass of juice, water, or soda. This had gone on for 7 years. Symptoms included fatigue, weakness, nausea, diarrhea, anorexia, weight loss, and declining school performance (Middleman, Emans, Cox, 1996).

Vitamin B$_{12}$ deficiency is associated with a variety of changes such as impaired neurological function, confusion, gait disturbance, position sense impairment, absent ankle reflexes, and reduced erythropoiesis (blood formation) (Stott et al., 1997).

Vitamin B$_{12}$ deficiency is a common problem in the aging population, with inadequate gastric acid production (achlorhydria) causing B$_{12}$ malabsorption in 10–30% of people aged 51 and older, and lack of intrinsic factor causing malabsorption in another 2% of older people (Ho, Kauwell, Bailey, 1999).

Pernicious anemia is the classic deficiency condition in which the bone marrow is unable to produce mature red blood cells, resulting in the development of large and immature blood cells, a condition known as *macrocytic* (megaloblastic) anemia. Symptoms include pallor, soreness of the mouth, prolonged bleeding time, anorexia, dyspnea, weight loss, fatigue, dizziness, hypotension, disorientation, numbness, confusion,

dimmed vision, and eventual psychosis. Gradually there is degeneration of the peripheral nerves, unsteadiness of gait, and mental depression. The anemia may not become evident for years, until liver stores have been depleted.

Vitamin B$_{12}$ deficiency may also be a risk factor for heart attack in that it is also associated with elevated levels of homocysteine as is folate and vitamin B$_6$, folate). B$_{12}$ is needed for the synthesis of methionine from homocysteine.

For those with achlorhydria, vitamin B$_{12}$ supplements and vitamin B$_{12}$ fortified foods are indicated. The synthetic forms are well absorbed in the absence of stomach acid. Those people who are lacking intrinsic factor are unable to absorb B$_{12}$ in any form and require vitamin B$_{12}$ injections.

Oral Implications of Vitamin B$_{12}$ Deficiency
Oral signs of deficiency, as with the other B-complex vitamins, include soreness of the mouth and atrophic glossitis resulting in bright red, sore, smooth, burning tongue.

Toxicity of vitamin B$_{12}$ has not been seen.

Summary and Implications for Dentistry of the Hematopoeitic Vitamins

* Older patients are at greatest risk for deficiency, which can cause neurological disorders and increased risk of heart attack in older adults (Chernoff, 2005).
* Deficiency of folic acid in pregnant women can cause irreversible birth defects. Intake of 400 IU/day of folic acid by food or supplement is particularly important for women of childbearing age.
* Oral signs of deficiency are seen, particularly burning tongue and glossitis.
* Daily multivitamin supplement containing folate is recommended for young women of childbearing age.
* Daily multivitamin containing folate and B$_{12}$ is recommended for older patients.
* Supplements of B$_6$ are usually *not* indicated, and excesses can cause harmful side effects.

Biotin

The name *biotin* derives from the fact that this vitamin was found to be one of the "bios" factors that yeast needed for growth. Biotin is a very active sulfur-containing vitamin, which is needed as a coenzyme for purine formation. Purine is needed for RNA and DNA synthesis.

Requirements and Range of Safety There is still not enough information to set a specific RDA or UL for biotin. Rather, an estimated safe and adequate daily dietary intake (AI) has been set. Biotin can be synthesized in the intestine, but may not be absorbed.

The AI for children ranges from 8 to 25 μg/day depending upon age.

The AI for adult men and women is 30 μg/day.

There is no UL.

Food Sources Food sources include liver, egg yolk, peanut butter, and soy flour (Table 9–13). Meat and fruit are poor sources.

Effects of Too Little Biotin Deficiency symptoms are general and vague, and mimic those of other B-complex deficiencies: anorexia, nausea, vomiting, dermatitis, depression, hair loss. Deficiencies have been seen only in infants given sulfa drugs and experimentally induced by feeding raw egg white. The protein avidin in raw egg white binds biotin and makes it unavailable for absorption. Cooking the egg will denature the avidin and prevent this effect. The deficiency occurs only with the consumption of large amounts of raw egg.

Oral Implications of Biotin Deficiency Oral signs of biotin deficiency include:

* glossitis (oral mucosa and tongue inflammation and swelling)
* painful tongue
* magenta (red colored) tongue

Effects of Too Much Biotin Biotin toxicity has not been shown.

TABLE 9–13 Food Sources of Biotin

Brewer's yeast (3.5 oz) = 85 μg
Beef liver (3 oz) = 82 μg
Almonds (1 oz) = 23 μg
Cooked soybeans (1/2 cup) = 22 μg
Canned clams (1/2 cup) = 20 μg
Peanut butter (2 Tbsp) = 12 μg
Cooked egg (1 large) = 11 μg
Salmon (3 oz) = 10 μg
Oat bran (1/3 cup) = 10 μg

Summary and Implications for Dentistry of Biotin Deficiencies of this vitamin are very rare. Because biotin is found commonly in food, supplementation is usually not needed.

Pantothenic Acid

This vitamin comes from the Greek word for "everywhere" because it is found widely in foods. It plays an important role in coenzyme A, which is involved in the release of energy from carbohydrates, proteins, and fats. It is needed for the release of ATP and for the synthesis of long-chain fatty acids. It is also involved in the synthesis of vitamin D, cholesterol and other steroids, and the porphyrin in hemoglobin. It is absorbed like the other water-soluble vitamins and occurs in free form in plasma. Pantothenic acid is found in all body tissues, but particularly in the liver. Vitamin status is measured by blood or urine levels.

Requirements and Range of Safety There is still not enough information to set a specific RDA for pantothenic acid, so an estimated safe and adequate daily dietary intake has been set.

The AI for children ranges from 2 to 4 mg/day depending upon age.

The AI for adult men and women is 5 mg/day.

No UL has been set as toxicity has not been shown.

Food sources Food sources are wide and varied, with a bioavailability of about 50% from foods (Table 9–14). Pantothenic acid is found particularly in yeast, meats, liver, eggs, whole grains, and legumes. Some may be synthesized by intestinal bacteria as well. Milk, fruits, and vegetables are only fair sources.

However, losses can be high in cooking and processing. Cooking red meat destroys 15–50% of the pantothenic acid. The milling of flour destroys about 50%. Sufficient pantothenic acid usually occurs with sufficient intake of the other B vitamins.

Effects of Too Little Pantothenic Acid It is difficult to separate out the effects of pantothenic acid deficiency from those of the other B-complex vitamins. Deficiency signs and symptoms are the same as with the other B-complex deficiencies and include burning of hands and feet, cramping of muscles, impaired coordination, fatigue and nausea.

Effects of Too Much Pantothenic Acid Toxicity of pantothenic acid has not been reported.

TABLE 9-14 Food Sources of Pantothenic Acid

Beef liver (3 oz) = 6.035 mg
Egg (1 med) = 1.1 mg
Avocado (1/2 med) = 1.1 mg
Canned mushrooms (1/2 cup) = 1 mg
Milk (1 cup) = 0.984 mg
Chicken (3 oz) = 0.765 mg
Cooked soybeans (1/2 cup) = 0.525 mg
Peanut butter (2 Tbsp) = 0.476 mg
Banana (1 med) = 0.45 mg
Orange (1 med) = 0.45 mg
Cooked collard greens (1/2 cup) = 0.425 mg
Potato (1 med) = 0.4 mg
Cooked broccoli (1/2 cup) = 0.315 mg
Brown rice (1/2 cup) = 0.3 mg
White rice (1/2 cup) = 0.15 mg
Cantaloupe (1/4 melon) = 0.3 mg
Whole wheat bread (1 slice) = 0.184 mg
White bread (1 slice) = 0.092 mg
Wheat germ (1 Tbsp) = 0.132 mg

Summary and Implications for Dentistry of Pantothenic Acid

- Pantothenic acid is very prevalent in foods.
- Deficiencies are rare.
- Toxicities have not been seen.
- Supplements are generally not needed.

Vitamin C (Ascorbic Acid)

The vitamin C deficiency disease, scurvy, was described as early as 1500 BC by French explorer Jacques Cartier, when 110 of his crew developed this potentially fatal scourge. He learned from native Indians that making a tea of boiled pine needles could prevent the disease. Later, in 1753, Dr. James Lind conducted the classic experiment onboard ship with 12 sailors who had scurvy. Their typical diet was watery cereal with sugar, mutton broth, biscuits with sugar, barley, raisins, and wine. He gave supplements of either vinegar, vitriol (sulfuric acid, alcohol, ginger, and cinnamon), salt water, a garlic-mustard-herb combination, or two oranges and one lemon to pairs of sailors. When those who received the fruit recovered, it became evident that something in these fruits prevented this disease and they were required aboard ship on long trips. This was the origin of the slang term *limey* for British sailors.

In 1932, the active compound that protected against scurvy was isolated, identified, and named *ascorbic acid* (vitamin C) (Carpenter, 2003a). Ascorbic acid has a chemical structure similar to glucose. Plants and most animals can synthesize vitamin C from glucose and do not need to obtain it directly from food. Several species—guinea pig, monkey, India fruit-eating bat, red-vented bulbal (bird), and humans—lack the enzyme l-gulonalactone oxidase that converts glucose to ascorbic acid in the liver. For them, vitamin C is an essential nutrient that must be obtained from food.

Of all the vitamins, vitamin C is the most easily destroyed by light, heat, air (oxygen), alkali, and the presence of minerals such as iron and copper. Losses occur over time with storage.

Functions

In contrast to the other water-soluble vitamins, vitamin C does not function directly in the release of energy from the macronutrients or act as a coenzyme. Its major role is as a potent antioxidant, functioning in a wide range of metabolic oxidation-reduction reactions. Vitamin C functions to maintain healthy cell function; hold cells together; heal wounds; build strong bones and teeth; form and maintain the cardiovascular, neurological, and digestive systems; keep the immune system intact to fight infection and disease; and detoxify medications and environmental pollutants (Jacob, 1999). Specific functions include the following:

- Serves as an electron donor for eight body enzymes including those needed for the formation of collagen, serotonin, norepinephrine, and bile.
- Protects vitamins A and E and polyunsaturated fatty acids (such as in cell membranes) from excessive oxidation.
- Quenches the free radicals thought to be important in aging and carcinogenesis.
- May be effective in preventing age-related opacities in the eye (Jacques et al., 1997).
- Facilitates calcium and nonheme (vegetable) iron absorption (helps counteract the effects of phytates and tannins, which decrease iron absorption) by increasing the solubility of nonheme iron.
- Synthesizes leukocytes and other immune system components (thus its role in resistance to infection).
- Detoxifies carcinogens or interferes with the carcinogenic processes via free radical scavenging, and enhancing immunocompetence.

Important Roles in Dentistry

Collagen Formation Vitamin C plays an essential role in collagen synthesis (Figure 9–8). Collagen is the most abundant (fibrous) protein in the body, with a wide variety of functions and characteristics. It is present in nearly all organs, and its structure varies to meet specific tissue needs. Collagen is responsible for the tensile strength of muscle and the viscosity of the vitreous of the eye. It is the intercellular cement that holds cells together in well-organized structural systems. Collagen is the primary organic component of the matrix of dentin, bone, and gingiva as well as for skin, tendons, and organs.

Collagen is composed primarily of four amino acids: glycine, proline, hydroxyproline, and hydroxylysine, which make up close to 70% of its composition and make collagen unique among proteins. The remaining third is composed of other amino acids. Vitamin C is needed for the hydroxylation of the amino acids proline and lysine to hydroxyproline and hydroxylysine. Both of these amino acids are unique to collagen and essential for optimal collagen synthesis and associated wound healing.

The fibroblast is the cell that forms collagen. In the fibroblast, proline and lysine are incorporated into a polypeptide chain, which is then hydroxylated by ascorbic acid into hydroxyproline and hydroxylysine. The polypeptide chains then combine to form a coiled helix and are secreted from the fibroblast. Three helices combine to form tropocollagen. These tropocollagen units combine in staggered arrangements to form collagen fibrils. The fibrils then combine to form the fiber that is functional collagen. These fibers have strong cross-linkages that provide collagen with its tensile strength. Mucopolysaccharide "ground substance" is also essential to the process. Ground substance is also secreted by the fibroblasts and helps arrange collagen fibrils in the order needed for developing stable connective tissue.

In the absence of sufficient vitamin C, lysine and proline are not hydroxylated, so hydroxylysine and hydroxyproline are not formed. The result is chaotically arranged fibers with weak cross-linkages. This defect is the foundation for the clinical signs and symptoms of deficiency.

Wound Healing When a wound begins to heal normally, mucopolysaccharide ground substance accumulates rapidly over the first few days to provide the foundation for the scab (Figure 9–9). As fiber formation

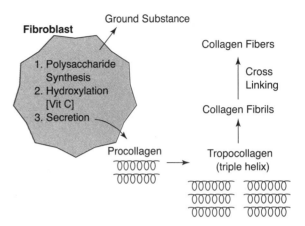

FIGURE 9–8 Collagen formation.

begins (around day 4), ground substance declines. Fiber formation continues until approximately day 11 when the scab is formed. In vitamin C deficiency, ground substance does not decline, continues to accumulate, and surrounds the fibrils preventing proper fiber synthesis. The scorbutic wound ends up with few, if any, collagen fibers, and has chaotically arranged tropocollagen fibrils surrounded by large masses of ground substance. This is a reversible phenomenon. If vitamin C is provided at any point in this process, the ground substance will decline and the fiber formation will proceed.

Metabolism

Most absorption of vitamin C is active, but some occurs by simple diffusion into the portal system. Normally, about 90% of the vitamin C consumed is absorbed in a diet containing from 30 to 180 mg, depending on body need. As vitamin C becomes depleted, absorption increases. As intake increases, absorption decreases and urinary excretion increases. Vitamin C is not stored in the body, but is concentrated in tissues with the greatest metabolic activity such as the glands, retina of the eye, and white blood cells. As discussed earlier, the amount of vitamin C contained in all body tissues at any time is called the body pool.

300 mg = scurvy risk
1500 mg = reasonable
4000 mg = highest possible pool

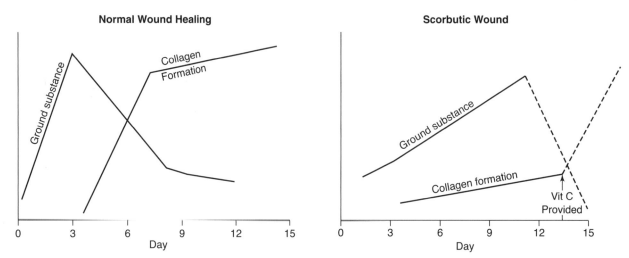

FIGURE 9-9 Wound healing: normal versus vitamin C deficiency. Straight line above represents scorbutic condition; dotted line represents vitamin C introduction and return to normal.

Healthy adults maintain a body supply (pool) of about 1500 mg of vitamin C on a diet of 100 mg/day. On an experimental diet devoid of vitamin C, healthy adults with a body pool of 1500 mg may show deficiency signs in about one month. A body pool of 300 mg of vitamin C or less is a risk for scurvy. The highest possible body pool is thought to be around 4000 mg. A body pool of 1500 mg or greater results in increased vitamin C excretion and catabolism. The kidneys excrete vitamin C and its breakdown products. Vitamin C repletion can reverse deficiency symptoms in weeks to months depending on the severity of the deficiency.

The best laboratory indicator of ascorbic acid status is either assessment of leukocyte ascorbic acid levels or a loading dose test. Excretion of less than 60% of the dose is an indication of tissue depletion.

Note: The lingual ascorbic acid test kit that has been marketed to dentists as an ascorbic acid status self-test, is *not* a reliable indicator of ascorbic acid status. It purports to show vitamin C status in saliva, as determined by the disappearance time of a dye placed on the tongue. This test has been proven to be invalid (Leggott et al., 1986).

Requirements and Range of Safety

The DRIs for vitamin C have increased from earlier recommendations:

The RDA for children ranges from 15 to 75 mg/day depending upon age and gender.

The RDA for adult men aged 19+ is 90 mg/day.

The RDA for adult women aged 19+ is 75 mg/day.

The UL ranges from 400 to 2000 mg/day depending upon age (Johnston, 1999), and supplementation up to this level is considered safe for most adults (Hathcock, et al., 2005).

An intake as low as 10 mg/day prevents scurvy. Intake over 100 to 200 mg/day results in increased urinary excretion. The average daily intake of vitamin C is from 70 to 80 mg/day (IOM, 2000; Levine, Rumsey, Daruwala, Park, Wang, 1999).

Those individuals with greater need for vitamin C above DRI levels may include (Ausman, 1999):

* People with infections such as pneumonia, rheumatic fever, and tuberculosis.
* People having higher demands for collagen synthesis, such as those with severe burns or fractures, or who are undergoing surgical procedures.
* Cigarette smokers. Cigarette smoking increases the vitamin C requirement by as much as 50%, or an increase of 35 mg/day. This may be due

to the increased oxidative stress produced by smoke, which depletes antioxidants (Jacob, 2000).

Food Sources

Most of the vitamin C in the Western world is from citrus and other fruits, potatoes, dark green and deep yellow vegetables, and other vegetables including tomatoes (Table 9–15). Five servings of fruits and vegetables per day will provide over 200 mg/day of vitamin C (but dried fruits contain little vitamin C). Today many processed foods are fortified with vitamin C, including fruit juices and drinks, breakfast cereals, and infant formulas. Human milk from healthy mothers supplies sufficient amounts of vitamin C for infants, but pasteurized milk contains only trace amounts.

Losses of vitamin C can vary greatly. Vitamin C is destroyed by heat and leaches out into cooking water, so foods are best prepared by microwave or by steaming quickly in small amounts of water. Keeping vegetables in steam tables (a common practice in restaurants, cafeterias, and health care facilities) causes vitamin C loss. Baking soda, an alkali sometimes added to green vegetables to retain color, destroys the vitamin C.

TABLE 9–15 Food Sources of Vitamin C

Green and red peppers, avocados, cabbage, turnip greens, kale, collards, parsley, sprouted alfalfa seeds, broccoli, tomatoes, lemons, orange peel, black currants, acerola cherries, cantaloupe, strawberries, citrus fruits, rose hips

Examples:
Guava (1 med) = 165 mg
Red bell pepper (1/2 cup) = 95 mg
Orange juice (3/4 cup) = 75 mg
Brussels sprouts (1/2 cup) = 68 mg
Strawberries (1/2 cup) = 66 mg
Orange (1 med) = 66 mg
Broccoli (1/2 cup boiled) = 52 mg
Cantaloupe (1/4 melon) = 32 mg
Tomato juice (6 oz) = 30 mg
Cabbage (1/2 cup) = 25 mg
Potato (1 small, baked, with skin) = 25 mg
Collard greens (1/2 cup boiled) = 25 mg
Asparagus (1/2 cup) = 19 mg
Green peas (1/2 cup) = 17 mg
Lima beans (1/2 cup) = 15 mg
Pineapple (1/2 cup) = 15 mg
French fries (8 fries) = 10 mg
Mashed potatoes (1/2 cup) = 10 mg
Corn on the cob (1 small) = 7 mg
Banana (1 med) = 6 mg
Carrots (1/2 cup) = 5 mg

Effects of Too Little Vitamin C

Scurvy is the classic vitamin C deficiency disease. Although scurvy has been eradicated as a public health problem, reports of isolated incidences still appear regularly in the literature. These are usually individuals who avoid all fruits and vegetables, usually by choice rather than some underlying health condition. Scurvy has also been reported in infants who have had a cow's milk formula for several months without vitamin C supplementation.

The signs and symptoms of scurvy derive from the well-documented defects that occur in collagen formation. Deficiency progresses in stages; the earliest effects are subclinical. They may include poor or slow healing, tissue friability, and decreased resistance to infection. As the deficiency progresses, symptoms of fatigue and hemorrhages from blood vessels may appear. There may be easy bruising and hemorrhaging of the skin, joint pain, and disruption of the cartilage that supports the skeleton. In infants, there may be extreme tenderness of the skin to touch. In children, deficiency can result in failure to grow, irritability, and soreness and swelling in joints. Radiographs show hemorrhages and bone changes. Classic signs of vitamin C deficiency include the development of small red hemorrhages around hair follicles (perifollicular petechiae) (Figure 9–10). Skin changes may be noted within the first month in a totally vitamin C devoid diet. Subsequently, oral signs may appear along with pains in joints, xerostomia, and hair loss (alopecia) (Hirschmann, Raugi, 1999).

Oral Implications of Vitamin C Deficiency

In tooth development, the rate of dentin formation is closely associated with vitamin C status. Deficiency can result in atrophy of odontoblasts, resulting in irregular or lacking dentin. The pulp may become dilated from increased blood volume (Alvares, Siegel, 1981) (Figure 9–11).

Deficiency is not always clinically evident and may not be manifest until stress of some type is imposed. For example, in edentulous individuals, there are no evident

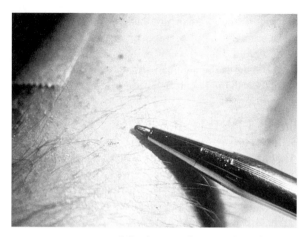

FIGURE 9–10 Perifollicular petechiae resulting from vitamin C deficiency.

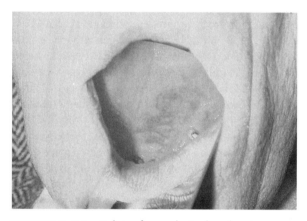

FIGURE 9–11 Palate of a scorbutic dental patient.

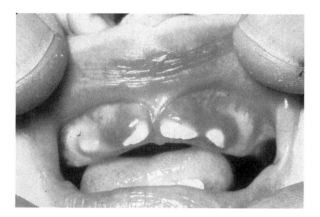

FIGURE 9–12 Scorbutic gingivae

mucosal changes. However, imposition of stress, such as placing a denture, can result in spontaneous bleeding.

In dentate individuals, signs include engorgement of the marginal gingiva with blood. The gingiva may increase to envelop the teeth. The gingiva will hemorrhage with the slightest provocation (Figure 9–12). The gingivae become bluish red in color. Reduced resistance can lead to oral infections. Characteristics are "punched out" interdental papillae and breath odor. Periodontal tissues are affected and teeth become loose and may be extruded. Histologically, there is evidence of periodontal fiber destruction, lack of fibroblasts and collagen fibrils, increased osteoclastic resorption, and impeded alveolar bone formation (Nizel, Papas, 1989). It is important to point out that vitamin C deficiency will not cause gingivitis and periodontal disease, but is a conditioning factor that exacerbates the disease process.

In older individuals, those with lower ascorbic acid levels had a higher prevalence of oral mucosal lesions (Tuovinen et al., 1992). Vitamin C is also an important factor in ensuring timely recovery after oral surgery. Vitamin C deficiency can delay the healing process and contribute to increased risk of infection (Leibson, 1997).

Many studies have shown an association between localized vitamin C levels and status of the gingival sulcular epithelium, which is a protective barrier against the invasion of periodontal bacteria. Early studies showed that when the concentration of vitamin C in the sulcal epithelium is low, epithelial permeability is increased (Vogel, Alvares, 1985). When monkeys were depleted in ascorbic acid to a subclinical level (no clinical signs), they had increased epithelial permeability and increased sulcular exudate (Alvares, Siegel, 1981). In a study that supplemented the diets of humans with vitamin C, the higher the vitamin C level in the gingival connective tissue and the sulcular epithelium, the lower the epithelial permeability. The conclusion was that increased vitamin C can help protect sulcular epithelium from bacterial permeation (Mallek, 1978).

More recent human studies have shown that people with the lowest dietary intakes of vitamin C (Grossi, 1998) or the lowest plasma ascorbic acid levels (Vaananen et al., 1993) were at the highest risk for periodontal disease, and the association is especially strong for smokers.

Effects of Too Much Vitamin C

Vitamin C is a popular supplement, and many healthy people regularly ingest more than the DRI, especially via supplements. Some take 1 to 5 g daily (20 to 80 times the RDAs), and reports of side effects appear periodically in the professional literature. Reported negative side effects of high doses include:

- nausea, vomiting, and diarrhea possible at levels greater than 1 g/day (Jacob, 1999)
- interference with the activity of anticoagulants such as heparin and coumadin
- increased excretion of uric acid, a problem for persons susceptible to gout
- false-negative test results for urinary glucose in patients with diabetes mellitus and for guiaic stool tests (tests blood in stool) (Johnston, 1999)
- formation of oxalate kidney stones in those individuals prone to stone formation
- possible systemic conditioning called rebound scurvy (the existence of this is controversial); scurvylike withdrawal symptoms have been reported when prolonged supplementation is abruptly stopped (Johnston, 1999); this may be first recognized by the dentist since the signs are evident in the oral cavity

Current Research on Vitamin C

Recent research has showed important effects of vitamin C in reducing the risk of developing cataracts (Jacques et al., 1997), and in slowing the progression of age-related macular degeneration. According to Ward (2004), vitamin C may be protective against heart disease as well. High blood levels of vitamin C also protect against infection with *H. Pylori*, the bacterium that increases the risk of stomach cancer and causes most ulcers (Ward, 2004).

Misconceptions about Ascorbic Acid

Several clinical trials have been conducted to determine the validity of the contention that increased vitamin C prevents colds. Results showed no preventive effect and only a mild reduction in length of symptoms. Consensus is that the effect is similar to that resulting from antihistamine medications, and supplementation is not warranted for cold prevention (Hemila, 1994).

Summary and Implications for Dentistry of Vitamin C

- Vitamin C is essential for formation and function of all tissues.
- It aids in the formation of bone, soft tissue, and teeth.
- It is needed for collagen formation and wound healing.
- It is needed for timely recovery after oral surgery.
- Deficiency is rare but seen in people with poor diets like elderly people subsisting on "tea and toast" diets.
- Deficiency signs are usually first seen in the oral cavity.
- RDA is about the amount found in one orange per day.
- Overconsumption is not innocuous and can cause serious problems in some people.
- Patients should be cautioned against taking doses larger than 500 mg/day.
- The lingual ascorbic acid test is not valid.
- Vitamin C does not prevent colds but may reduce their severity and symptoms.

SUMMARY AND IMPLICATIONS FOR DENTISTRY OF THE WATER-SOLUBLE VITAMINS

Table 9–16 summarizes the water-soluble vitamins. Deficiencies of most B-complex vitamins are uncommon with the exception of folic acid and vitamin B_{12}. The greatest risk of deficiency of these vitamins is in older patients, and can result in neurological disorders and increased risk of heart attack. A daily multivitamin containing folate and B_{12} is recommended for older patients. Deficiency of folic acid in pregnant women can cause irreversible birth defects, so intake of 400 IU/day of folic acid by food or supplement is particularly important for women of childbearing age. Recent supplementation of bread with folic acid should be helpful.

The most common oral signs and symptoms of B-complex vitamin deficiencies are glossitis (swollen red tongue), angular cheilosis (cracks in the corners of the mouth), and burning tongue. Angular cheilosis can result from loss of vertical dimension and from fungal infections as well, so cheilosis is not a definitive diagnosis for vitamin deficiency.

TABLE 9-16 Summary of Water-Soluble Vitamins

Vitamin, Requirements, and Food Sources	Metabolism and Function	Deficiency or Excess	Oral Implications
Thiamin Vitamin B_1 *RDA:* Men: 1.2 mg; women: 1.1 mg; UL not set *Sources:* Found widely in foods such as pork, liver, meats, poultry, dry beans and peas, peanut butter, enriched and whole grains (breads, cereals, rice), milk, eggs, butter; lost in cooking; removed in refining, replaced in enriched grain products	*Metabolism:* Absorbed in portal circulation; no specific storage location, excreted in urine, short half-life of 9–18 days so a constant supply is needed *Functions:* Component of coenzyme thiamine pyrophosphate (TPP) which catalyzes glucose, protein, and fat breakdown for energy, and is needed for formation of DNA and RNA; needed for synthesis of acetylcholine for healthy nerves	*Deficiency:* Classic disease is beriberi: fatigue, poor appetite, constipation, mental depression, edema, polyneuritis, heart failure *Excess:* Toxicity not seen	*Deficiency:* Leads to taste loss; burning tongue; ↑ sensitivity of oral mucosa; rare in developed countries
Riboflavin Vitamin B_2 *RDA:* Men: 1.3 mg; women: 1.1 mg; UL not set *Sources:* Milk and other animal products (cheese, meat, poultry, fish), enriched and whole grains (breads, cereals, rice)	*Metabolism:* Yellow-green fluorescent pigment; exists in free state or in compounds; no specific storage location *Functions:* Part of enzymes riboflavin monophosphate (FMN) and flavin adenine dinucleotide (FAD) that help form ATP; ATP helps release energy from carbohydrate, protein, and fat; B_2 also needed for fatty acid and amino acid synthesis—cellular growth cannot occur without B_2	*Deficiency:* Growth failure, greasy skin scaliness around nose and ears, burning, itching, sensitive eyes; delayed wound healing *Excess:* Toxicity not seen	*Deficiency:* Leads to angular cheilosis; atrophy of filiform papillae; enlarged fungiform papillae; shiny red, cracked lips; sore, magenta tongue; taste loss or distortion, halitosis

Niacin

Vitamin B$_3$

Nicotinic acid

Niacinamide

RDA: Men: 16 mg; women: 14 mg; UL of 35 mg/day for adults based on supplement use

Sources: Meat, poultry, fish, dark, green leafy vegetables, enriched grains (breads, cereals, rice); niacin in whole grains is mostly unavailable; stable in heat, acid, light, air, but leeches out into cooking water

Metabolism: Tryptophan precursor: 60 mg = 1 mg niacin; food sources almost completely absorbed

Functions: Needed for all cell functioning; constituent of nicotinamide adenine dinucleotide (NAD) and nicotinamide adenine dinucleotide phosphate (NADP) needed for energy release from carbohydrates, proteins, and fats; also for steroid formation; red blood cell formation; drug metabolism

Deficiency: Classic disease is pellagra: dermatitis, diarrhea, mental depression, disorientation, delirium

Excess: Toxicity not seen from food sources; use of nicotinic acid in elevated blood cholesterol treatment involves high doses, and must be under a physician's supervision; side effects can include skin flushing, redness, gastric ulcers, ↑ blood glucose, risk of liver damage

Vitamin B$_6$

Pyridoxine (plants)

Pyridoxal (animals)

Pyridoxamine (animals)

RDA: Adult men: 1.3 mg 19–50 yr, 1.7 mg 51+ yr; women: 1.3 mg 19–50 yr, 1.5 mg 51+ yr; UL 100 mg/day; requirements based on protein intake

Sources: All foods except fat and sugar; best from animal sources and minimally processed food: poultry, beef, noncitrus fruits, whole grain cereals, dark green vegetables, potatoes; binds with fiber, lost in milling, and not added to enriched grains

Metabolism: Bound in food, released during digestion; stored mostly in liver and muscles

Functions: Primarily involved in protein as component of coenzyme pyridoxal phosphate (PLP) functions in protein amination, deamination, and transamination, and in red blood cell and hemoglobin synthesis; also functions in conversion of tryptophan to niacin, conversion of glycogen to glucose, and in selenium function

Deficiency: Depression, irritability, nervousness, convulsions, impaired immune function, dermatitis, peripheral neuritis, increased risk of heart attack (along with folate and B$_{12}$ in homocysteine metabolism); several drugs can affect absorption and/or metabolism

Excess: From supplement doses over 200 mg/day, poor muscle coordination, tingling and numbness of fingers and toes, irreversible nerve tissue degeneration

Deficiency: Leads to angular cheilosis; mucositis; stomatitis; oral pain; ulceration; denuded tongue; glossitis; glossodynia (tip of tongue is red, swollen, beefy; dorsum smooth and dry); ulcerative gingivitis

Deficiency: Leads to angular cheilosis; atrophy of fili-form papillae; sore, burning mouth; glossitis; glossodynia; magenta tongue

(continued)

223

TABLE 9–16 Summary of Water-Soluble Vitamins (Continued)

Vitamin, Requirements, and Food Sources	Metabolism and Function	Deficiency or Excess	Oral Implications
Biotin *AI:* Men and women: 30 µg; UL not set *Sources:* Organ meats, egg yolk, legumes, nuts, yeast	*Metabolism:* Some synthesis in intestine; avidin, a protein in raw egg white, interferes with absorption *Functions:* Component of coenzyme for purine formation for RNA and DNA synthesis	*Deficiency:* Occurs only when large amounts of raw egg whites are eaten; vague symptoms such as anorexia, nausea, vomiting, dermatitis, depression, and hair loss *Excess:* Toxicity not seen	*Deficiency:* Leads to glossitis; painful tongue; magenta tongue; deficiencies occur rarely
Pantothenic Acid *AI:* Men and women: 5 mg; UL not set *Sources:* Found widely in foods such as liver, eggs, yeast, poultry, milk, legumes, whole grains	*Metabolism:* Found in all body tissues, particularly liver, and in free form in plasma *Functions:* Component of coenzyme A; for energy release from carbohydrates, proteins, and fats; also synthesis of vitamin D, long-chain fatty acids, cholesterol and other steroids, and for hemoglobin synthesis of sterols, fatty acids, and heme	*Deficiency:* Neuritis of arms and legs, burning sensation of feet; muscle cramps, impaired coordination, fatigue, and nausea; deficiencies occur rarely *Excess:* Toxicity not seen	*Deficiency:* Leads to no specific oral implications; deficiency symptoms are same as for other B-complex vitamins
Folate Folic acid Folacin *RDA:* Men and women: 400 µg; UL: 1000 µg *Sources:* Dark green leafy vegetables, fortified grains, legumes	*Metabolism:* Most is retained once absorbed; mainly stored in liver *Functions:* Maturation of red blood cells; synthesis of DNA and RNA; not a substitute for vitamin B_{12}	*Deficiency:* Birth defects (spina bifida), macrocytic anemia; heart disease *Excess:* Toxicity not seen; masks B_{12} deficiency	*Deficiency:* Leads to angular cheilosis; mucositis; stomatitis; sore or burning mouth; ↑ risk of candidiasis; inflamed gingiva; glossitis

Vitamin B$_{12}$
Cobalamin
RDA: Men and women: 2.4 µg; UL not set
Sources: Animal foods only: milk, eggs, meat, poultry, fish

Metabolism: Requires intrinsic factor from stomach for absorption
Functions: Formation of mature red blood cells; synthesis of DNA and RNA

Deficiency: Pernicious anemia—lack of intrinsic factor, or after gastrectomy; macrocytic anemia—leads to neurologic degeneration; delayed wound healing
Excess: Toxicity not seen

Vitamin C
Ascorbic Acid
RDA: Men: 90 mg; women: 75 mg; UL 1800–2000 mg
Sources: Citrus fruits, strawberries, cantaloupe, tomatoes, broccoli, raw green vegetables

Metabolism: Not stored in the body, but concentrated in tissues with the greatest metabolic activity
Functions: Collagen formation; keeps teeth firm in gums; hormone synthesis; wound healing; resistance to infection; improves iron absorption

Deficiency: Poor wound healing; poor bone and tooth development; scurvy: bruising and hemorrhage, bleeding gums, loose teeth
Excess: Chronic overdosing can increase vitamin C metabolism as an adaptation; rebound scurvy may occur after dose normalization

Deficiency: Leads to angular cheilosis; sore, burning mouth; stomatitis; hemorrhagic gingiva; halitosis; epithelial dysplasia of oral mucosa; oral paresthesia; detachment of periodontal fibers; loss or distortion of taste; glossitis; glossodynia; xerostomia; aphthous-type ulcers

Deficiency: Leads to ?↑ risk of infection; blood vessel fragility; ↑ periodontal signs and symptoms; delayed wound healing
Severe deficiency: Leads to red, swollen gingiva; gingival friability and bleeding on provocation; interdental papillary infusions; petechiae; sore, burning mouth; ↑ risk of candidiasis; subperiosteal hemorrhage; periodontal destruction; ↑ tooth mobility and exfoliation; soft tissue ulceration; malformed enamel; inadequate dentin

Vitamin C is essential for the formation and function of all tissues. As such it is important for oral tissue and structure formation and continued regeneration. Vitamin C deficiency can result in delayed wound healing and recovery after oral surgical interventions. Deficiency signs are usually first seen in the oral cavity, and include bleeding upon provocation, blood-engorged interdental papillae, and petecchiae on arms, legs, and chest. Vitamin C deficiency is rare but is seen periodically, usually in people choosing to eliminate all vitamin C sources from their diets.

QUESTIONS PATIENTS MIGHT ASK

Q. Shouldn't I take extra vitamins to provide energy for my workouts at the gym?

A. No. Vitamins don't supply energy. Carbohydrates, proteins, and fats do. If you are already eating an adequate diet to meet your energy needs, you shouldn't need vitamin supplements. The small amount of extra vitamins you may need to produce energy from more servings of the foundation foods comes packaged with the foods themselves.

Q. Won't I lose the vitamins from my foods by cooking them?

A. It is true that some of the vitamins dissolve in water and can be destroyed by heat. However, if you steam the foods, they do not come in contact with the cooking water. If you use the microwave, the cooking is fast and vitamin losses are minimal. Add lemon or vinegar to retain color, but do *not* add baking soda as it destroys some vitamins. If you must cook in water for longer periods, use the water for gravy or soup to reclaim the vitamins and minerals that have leeched into the water.

Q. Is it true that even a balanced diet may not meet the vitamin needs of older people?

A. As we age, a variety of factors help undermine our ability to get an adequate diet and utilize the nutrients we do get. For these reasons, a daily multivitamin/mineral supplement (at the level of $1\times$ the RDA only) is recommended for adults as an adjunct to a healthy diet.

CASE STUDY

A 60-year-old male executive was seen in the dental faculty practice for a second opinion concerning lesions on his hard palate. He had been recently told by a physician in Florida that the lesions were Kaposi's sarcoma and he needed to be tested for AIDS. Frightened, he came to the dental school to seek a second opinion from a dental faculty member who was a close relative.

Upon oral examination, the dentist found what appeared to be red dots on the patient's arms and chest, and on his hard palate. The gingiva bled spontaneously during gingival probing. The dentist sent him for a complete physical examination. The medical history was found to be unremarkable, blood tests were normal, and systemic disease was ruled out.

When asked about his diet, the patient responded that he was a "meat and potatoes man."

He didn't particularly like fruits and vegetables, so he eliminated them from his diet. His diet consisted primarily of bread and butter, meat and potatoes, and was virtually devoid of fruits, vegetables, and dairy products. He lived alone and was responsible for his own meal planning and cooking.

Questions:
1. What is the most likely cause of this executive's oral condition?
2. What are the red dots on the patient's hard palate, arms, and chest?
3. Why would the gingiva bleed profusely on provocation?
4. What underlying mechanism caused these signs?
5. What diet suggestions would you make?

REFERENCES

Alvares O, Siegel I: Permeability of the gingival sulular epithelium in the development of scorbutic gingivitis. *J Oral Pathol* 1981; 10:40.

Anzano MA, Lamb AJ, Olson JA: Impaired salivary gland secretory function following the induction of rapid, synchronous vitamin A deficiency in rats. *J Nutri* 1981; 111 (3):496–504.

Ausman L: Criteria and recommendations for vitamin C intake. *Nutr Rev* 1999; 57:222–24.

Bailey LB: Dietary reference intakes for folate: The debut of dietary folate equivalents. *Nutri Rev* 1998; 56:294–99.

Binkley N, Krueger D: Hypervitaminosis A and bone. *Nutri Rev* 2000; 58(5):138–44.

Blank S, Scanlon KS, Sinks TH, Lett S, Falk H: An outbreak of hypervitaminosis D associated with the overfortification of milk from a home-delivery dairy. *Am J Public Health* 1995; 85:656–59.

Booth SL, Centurelli M: Vitamin K: A practical guide to the dietary management of patients on warfarin. *Nutri Rev* 1999; 57:288–96.

Booth SL, Tucker KL, Chen H, Hannan MT, Gagnon DR, Cupples LA, et al.: Dietary vitamin K intakes are associated with hip fracture but not with bone mineral density in elderly men and women. *Am J Clin Nutr* 2000; 71(5):1201–8.

Calvo M, Whiting SJ, Barton CN: Vitamin D intake: A global perspective of current status. *J Nutr* 2005; 135:310–16.

Carpenter KJ: A short history of nutritional science: Part 1 (1785–1885). *J Nutr* 2003a; 133:638–45.

Carpenter KJ: A short history of nutritional science: Part 2 (1885–1912). *J Nutr* 2003b; 133:975–84.

Carpenter KJ: A short history of nutritional science: Part 3 (1912–1944). *J Nutr* 2003c; 133:3023–32.

Carpenter KJ: A short history of nutritional science: Part 4 (1945–1985). *J Nutr* 2003d; 133:3331–42.

Chasan-Taber L, Willett WC, Seddon JM, Stampfer MJ, Rosner B, Colditz GA, et al.: A prospective study of carotenoid and vitamin A intakes and risk of cataract extraction in US women. *Am J Clin Nutr* 1999; 70 (4):509–16.

Chernoff R: Micronutrient requirements in older women. *Am J Clin Nutr* 2005; 81(5):1240S–45S.

Daly S, Mills JL, Molloy AM, Conley M, Lee YJ, Kirke PN, et al.: Minimum effective dose of folic acid for food fortification to prevent neural-tube defects. *Lancet* 1999; 350(9092):1666–69.

Dawson-Hughes B, Harris SS, Krall EA, Dallal GE: Effect of calcium and vitamin D supplementation on bone density in men and women 65 years of age or older. *N Engl J Med* 1997; 337:670–76.

De Menezes AC, Costa IM, El-Guindy MM: Clinical manifestations of hypervitaminosis A in human gingiva: A case report. *J. Periodontol* 1984; 55 (8):474–76.

Duyff, RL: *American Dietetic Association Complete Food and Nutrition Guide*, 2nd Ed., Hoboken, NJ, John Wiley, 2002.

Dwyer JT, Dietz WH Jr, Hass G, Suskind R: Risk of nutritional rickets among vegetarian children. *A J Dis Child* 1979; (133):134–40.

Feskanich D, Singh V, Willett WC, Colditz GA: Vitamin A intake and hip fractures among postmenopausal women. *J Am Med Assoc* 2002; 287(1):47–54.

Forman JP, Rimm EB, Stampher MJ, Curham GC: Folate intake and the risk of incident hypertension among US women. *JAMA* 2005; 293(3):320–29.

Gauthier G, Keevil JG, McBride PE: The association of homocysteine and coronary artery disease. *Clin Card* 2003; 26(12):563–68.

Giunta JL: Dental changes in hypervitaminosis D. *Oral Surg Oral Med Oral Pathol Oral Radiol Endodont* 1998; 85(4):410–13.

Golebiewska M, Bielaczyc A: Scanning electron microscopy of the influence of dietary calcium and vitamin D deficiency on the periodontium in the adult rat. *Rocz Akad Med Bialymst* 1997; 42(Suppl 2):159–65.

Grossi S: *Low Dietary Calcium, Low Vitamin C Linked to Increased Risk of Gum Disease*. Nice, France: IADR, 1998.

Hanley DA, Davison KS. Vitamin D insufficiency in North America. *J Nutr* 2005; 135:3332–37.

Harris S, Dawson-Hughes B: Seasonal changes in plasma 25-hydroxyvitamin D concentrations of young American black and white women. *Am J Clin Nutr* 1998; 67:1232–36.

Hathcock, JN, Azzi A, Blumberg J, Bray T, Dickinson A, Frei B, et al.: Vitamins E and C are safe across a broad range of intakes. *Am J Clin Nutr* 2005; 81(4):736–45.

Hathcock JN, Hattan DG, Jenkins MY, McDonald JT, Sundaresan PR, Wilkening VL: Evaluation of vitamin A toxicity. *Am J Clin Nutr* 1990; 52:183–202.

Hemila H: Does Vitamin C alleviate the symptoms of the common cold? A review of current evidence. *Scand J Infect Dis* 1994; 26:1–6.

Hirschmann JV, Raugi GJ: Adult scurvy. *J Am Acad Dermatol* 1999; 41(6):895–906.

Ho C, Kauwell GP, Bailey LB: Practitioners' guide to meeting the vitamin B_{12} recommended dietary allowance for people aged 51 and older. *J Am Diet Assoc* 1999; 99:725–27.

Holick MF: Vitamin D requirements for humans of all ages: New increased requirements for women and men 50 years and older. *Osteoporos Int* 1998; 8(Suppl 2):S24–S29.

Hopkin K: Bioavailability and biokinetics of vitamin E. *Ann NY Acad Sci* 1031:449–54.

Jacob RA: Passive smoking induces oxidant damage preventable by vitamin C. *Nutri Rev* 2000; 58(8):239–41.

Jacob RA: Vitamin C. In Shils M, Olsen JA, Shike M, Ross AC (eds): *Modern Nutrition in Health and Disease*, 9th ed. Baltimore: Williams & Wilkins, 1999.

Jacobus CH, Holick MF, Shao Q, Chen TC, Holm IA, Kolodny JM, et al.: Hypervitaminosis D associated with drinking milk. *N Engl J Med* 1992; 326(18):1173–77.

Jacques PF, Taylor A, Hankinson SE, Willett WC, Mahnken B, Lee Y, et al.: Long-term vitamin C supplement use and prevalence of early age-related lens opacities. *Am J Clin Nutr* 1997; 66:911–16.

Johnston S: Biomarkers for establishing a tolerable upper intake level for vitamin C. *Nutri Rev* 1999; 57:71–7.

Krinsky N: Human requirements for fat-soluble vitamins, and other things concerning these nutrients. *Mol Aspects Medi* 2003; 24(6):317–24.

Leggott PJ, Robertson PB, Rothman DL, Murray PA, Jacob RA: Response of lingual ascorbic acid test and salivary ascorbate levels to changes in ascorbic acid intake. *J Dent Res* 1986; 65(2):131–34.

Leibson L: Notes from the Academy of General Dentistry: Vitamin C and diet speeds recovery from oral surgery wounds. *DentalNotes* 1997; 2:4.

Levine M, Rumsey SC, Daruwala R, Park JB, Wang Y: Criteria and recommendations for vitamin C intake. *JAMA* 1999; 281:1415–23.

Li E, Tso: Vitamin A uptake from foods. *Curr Opin Lipidology* 14(3):241–47.

Liede KE, Haukka JK, Saxen LM, Heinonen OP: Increased tendency towards gingival bleeding caused by joint effect of alpha-tocopherol supplementation and acetylsalicylic acid. *An Med* 1998; 30(6):542–46.

Low levels of Vitamin B_6 tied to artery disease: *Tufts Univ Health Nutr Lett* 2004; 22:5.

Lyle BJ, Mares-Perlman JA, Klein BE, Klien R, Greger JL: Antioxidant intake and risk of incident age-related nuclear cataracts I: The Beaver Dam Eye Study. *Am J Epidemiol* 1999; 149(9):801–9.

Lyle BJ, Mares-Perlman JA, Klein BE, Klein R, Palta M, Bowen PE, et al.: Serum carotenoids and tocopherols and incidence of age-related nuclear cataract. *Am J Clin Nutr* 1999; 69(2):272–77.

Mallek H: An investigation of the role of ascorbic acid and iron in the etiology of gingivitis in humans. PhD dissertation, Massachusetts Institute of Technology, 1978.

Malouf R, Grimley Evans J. The effect of vitamin B_6 on cognition. Cochrane Database Syst Rev. 2003; (4):CD004393. Review. PMID: 14584010 [PubMed - indexed for MEDILINE].

Mason JB, Levesque T: Folate: effects on carcinogenesis and the potential for cancer chemoprevention. *Oncology* 1996; 10(11):1727–36, 1742–43, discussion 1743–44.

McDonald JB, Gibbons RJ: The relationship of indigeinous bacteria to periodontal disease. *J Dent Res* 1962; 41:320.

Mellanby E: Experimental rickets, *Med Res Council, Spec. Rept. Ser.* 1921; 61:1–78.

Meydani SN, Meydani M, Blumberg JB, Leka LS, Siber G, Loszewski R, et al.: Vitamin E supplementation and in vivo immune response in healthy elderly subjects. *JAMA* 1997; 277:1380–86.

Middleman AB, Emans SJ, Cox J: Nutritional vitamin B_{12} deficiency and folate deficiency in an adolescent patient presenting with anemia, weight loss, and poor school performance. *J Adolesc Health* 1996; 19(1):76–9.

Morita R, Yamamoto I, Takada M, Ohnaka Y, Yuu I: Hypervitaminosis D. *Nippon Rinsho* 1993; 51:984–88.

Morrison HI, Schaubel D, Desmeules M, Wigle DT: Serum folate and risk of fatal coronary heart disease. *JAMA* 1996; 275(24):1929–30.

Institute of Medicine, National Academy of Sciences: *Dietary Reference Intakes for Calcium, Phosphorus, Magnesium, Vitamin D, and Fluoride*. Washington, DC: National Academies Press, 1997.

Institute of Medicine, National Academy of Sciences: *Dietary Reference Intakes for Thiamin, Riboflavin, Niacin, Vitamin B_6, Folate, Vitamin B_{12}, Pantothenic Acid, Biotin, and Choline*. Washington, DC: National Academies Press, 1998.

Institute of Medicine, National Academy of Sciences: *Dietary Reference Intakes for Vitamin C, Vitamin, Selenium, and Carotenoids*. Washington, DC: National Academies Press, 2000.

Institute of Medicine, National Academy of Sciences: *Dietary Reference Intakes for Vitamin A, Vitamin K, Arsenic, Boron, Chronium, Copper, Iodine, Iron, Manganese, Molybdenum, Nickel, Silicon, Vanadium, and Zinc*. Washington, DC: National Academies Press, 2001.

Nizel AE, Papas A: *Nutrition in Clinical Dentistry*, 3rd ed. Philadelphia: WB Saunders, 1989.

Olson JA: Hypovitaminosis A: Contemporary scientific issues. *J Nutri* 1994; 124(8 Suppl):1461S–66S.

Pennington JAT, Douglass JS: *Bowes & Churchs Food Values of Portions Commonly Used*, 18th ed. Philadelphia: Lippincott Williams & Wilkins, 2004.

Pfeiffer CM, Rogers LM, Bailey LB, Gregory JF: Absorption of folate from fortified cereal-grain products and of supplemental folate consumed with or without food determined by using a dual label stable-isotope protocol. *Am J Clin Nutr* 1997; 66:1388–97.

Pindborg JJ: *Pathology of the Dental Hard Tissues*. Philadelphia: WB Saunders, 1970.

Powers H: Riboflavin (vitamin B_2) and health. *Am J Clin Nutr* 2003; 77 (6):1352–60.

Rimm EB, Stampfer MJ, Ascherio A, Giovannucci E, Colditz GA, Willet WC: Vitamin E consumption and the risk of coronary disease in women. *N Engl J Med* 1993; 328:1450–56.

Robinson K, Arheart K, Refsum H, Brattstrom L, Boers G, Ueland P, et al.: Low circulating folate and vitamin B_6 concentration. Risk factors for stroke, peripheral vascular disease, and coronary artery disease. *Circulation* 1998; 97:437–43.

Rock CL, Jacob RA, Bowen PE: Update on the biological characteristics of the antioxidant micronutrients: Vitamin C, vitamin E, and the carotenoids. *J Am Diet Assoc* 1996; 96:693–702.

Rosenberg I: B vitamins, homocysteine, and neurocognitive function. *Nutri Rev* 2001; 59(8, Part II):S69–S73.

Ross A: Vitamin A and retinoids. In Shils M, Olsen JA, Shike M, Ross AC (eds): *Modern Nutrition in Health and Disease*, 9th ed. Baltimore: Williams & Wilkins, 1998.

Sommer A, West KP Jr: *Vitamin A Deficiency: Health, Survival, and Vision*. New York: Oxford University Press, 1996.

Steiner M: Vitamin E: A modifier of platelet function: Rationale and use in cardiovascular and cerebrovascular disease. *Nutr Rev* 1999; 57:306–9.

Stott DJ, Langhorne P, Hendry A, McKay PJ, Holyoake T, Macdonald J, et al.: Prevalence and haemopoietic effects of low serum vitamin B_{12} levels in geriatric medical patients. *Br J Nutri* 1997; 78(1):57–63.

Suttie IW: The importance of menaquinones in human nutrition. *Annu Rev Nutr* 1995; 15:399–417.

Tuovinen V, Vaananen M, Kullaa A, Karinpaa A, Markkanen H, Kumpusalo E: Oral mucosal changes related to plasma ascorbic acid levels. *Proc Finn Dent Soc* 1992; 88(3–4): 117–22.

Vaananen MK, Markkanen HA, Tuovinen VJ, Kullaa AM, Karinpaa AM, Kumpusalo EA: Periodontal health related to plasma ascorbic acid. *Proc Finn Dent Soc* 1993; 89(1–2):51–59.

Venning G: Recent developments in vitamin D deficiency and muscle weakness among elderly people. *Br Med J* 2005; 330(7490):524–26.

Vermeer C, Shearer MJ, Zitterman A, Bolton-Smith C, Szulc P, Hodges S, et al.: Beyond deficiency potential benefits of increased intakes of vitamin K for bone and vascular health. *Eur J Nutr* 2004; 46(6):325–35.

Vieth R: Vitamin D supplementation, 25-hydroxyvitamin D concentrations, and safety. *Am J Clin Nutr* 1999; 69:842–56.

Vogel RI, Alvaresz OF: Nutrition and peridontal disease. In Pollack RL, Kravitz E (eds): *Nutrition in Oral Health and Disease*. Philadelphia: Lea & Febiger, 1985.

Vogel RI, Deasy MH: The effect of folic acid on experimentally produced gingivitis. *J Prevent Dent* 1978; 5:30.

Ward E: Vitamin C: Still key for immunity, cancer, heart disease, eye health. *Environmental Nutrition Newsletter*, 2004; 27:3.

Weaver C, Fleet, JC. Vitamin D requirements: Current and future. *Am J Clin Nutr* 2004; 80(6):1735S–39S.

Weigley E, Mueller D, Robinson C: *Robinson's Basic Nutrition and Diet Therapy*, 8th ed., Upper Saddle River, NJ: Prentice Hall, 1997:162–86.

Whiting SJ, Lemke B: Excess retinol intake may explain the high incidence of osteoporosis in northern Europe. *Nutri Rev* 1999; 57(6):192–98.

Wilkinson J, Hanger HC, Elmslie J, George PM, and Sainsbury R: The response to treatment of subclinical thiamine deficiency in the elderly. *Am J Clin Nutr* 1997; 66:925–28.

Yates A, Schlicker S, Suitor C: Dietary Reference Intakes: The new recommendations for calcium and related nutrients, B vitamins and choline. *J Am Diet Assoc* 1998; 98:699–706.

Zhang SM: Role of vitamins in the risk, prevention, and treatment of breast cancer. *Curr Opinion Obstet Gynecol* 2004; 16(1):19–25.

Chapter **10**

Dietary Supplements

Marla Scanzello and Carole A. Palmer

OBJECTIVES
The student will be able to:
- Recognize the different types of dietary supplements.
- Understand the regulatory aspects of supplements.
- Distinguish between appropriate and inappropriate use of dietary supplements.
- Discuss the potential benefits and risks of dietary supplements.
- Describe dietary supplements with particular effects on dental health.
- Take a dietary history that includes information on dietary supplement use.
- Access reliable resources for more information.

INTRODUCTION

A dietary supplement is a product containing a "dietary ingredient" (distinct from a drug) that is taken by mouth and intended as a supplement to the diet (FDA, 2004). The dietary ingredient may include:

- a vitamin
- a mineral
- an herb or other botanical
- an amino acid
- a dietary substance to supplement the diet by increasing the total dietary intake (e.g., enzymes or tissues from organs or glands)
- a concentrate, metabolite, constituent, or extract

Dietary supplements can come in many forms: tablets, capsules, softgels, gelcaps, liquids, powders, or bars.

In the 1990s, along with the increasing popularity of alternative medicine, there was a sharp increase in the sales of dietary supplements in the United States (Harvard, 2004). Today, supplements are a multibillion-dollar industry; consumers spent over $18 billion on supplements in 2003 (Briefel, Johnson, 2004). About 57% of adult females and 47% of adult males reported using dietary supplements according to the 1999–2000 National Health and Nutrition Examination Survey (NHANES) (Balluz, Kieszak, Philen, Mulinare, 2000; Briefel, Johnson, 2004). Research indicates that supplement use is most common among whites, women, older individuals, and people with more education and higher income levels (Hunt, Dwyer, 2001; Kelly et al., 2005). Indeed, nutritional supplement users may have higher nutrient intakes from foods than nonusers (Hunt, Dwyer, 2001).

People take supplements for many reasons. Supplements may be indicated and/or prescribed for certain documented health conditions or life stages (see Table 10–1). However, many people take supplements for unproven reasons such as for pep and energy, nutrition insurance against poor eating habits, cold

TABLE 10–1   Populations among Which Dietary Supplementation May Be Required

Population Subgroup	Dietary Supplementation	Rationale
Elderly	B vitamins Antioxidants Vitamin D	Low intake, anemias Suppressed immunity Poor overall intake, bone health
Adolescents	Micronutrients	Energy-dense, but nutrient-deficient dietary selections
Adults (adolescents)	Calcium (possibly magnesium, vitamins D and K)	Bone health
Heavy alcohol consumers	Thiamin, folate, other B vitamins, vitamin K	Inadequate diet, altered metabolism
Risk or history of cardiovascular disease	Vitamin E Folate, B_{12}, riboflavin	Low-fat diet can reduce intake Reduce homocysteine among those with elevated levels
Reproductive history of neural tube defect	Folate	Reduced risk for NTD
Risk for prostate cancer	Vitamin E, selenium	Deficiencies described; reduced risk reported
Risk for colon cancer	Calcium, folate	Reduced DNA damage, favorable bowel pH, reduced risk reported
Patients with hypertension	Calcium, potassium	If diet is inadequate, these nutrients can modulate blood pressure

Source: Adapted from Thomas, 2005.

prevention, stress reduction, protection from serious diseases, prolonging of the aging process (Johnson, 2000; *Prevention*, 2000), weight loss, increased strength, and improved fitness and performance (Morrison, Gizis, Shorter, 2004).

The top-selling dietary supplements are multivitamins, with an estimated one-fourth of American adults taking them (Harvard, 2004; Kaufman et al., 2002). Individual vitamin and mineral supplements, such as calcium, iron, and vitamins E and C, also lead supplement sales. Other types of top-selling dietary supplements include glucosamine and chondroitin, and herbal supplements such as ginkgo biloba, garlic, echinacea, and ginseng (Harvard, 2004). Fish oil, flaxseed, black cohosh, antioxidants, and amino acids are among the supplements with the greatest increases in sales in recent years (Marra, 2002). Sales of plant-derived products reached $4.2 billion in 2001 with an estimated 45 million users (Kostka-Rokosz, Dvorkin, Vibbard, Couris, 2005).

Some dietary supplements, such as folic acid for the prevention of birth defects, are considered conventional medicine; others, such as herbals and other supplements that have not been scientifically proven to be effective therapies, are considered complementary and alternative medicine (National Center for Complementary and Alternative Medicine) (http://nccam.nih.gov/health/bottle).

Although some supplements do play an important role in health, *misuse* (improper use due to false expectations) and *abuse* (i.e., overuse) are common. It is extremely important, therefore, that the dental team becomes familiar with the supplements commonly taken by the public and has access to resources to help determine their potential benefits or risks (Nesheim, 1999).

This chapter will review the spectrum of dietary supplements commonly used today.

HOW SUPPLEMENTS ARE REGULATED

In 1994, the Dietary Supplement Health and Education Act (DSHEA) was signed into law, amending the federal food, drug, and cosmetic act, and creating a new regulatory framework for the oversight and labeling of dietary supplements. Differing from the regulation of drugs, under DSHEA, dietary supplements do *not* need approval from the Food and Drug Administration (FDA) before they are marketed, *nor* must they be proven safe *or* effective to be allowed on the market.

Under DSHEA, the manufacturer or distributor is responsible for determining that the dietary supplements are safe, that any representations or claims made about them are substantiated by adequate evidence, and that the product contains the ingredients listed on the label. (Table 10–2 describes the regulation of drugs versus dietary supplements.) Note that it is only after the fact, when adverse events occur and are reported, that the FDA has the authority to investigate and perhaps remove the product from the market.

DSHEA requires that every supplement be labeled properly following specific regulated guidelines (FDA, 1994), and must not represent the product as a conventional food or as the only item of a meal or diet. Table 10–3 shows the information required on a supplement label.

Unless the supplement contains vitamins and/or minerals, there are no Dietary Reference Intake (DRI) standards for dietary supplements to indicate safe or effective doses (Thomas, 2005).

DSHEA also regulates the types of claims that can be made on dietary supplement labels. Supplement labels may not claim that their product will diagnose, cure, mitigate, treat, or prevent a disease. The label may contain one of three types of claims: a health claim, a nutrient content claim, or a structure/function claim (http://www.cfsan.fda.gov/~dms/hclaims.html).

- Health claims describe a relationship between a food, food component, or dietary supplement ingredient and reducing risk of a disease or health-related condition.
- Nutrient content claims describe the relative amount of a nutrient or dietary substance in a product. (See Figure 10–1 and Table 10–3.)
- Structure/function claims are statements describing how a product may affect the organs or systems of the body and it cannot mention any specific disease. Structure/function claims do not require FDA approval, but the manufacturer must provide the FDA with the text of the claim within 30 days of putting the product on the market (FDA Center for Food Safety and Applied Nutrition, http://www.cfsan.fda.gov/~dms/ds-labl.html#structure). Product labels containing such claims must also include a disclaimer that reads, "This statement has not been evaluated by the FDA. This product is not intended to diagnose, treat, cure, or prevent any disease."

TABLE 10–2 Regulation of Drugs versus Dietary Supplements

	Drugs	*Dietary Supplements*
FDA approval	*Required*	*Not required*
Evidence of safety and efficacy	Manufacturers must provide FDA with evidence of product's safety and efficacy based on clinical trials.	The manufacturer is responsible for determining the safety of the product but does not have to provide evidence of safety and efficacy to FDA.
Risk disclosure	Labels and inserts must list all potential adverse effects and interactions.	Not required to have safety warnings on labels.
Product quality	Must follow strict Good Manufacturing Practice (GMP) regulations to ensure purity and accurate labeling.	No current GMP regulations for supplements; must follow food GMPs, which do not ensure all aspects of supplement quality.
Adverse event reporting	Drug companies required to report all adverse events to the FDA.	Manufacturers not required to record or investigate adverse events. Reporting of adverse events to the FDA is voluntary.

Sources: Dangerous supplements, 2004; National institutes of Health, Office of Dietary Supplements: Dietary supplements: Background information. Retrieved April 28, 2005, from http://dietary-supplements.nih.gov/factsheets/Dietarysupplements_pf.asp; U.S. Food and Drug Administration: Overview of dietary supplements. January 3, 2001. Retrieved from http://www.cfsan.fda.gov/~dms/ds-oview.html.

TABLE 10–3 Required Information on Dietary Supplement Labels

General Information
- Name of product (including the word "supplement" or a statement that the product is a supplement)
- Net quantity of contents
- Name and place of business of manufacturer, packer, or distributor
- Directions for use

Supplement Facts Panel
- Serving size, list of dietary ingredients, amount per serving size (by weight), percent of Daily Value (%DV), if established
- If the dietary ingredient is a botanical, the scientific name of the plant or the common or usual name standardized in the reference *Herbs of Commerce,* 2nd ed. (2000 edition) and the name of the plant part used
- If the dietary ingredient is a proprietary blend (i.e., a blend exclusive to the manufacturer), the total weight of the blend and the components of the blend in order of predominance by weight

Other Information That Must Be Included
- Fillers, artificial colors, sweeteners, flavors, or binders—listed by weight in descending order of predominance and by common name or proprietary blend
- The source of dietary ingredients not identified in the "Supplement Facts" panel (e.g., rose hips as the source of vitamin C)
- Other food ingredients (e.g., water and sugar)
- Technical additives or processing aids (e.g., gelatin, starch, colors, stabilizers, preservatives, and flavors)

Source: For more details, see the *Federal Register* 1997; 62(184): 49825–858. Retrieved from http://www.cfsan.fda.gov/~lrd/fr97923a.html.

Supplement Facts

Serving Size 1 Capsule

Amount Per Capsule	% Daily Value
Calories 20	
Calories from Fat 20	
Total Fat 2 g	3%*
Saturated Fat 0.5 g	3%*
Polyunsaturated Fat 1 g	†
Monounsaturated Fat 0.5 g	†
Vitamin A 4250 IU	85%
Vitamin D 425 IU	106%
Omega-3 fatty acids 0.5 g	†

* Percent Daily Values are based on a 2,000 calorie diet.
† Daily Value not established.

Ingredients: Cod liver oil, gelatin, water, and glycerin.

FIGURE 10–1 Supplement label.
Source: From http://www.cfsan.fda.gov/~dms/ds-savv2.html.

The Federal Trade Commission (FTC) is responsible for regulating health claims made in advertising dietary supplements. The FTC can require companies to show evidence to support claims suspected of being false or misleading and can remove products from the market if their advertising is unsubstantiated (Art and Law, 2004). For example, when the FTC evaluated 300 weight-loss advertisements that appeared in 2001, the majority of them for dietary supplements, it found that most represented their products in ways that were almost certainly false or at least lacked adequate substantiation. Among the most frequent misrepresentations were that the product caused rapid and long-term weight loss, was clinically proven or doctor approved, was "all natural" and therefore safe, and that success did not require dieting or exercise (Thomas, 2005).

TYPES OF SUPPLEMENTS

Vitamin and Mineral Supplements

Many consumers assume that they do not need to rely on a healthy diet to provide nutrients if they take dietary supplements. However, this is an important misconception.

Foods contain much more than just vitamins and minerals. New health benefits of compounds such as fiber and phytochemicals are being actively researched, and may play important roles in health promotion and disease prevention.

Potential Benefits

Although nutrients such as vitamins and minerals should be obtained primarily from foods, supplements may be appropriate in some circumstances. Traditionally, supplements are used to treat clinically proven vitamin and mineral deficiencies. Supplements also may be helpful for the specific types of individuals shown in Table 10–1 (Ervin, Kennedy-Stephenson, 2002).

- **Multivitamin with minerals:** These supplements contain 100% of the daily value for most vitamins and several minerals (Dickinson, 2002). People should take a multivitamin supplement daily if they are over age 50 or on weight-loss diets and consume less than 1200 kcal/day (Hunt, Dwyer, 2001). In addition, prenatal multivitamins may be recommended for pregnant women to ensure that they meet their increased nutrient needs (Forman, Altman, 2004).
- **Folate:** Women of childbearing age should consume 400 µg/day of folic acid to help prevent birth defects in unborn children (Hunt, Dwyer, 2001). A multivitamin supplement with folate will supplement food sources of folate that include green leafy vegetables and fortified grain products.
- **Vitamin B_{12}:** Many people over age 50 cannot produce enough stomach acid to absorb vitamin B_{12} adequately. A vitamin B_{12} supplement or multivitamin containing vitamin B_{12} can help overcome this problem. A vitamin B_{12} supplement is also recommended for vegans who consume no animal products (Hunt, Dwyer, 2001).
- **Vitamin D:** Lack of sun and age-related changes can impair the body's ability to synthesize vitamin D. For older adults and those who have little exposure to sun, a multivitamin or calcium supplement containing vitamin D is appropriate in addition to dietary sources to meet the recommended 200 international units (IU) for those under age 50, 400 IU for ages 51–70, and 600 IU for those over 71 (see DRI tables in the Appendix).
- **Calcium:** People who are lactose intolerant and/or do not include liberal amounts of dairy

products in their diets may need to take calcium supplements. Postmenopausal and older women, for whom the DRI is over 1000 mg/day, may find it difficult to obtain sufficient calcium from food alone and may need calcium and vitamin D supplements as well.

- **Iron:** Iron supplementation is routinely recommended for pregnant women who may not be able to meet their increased needs for this nutrient through food sources alone (Hunt, Dwyer, 2001).

Potential Risks

Because the use of supplements in addition to food sources results in increased total vitamin and mineral intake, vitamin and mineral safety becomes an important concern (Krone, Ely, Harms, 2004). Dangers of excess intake of vitamins and minerals led to the development of the Upper Limit of Intake (UL) category for the most recent release of the Dietary Reference Intakes. The following are some of the real dangers related to vitamin and mineral supplement overuse. (See also Chapters 8 and 9 for specifics).

Toxicity As with all foods and drugs, excess as well as deficiency can be harmful. The known range of safety differs among vitamins and minerals. Some, such as vitamin A or D, have a very narrow range of safety. As a general rule, minerals have a narrower range of safety than do vitamins. Toxicity of iron (Hunt, Dwyer, 2001), selenium (Clark, Strukle, Williams, Manoguerra, 1996), and chromium (Steams, Wise, Patierno, Wetterhann, 1995) have been reported. Fluoride can be toxic if consumed in excess (Duyff, 2002). (See Chapters 8 and 9 on vitamins and minerals.)

The DRI and the UL provide good monitors of safe and unsafe levels of nutrient intake. One rule of thumb is that supplements at the level of 100% of the DRI are generally considered safe (the amount in a one-a-day type multivitamin). As intake increases above this level, so does risk. Thus higher intakes should be undertaken only under the supervision of a physician. Harmful effects of *megadoses* (very large doses, 10 times the DRI or more) continue to appear in the literature, often as a result of misguided individuals who think that "if a little is good, a lot will be even better."

Contamination Contamination of mineral supplements is another potential risk as some natural calcium supplements have been found to contain high levels of heavy metals. For example, bone meal, dolomite, or calcium carbonate supplements may be contaminated with lead (Roberts, 2000; Ross, Szabo, Tebbet, 2000). When selecting vitamin and mineral supplements, look for those with the USP (United States Pharmacopoeia) "Dietary Supplement Verified" logo on the label, meaning that the supplement has undergone voluntary testing and meets the USP standards for purity and potency. A list of products that have been tested and meet USP standards can be accessed at http://www.uspverified.org. Supplements with the NSF (National Sanitation Foundation) mark have also undergone voluntary testing and meet NSF international standards for quality (Klausner, 2004).

Contraindications for Certain Populations Some supplements may pose additional health risks for certain groups of people. For example iron oversupplementation may be dangerous for individuals (particularly men) with hemochromatosis, a condition characterized by excess iron storage. People with impaired kidney function are at increased risk of toxicity from magnesium supplements.

Herbal or Botanical Supplements

Close to $300 million was spent on herbals in the United States in 2002, although sales of many herbal supplements have slowed due to public awareness of issues such as efficacy and herb–drug interactions (Harvard, 2004; Marra, 2002) (Table 10–4).

An herb is a type of botanical, defined as "a plant or plant part valued for its medicinal or therapeutic properties, flavor, and/or scent" (NIH Office of Dietary Supplements, http://ods.od.nih.gov/factsheets/ BotanicalBackground.asp). Plant parts include leaves, roots, stems, bark, seeds, whole flowers, pollen, petals, pistils, stamen, and their extracts. Herbal supplements come in many different forms and their action ranges from mild to very potent. Herbs may be purchased fresh or dried, as extracts, capsules, tablets, powders, or teas. The process of extraction obtains the active compound(s) from a crude, natural source by using a solvent such as water, fat, oil, or alcohol. The form in which an herb is taken may affect its potency. For instance, although peppermint tea is generally safe, peppermint taken as a more concentrated oil may be toxic. Some

TABLE 10–4   Popular Supplements and Herbal Remedies

Legend:
↔ means uncertain or conflicting data
↑? = some preliminary evidence
↑ = good evidence
↓ = not supported
NR = no sufficient good research

Supplement	Unproven Claims for Usage	Precautions/Risks of Adverse Effects
Bee pollen	• nature's perfect food ↓ • increases vitality, memory, well-being **NR** • improves exercise performance **NR** • fights respiratory tract infections, endocrine disorders, allergies **NR**	• not recommended for people with asthma or allergies to honey or bee stings • not "perfect food"—made up of nutrients found naturally in foods such as starch, sugar, protein, fat
Carnitine	• helps heart ↑? • improves aerobic power ↓ • improves immune function **NR** • enhances energy **NR** • burns fat **NR**	• no harmful effects seen in doses up to 6 g/day • larger doses associated with nausea and diarrhea • may cause weight gain or water retention • may be harmful for people with kidney conditions
Creatine	• increases muscle strength ↑? • delays fatigue **NR** • increases muscle mass **NR** • burns fat **NR** • increases strength in people with muscular diseases ↑? • increases strength in the elderly **NR**	• avoid doses over 5 g
DHEA	• boosts energy, **NR** • slows aging **NR** • enhances immunity↔ • improves heart function↔	• self-supplementation not recommended • may increase risk of breast and prostate cancer • can cause acne and excess hair growth on face and body Note: Coenzyme Q10 is synthesized in the body and aids in production of energy and serves as an antioxidant. There is no agreement that taking added coenzyme Q10 has benefit.

Echinacea	• boosts the immune system ↑?
	• protects against the common cold or flu ↓
		• loses effectiveness with continued use
		• may cause allergic reactions in people with asthma or sensitivity to grass pollen
		• may cause headache, dizziness
		• topical use may cause skin irritation
		• contraindications:
		  • people with reduced immunity
		  • people taking corticosteroids or anabolic steroids

Ephedra **Taken off the market by the FDA due to proof of danger**	• ephedrine (main active ingredient) functions as a vasoconstrictor ↑? • stimulates the central nervous system (CNS) ↑? • acts as a diuretic (used in weight-loss products) ↑?	• misuse has caused deaths • can cause hypertension, heart attack, stroke, death • can cause CNS stimulation (nervousness, insomnia, palpitations, tremors) • may increase the toxic effects of the depression medication Elavil

	• provides a sense of Euphoria **NR**	• can exacerbate the toxic effects of caffeine products Caffedrine, No Doz, Vivarin • can exacerbate the rapid heart rate, anxiety, and high blood pressure associated with the use of the asthma medication Theo-Dur (Golub, 1999) • can cause hyperglycemia
Evening primrose oil	• helps PMS and other women's disorders ↔ • eliminates pain of rheumatoid arthritis ↔ • helps allergic skin conditions and clears up acne ↔ • improves heart disease and diabetes **NR** • prevents hair loss **NR**	• may be contaminated with other oils that alter its activity (non-GRAS*; Craig, 1997) • not to be used with trycyclic antidepressants or anticonvulsants • may cause nausea, diarrhea, indigestion, headache • may increase risk of pregnancy complications
Feverfew	• prevents migraines • relieves fever, arthritis, tinnitue, and vertigo • relieves toothaches (used topically)	• may cause indigestion, diarrhea • possibly increases headache, insomnia, joint pain with long-term use • interferes with anticoagulant and antiplatelet agents and NSAIDS (nonsteroidal antiinflammatory drugs)
Garlic	• lowers LDL, raises high-density lipoprotein (HDL) cholesterol ↑? • improves circulation (antithrombic) ↑? • contains antibiotic, antifungal properties ↔	• may increase bleeding by interacting with anticoagulants • long-term use of extract effect unknown • high doses can irritate stomach lining • avoid taking within 7 days of surgery • topical can cause dermatitis and burns with long-term use
Ginkgo biloba	• improves cognitive performance and social functioning in patients with dementia or Alzheimer's disease ↔ • improves memory in healthy people **NR** • improves circulation ↑?	• may increase bleeding: monitor if taking anticoagulant medications • avoid during pregnancy/lactation • avoid taking within 36 hours of surgery • can cause bleeding, GI upset, headaches • can cause allergic skin reactions
Ginseng	• enhances exercise ability ↓ • boosts energy and mood **NR** • serves as an aphrodisiac **NR**	• can cause nervousness/excitation, headache, insomnia, palpitations • a danger to hypertensives • may interact with antidepressants, warfarin • topically can cause rash, exacerbate photosensitivity • may adversely affect blood glucose levels • avoid taking within 7 days of surgery
Glucosamine	• relieves arthritis pain ↑? • heals tendons and ligaments **NR** • improves symptoms of tendonitis and bursitis **NR**	• no harmful effects in short-term studies • may affect glucose levels so people with diabetes should closely monitor blood glucose levels
Goldenseal	• soothes sore mouth and throat **NR** • protects against traveler's diarrhea **NR** • masks drug use in urine tests **NR**	• avoid if pregnant • high doses may cause nausea, vomiting, diarrhea, CNS stimulation, respiratory failure • no scientific evidence to evaluate safety
Green tea	• serves as a strong antioxidant ↑	• some may contain caffeine
Kava	• acts as an antidepression ↑? • enhances sleep **NR**	• dangerous interactions with antianxiety medicines • increases effects of alcohol, other CNS depressants

(continued)

TABLE 10–4 Popular Supplements and Herbal Remedies (Continued)

Supplement	Unproven Claims for Usage	Precautions/Risks of Adverse Effects
		• high doses cause muscle weakness • may be associated with liver toxicity • chronic use causes irreversible skin discoloration and eye disturbances • avoid if pregnant, lactating, or depressed
Saw palmetto	• remedies enlarged prostate ↑? • prevents prostate cancer **NR**	• may cause stomach upset, headache, diarrhea at high doses, • avoid if pregnant • may aggravate estrogen-sensitive tumors • avoid use with anticoagulants
Shark cartilage	• acts as a cancer cure **NR**	• insufficient data to assess safety • may be linked to hepatitis
Spirulina/ blue-green algae	• boosts immunity **NR** • lowers cholesterol **NR** • reduces cancer risk **NR**	• no reported adverse effects
St. John's wort	• relieves depression ↑?	• dangerous when combined with antidepressant medications • may cause rash; exacerbates photosensitivity to tetracycline • may cause side effects with use and rapid withdrawal: anxiety, nausea, dry mouth, headache, dizziness, photosensitivity
Valerian	• functions as a sedative for antianxiety **NR** • helps insomnia ↑?	• can cause drowsiness, headaches, anxiety • harmful with barbiturates or other sleep medications • harmful for people with liver disorders
Yohimbine	• increases sex drive ↓ • aids weight loss **NR** • builds muscle **NR**	• potentially harmful • doses from 4 to 20 mg/day associated with abnormal heartbeat, low blood pressure, tremors • may increase toxicity in those taking phenothazines (used for mental disorders) • harmful for people with high or low blood pressure, liver disease, kidney disease, or bipolar disorders

*GRAS-Generally Regarded as Safe, an FDA classification.
Sources: Table is adapted from:
Duyff, 2002, pp. 593–598.
Kostka-Rokosz et al., 2005, pp. 17–28.
Foster S, Tyler E: *Tyler's Honest Herbal: A Sensible Guide to the Use of Herbs and Related Remedies,* 4th ed. New York: Haworth Herbal Press, 1999.
Thomas, 2005, pp. 6–12.
Turner, Bauer, Woelkart, Hulsey, Gangemi, 2005.

herbals may have immediate effects, whereas milder botanicals may take several weeks or even months before having an effect. For example, kava may have an immediate and strong effect on muscle relaxation, whereas valerian may not have an effect as a sleep aid until it has been taken for a number of days (NIH Office of Dietary Supplements, http://ods.od.nih.gov/factsheets/BotanicalBackground.asp).

Historically, every culture has used herbal remedies. For example:

• Opium and belladonna were used mostly as poisons.
• Foxglove is the source of digitalis.
• Salicin, the basis for aspirin, comes from willow bark.

- Indian snakeroot was the source of reserpine, used to control blood pressure.
- The autumn crocus provided colchicine, a drug for gouty arthritis. (Ellenhorn, Schonwald, Ordog, Wassenberger, 1997; Stone, 1997)

Potential Benefits

Today, several billion dollars' worth of prescription drugs are derived from plants each year. Plants have developed defenses against bacteria, fungi, insect pests, and other natural enemies, so they are sources of antibiotics, fungicides, pesticides, and other substances useful to humans. However, many natural plant materials are too toxic for human use (Ellenhorn et al., 1997; Stone, 1997). Some plant cytotoxins have anticancer effects (e.g., taxol, vincristine), but natural plant substances can also cause cancer, especially tobacco.

In addition to prescription drugs derived from plants, there are a number of dietary supplements derived from plants that are currently used in hopes of preventing or treating a variety of conditions. Although there is not sufficient evidence to prove the efficacy of the majority of herbal supplements that are used today, there are some that may have potential benefits. For example, systematic reviews have found evidence that garlic may lower cholesterol, saw palmetto may be beneficial for benign prostatic hyperplasia, St. John's wort may alleviate mild to moderate depression, and ginkgo biloba may improve Alzheimer's, vascular dementia, and claudication (Bent, Ko, 2004; Duyff, 2002; Harvard, 2004). Fiber supplements (psyllium, bran tablets, or other forms) can help improve constipation, but they have not been proven effective for weight loss. Conversely, taking fiber supplements may result in excessive fiber consumption that can inhibit absorption of certain nutrients and cause gastrointestinal discomfort (Duyff, 2002). See Table 10–4.

Potential Risks

The major issues facing consumers concerning herbal supplements currently on the market are as follows:

- **Adverse effects:** Herbal and botanical products have a wide variety of possible side effects, depending on the product and the individual taking it, that can range from headaches, rashes, and gastrointestinal distress to more severe side effects such as liver damage or even death. Serious harm has been reported from the use of several herbals

(Betz, 1998; Chung, 2004; Herbal, 1996, 1999; Shekelle et al., 2003). The herb *Aristolochia fangchi*, for example, was found to be nephrotoxic and carcinogenic, and was shown to cause nephropathy, and even some cases of end-stage renal disease, in over 100 women who took weight-loss supplements containing this herb (Bent, Ko, 2004). See Table 10–5 for a list of dietary supplements on the FDA's warning list because of serious safety concerns (http://www.cfsan.fda.gov/~dms/ds-ill.html).

- **Surgical complications:** Because herbal supplements such as garlic, ginger, ginseng, and ginkgo biloba may increase the risk of bleeding, patients should discontinue using such supplements for up to 2 or 3 weeks before surgery or other dental procedures (Bent, Ko, 2004; Duyff, 2002; Harvard, 2004).

- **Possibility of adulteration of products with potent standard drugs (including prescription drugs) and other potentially harmful substances:** Some products have been found to be adulterated with toxic substances, or to contain synthetic drugs without warnings of possible side effects. For example, the herbal supplement PC-SPES used for prostate cancer was taken off the market after it was found to contain the drug warfarin. Some herbals also have been found to contain toxic heavy metals such as lead, arsenic,

TABLE 10–5 Examples of Dietary Supplements and Ingredients on FDA's Warning List

- Androstenedione
- Aristolochic acid
- Comfrey
- Ephedrine alkaloids
- Kava
- Tiractricol
- Gamma butyrolactone (GBL)
- Gamma hydroxybutyric acid (GHB)
- 1,4 butanediol (BD)
- L-tryptophan
- LipoKinetix
- PC SPES and SPES
- Chaso diet capsules and Chaso Genpi
- Herbal Fen-Phen

Source: U.S. Food and Drug Administration, http://www.fda.gov.

and mercury (Bent, Ko, 2004; Harvard, 2004; Huang, Kuo-Ching, Mei-Ling, 1997; Ko, 1998).

- **Drug interactions:** The greatest health risk posed by herbal medicines involves their potential interaction with prescription drugs. For example, St. John's wort can render several life-saving drugs ineffective. See Table 10–6 for some common herb–drug interactions. These potential interactions are of great concern because about 16% of those who take prescription drugs also take at least one type of herbal or dietary supplement (Kaufman et al., 2002).

- **No standardization of product names:** Herbs are often sold under a variety of names, which can make it confusing for consumers to know exactly what a product contains. For instance, the dangerous herb *Aristolichia* is also called aristolochic acid, birthwort, snakeroot, snakeweed, sangree root, sangrel, serpentary, serpentaria, *Asarum canadense*, and wild ginger (Dangerous Supplements, 2004).

TABLE 10–6   Herb–Drug Interactions with Some Commonly Used Herbs

Herb	*Drug*	*Interaction*
Garlic	Warfarin	Bleeding, increase in international normalized ratio
	Chlorpropamide	Hypoglycemia
Ginkgo biloba	Warfarin	Bleeding
	Aspirin	Bleeding
	Thiazide diuretic	Increase in blood pressure
	Trazodone	Increased sedation
Ginseng	Warfarin	Decrease in international normalized ratio
	Phenelzine	Insomnia, headache, tremulousness, mania
St. John's wort	Amitriptyline	Reduced plasma concentrations
	Cyclosporine	Reduced plasma concentrations
	Digoxin	Reduced plasma concentrations
	Indinavir	Reduced plasma concentrations
	Nefazodone	Symptoms of central serotonin excess
	Oral contraceptives	Altered menstrual bleeding
	Paroxetine	Symptoms of central serotonin excess
	Phenprocoumon	Reduced plasma concentrations
	Sertraline	Symptoms of central serotonin excess
	Theophylline	Reduced plasma concentrations
	Warfarin	Decrease in international normalized ratio
Echinacea	Anabolic steroids	Increased liver damage
	Amiodarone	
	Methotrexate	
	Ketoconazole	
	Antihypertensives	
	Antiarrhythmics	
Licorice	Digoxin	Increased salt and water retention and increased blood pressure
	Diuretics	Increased risk of abnormal heart
	MAOIs	Decreased potassium
		Decreased potassium
		Decrease effectiveness of drug

Source: From Bent and Ko, 2004.

- **No standardization of dosages:** The strength of pharmacological substances can vary widely among herbal products. For example, the *Los Angeles Times* commissioned an analysis of 10 brands of St. John's wort. Three were found to have no more than half the potency listed on the label, and another four had less than 90% of the labeled amount. The USP is now setting standards for more than 50 different herbal products in the *National Formulary* (*NF*) (*The Pharmacist's Letter*, 1998, 1999).
- **Failure to provide information for proper use by consumers:** Herbal products intended for medicinal use often do not contain the information consumers need to be able to use them properly. In comparison, U.S. drug labels require (1) description and clinical pharmacology, (2) ingredients, (3) indications, (4) contraindications, (5) warnings and precautions, (6) adverse reactions, (7) dosage and administration, and (8) overdosage levels.
- **Failure to track product use for unanticipated adverse effects:** Unlike with drugs, manufacturers of herbal products are not required by law to keep record of or to report adverse effects to the FDA. The surveillance system for tracking adverse effects of herbal products identifies less than 1% of such events (Bent, Ko, 2004).

Sports Nutrition and Ergogenic Aids

A wide variety of dietary supplements have been promoted as ergogenic aids that are claimed to enhance athletic performance; some surveys have found that as many as 76–100% of those participating in certain athletic activities may use supplements. Sports nutrition supplements include certain herbals as well as amino acids, whey protein, carnitine, creatine, chromium picolinate, glutamine, dehydroepiandrosterone (DHEA), and other products.

Potential Benefits

Although there are sports nutrition supplements that may have some potential benefits, athletic performance is determined largely by genetic potential, training, and nutritional status (Eschbach, 2000). Research suggests that supplemental creatine may be beneficial for anaerobic exercise involving high-intensity, repetitive activity

in some individuals, but it has not been found to improve endurance activity. The long-term safety of creatine is unknown (Ahrendt, 2001; Bell, Dorsch, McCreary, Hovey, 2004; Duyff, 2002; Eschbach, 2000; Froiland, Koszewski, Hingst, Kopecky, 2004).

Potential Risks

Many products sold as ergogenic aids do not increase performance and may have serious side effects. People commonly take protein supplements because the fact that muscles are composed largely of protein has led to the simplistic notion that eating extra protein will build extra muscle. In truth, muscular hypertrophy is largely dependent on stimulation of the muscles through high-resistance exercise. High-performance athletes engaged in endurance work or body building have increased protein needs, but these are not extreme and supplementation is unnecessary in meeting that need. High-protein diets can cause abnormal strain on the kidneys trying to excrete the breakdown products of excessive protein intake. High-protein liquid diets also carry health risks and should not be used except under a physician's guidance. These diets are reviewed in Chapter 3. In addition to the risk of adverse effects, use of certain supplements in competition may also have legal and ethical issues. Hormonal supplements, such as anabolic steroids and DHEA are associated with potentially dangerous adverse effects, are strongly contraindicated for children and adolescents, and are banned by organizations such as the International Olympic Committee (IOC).

Specialty Supplements

This category includes supplements that do not fall into the above categories, such as glucosamine, melatonin, and other hormones; amino acids; lecithin; and fish oils. Some of these specialty supplements may have potential benefits, whereas others have been found ineffective. Because research has shown the benefits of omega-3 fatty acids on cardiovascular disease, fish oil or other omega-3 fatty acid supplements may have beneficial effects (Dickinson, 2002). Like the other categories of dietary supplements, specialty supplements also pose the same risks of potential adverse effects, possible contamination, and contraindications for certain individuals. The amino acid L-tryptophan, for example, was a popularly promoted sleep aid supplement until it caused harm to several users and was taken off the market (Das, Bagchi, Bagchi, Preuss, 2004).

Liquid Nutritional or Meal Replacement Supplements

Liquid nutritional supplements were originally developed for medically compromised hospital patients who were unable to obtain adequate nutrition via regular foods and meals. They were used either to augment the diet, or serve as total food replacements. If used as total food replacements, a specific number of daily servings would meet all of an individual's nutritional needs (Table 10–7).

Liquid nutritional supplements were designed for patients with special health requirements (e.g., high calorie, high protein, high fiber, lactose free). These products are lifesavers for many patients such as those with cancer, anorexia, or other disorders that interfere with the ability to consume a normal nutritious diet. Surgery patients, cancer patients on chemotherapy, patients with swallowing disorders, patients with AIDS, and frail nursing home patients have been the primary users of liquid nutritional supplements. However, individuals with oral impairments, poor appetites, or the ability to consume only small amounts of food may also benefit from additional calories and protein that can be obtained from a liquid supplement.

Liquid supplements are made up of water, milk, protein, soy, sugar, oil, vitamins, and minerals. They may be milk-based, lactose-free casein-based, low carbohydrate, or concentrated with added calories and protein, depending on intended use. Liquid supplements as diet adjuncts are helpful for frail elderly people to improve weight and reduce falls (Gray-Donald, Payette, Boutier, 1995; Schurch et al., 1998).

In recent years variations of the complete liquid supplement have been "repackaged" for new markets as:

- A breakfast alternative for healthy people on the run, who might otherwise skip breakfast. These Instant Breakfast type drinks were designed to be mixed with milk and provide about one-third of the DRIs for the day and about 250 calories (including the milk).
- A meal supplement for healthy older individuals allegedly to improve vitality, energy, well-being, and longevity.
- A meal replacement for those with a fast-paced lifestyle.
- A healthy, convenient alternative to high-fat snacks and fast-food meals for the health-conscious adult.
- A nutritional supplement that will improve performance in athletes.

All of the liquid supplements are similar in composition. They provide from 200 to 300 calories and about one-third of the total daily nutrient requirement per serving. (See Table 10–7.)

The majority of complete nutritional supplements are costly. Instant breakfasts made with whole or lactose-reduced milk provide similar nutritional benefits at a lower price. These products are promoted as good as or better than whole foods such as grains, fruits, and vegetables. Yet the lack of some essential nutrients, fiber, and phytochemicals in these liquid supplements means that the consumer is missing some of the protective nutritional components of food.

Liquid nutritional supplements may be beneficial for dentally impaired people, frail older people, and

TABLE 10–7 Liquid Nutrition Supplements: Comparison of Nutrient Composition of Eight-Ounce Liquid Nutrition Supplements

	Calories	*Protein (g)*	*Fat (g)*	*CHO (g)*
Ensure	250	9	6	40
Ensure Plus	360	13	11	50
Boost	240	10	4	41
Boost Plus	360	14	14	45
Instant Breakfast with whole milk	280	13	8	39

very sick patients. They are an alternative to not eating at all, a way to improve nutrient intake in addition to meals, and an alternative to soda and cookies for breakfast. On the other hand, the brand name products are costly, and they are often marketed on the basis of unrealistic expectations to vulnerable populations such as elders, who may least afford them and would be better off eating nutritious whole foods.

SOUND VERSUS UNSOUND CLAIMS

Health professionals need to know if claims made for dietary supplements and other nutritional products are based on sound evidence. Many of the studies on dietary supplements have not been well designed, executed, or analyzed, and often little is known about the long-term efficacy and safety of these products (Thomas, 2005). See Table 10–4.

The FTC has found many claims made for weight-loss supplements to be false and unsubstantiated and has taken legal action against several popular products. Some of the most common misleading claims for weight-loss supplements are that they are doctor approved or clinically proven and cause rapid, long-term weight loss. Because the FTC does not have the resources to evaluate the abundance of health claims for all dietary supplements, consumers are still exposed to misleading advertisements not based in sound science. Many herbal and other supplements are promoted and sold on the Internet, a source of health information that many people believe to be credible. Although manufacturers are not allowed to claim that dietary supplements can treat, prevent, diagnose, or cure a specific disease, almost half of the websites evaluated for eight common herbs were found to make such claims. Patients may be at risk for harm if they rely on false medical information and choose to take a supplement in place of a scientifically proven treatment for their condition (Morris, Avorn, 2003). Several "red flags" or common themes indicate unfounded nutritional products or approaches. They are detailed in Table 10–8.

The promoters of unfounded products or approaches often use the natural course of disease to their advantage in claiming cures. For example:

- **The placebo effect:** The act of treatment alone is enough to elicit a positive response in many people. Marketers attribute "placebo effect" to their product.

- **Natural remission:** Remission often occurs naturally in illness, but marketers attribute the improvement to their product.
- **Misinterpretation:** When patients fail to improve or become worse off, adverse symptoms are explained as "poisons coming out of the body." Thus, apparent failures are explained as clinical successes. People who believe such explanations will interpret failures as successes.

RELIABLE RESOURCES ON DIETARY SUPPLEMENTS

Much more research on the safety of dietary supplements as well as improved regulation is necessary to protect consumers. The Office of Dietary Supplements (ODS) was established at the National Institutes of Health (NIH) in 1995 to promote and disseminate scientific research on dietary supplements (http://dietary-supplements.info.nih.gov). ODS is a reliable source of information on the safety and efficacy of botanicals and other dietary supplements. A wealth of information is accessible from its website, including a comprehensive database of research studies as well as fact sheets appropriate for consumers on various dietary supplements.

The NIH established the National Center for Complementary and Alternative Medicine (NCCAM) in 1998, which also supports research for botanicals and other dietary supplements (http://nccam.nih.gov).

The FDA (www.fda.gov) is taking steps to improve the regulation of dietary supplements (including a system of evaluating safety issues and adverse events). The following is a list of sound dietary supplement resources.

http://www.consumerlab.com (tests herbs, vitamins, other dietary supplements)

http://www.cfsan.fda.gov/~dms/supplmnt.html (Food and Drug Administration)

http://dietary-supplements.info.nih.gov (NIH Office of Dietary Supplements home page)

http://ods.od.nih.gov/databases/ibids.html (ODS International Bibliographic Information on Dietary Supplements)

http://nccam.nih.gov/health/supplements.htm (National Center for Complementary and Alternative Medicine)

TABLE 10–8 Hallmarks of Sound and Unsound Nutrition Information

Unsound	*Sound*
• Supplements are cure-alls. • Promises are too good to be true. • The concept that many health conditions can be cured by nutritional supplements. • Amount of money spent on supplements usually turns out to be substantial. • Claims of being persecuted by the traditional medical community. • The concept that traditional health care providers are threatened or jealous of their recommendations. Appeals to the public who identify with the "underdog." • Supportive "evidence" relies on anecdotal data and individual reports. • Use of invalid methods of health assessment to convince their clients that they have special needs. Such "tests" provide the rationale for prescribing supplements. • Supportive data are published in the popular press and non-peer-reviewed journals. • There is something for sale. This could be supplements, books, devices, potions, etc. • Special brands are promoted. • The practitioner sells the items directly. • The practitioner tries to enlist the client as a salesperson. • They are sent to something other than a regular prescription counter. • Promotion by unqualified providers (e.g., diploma mill graduates, salespersons).	• Only diagnosed nutrients deficiencies can be cured by nutritional supplements. • Sound nutrition avoids grandiose promises that can't be kept. • Emphasize making basic changes in lifestyle, such as better food choices, improved eating patterns, or exercise, as well as indicated supplements. • The traditional medical community is unlikely to reject anything that has been proven effective after research using accepted methodologies (i.e., double-blind studies). • Supportive evidence is required through sound research, and replicated by others before being accepted as fact. • Assessment methods are proven and accepted by the professional community. • Before accepted as true, research is subjected to peer review, published in peer reviewed journals, and replicated by more than one researcher. Publication in lay publications requires none of this and does not even require that the data be true. • Trustworthy health professionals try to avoid commercialism (ADA Code of Ethics, 1998). • Needed supplements are usually available in generic or store brands as well as name brands. • Recommendations by qualified health professionals such as physicians, registered dietitians.

http://www.herbalgram.org (American Botanical Council)

http://www.supplementwatch.com (Supplement Watch)

http://www.fda.gov/medwatch/report/hcp.htm (MedWatch, the FDA website for reporting harmful effects of supplements)

http://www.cfsan.fda.gov/~dms/ds-savvy.html (FDA website on navigating the Internet for dietary supplement information)

SUMMARY AND IMPLICATIONS FOR DENTISTRY OF SUPPLEMENTS

The dietary supplement industry is a multibillion-dollar business. Although herbal remedies have been used for centuries, sound research on the safety and efficacy of most of them has lagged behind their public embrace and commercial marketing. There are many different types of dietary supplements that are promoted for a wide range of uses, only some of which are appropriate for the intended use. Information is trickling in as to the

TABLE 10–9 Questions to Ask in Taking a Dietary Supplement History

1. Do you take any over-the-counter or prescribed dietary supplements?*
2. What kind of supplement(s) do you use (vitamin, mineral, herbal, amino acid, fiber, liquid nutritional, etc.)?
3. What is the brand or manufacturer of the supplement(s)?
4. How long have you been taking the supplement(s)?
5. How long do you plan to use the supplement(s)?
6. What are your primary reason(s) for taking the supplement(s)?
7. What amount or dose of the supplement(s) do you take?
8. How often do you take the supplement(s)?

*Note that people do not always regard a supplement as such, so listing examples or calling them "minerals or vitamins" is needed.

possible efficacy of some products, as well as harmfulness of others. Dental professionals need to:

- Ask patients about dietary supplement usage (see Table 10–9 for taking a dietary supplement history).
- Realize when some vitamin and mineral supplementation is appropriate and indicated for some groups of people.
- Have access to resources to tell whether there may be risk for interaction with drugs used in the dental office (see Chapter 16).
- Be aware of the hallmarks of unfounded nutrition promotion and its purveyors to determine the validity of supplement recommendations.
- Be able to answer patients' questions about dietary supplements or steer them to reliable nutrition resources (see Chapter 23).
- Report any adverse events that may be related to dietary supplement usage by their patients to the FDA MedWatch program. Adverse events can be reported by calling the MedWatch hotline at 1-800-FDA-1088, by fax at 1-800-FDA-0178, or online at http://www.fda.gov/medwatch/report/hcp.htm.

QUESTIONS PATIENTS MIGHT ASK

Q. Are brand-name multivitamins better than generic?

A. Generic or store-brand multivitamins are generally comparable to brand-name multivitamins. In addition, generic vitamins are usually less expensive (Forman, Altman, 2004).

Q. Are natural vitamins better than synthetic?

A. For most nutrients, chemical forms and natural forms are equally well absorbed and utilized. Exceptions are vitamin E, which is better absorbed in its natural form and vitamin B_{12}, which is better absorbed in the synthetic form (Golub, 1999).

Q. Are chelated (combined with other compounds for alleged improved absorption) vitamins better than nonchelated?

A. Chelated vitamins do not offer superior absorption ability. Stomach acid breaks down chelates and nutrients are absorbed as any others (Golub, 1999).

Q. Are time-release vitamins better than regular ones?

A. There is no value of time release for multivitamins. To improve absorption of nutrients, take them with foods. For example, Nicotinic acid may be prescribed—under careful medical supervision—as time release, due to toxicity risks (Golub, 1999).

Q. Do children's multivitamin supplements have fluoride in them?

A. Most children's multivitamins do not contain fluoride. This is because supplemental fluoride may increase the risk of fluorosis (Bowen, 2002). Separate fluoride supplements, however, may be recommended for children who do not receive adequate fluoride through drinking water and other dietary sources.

Q. Are children's multivitamin supplements cariogenic?

A. Children's chewable and liquid vitamin supplements may be cariogenic if they are sweetened with sugar. It may be advisable for children who are at high risk for dental caries to take a vitamin sweetened with sorbitol instead (Soxman, 2005). Children should rinse their mouth with water after taking a liquid vitamin supplement that contains added sugars.

Q. Are "natural" supplements always safe?

A. Just because a product is natural does not mean that it has milder effects or is always safe. For example, some natural wild mushrooms are poisonous. Dietary supplements that are claimed to be natural may still be harmful to certain individuals, interact with certain drugs, and have possible contamination (National Center for Complementary and Alternative Medicine, http://www.cfsan.fda.gov, http://nccam.nih.gov/health/bottle/)

CASE STUDY

Altagracia Garcia is a 25-year-old woman who came to the dental office for a routine checkup. She is in good health except for high blood pressure, which she controls with medication. She enjoys running short marathons and considers herself to be fit. She is very conscientious of her diet, and follows the types and amounts of foods recommended on the food guide pyramid carefully. She also takes a variety of supplements that she buys at her local health food store. She takes 4000 μg/day of vitamin A, 3 g/day of vitamin C, 300 mg/day of vitamin B$_6$, as well as various amounts of herbal supplements such

as creatine, ginkgo biloba, and St. John's wart for energy, stamina, and mood improvement. She was married in the past 6 months and is planning to start a family soon.

Questions:
1. What would you say to Altagracia about her supplement usage?
2. What issues are of concern regarding her supplement usage?
3. What recommendations would you make to her?

REFERENCES

Ahrendt DM: Ergogenic aids: Counseling the athlete. *Am Fam Physician* 2001; 63:913–11. Retrieved February 25, 2005, from http://www.aafp.org/afp/20010301/913.html.

Art and law of supplement labels: ConsumerReports.org. 2004. Retrieved April 28, 2006. Available at http://www.consumerreports.org.

Balluz LS, Kieszak SM, Philen RM, Mulinare J: Vitamin and mineral supplement use in the United States. Results from the Third National Health and Nutrition Examination Survey. [Erratum appears in *Arch Fam Med* 2000; 9(7):652]. *Arch Fam Med* 2000; 9(3):258–62.

Bell A, Dorsch KD, McCreary DR, Hovey R: A look at nutritional supplement use in adolescents. *J Adolesc Health* 2004; 34(6):508–16.

Bent S, Ko R: Commonly used herbal medicines in the United States: A review *Am J Med* 2004; 116(7):478–85.

Betz W: Epidemic of renal failure due to herbals. *Sci Rev Alternative Med* 1998; 2(2):12.

Bowen WH: Fluorosis: Is it really a problem? *J Am Dent Assoc* 2002; 133(10):1405–7.

Briefel RR, Johnson CL: Secular trends in dietary intake in the United States. *Annu Rev Nutr* 2004; 24:401–31.

Chung MK: Vitamins, supplements, herbal medicines, and arrhythmias. *Cardiol Rev* 2004; 12(2):73–84.

Clark RF, Strukle E, Williams SR, Manoguerra, AS: Selenium poisoning from a nutritional supplement. *JAMA* 1996; 275(14):1087–88.

Cook TF, Frighetto L, Marra CA, Jewesson PJ: Patterns of use and patients' attitudes toward complementary medications: A survey of adult general medicine patients at a major Canadian teaching hospital. *Can J Clin* Pharmacol 2002; 9(4):183–89.

Dangerous supplements: Still at large: ConsumerReports .org. May 2004. Retrieved April 28, 2005, from http://www.consumerreports.org.

Das YT, Bagchi M, Bagchi D, Preuss HG: Safety of 5-hydroxy-L-tryptophan. *Toxicol Lett* 2004; 150(1):111–22.

Dickinson A: *The Benefits of Nutritional Supplements.* Council for Responsible Nutrition. 2002. Retrieved March 1, 2005, from http://www.crnusa.org/benpdfs/CRN000benefits_ExecSumm.pdf.

Duyff RL: *American Dietetic Association Complete Food and Nutrition Guide.* Hooken, NJ: Wiley & Sons, 2002.

Ellenhorn MJ, Schonwald S, Ordog G, Wassenberger J: *Ellenhorn's Medical Toxicology. Diagnosis and Treatment of Human Poisoning,* 2nd ed. Baltimore: Williams & Wilkins, 1997.

Ervin RB, Kennedy-Stephenson J: Mineral intakes of elderly adult supplement and nonsupplement users in the Third National Health and Nutrition Examination Survey. J Nutr 2002; 132(11):3422–27.

Eschbach LC: Protein and creatine: Some basic facts. American College of Sports Medicine's Fit Society 2000. Retrieved February 25, 2005, from http://www.acsm.org/pdf/0080FS44.pdf.

FDA Center for Food Safety and Applied Nutrition: Fact sheet on FDA's regulatory strategy for dietary supplements. November 2004. Retrieved February 25, 2005, from http://www.fda.gov.

FDA Center for Food Safety and Applied Nutrition. Fact sheet on claims that can be made for conventional foods and dietary supplements. September 2003. Retrieved May 19, 2006 from http://www.cfsan.fda.gov/~dms/hclaims.html.

Forman D, Altman D: Vitamins to prevent cancer: Supplementary problems. *Lancet* 2004; 364(9441):1193–94.

Froiland K, Koszewski W, Hingst J, Kopecky L: Nutritional supplement use among college athletes and their sources of information [Erratum appears in *Int J Sport Nutr Exerc Metab* 2004; 14(5):following 606]. *Int J Sport Nutr Exer Metab* 2004; 14(1):104–20.

Golub C: Making sense of supplement scene. *Environ Nutr* 1999; 22(11):1, 4, 5.

Gray-Donald K, Payette H, Boutier V: Randomized clinical trial of nutritional supplementation shows little effect on functional status among free-living frail elderly. *J Nutr* 1995; 125:2965–71.

Harvard Medical School: *Buyer's Guide to Herbs and Supplements Special Health Report*. Cambridge, MA: Harvard Health Publications, 2004.

Herbal, Rx: The promises and pitfalls. *Consum Rep* 1999; 64(3):47.

Huang WF, Kuo-Ching W, Mei-Ling H: Adulteration by synthetic therapeutic substances of traditional Chinese medicines in Taiwan. *J Clin Pharmacol* 1997; 37:344–50.

Hunt J, Dwyer J: Position of the American Dietetic Association: Food fortification and dietary supplements. *J Am Diet Assoc* 2001; 101:114–25.

Johnson BA: Prevention magazine assesses use of dietary supplements. *HerbalGram* 2000; 48:65.

Kaufman DW, Kelly JP, Rosenberg L, Anderson TE, Mitchell AA: Recent patterns of medication use in the ambulatory adult population of the United States: The Slone Survey. *JAMA* 2002; 287(3):337–44.

Kelly JP, Kaufman DW, Kelley K, Rosenberg L, Anderson TE, Mitchell AA: Recent trends in use of herbal and other natural products. *Arch Int Med* 2005; 165(3):281–86.

Klausner A: New supplement seal better assures quality, but not effectiveness. *Environ Nutr.* November 2004: Retrieved February 25, 2005, from http://www. environmentalnutrition.com

Ko RJ: Adulterants in Asian patent medicines. *N Engl J Med* 1998; 339(12):847.

Ko RJ: A U.S. perspective on the adverse reactions from traditional Chinese medicines. *J Chin Med Assoc* 2004; 67(3):109–16.

Ko RJ: Causes, epidemiology, and clinical evaluation of suspected herbal poisoning. *J Toxicol Clin Toxicol* 1999; 37(6):697–708.

Kostka-Rokosz MD, Dvorkin L, Vibbard KJ, Couris RR: Selected herbal therapies: A review of safety. *Nutr Today* 2005; 40(1):17–28.

Krone C, Ely J, Harms L: Nutritional supplements: Friend or foe? *New Zealand Med J* 2004; 117(1196):U937.

Marra J: The state of dietary supplements. *Nutraceut World* 2002.

Morris CA, Avorn J: Internet marketing of herbal products. *JAMA* 2003; 290(11):1505–10.

Morrison LJ, Gizis F, Shorter B: Prevalent use of dietary supplements among people who exercise at a commercial gym. *Int J Sports Nutr Exer* 2004; 14(14):481–92.

National Center for Complementary and Alternative Medicine, National Insitutes of Health. Fact sheet on "What's in a bottle? An introduction to dietary supplements." March 2006. Retrieved May 19, 2006 from http:// www.nccam.nih.gov/health/bottle.

Nesheim MC: What is the research base for the use of dietary supplements? *Public Health Nutri* 1999; 2:35–38.

Office of Dietary Supplements, National Institutes of Health. http://dietary-supplements.info.nih.gov.

Prevention Magazine assesses dietary supplement use. *NCRHI Newsletter* 2000; 23(3):1.

Roberts HJ: Lead in calcium supplements. *JAMA* 2000; 284:3126–27.

Ross EA: Vitamin A and retinoids. In Shils M, Olsen JA, Shike M, Ross AC (eds.): *Modern Nutrition in Health and Disease*, 9th ed. Baltimore: Williams & Wilkins, 1999.

Ross EA, Szabo NJ, Tebbet IR: Lead content of calcium supplements. *JAMA* 2000; 284:1425–29.

Schurch MA, Rizzoli R, Slosman D, Vadas L, Vergnaud P, Bonjour JP: Protein supplements increase serum insulin-like growth factor-I levels and attenuate proximal femur bone loss in patients with recent hip fracture. A randomized, double-blind, placebo-controlled trial. Ann *Intern Med* 1998; 128(10):801–9.

Shekelle PG, Hardy ML, Morton SC, Maglione M, Mojica WA, Suttorp MJ, et al.: Efficacy and safety of ephedra and ephedrine alkaloids for weight loss and athletic performance: A meta-analysis. *JAMA* 2003; 289(12):1537–45.

Stearns DM, Wise JP, Patierno SR, Wetterhahn KE: Chromium (III) picolinate produces chromosome damage in Chinese hamster ovary cells. *FASEB J.* 1995; 9(15):1643–48.

Stone F: *Know Your Plants . . . Safe or Poisonous?* San Francisco: California Poison Control System, 1997.

The Pharmacist's Letter: Standardized herbal products. November 1998. Retrieved from www.pharmacistsletter .com May 19, 2006.

The Pharmacist's Letter: The United States Pharmacopeia (USP) is now setting standards for herbal products. March 1999. Retrieved from www.pharmacistsletter.com March 1999.

Thomas P: Dietary supplements for weight loss? *Nutr Today* 2005; 40(1):6–12.

Turner RB, Bauer R, Woelkart K, Hulsey TC, Gangemi JD: An evaluation of *Echinacea angustifolia* in experimental rhinovisus infections. *New Eng J Med* 2005; 353(4):341–48.

Chapter **11**

Nutritional and Oral Implications of Common Chronic Health Conditions: Hypertension, Osteoporosis, and Immune-Compromising Conditions

Linda Boyd and Carole A. Palmer

OUTLINE

OBJECTIVES

The student will be able to:

- List at least two clinical signs or symptoms for each chronic condition.
- List the major risk factors for each chronic condition.
- Describe known associations between each chronic condition and oral health status.
- Outline the general dietary principles for prevention and management of each condition.
- Describe the roles of nutrition in immunity.
- Discuss the major nutritional factors involved in cancer etiology and progression, particularly oral cancer.
- Discuss the oral and nutritional implications of cancer and immune-compromising disorders.
- Describe oral manifestations encountered and palliative treatment recommendations for cancers and other immune-compromising conditions.
- Suggest basic dietary recommendations for those with oral manifestations that jeopardize adequate nutrient intake.
- Discuss the nutritional implications of oral lesions.

INTRODUCTION

The documented associations between oral health and systemic disease in humans demonstrates the need for dental professionals to become more knowledgeable about the prevention, pathogenesis, and standards of care for treatment of systemic, as well as oral diseases (Glick, 1998).

This chapter provides an overview of the most common chronic conditions and their implications for nutrition. Many patients with chronic diseases should be referred to a registered dietitian for nutrition counseling, as their needs are beyond the scope of practice for a dental office. However, the dental staff can and should provide support to the patient for behavioral and dietary changes that will help in the prevention of chronic disease.

HYPERTENSION

Hypertension is defined as "systolic blood pressure of 140 mm Hg or greater, and/or a diastolic blood pressure of 90 mm Hg or greater, and/or the use of antihypertensive medications" (He, Welton, 1997) (Table 11–1). At least 50 million (28%) adults in the general population of the United States have hypertension or elevated blood pressure and 30% of those people have not been diagnosed (AHA, 2005). Of those people being treated for hypertension, 34% are well controlled (AHA, 2005). Hypertension is a contributing and modifiable risk factor in coronary heart disease, stroke, congestive heart failure, and end-stage renal disease (He, Welton, 1997).

Nonmodifiable risk factors include heredity, age, gender (men have a higher overall prevalence and incidence of hypertension than women) (AHA, 2005),

diabetes, and ethnicity. The incidence of hypertension is 36.8 to 39.4% in African American men and women, respectively, and 23% in Caucasians and Mexican Americans (AHA, 2005). Modifiable risk factors for hypertension include physical inactivity, obesity, alcohol consumption, smoking, and sodium intake (Appel et al., 1997).

Hypertension is due to an increase in peripheral resistance in the blood vessels resulting from either vasoconstriction or narrowing of the peripheral blood vessels (Thomas, 1993). This increase in pressure tends to increase left ventricular wall stress, which may affect the efficiency of heart function as well as exacerbating ischemia. Ischemia occurs during diastole when the increased pressure prevents the heart from filling with blood, reducing the supply of oxygen and nutrients to the heart muscle. It is difficult to determine a specific etiology for hypertension. Approximately 95% of cases of hypertension have an unknown cause and are referred to as *essential* or *primary* hypertension (Thomas, 1993). The remaining 5% of those with high blood pressure have *secondary* hypertension, arising from an identifiable disorder. The most common cause of secondary hypertension is a narrowing of the artery to one or both kidneys.

Diagnosis

Updated guidelines from *The Seventh Report of the Joint National Committee on Prevention, Detection, Evaluation and Treatment of High Blood Pressure* are much stricter than previous versions. Normal blood pressure is now considered to be below 120/80 and data suggest that 115/75 should be the new gold standard. The new category of prehypertension is diagnosed

TABLE 11–1 Blood Pressure Classification for Adults Aged 18 Years or Older

Category	Systolic Blood Pressure (mm Hg)		Diastolic Blood Pressure (mm Hg)
Normal	≤120	and	<80
Prehypertension	120–139	or	80–89
Stage 1 hypertension	140–159	or	90–99
Stage 2 hypertension	>160	or	>100

Source: National Cholesterol Education Program: *Third Report of the Expert Panel on Detection, Evaluation, and Treatment of High Blood Cholesterol in Adults.* Bethesda, MD: National Institutes of Health, National Heart, Lung, and Blood Institute, 2002.

when the systolic pressure is between 120 and 139 and a diastolic pressure between 80 and 89 (USDHHS, 2004). Diagnosis of hypertension requires a systolic blood pressure of 140 millimeters of mercury (mm Hg) or greater, and/or a diastolic blood pressure of 90 mm Hg or greater on two or more occasions. The current recommendation is to measure blood pressure yearly after the age of 3 years (Sinaiko, 1996).

Management

Management of hypertension usually requires a multifaceted approach including lifestyle changes, diet changes, and perhaps drug therapy. The dental team contributes to the diagnosis of hypertension in dental patients through the common practice of taking blood pressure readings as part of the initial examination and at each appointment when local anesthesia may be required. This blood pressure screening provides a valuable screening service for patients, particularly those who may be unaware of their high blood pressure or who are poorly controlled (Glick, 1998). For those hypertensive patients with diabetes, the lower the blood pressure, the greater the reduction of risk for stroke and heart attack.

Lifestyle modifications should include the following:

- Regular physical activity: Regular aerobic activity can reduce both systolic and diastolic blood pressure independent of body weight. The recommendation is for 30 minutes per day on most days of the week (Arroll, Beaglehole, 1992; USDDHS, 2004).
- Weight control: Overweight individuals have a 50–300% higher incidence of hypertension. Even modest weight loss of 8 to 10 pounds produced a 34% reduction in the incidence of hypertension (Stevens et al., 1993).
- Healthy eating: Dietary Approaches to Stop Hypertension (DASH) is often recommended and is high in fruits, vegetables, whole grains, and low-fat dairy products. These foods tend to be high in potassium, magnesium, and calcium while being low in saturated fat, total fat, and sodium. The average reduction in blood pressure with this eating plan is 5–11 mm Hg (Sacks et al., 2001; USDHHS, 2004).

- Alcohol reduction: Modification of alcohol use is an important means of preventing and/or reducing hypertension. A reasonable limit should be no more than two alcohol-containing drinks per day and preferably less than 1 oz of ethanol per day for men and 0.5 oz for women (Marmot et al., 1994; Moore, McKnight 1995)
- Sodium restriction: Some individuals appear to be salt sensitive and may benefit from sodium restriction, but for others with hypertension, sodium restriction produces little benefit (Law, Frost, Wald, 1991). Those whose hypertension responds to salt restriction should limit sodium intake to 2000 to 2400 mg/day. Table 11–2 shows dietary sources of sodium.
- Stress management.
- Tobacco cessation.

Oral Implications

People with a poor dentition and the edentulous (those lacking teeth) tend to have diets high in fat, sodium, and simple carbohydrates and low in fruits and vegetables (Carlos, Wolfe, 1989). Many patients with hypertention are also prescribed calcium channel blockers that can cause gingival hyperplasia. This gingival overgrowth makes it more difficult to maintain periodontal health, and may affect food choices and eating desire and ability.

TABLE 11–2 Avoiding Excess Sodium in Foods

- Use mostly fresh foods.
- Avoid added salt (sodium chloride).
- Avoid canned vegetables and meat or rinse thoroughly.
- Avoid canned soups, broths, and brine.
- Avoid preserved foods, as sodium is often used as a preservative.
- Watch for ingredients and additives that contain sodium such as:
Baking powder
Baking soda (sodium bicarbonaate)
Monosodium glutamate (MSG)
Sodium sulfite
Sodium citrate
Sodium acetate
Sodium algenate
Sodium proprionate
Sodium benzoate

OSTEOPOROSIS

Osteoporosis is a crippling and debilitating chronic bone disease, which is potentially preventable. Osteoporosis is sometimes called a "silent" disease because the first symptom is usually a bone fracture. Osteoporosis results in approximately 1.5 million fractures annually in the United States. With the rising age of the population, the incidence of hip fracture is expected to increase in coming years (IOM, 1997). An estimated 10 million Americans over 50 have osteoporosis and another 34 million are at risk for developing osteoporosis. The prevalence of osteoporosis is lower in men, but still affects 13% of Caucasian men in the United States. (USDHHS, 2004).

In osteoporosis, there is a quantitative decrease in the total amount of bone in the body, but the bone's composition is normal. With age, both cortical and trabecular bone are lost, but the trabecular bone is lost at a faster rate. The loss of bone is associated to some extent with normal aging. People often become "bent over" and complain that they have "gotten shorter." The bone loss becomes the condition "osteoporosis" when there is a reduction in bone mass and increased bone fragility to the point where the skeleton is unable to withstand ordinary stresses, and it fractures (USDHHS, 2004).

Throughout life, bone is undergoing active remodeling. Remodeling is defined as bone breakdown by osteoclasts followed by rebuilding by osteoblasts. During normal growth, total osteoblastic activity exceeds osteoclast activity. However, when osteoclastic activity (bone breakdown) exceeds osteoblastic activity (bone synthesis), osteoporosis can result. Bone strength is determined by the trabecular microstructure. In osteoporosis the porosity of the trabecular bone increases and the cortical bone thins (Figure 11–1). Extensive resorption, as seen in osteoporosis, results in microfracture of the trabecula, which further weakens the bone, making it more susceptible to fracture.

Ninety percent of peak bone mass is attained by age 16.9 + 1.3 years, and 99% of peak bone mass is reached by age 26.2 years + 3.7 years. Inadequate calcium intake prior to attainment of peak bone mass may account for as much as 50% of the hip fractures in women in the postmenopausal years. Even more importantly, a low bone mineral density (BMD) may also predict fractures in children (Weaver, Peacock, Johnston, 1999).

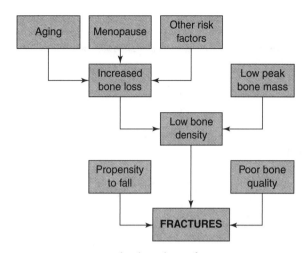

FIGURE 11-1 Pathophysiology of osteoporosis.

Risk Factors

Risk factors for developing osteoporosis include race, female gender, advancing age, slight body build, low estrogen status, family history, suboptimal peak skeletal mass, history of poor calcium/vitamin D intake, physical inactivity, certain medical conditions and medications, excessive intake of caffeine and alcohol, and tobacco use (USDHHS, 2004) (Table 11–3). Petite women of Asian or northern European descent are at greatest risk for osteoporosis.

Peak bone mass is determined by genetics, physical activity, and adequacy of calcium and vitamin D intake in adolescence and young adulthood (Barr, McKay, 1998). Genetics exerts 60–75% of the control of peak bone mass density, but peak bone mass attained between 19 and 30 years of age is greatly influenced by physical activity and nutrition (Anderson, Rondano, 1996). Unfortunately, the average calcium intake in females 9 to 13 years is only 889 mg/day (69% of the RDA) and in females 14–18 years is only 713 mg/day (55% of the RDA), whereas the Dietary Reference Intake (DRI) is 1300 mg/day (IOM, 1997). Thus, many young women are in negative calcium balance for the majority of their lives. Of even more concern is the people who are lactose intolerant because the intake for those with self-diagnosed lactose intolerance is approximately 320 mg/day (25% of the RDA) (Carroccio et al., 1998).

Low levels of estrogen result in a reduction in the efficiency of calcium absorption in the intestine as well

TABLE 11–3 Factors Associated with Osteoporosis Risk

Factors Increasing Risk
- Family history of osteoporosis
- Race: Asian or northern European descent
- Gender: women more than men
- Advancing age
- Body build: small boned greater risk
- Estrogen status: postmenopausal without hormone replacement
- Suboptimal peak skeletal mass
- History of poor calcium/vitamin D intake
- Physical inactivity
- Some medical conditions (e.g., hyperthyroidism, hyperparathyroidism)
- Some medications
- Excessive caffeine, alcohol, protein intake
- Tobacco use

Factors Decreasing Risk
- Estrogen replacement therapy
- Family history of large bone mass
- Black race
- Physical activity/weight-bearing exercise
- Adequate dietary calcium and vitamin D status
- Overall adequate diet
- Attaining peak bone mass at early age
- Nonsmoking

as an increased rate of bone turnover (IOM, 1997). Bone loss accelerates in the early years of menopause, but can be slowed with the initiation of hormone replacement therapy. The use of estrogen protects against osteoporosis and maintains bone mineral density (Moore, Bracker, Sartoris, Saltman, Strause, 1990). Unfortunately, recent studies have also found that hormone replacement therapy may increase the risk for cardiovascular disease and for invasive breast cancers, so estrogen plus progestin is generally not the best choice for prevention of bone loss (Rossouw et al., 2002).

Caffeine may cause accelerated bone loss, but this appears to be a problem only in postmenopausal women consuming less than 800 mg of calcium per day (Harris, Dawson-Hughes, 1994).

Tobacco use puts patients at greater risk for osteoporosis (Krall, Dawson-Hughes, 1999). It is unclear if

this is due to toxic effects of the smoke, or because of decreased absorption of calcium.

Diagnosis

Bone mineral density (BMD) is the most easily measured and most accurate predictor of fracture risk (Center, Eisman, 1997). BMD can be measured by dual-energy x-ray absorptiometry (DXA). DXA can measure changes in total body BMD as well as at specific high-risk sites, such as the spine, hip, and forearm (IDM, 1997). A BMD test is recommended for people over 65 years, postmenopausal women with one or more risk factors, postmenopausal women who have had a fracture, and perhaps younger people with significant risk factors to assess baseline bone levels (National Osteoporosis Foundation, 2003).

Prevention and Management

Prevention of osteoporosis is a lifelong process that includes attaining optimal peak bone mass, maintaining bone mass through middle adulthood, and minimizing postmenopausal bone loss (see Table 11–4). People of all ages need to have adequate intakes of calcium and vitamin D; consume moderate amounts of sodium and protein; do regular weight-bearing exercise such as walking, jogging, cycling, and weightlifting; and avoid tobacco use.

Most adults require three to four servings of dairy foods daily to meet calcium and vitamin D requirements. Vegetable sources like legumes and green leafy vegetables provide only limited amounts of calcium, because the calcium is bound and unavailable for absorption. For those who cannot tolerate milk products, calcium-processed soy products (tofu) and calcium-

TABLE 11–4 Recommendations for Osteoporosis Prevention

- Be active and do weight-bearing exercise regularly.
- Don't smoke.
- Keep alchohol intake moderate.
- Start young getting sufficient calcium and vitamin D daily (this means 3–4 servings of vitamin D fortified dairy products or its equivalent per day).

fortified orange juice are good options, as are lactose-reduced dairy products. For older persons who may have ahydrochloria (reduced stomach acid), the acidity of the orange juice may aid in calcium absorption (see Chapter 8). If food sources are not sufficient to meet requirements, supplements may be indicated. Calcium citrate malate has the highest absorption rate followed by calcium carbonate (IOM, 1997). Calcium supplements should be approached with caution because analysis of 21 formulations, including natural sources of calcium such as oyster shell and synthetic calcium such as that found in antacids, found measurable lead content in 38% of supplements (Ross, Szabo, Tebbett, 2000). This is allowed to occur because there is little regulation or oversight of the manufacture of supplements under the current Dietary Supplement Health Education Act (DSHEA). If supplements are the preferred source of calcium, absorption can be enhanced by taking the calcium in doses divided throughout the day and should not exceed 500 mg/dose. (IOM, 1997). Calcium supplements containing Vitamin D may also improve calcium absorption. Caution should be used with supplements containing additional magnesium should be used with caution. The upper limit of intake (above which toxicity may occur) is 320 mg/day, a level easily exceeded with supplements. High levels of magnesium may also cause diarrhea (IOM, 1997).

Oral Implications

The age-related bone loss that occurs throughout the skeleton may also increase the risk of tooth loss and edentulism (Krall, Dawson-Hughes, Papas, Garcia, 1994). Also, men and women with few remaining teeth tend to have low BMD at skeletal sites such as the forearm, spine, hip, and whole body (Krall, Dawson-Hughes, 1999; Wactawski-Wende et al., 1996). Research suggests that the number of teeth with progression in alveolar bone loss over a 7-year study period was significantly lower among men whose calcium intake was at least 1000 mg/day (Krall, 2001). Animal studies that promoted osteoporosis found that bone loss in the maxilla was twice as pronounced as that found in the tibia, a finding that may have implications for alveolar bone loss in humans (Teofilo, Azevedo, Petenusei, Mazaro, Lamano-Carvalho, 2003). Dental radiographs may be able to detect altered trabecular patterns or changes in width of the mandible that suggest a patient may need further evaluation of his or her bone status (Horner, Devlin, 1998; Jeffcoat, 2005; Mohammad, Alder McNally, 1996; White, Rudolph, 1999).

Frequent consumption of chewable calcium supplements can increase caries risk, especially in people with xerostomia (dry mouth), because they contain sugars. Wherever possible, patients should be encouraged to incorporate food sources of calcium into their diets rather than relying on calcium supplements.

Summary Principles for Osteoporosis Prevention

Dental professionals can be instrumental in encouraging patients to attain and maintain an adequate bone density. If the patient has expressed a problem, such as self-diagnosed lactose intolerance, the dental practitioner should encourage the patient to see his or her physician for a definitive diagnosis. The patient should also be informed about sources of calcium and the importance of a lifelong adequate intake. The following principles should be stressed:

- Consume three to four daily servings of foods rich in calcium and vitamin D, especially in adolescence and young adulthood.
- Moderate intake of protein, sodium (processed foods), and phosphorus (soda).
- Minimize the use of non-calcium-based antacids that may reduce absorption of calcium.
- If unable to obtain adequate calcium from food sources, see your physician about supplementation. Usual recommendations are:
  - Calcium supplementation to achieve 1000 to 1300 mg/day (calcium citrate malate or calcium carbonate are good choices).
  - Vitamin D supplements of 200 to 600 IU/day for those who avoid milk, live in northern latitudes, or get little or no sun exposure.
- Stop smoking.
- Do regular daily weight-bearing exercises such as walking, jogging, cycling, or weightlifting.
- For postmenopausal women who have not had a baseline DXA to assess bone health, see your physician.

IMMUNE SYSTEM DISORDERS

How the Immune System Functions

A healthy immune system is the body's indispensable defense system. Immune function is central to normal tissue repair, healing, and body response to pathogens such as the bacterial challenge in periodontal disease. Converesly, the immunocompromised patient has impaired ability to fight infection. The mechanisms responsible for decreased resistance include production of humoral antibodies and mucosal secretory antibodies, cell-mediated immunity, phagocytic capacity, complement formation, numbers of T lymphocytes and T cells (helper, suppressor-cytotoxic, and natural killer cells), and nonspecific defense mechanisms. Nonspecific defense mechanisms include the skin, mucosa, and epithelium; intestinal flora; secretions such as lysozymes, mucus, and gastric acid; and the febrile response (Scrimshaw, Sangiovanni, 1997). Figure 11–2 shows the importance of the immune system.

The immune system can become compromised in a number of ways. Primary immune-compromising conditions are rare. The majority of problems are caused by secondary immunodeficiencies in which underlying

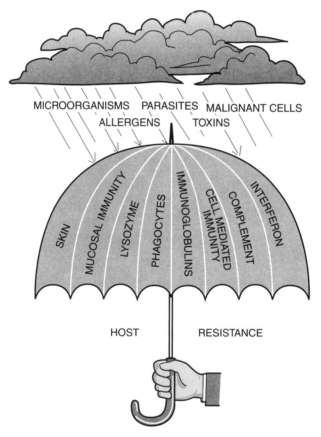

FIGURE 11–2   Host resistance. A simple view of host defenses as a protective umbrella, consisting of physical barriers (skin and mucous membranes), nonspecific mechanisms (complement, interferon, lysozyme, and phagocytes), and antigen-specific processes (antibodies of five immunoglobulin isotypes and cell-mediated immunity).

Source: From Chandra RK (ed): *Nutrition and Immunology.* St. John's Canada: ARTS Biomedical, 1992; reprinted as Chandra RK: Nutrition and the immune system. *Am J Clin Nutr* 1997; 66:460S–63S.

illness or its treatment cause depressed immunity in previously healthy people. Immune depression commonly occurs in malnutrition, acquired immunodeficiency syndrome (AIDS), cancer, organ transplant, autoimmune diseases, and from the drugs used to treat these conditions (e.g., corticosteroids, azathioprine, methotrexate, and cyclosporine) (Moons et al., 1998; Thomas, 1993). Immune depression can also occur in patients hospitalized with acute disease and those with chronic inflammatory disorders. The immune system also declines in function with the aging process (Hakim, 2004). This immune depression poses a greater risk for morbidity due to oral infections (USDHHS, 2000).

Patients with compromised immune systems are seen with increasing frequency in private dental practice owing to the many advances in treatment that allow people to live much longer. Because oral tissues have a rapid turnover, the oral cavity is one of the first places where manifestations of systemic disease or changes in metabolism are observed. Diseases and medications affecting the immune system often result in oral manifestations, including xerostomia, mucositis, esophagitis, stomatitis, and candidiasis.

Deterioration of oral health is highly correlated with deterioration of general health, and this may in part be due to the role of the mouth as a "portal of entry for infection" (Hollister, Weintraub, 1993; USDHHS, 2000, p. 133). The interrelationship of general health, dental health, and adequate nutritional intake is especially important in the immunocompromised patient. A healthy oral cavity is essential to keep the patient well nourished and maintain an acceptable quality of life. This chapter describes the nutritional implications in immunity and reviews the oral and nutritional implications of cancers and other immune-compromising conditions.

Nutrition Interrelationships with Immunity

Nutrition plays an important role in maintaining optimal functioning of the immune system (Figure 11–3). Individuals who are undernourished have impaired immune responses including abnormalities in cell-mediated immunity, phagocytosis, and antibody function. In the United States, the Nutrition Screening Initiative estimates that 40 to 60% of hospitalized adults are malnourished or at risk for malnutrition, and that 40 to 85% of nursing home residents are malnourished

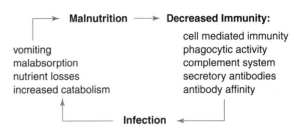

FIGURE 11–3 Relationship of nutrition to infection and immunity.

(National Screening Initiative [NSI], 2002). Furthermore, worldwide, approximately 30% of elders in industrialized countries suffer from some level of malnutrition. Nutrients that affect immune function include vitamins A, C, D, E, B-complex, beta-carotene, iron, copper, zinc, and protein, as well as total calories (Chandra, 2004). Deficiencies of nutrients that protect skin, such as vitamin A and zinc, can facilitate the invasion of harmful microorganisms. Vitamin A, protein, and many other nutrients are also needed for the health of the intestine, as well as for the formation of antibodies that protect the intestines. The phagocytes (neutrophils and macrophages that engulf and kill invading organisms) live for only a few days and must be constantly replenished. Their optimal development and function require vitamins C, E, A, B_6, B_{12}, and folic acid, protein, zinc, copper, and iron. Deficiencies of any of these nutrients can result in decreased cell-mediated immunity (Chandra, 2004).

Conversely, nutrient toxicities can impede immune function. There is also some evidence that obesity may affect the incidence and severity of certain infections and illnesses through an effect on immune function (Marti, Marcos, Martinez, 2001).

Infections, even mild ones, can in turn adversely affect nutritional status. Factors that determine the effect of infection on nutritional status may include:

- nutrient adequacy before infection
- the severity and duration of the infection or disease
- dietary intake during recovery (Chandra, 1997)

The general principles regarding the role of nutrition in immune function are as follows (Chandra, 2004):

- Changes in immune response happen early in the process of nutrient deficiency.

- The degree of immunological impairment is determined by the type of nutrient involved, its interaction with other nutrients, the severity of the deficiency, the presence of infection, and the age of the person.
- The immunological abnormalities predict the outcome, such as the risk of infection and mortality.
- Excessive intake of many micronutrients (vitamins and minerals) results in impaired immune response.

Cancer

Cancer is defined as uncontrolled growth of cells derived from normal tissues (Thomas, 1995). This uncontrolled, unorganized, unregulated cell proliferation is able to kill the host by the spread of cells from the site of origin to distant sites or by local spread. There are an estimated 200 different kinds of cancer. In 2001, it was estimated that 9.8 million Americans had a history of invasive cancer (National Cancer Institute [NCI], 2004). It was estimated that in 2004, over 1.3 million Americans received a new diagnosis of invasive cancer and that number is expected to double in the next 50 years (NCI, 2005). The incidence and death rate from cancer is higher in blacks than in whites, Hispanics, or Asian/Pacific Islanders (NCI, 2005).

The most common cancer overall is skin cancer. In American men, the most common invasive cancers are prostate, lung, and colorectal, respectively (NCI, 2004). In women, breast, lung, and colorectal cancer, respectively, are the most common in the United States. (NCI, 2004).Worldwide, there is a fivefold difference in male cancer incidence rates and a fourfold difference in female rates (Ferlay, Bray, Pisani, Parkin, 2004). Japan is often considered as a low-risk country for breast, colon, and prostate cancer when compared with the United States. However, studies of Japanese migrants to the United States have shown that within two generations, the Japanese immigrants have the same mortality rate for these cancers as the general U.S. population. Japan has also been observing an increase in breast, colon, and prostate cancer rates. Breast cancer incidence more than doubled from 1960 to the late 1980s (Deapen, Liu, Perkins, Bernstein, Ross, 2002). This has been attributed to a change in diet to the more Western style, which is high in fat and total calories, low in fruits and vegetables, with little consumption of soy products (Deapen et al., 2002).

Oral Cancer

Although oral cancers account for only about 3–4% of all cancers in the United States, they generally have a poor long-term prognosis in comparison to other cancers. Ninety-five percent of oral cancers are diagnosed in individuals over 40, and the average age of diagnosis is 60 years. Males are twice as likely to have oral cancer than females, and the incidence in black males is 1.6 times higher than than the rate of white males, but the death rate for black males is 2.5 times higher. The 5-year survival rate for oral cancer is 35% for blacks and 55% for whites (CDC, 1998, 2001).

High-risk sites for cancer include the oropharynx, which includes the soft palate, anterior tonsillar pillar, and retromolar trigone; tongue; floor of the mouth; mandibular gingiva; and lower lip. Complications associated with oral cancer and its treatment include chronic pain, impaired swallowing and chewing resulting in weight loss, caries, osteonecrosis, trismus, speech difficulties, mucositis, xerostomia, and physical disfigurement.

Cancer Etiology (Carcinogenesis) and Risk Factors

Cancer development is a stepwise process. When the body is exposed to carcinogenic agents, a variety of potential effects can result, which may (or may not) lead to cancer. The changes that do occur happen over a long period and are modulated by many factors, including diet. Table 11–5 shows the general process of carcinogenesis. Although much is known about the causes and development of cancer, many of the steps involved are still not well understood. Risk factors include:

- **Genetics:** This includes both genetics and complex gene–environment interactions. However, genetic factors alone are not an accurate predictor of cancer incidence (Greenwald, 1996).
- **Environmental factors:** These include air and ground pollution, exposure to chemicals, and excess radiation. Environmental factors and exposure to sunlight may be responsible for 75% of cancers (CDC, 1998). Basal cell and squamous cell cancers of the skin are the most prevalent, making sunlight the most significant environmental carcinogen.
- **Alcohol and tobacco:** Smoking is the leading cause of preventable cancer death in the United States accounting for approximately one-third of

TABLE 11–5 The Process of Carcinogenesis

- **Initiation:** Carcinogen binds to DNA. This is rapid and irreversible.
- **Promotion:** Period between initiation and premalignancy. (Generally, gene activity rather than structure is regulated.) This is generally reversible, and may be very prolonged.
- **Progression:** Period between premalignant and malignant disease. (Generally involves genetic alteration.) This is generally irreversible and may be very prolonged.

all cancer deaths. Alcohol and tobacco use is associated with 75% of the incidence of squamous cell carcinomas of the mouth, oral pharynx, larynx, and esophagus (CDC, 1998).

- **Dietary and nutritional factors:** Dietary and nutritional factors are estimated to account for between 20 and 30% of cancer incidence (Key et al., 2004), and may participate in any or all of the steps involved in carcinogenesis. Dietary factors include carcinogens in food; food preparation methods; obesity; high-fat, low-fiber, low-fruit and vegetable intake; high red and processed meat intake (Chao et al., 2005); and excessive alcohol intake. Relationships between specific dietary factors and cancers are difficult to delineate because factors often occur together. For example, consumers of high-fat diets are often overweight or obese, have low-fiber intake, and consume few fruits and vegetables. Table 11–6 shows the food sources of carcinogens. Contaminants in food, such as the insecticide DDT, that may enter food before processing, and

trichloroethylene or methylene chloride, introduced during processing, are carcinogens as well.

Among all of these factors, exposure to sunlight, tobacco use, physical inactivity, and poor dietary choices are most likely to impact personal cancer risk.

Protective Effects of Nutrition in Cancer Prevention

Several nutrients and foods have also been associated with helping prevent cancers (Table 11–6). The major protective factors are fruits and vegetables, antioxidants, and plant components (isoflavenoids and lignins). Fruits and vegetables are the best sources of the antioxidant vitamins E and C, carotenoids, retinoids, flavones, and selenium. Cruciferous vegetables (e.g., cabbage, Brussels sprouts) also increase detoxifying liver enzymes (Block, Patterson, Subar, 1992; Riboli, 2003). Soy products (especially tofu) are the best sources of isoflavonoids that may help account for the low breast and prostate cancer rates of the Asian populations in addition to their low-fat, high-fiber intake (Badger, Ronis, Simmen, Simmen 2005).

Deficiencies of vitamins A, E, C, B_{12}, folate, and beta-carotene may interact with tobacco use and potentially increase the risk of oral precancerous lesions (Ramaswamy, Rao, Kumaraswamy, Anantha, 1996). Conversely, high dietary folate intake may help reduce risk of oral and pharyngeal cancer.

Recent research has shown that green tea can destroy oral and other cancer cells (Schwartz, Baker, Larios, Chung, 2005). The polyphenols in green tea eliminate free radicals that can combine with DNA to cause cells to mutate. This effect is not seen in black tea,

TABLE 11–6 Links between Cancers and Dietary Factors

Dietary Factors That INCREASE Cancer Risk	*Dietary Factors That DECREASE Cancer Risk*
• Low intake of antioxidants • High fat intake • High nitrate and salt intake • Increased alcohol consumption (oral cancer) • High red meat and processed meats consumption	• Low-fat/high-fiber intake • High intakes of fruits and vegetables • Antioxidants like vitamins E, C, retenoids, flavones, and seleniun • Plant components like isoflavenoids and lignins • Cruciferous vegetables like cabbage, Brussels sprouts

the type most commonly consumed in the United States and Canada (Hsu, 2001; Khafif, Schantz, al-Rawi, Edelstein, Sacks, 1998).

Nutritional Implications of Cancer and Its Treatment

Both cancer and its treatment have side effects that compromise nutritional and oral status, contribute to malnutrition, undermine recovery, and diminish the quality of life (American Cancer Society, 1999). Significant malnutrition accounts for approximately 30% of deaths in cancer patients overall (Palesty, Dudrick, 2003). Overt malnutrition leads to 30–50% of deaths in patients with gastrointestinal cancers and up to 80% of deaths in those with advanced pancreatic cancer (Palesty, Dudrick, 2003). Both the disease process and treatment often lead to the protein-calorie malnutrition that is a major cause of morbidity and mortality (NCI, 1999).

The outcomes of treatment are significantly affected by the patient's nutritional status before diagnosis, stage and site of the cancer, and the aggressiveness of therapy required to treat the cancer.

Nutritional Effects of Cancer Itself

The cancer itself (independent of its treatment) may initiate a syndrome of weight loss and wasting (cachexia), which leads to abnormal tissue and electrolyte losses. This cancer cachexia syndrome involves disturbances in protein, fat, carbohydrate, and mineral metabolism; early satiety; anorexia; anemia; weight loss; and wasting. Loss of 40 of body cell mass results in death. In addition, when patients have lost lean body mass, their calorie and protein needs increase. Calorie and protein requirements in persons with cancer (and AIDS) may be 40 to 100% higher than normal. Even a normally adequate diet may be insufficient to counteract the effects of cachexia, and just maintaining weight often presents a major challenge (Palesty, Dudrick, 2003). Currently the goals in treating patients with cancer cachexia are to minimize adverse effects or complications from the malignancy and/or therapy, and increase appetite and food intake to enhance the patient's quality of life and improve chances for survival (Palesty, Dudrick, 2003).

Nutritional Effects of Cancer Treatments

Side effects of treatment vary with the location of the cancer being treated and the type, length, and dose of treatment (NIH, 1994). Side effects that affect the oral cavity and gastrointestinal tract have the greatest impact on nutritional status and are of primary concern to improve treatment outcomes (Daly, Shinkwin, 1995). Patients may experience anorexia (loss of appetite); foods may taste odd, salty, bitter or "tinny" (metallic); and sense of smell may decrease. Early satiety may make it difficult to eat sufficient calories. Nausea can reduce the desire to eat. Changes in the oral cavity can make it difficult to masticate and swallow. The physical disfigurement, speech problems, eating difficulties, and psychological and emotional problems associated with some cancers and their treatment can contribute to social withdrawal and further declines in nutritional status (Rosenthal et al., 1990). Malnutrition, in turn, undermines response to treatment, increases disease severity, and decreases immune status. Decreased immunity increases the risk of infection. Nutritional status also appears to influence cancer prognosis in that the greater the preoperative weight loss, the higher the mortality (Williams, Meguid, 1989).

Surgical resection of head and neck neoplasms can severely impair oral intake for considerable periods. If salivary gland function is affected, the resulting xerostomia can make it extremely difficult to chew, move food around in the mouth, and swallow. People who lack saliva often complain that food tastes like "cotton" to them. When part of the tongue is lost, it becomes difficult to move food around in the mouth and to the back of the mouth to be swallowed. If there is jaw or palate excision or resection, food can become trapped in resected areas, making it hard to swallow and potentially contributing to infection. When the surgery includes the palatal area or nasal cavity, food may become inhaled into the naval cavity during swallowing attempts.

Large lesions of the tongue that require extensive resection result in problems with speech, difficulty in swallowing, and potential problems aspirating liquids and food. More advanced lesions with bone involvement may involve extensive resection of the mandible or maxilla, which can make speech and eating difficult.

Postoperative complications, such as infection, fistulas, and wound dehiscence, can increase nutrient requirements while further contributing to decreased oral intake (Johns, 1988; Wood, Lander, Mosloy, Hiatt, 1989).

Surgery in other parts of the gastrointestinal tract can have major effects on digestion, absorption, and utilization of foods. For example, cancer in the gastrointestinal tract can interfere with nutrient absorption. Cancer of the esophagus can interfere with swallowing. Cancer in the liver or pancreas will interfere with digestion, utilization, and storage of nutrients. Because of the vast array of possible side effects, the nutrition team must determine specific problems early and institute appropriate nutritional interventions.

Radiation therapy can affect nutritional status systemically and locally (Wilson, Herman, Chubon, 1991). The location and dosage of radiation treatment determine the type and severity of complications (Levene, Harris, 1982). Radiation can result in generalized nausea, vomiting, and malabsorption. Radiation in the oral cavity affects oral tissues directly. The gingival tissues and palate become inflamed (stomatitis). Hemorrhages and ulcers or white patches may develop. Pain and lack of salivary lubrication make eating painful and difficult. As a result, eating, drinking and oral hygiene become difficult. Hot or cold foods, spicy foods, and hard foods may be intolerable. Toothbrushing is also painful and may be avoided (Marques, Dib, 2004). If the pharynx is in the field of radiation, the patient may experience severe pain when swallowing and become dysphagic (unable to swallow).

Decreased immunity caused by the radiation can lead to infection. Oral infections, if allowed to progress untreated, can result in necrosis of the jawbone (osteoradionecrosis), a serious and potentially fatal complication (Figure 11–4).

Chemotherapeutic agents adversely affect healthy tissue cells with a rapid turnover, especially the epithelium of the mouth and gastrointestinal intestinal tract. Common side effects are nausea, diarrhea, prolonged periods of anorexia, anemia, neutropenia, mucositis/stomatitis, changes in taste, abdominal pain, ulceration, vomiting, and weight loss (Charuhas, 1990; Shils, Olsen, Moshe, 1994).

Most of the conditions or medications that result in immunosuppression have similar side effects such as xerostomia, oral lesions (mucositis, stomatitis, and esophagitis), increased incidence of fungal infections, anorexia, nausea or vomiting, and diarrhea. All of these can have considerable impact on the ability and desire to eat.

Nutrition Management of the Side Effects of Cancer and Its Treatment Health professionals need to work together to attempt to minimize the impact of cancer and its side effects on nutritional status, oral health, overall health, and quality of life. Nutrition monitoring is especially critical in cancer patients. Nutrition support is essential throughout the cancer process to help maintain healthy weight, protect against unnecessary weight loss, promote resistance, prevent infection, provide palliation, and manage the side effects of cancer and its treatment. Nutrition goals are to maintain a high level of nutriture in the face of major barriers to ingestion. Nutritional support can range from general counseling on helpful food selection to aggressive therapies such as enteral (feeding tubes) and parenteral (intravenous) nutrition care.

The major nutritional issue in cancer patient management is maintaining weight. The most important question to ask cancer patients is "How has your weight been?" Unplanned weight loss of more than 10 pounds in the last 6 months is a major indicator of cachexia. Appropriate dietary recommendations often include small, frequent meals that are high in calories that may include high levels of sugar and fat. Although cariogenicity is an important consideration, it is not as important as maintaining weight. The dental team should know what the nutrition recommendations have been and not contradict them by advising people to reduce the frequency of eating, if frequent meals have been prescribed. Rather, they may need to compensate for the increased caries risk presented by frequent meals and snacks by showing patients how to clean the mouth thoroughly after each eating episode and by prescribing appropriate fluoride therapy. On the other hand, medical/nutritional care teams should be cautioned not to recommend hard candies to increase saliva (as was done in the past). This is just one reason why the dental professional must work closely with physicians

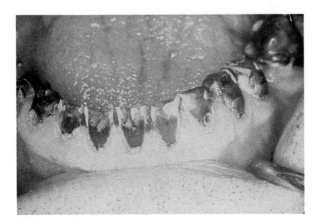

FIGURE 11–4 Radiation-induced dental caries.

and nutritionists to ensure that integrated comprehensive care is provided that will optimize both oral and general health. Table 11–6 provides general suggestions for managing cancer side effects. Table 11–7 provides specific food suggestions for managing these conditions.

Autoimmune Diseases and Their Nutritional Implications

The term *autoimmune diseases* refers to a group of chronic illnesses that affect a variety of organ systems. An ever increasing number of autoimmune diseases

TABLE 11–7   General Nutrition Tips for Side Effects of Cancer and Its Therapy

Problem	*Nutrition Suggestions*
Cachexia and weight loss	• Have small, frequent meals (e.g., every 1–2 hours). • Determine the patient's food preferences and offer only those. • Have calorie-dense and nutrient-dense foods and avoid empty calories. • Add powdered milk to any milk beverages to increase protein, calories, vitamins, and minerals. • Use low-lactose milk product if milk cannot be tolerated. • Use instant breakfast-type beverages made with milk. • If tolerated, use whole milk and cream whenever possible. • Add cheese and cream sauces to vegetables, casseroles, and so on. • Have milkshakes or ice cream sodas instead of soda. • Add whipped cream or ice cream to desserts like pies, cakes, or fruit. • Add butter, margarine, or gravy to potatoes, meats, noodles, vegetables. • Add cream to soups, cereal, custard, or puddings. • Use cream cheese on bagels, muffins, or crackers. • Add sour cream to soups, baked potatoes, salad dressing. • Take medications with high-calorie fluids. • Determine the patient's food preferences and offer only those.
Anorexia	• Eat solid foods before liquids at meals. Liquids may cause early satiety. • If eating solid food is unappealing to the patient, use liquid supplements. • Prepare and store small portions of favorite foods so they are ready to eat when the patient is hungry. • Time meals so that they coincide with the times during the day when the patient is feeling the best. Generally, patients have a better appetite early in the day. • Stimulate the appetite with light exercise. • Make surroundings attractive, try new recipes, eat with friends, and so on. • Choose foods with fewer odors. Strong odors can be avoided by cooking outside on a grill, using fans to blow food odors away from patient, serving cold food instead of hot, taking off food covers to release odors before entering the patient's eating area, or by ordering take-out food. • Choose and prepare foods that look and smell good to the patient. • Mealtime is not a time to discuss the patient's food intake or lack thereof. • Serve foods at room temperature. • Help the flavor of meat, chicken, or fish by marinating it in sweet fruit juices, sweet wine, Italian dressing, or sweet and sour sauce. • Try using small amounts of flavorful seasonings such as basil, oregano, or rosemary.

Nausea and vomiting	• Try these foods:
	    Crackers and toast, pretzels
	    Clear liquids (e.g., ginger ale)
	    Yogurt, sherbet, Italian ices

> Oatmeal, dry cereal
> Boiled or baked potatoes, plain rice
> Skinned chicken (baked or broiled, not fried)
> Soft and bland fruits, such as peaches

- Eat slowly and serve small portion sizes.
- Eat small, frequent meals and snacks.
- Eat solid foods before drinking liquids at meals.
- Sip liquids throughout the day, except at mealtime.
- Drink cool beverages.
- Eat foods cool or at room temperature.
- Rest sitting up for about an hour after meals.
- Rinse out the mouth before and after eating.
- Suck on *sugarless* hard candies if the mouth has a bad taste.
- Avoid eating in a room that has cooking odors or that is overly warm.
- Wear loose-fitting clothes.
- Avoid eating 1 to 2 hours before treatment or taking a medication that causes nausea.

Xerostomia

- Have frequent sips of water to lubricate and moisten the mouth to alleviate dryness and make swallowing and talking easier. For convenience, try carrying a water bottle or insulated cup with cool water.
- When you can't brush and floss after a meal, end the meal with a dairy product or rinse thoroughly with water.
- Include at least 2–4 servings of dairy products daily.
- Add cream sauces and gravies to foods to make them moist and easier to swallow.
- Take small bites and chew thoroughly.
- Use sugarless gum and sugar-free candies to stimulate saliva and help moisten the mouth.
- Eat frozen desserts (such as frozen grapes and ice pops) or ice chips.
- Avoid mouth rinses that contain alcohol.
- Discuss saliva substitutes or salivary stimulants if the xerostomia symptoms are severe.
- Continue with regular professional dental care along with daily home care and use of topical fluorides.

Oral lesions

- Eat soft foods that are easy to chew and swallow, such as:
  > Milkshakes
  > Instant breakfast-type drinks with whole milk
  > Bananas, applesauce, and other soft fruits
  > Peach, pear, and apricot nectars
  > Mashed potatoes, macaroni and cheese
  > Custards, puddings, and gelatin
  > Scrambled eggs
- Avoid foods that irritate the mouth, such as citrus fruit or juice, spicy or salty foods, and rough, coarse, or dry foods.
- Cook foods until they are soft and tender.
- Increase the fluid content of foods by adding gravy, broth, or sauces.
- Supplement meals with high-calorie, high-protein drinks.
- Numb the mouth with ice chips or flavored ice pops.
- Mix food with butter, thin gravies, and sauces to make them easier to swallow.
- Use a straw to drink liquids.
- Experiment with temperatures of foods; usually cold foods or those at room temperature are well tolerated.
- Rinse mouth often to help remove food debris.

Sources: From the NCI, 2005; NIH, 1994; Boyd, Dwyer, Papas, 1997.

has been identified. The underlying problem in all of these diseases is similar: the body's immune system can no longer distinguish "self" from "non-self," and attacks body cells and organ systems.

Sjögren's Syndrome

Sjögren's syndrome is the autoimmune disease with the greatest oral health implications. It occurs primarily in women (Atkinson, Wu, 1994) and is characterized by lymphocytic infiltration and destruction of the exocrine glands (primarily the lacrimal [tear] and salivary glands) (Linardaki, Moutsopoulos, 1997). (See Table 11–8.)

Due to the severe xerostomia of Sjögren's syndrome, the patient may have trouble chewing and swallowing food, which may compromise adequate nutrient intake. The prolonged swallowing time may also lead to choking or food aspiration, leading to aspiration pneumonia (Hensel et al., 1997).

Generally the side effects of the drugs used to treat autoimmune diseases cause side effects such as nausea, vomiting, anorexia, stomatitis, and esophagitis, all of which may compromise nutritional status. Long-term steroid use may cause fracture and collapse of the temporomandibular joint, resulting in severe malocclusion and impaired masticatory function, and further compromising oral hygiene and adequate nutritional intake.

Human Immunodeficiency Virus (HIV) and Acquired Immunodeficiency Syndrome (AIDS)

The HIV virus is a retrovirus that infects the host immune cells (CD4) and interferes with the normal functioning of the immune system. AIDS is characterized by an array of opportunistic infections that occur in the final stage of infection by the HIV. These include candidiasis, herpes simplex, herpes varicella zoster, cytomegalovirus, *Pneumocystis carinii*, cryptococcus, toxoplasmosis, salmonella, and Kaposi's sarcoma (Thomas, 1995). Oral lesions associated with HIV infection include Kaposi's sarcoma, oral candidiasis, hairy leukoplakia, xerostomia, and recurrent oral ulcers. These oral lesions may interfere with speech, swallowing, and chewing and can lead to extensive weight loss, as seen with the metabolic changes discussed earlier.

HIV treatments may have a variety of nutritional effects. Changes in taste and smell are common, as are inadequate oral intake, malnutrition, weight loss, and ultimately wasting (Heald et al., 1998). The use of protease inhibitors also leads to a syndrome of peripheral lipodystrophy in susceptible individuals (USDHHS, 2005). Other side effects may include diarrhea, nausea, vomiting, anorexia, headaches, strength loss, fatigue, taste disturbances, gastroesophageal reflux disturbances of fat metabolism, insulin resistance, hyperlipidemia, and even osteoporosis (Madeddu et al., 2004; USDHHS, 2005).

For those individuals who progress to full-blown AIDS, dealing with opportunistic infections can lead to a downward spiral of weight loss, malabsorption, diarrhea, anorexia, and increased risk for morbidity and mortality. The causes of weight loss in the AIDS patient include metabolic disturbances, malabsorption of fat and protein, and anorexia/cachexia. With each infection, weight is lost, followed by an incomplete recovery. Large amounts of weight loss, particularly lean body mass, worsen the prognosis for survival and further weaken the immune system (Evans, Roubenoff, Shevitz, 1998).

Dietary recommendations for oral lesions that interfere with nutrient intakes are mainly palliative. The goal is to maintain lean body mass and an adequate nutritional status until the oral lesions subside. A high-calorie, high-protein diet that provides substantial calories and protein in small volumes of food is the usual recommendation.

In addition to managing the cachexia and eating impediments, HIV and AIDS patients must be particularly concerned with food sanitation. Because of their reduced immunity, these individuals are at high risk for foodborne infections.

Erosive Oral Lesions

Erosive oral lesions, such as recurrent aphthous stomatitis, recurrent herpetic lesions, and erosive lichen planus, are commonly seen in everyday dental practice and can

TABLE 11–8 Functions of Saliva

- Lubricates to aid in chewing and swallowing
- Maintains the integrity of the mucous membranes, which are the first line of defense in innate immunity
- Aids in remineralization of the teeth
- Buffers acids and maintains the pH near neutral
- Has an antimicrobial effect on bacterial growth
- Cleanses the mouth
- Dissolves food to allow the sensations of sweet, sour, salty, and bitter tastes
- Aids in swallowing and speaking

have a significant impact on food intake. However, a direct role of nutrition in the etiology and/or prevention of these lesions has not been well defined. Anemias resulting from deficiencies of vitamin B_{12}, folic acid, and iron have been associated with increased incidence of recurrent aphthae (American Academy of Periodontology, 1994; Haisraeli-Shalish, Livneh, Katz, Doolman, Sela, 1996; Weusten, van de Wiel, 1998; Wray, Ferguson, Hutcheon, Dagg, 1978). Patients with recurrent apththous ulcers may also be deficient in vitamin B_1, calcium, and vitamin C as well as iron (Ogura et al., 2001). A number of studies have demonstrated the effectiveness of L-lysine in suppressing recurrent herpetic lesions (American Academy of Periodontology, 1994; Griffith et al., 1987; Thein, Hurt, 1984). There are no reported nutritional factors that predispose people to oral lichen planus.

The primary nutritional goal for each of these conditions is to ensure adequate hydration and nutrient intake while the erosive lesions remain symptomatic. As with the lesions associated with immune-compromising conditions, nonirritating food choices should be made that will be well tolerated and meet nutrient and calorie requirements (see Table 11–9).

ALTERNATIVE THERAPIES

Medicine's inability to cure many cancers and the challenging side effects of chemotherapy and radiotherapy have lead many people to look to alternative medicine for options. Alternative therapies include use of herbs and related products, and other nontraditional approaches to health and healing (Spaulding-Albright, 1997). In a recent study in the United Kingdom, 29% of cancer patients reported using complementary and alternative medicine (CAM) therapies (Scott, Kearney, Hummerston, Molassiotis, 2005). A study in Europe found 35.9% of patients used some form of CAM therapy and that use of herbal medicine tripled after the cancer diagnosis was made (Molassiotis et al., 2005). In a survey of newly diagnosed cancer patients in New York, 91% reported using at least one form of CAM and 57% reported using CAM therapies after having discussed it with their oncologist or primary care physician (Yates et al., 2005). The majority of patients used CAM therapies because they felt it increased the body's ability to fight cancer or improve physical and emotional well-being (Cassileth, 2000; Molassiotis et al., 2005; Richardson, Masse, Nanny, Sanders, 2004).

Many of these therapies have not been tested to determine their safety or effectiveness. The National Institute of Health's National Center for Complementary and Alternative Medicine (NCCAM) came into being in 1999 and funds research to identify, investigate, and validate CAM therapies that benefit the health and well-being of the public. When patients express interest in pursuing alternative therapies, the dental team needs to encourage them to consult reliable resources to determine their safety and efficacy.

SUMMARY AND IMPLICATIONS FOR DENTISTRY

Cancer and other immune-compromising conditions and their treatment can have major effects on nutritional status and oral health. The oral condition, in turn, is a major factor in determining nutritional status. Nutrition interventions can help prevent cancer and counteract the debilitating effects of immune-compromising conditions and their treatment. The result will be to help improve chances of survival and enhance quality of life.

The challenge for the dental professional is to partner with the patient, physician, and registered dietitian to achieve the highest quality of life through maintaining optimal oral health. The dental professional should screen patients for cancer risk, provide appropriate oral management before and during treatment, and be familiar with nutritional concerns and management strategies. The dental team needs to remember that the major nutritional issue in the management of immune-compromised patients and those with other oral lesions is maintaining weight and lean body mass. The most important question to ask the patients is "What changes in weight have you had in the last 6 months?"

Proper patient nutrition should be individualized to target specific patient concerns. The dental team should:

- Screen patients for nutritional risk and monitor weight and diet changes carefully.
- Refer patients to a registered dietitian for comprehensive nutrition care when indicated.
- Be aware of the many challenging side effects associated with immune-compromising conditions and oral lesions and their management.
- Provide appropriate preventive oral care.
- Provide effective education and referral for smoking cessation and alcohol dependence management.

(Continued on p. 266)

TABLE 11-9 Food Choice Suggestions for Patients with Oral Complications of Immune-Compromising Conditions or Their Treatment

Food Group	Xerostomia	Weight-Loss Cachexia	Dysphagia	Nausea/ Vomiting	Mucositis
Dairy products At least 2 servings (Double-strength milk mix: 1 cup nonfat dry milk powder and 1 quart whole milk; provides twice the protein, vitamins, and minerals and 1½ times the calories.)	Instant breakfast, egg-nogs, frappes, custards, puddings, hot cereals, creamed soups, cheese sauces (all made with double-strength milk when possible); ice cream, cottage cheese, fruited yogurt	See Xerostomia column, and: use cheese liberally (sandwiches, sauces, toppings, and in baking), cream and cream cheese when not contraindicated	See Xerostomia column, and: avoid hard, unmelted cheese	See Xerostomia column, and: encourage plain yogurt if tolerated	See Xerostomia column, and: tilt head or use straw to swallow
Protein sources At least 2 servings No raw eggs.	Hearty meat, fish, poultry, beans, tofu, peanut butter, stews, soups and chowders, meat sauces, pot roasts; gravies and sauces added to most fish and poultry; eggs added to soups, sauces, and hot cereal	See Xerostomia column, and: peanut butter added to frappes, fruit, and bread	See Xerostomia column, and: pureed or blenderized meat, fish, poultry; beans and tofu added to soups and to mashed or pureed vegetables	See Xerostomia column, and: avoid spicy, highly seasoned foods; for acute phase, encourage salty soups (miso, chicken)	See Xerostomia column, and: avoid spicy foods
Fruit 2–3 servings as tolerated	Soft, ripe fruits and fruit juices, applesauce, cooked and canned fruits, chopped meat mixed with fruit juices, frozen fruit/fruit juice popsicles	All fruit, especially bananas, grapes, and pineapple juice; cooked fruit with cream or liquid supplement	Pureed fruits, all fruit and vegetable juices as tolerated, apple-sauce or banana blended with tofu, frozen fruit juice popsicles	All fruits and juices as tolerated; lemon wedge or juice in carbonated beverages	See Xerostomia column, and: avoid all citrus fruits, tomatoes, and acid fruits
Vegetables 3–5 servings as tolerated	Soft, cooked vegetables; hearty vegetable soups, stews; vegetable juices	All vegetables with sauces and gravies; starchy vegetables such as potatoes, winter squash, creamed corn	Pureed or mashed potatoes and all vegetables (carrots, beets, corn, etc.) and vegetable juices as tolerated	Only as tolerated; avoid vegetables with strong odors; vegetable juices as tolerated	See Xerostomia column, and:
Grain products 6–11 servings	Creamy, hot cereals; noodles, pasta, bread; dry cereals added to soups and sauces;	All breads (sandwiches, bread puddings, cereals, cakes, cookies, pies);	See Xerostomia column, and:	All breads and cereals as tolerated; encourage dry toast,	See Xerostomia column, and:

				instruct patient to brush thoroughly after eating sweets	salted crackers before getting out of bed or before a meal
Fats For added calories use as tolerated if not contraindicated by obesity or diarrhea	Oil, cream, margarine, or butter used liberally in hot cereals, soups, sauces, gravies, and on vegetables; cream cheese; sour cream, mayonnaise; avocados	wheat germ added to cereals, breakfast drinks, custards, frappes, yogurt, etc.; French toast, pancakes, bread pudding; avoid dry toast and hard, crusty bread unless soaked in beverage or soup	See Xerostomia column, and: use liberally except when contraindicated by heart or weight issues	See Xerostomia column, and: use liberally except when contraindicated by heart or weight issues	See Xerostomia column, and: use liberally except when contraindicated by heart or weight issues
Complete nutritional supplements (for added calories, protein, vitamins, and minerals) Powdered breakfast beverage: • Readily available • Inexpensive • Many flavors • About 280 cal with whole milk • Use lactose-free milk if needed Ensure, Sustacal, Boost • More expensive • Lactose and milk free • Average 250 cal/can	All supplements are high in sugar, therefore stress toothbrushing after eating Add to, or use to replace milk in beverages, French toast, puddings, sodas, etc.	Use as needed	Use as needed	Use as needed	Use as needed and tolerated

265

- Educate nondental colleagues about the oral implications of immune-compromising conditions and oral lesions and become an active team member.
- Provide appropriate diet suggestions for managing specific oral problems.
- Provide appropriate oral care that complements rather than contradicts nutritional care.

QUESTIONS PATIENTS MIGHT ASK

Q. Can I prevent hypertension by having a low-sodium diet?

A. Not necessarily. Some people with high blood pressure and a high sodium diet can reduce their blood pressure by reducing the dietary sodium alone. These people are considered "salt sensitive." For others, reducing dietary sodium is not sufficient to reduce hypertension and they require medications as well. Because nobody knows who will and will not respond to sodium reduction, it is prudent for everyone to keep sodium intake in the range of 2–3 grams a day as recommended by the *Dietary Guidelines for Americans*.

Q. How can I help protect myself against osteoporosis if I have a family history?

A. There is no one foolproof solution, but a variety of lifestyle factors can play an important role. Try to get sufficient weight-bearing exercise like walking. Eat liberal amounts of calcium and vitamin D containing foods. If you can't tolerate dairy products, try vitamin D fortified lactose-free foods. You may also need a daily calcium/vitamin D supplement. Adults need to get at least 1 gram of calcium a day.

Q. I am recuperating from cancer treatment and have lost my appetite. Some of my friends have said that there are a lot of supplements available at the health food store that will help me boost my immunity and help cure the cancer. Do you think I should invest in them?

A. I wouldn't suggest it. Nutrition alone cannot cure cancer. Good nutrition is important for good immunity, but these benefits come from the many substances in foods themselves, not individual supplements. Since supplements do not have to be proven effective to be on the market, you may be wasting money on products of questionable value. A better approach would be to see a registered dietitian who can make nutrient-packed food suggestions to help you overcome your problems and support your recovery. If he or she recommends supplements, you will know that they are appropriate and helpful.

CASE STUDY

Dental history: The patient has a history of "deep cleanings" on all four quadrants of his mouth 15 years ago. He has not been seen for any treatment since then.

Medical history: The medical history indicates he has a history of hypertension, hyperlipidemia, depression, and angina. He takes hydrochlorathiazide for hypertension, Lipitor for his high cholesterol, Prozac for depression, and carries nitroglycerin for anginal episodes. The last episode of angina was 2 weeks ago when he was going out to get the newspaper in the morning. The patient reports he had excessive thirst for the last couple of weeks and feels the need to urinate frequently. He drinks three to four shots of bourbon every evening. His tobacco history is 50-pack years; he is in the process of

trying to quit again. His father and grandmother had diabetes, and his father died of a heart attack at age 50.

Nutrition status: Diet screening identifies that the patient avoids dairy because it is too high in fat. He is a "meat and potatoes man" and likes a big piece of red meat for dinner. He likes fruits and vegetables, but just never thinks of eating them. His physician told him to lose weight and eat less, and handed him a relevant pamphlet at his last appointment, but he has had no formal diet instruction.

Clinical findings: On clinical examination his blood pressure is 170/105. His periodontal diagnosis is generalized moderate to severe chronic adult periodontitis. There are also extensive cervical caries.

Questions:

1. What aspects of this patient make you feel that a consultation with his physician is necessary?
2. What dietary recommendations might you make to this patient?
3. What is the dental professional's role in assisting this patient with tobacco cessation?
4. What concerns do you have for this patient regarding his healing response to initial periodontal therapy?

CASE STUDY

Rose Jackson, a 57-year-old attorney, came to the office complaining that her teeth "seem to be falling apart." She complains that the enamel is flaking off, and she is experiencing sensitivity to hot and cold.

Rose recently completed radiation therapy at a local hospital for a neoplasm on the lateral border of her tongue. She says that it was caught early and the prognosis is good. Since then, she has had difficult eating and swallowing, and she eats more slowly than the rest of her family. Her appetite has been declining and she has lost 15 pounds in the last month. She complains that she has lost her taste for meat and many foods taste "off" to her. She says sometimes food tastes like "cotton." During the day, she eats on the run, consuming lots of liquids such as coffee and buying meals at fast-food restaurants.

Dental examination reveals extensive generalized carious lesions and a plaque-free index of 45%. She brushes her teeth on the run in the morning (but it hurts) and uses a fluoride dentifrice.

24-Hour Diet Recall

B: $1/2$ cup oatmeal
$1/2$ cup milk
2 tsp. honey
$1/2$ cup apple juice
1 cup coffee
1 tsp. creamer or instant breakfast

L: 1 cheeseburger
fries

$1/2$ cup chocolate pudding
1 soda

D: 1 cup macaroni & cheese
$1/2$ cup green beans
2 bananas
1 cup coffee
2 tsp. creamer

Snacks:

Morning: 1 plain donut
1 cup coffee
2 tsp. creamer

Evening: 1 cup. cocoa before bed
1 dish vanilla ice cream

All Day: 10–12 cups coffee with 2 tsp. creamer each
6–7 lemon drops

Questions:

1. What are the potential side effects of radiation therapy? How do these side effects affect the oral cavity?
2. What factors may have contributed to Rose Jackson's extensive caries problem?
3. How does cancer affect nutritional status? What is the *most important nutritional* issue?
4. What would your dental care plan be to ameliorate her current dental problem and prevent future problems?
5. What should the nutrition care rationale be?
6. How should the dental therapy and nutrition care be coordinated?

CASE STUDY

A 35-year-old black man presents for dental treatment.

Medical history: Patient reports he has just been diagnosed with non-Hodgkin's lymphoma (NHL) and is presently not undergoing any treatment for it. He plans to start induction therapy (high-dose chemotherapy and total body irradiation) for a bone marrow transplant in 4 weeks. On meeting the patient, you note that he is extremely thin and appears weak.

Dental history: The patient does not have regular dental care. He came today only because his physician has recommended he have his entire dental treatment completed before he begins chemotherapy.

Nutrition status: The patient reports that he has lost 20 pounds in the last 2 months because his appetite has been poor. He was previously at a good weight and now is worried about becoming too thin. Since being diagnosed with NHL, he has stopped eating meat and has become a vegetarian. He also doesn't consume dairy products because he says "it causes him to have more phlegm." On further questioning, you find that the patient is eating basically fruits and vegetables and few sources of plant proteins.

Clinical examination: His periodontal diagnosis is generalized moderate adult periodontitis. He has few pockets over 3 mm at this time, but has 2 to 3 mm of generalized gingival recession. His home care is good, with a plaque score of 15%. He has only two small recurrent caries.

Questions:
1. Why is a consultation with the patient's physician necessary?
2. What general dietary recommendations would you make to this patient?
3. What are some of the potential oral side effects of his treatment protocol?
4. What is the role of the dental office in the patient's treatment?

REFERENCES

Hypertension

American Heart Association: *Heart Disease and Stroke Statistics—2005 Update.* Dallas, TX: American Heart Association, 2005.

Apple LJ, Moore TJ, Obarzanek E, Vollmer WM, Svetkey LP, Sacks FM, et al.: A clinical trial of the effects of dietary patterns on blood pressure. DASH Collaborative Research Group. *N Engl J Med* 1997; 336(16):1117–24.

Arroll B, Beaglehole R: Does physical activity lower blood pressure: A critical review of the clinical trials. *J Clin Epidemiol* 1992; 45:439–47.

Carlos JP, Wolfe MD: Methodological and nutritional issues in assessing the oral health of aged subjects. *Am J Clin Nutr* 1989; 50:1210–18.

Glick M: New guidelines for prevention, Detection, evaluation, and treatment of high blood pressure. *J Am Dent* 1998; 129(11):1588–95.

He J, Welton PK: Epidemiology and prevention of hypertension. *Med Clin North Am* 1997; 81(5):1077–97.

Law MR, Frost CD, Wald NJ: By how much does dietary salt reduction lower blood pressure? III: Analysis of data from trials of salt reduction. *Br Med J* 1991; 302:819–24.

Marmot MG, Elliott P, Shipley MJ, Dyer AR, Ueshima HU, Beevers DG, et al.: Alcohol and blood pressure: The INTERSALT study. *Br Med J* 1994; 308(6939):1263–67.

Moore TJ, McKnight JA: Dietary factors and blood pressure regulation. *Endocrinol Metab Clin North Am* 1995; 24(3):643–55.

Sacks FM, Svetkey LP, Vollmer WM, Appel LJ, Bray GA, Harsha D, et al.: Effects on blood pressure of reduced dietary sodium and the Dietary Approaches to Stop Hypertension (DASH) diet. *N Engl J Med* 2001; 344:310.

Sinaiko AR: Hypertension in children. *N Engl J Med* 1996; 335(26):1968–73.

Stevens VJ, Corrigan SA, Obarzanek E, Bernauer E, Cook NR, Hebert P, et al.: Weight loss intervention in phase I of the Trials of Hypertension Prevention. The TOHP Collaborative Research Group. *Arch Intern Med* 1993; 153(7):849–58.

Thomas CL: *Taber's Cyclopedic Medical Dictionary.* Philadelphia: FA Davis, 1993.

U.S. Department of Health and Human Services, National Institutes of Health, National Heart, Lung, and Blood Institute: *The Seventh Report of the Joint National Committee on Prevention, Detection, Evaluation, and Treatment of High Blood Pressure 2004.* Bethesda, MD: National Institutes of Health, 2004.

Osteoporosis

Anderson JJ, Rondano PA: Peak bone mass development of females: Can young adult women improve their peak bone mass? *J Am Coll Nutr* 1996; 15(6):570–74.

Barr SI, McKay HA: Nutrition, exercise, and bone status in youth. *Int J Sport Nutr* 1998; 8(2):124–42.

Carroccio A, Di Prima L, Di Grigoli C, Soresi M, Farinella E, Di Martino D, et al.: Exocrine pancreatic function and fat malabsorption in human immunodeficiency virus-infected patients. *Scand J Gastroenterol* 1999; 34(7):729–34.

Center J, Eisman J: The epidemiology and pathogenesis of osteoporosis. *Baillieres Clin Endocrinol Metab* 1997; 11(1):23–62.

Harris SS, Dawson-Hughes B: Caffeine and bone loss in healthy postmenopausal women. *Am J Clin Nutr* 1994; 60(4):573–78.

Horner K, Devlin H: The relationship between mandibular bone mineral density and panoramic radiographic measurements. *J Dent* 1998; 26(4):337–43.

Institute of Medicine, National Academy of Sciences: *Dietary Reference Intakes for Calcium, Phosphorus, Magnesium, Vitamin D, and Fluoride*. Washington, DC: National Academies Press, 1997: 71–145.

Jeffcoat MK: Osteoporosis: A possible modifying factor in oral bone loss. *Ann Periodontol* 1998; 3(1): 312–21.

Jeffcoat MK, The association between osteoporosis and oral bone loss. *J Periodontol* 2005 Nov; 76(11 Suppl):2125–32. Review.

Krall EA, Dawson-Hughes B: Smoking increases bone loss and decreases intestinal calcium absorption [Process Citation]. *J Bone Miner Res* 1999; 14(2):215–20.

Krall EA, Dawson-Hughes B, Papas A, Garcia RI: Tooth loss and skeletal bone density in healthy postmenopausal women. *Osteoporosis Int* 1994; 4:104–9.

Mohammad AR, Alder M, McNally MA: A pilot study of panoramic film density at selected sites in the mandible to predict osteoporosis. *Int J Prosthodont* 1996; 9(3):290–94.

Moore M, Bracker M, Sartoris D, Saltman P, Strause L: Long-term estrogen replacement therapy in postmenopausal women sustains vertebral bone mineral density. *J Bone Miner Res* 1990; 5(6):659–64.

National Osteoporosis Foundation: *Physician's Guide to Prevention and Treatment of Osteoporosis*. Washington, DC: National Osteoporosis Foundation, 2003.

Ross EA, Szabo NJ, Tebbett IR: Lead content of calcium supplements. *JAMA* 2000; 284:1425–29.

Rossouw JE, Anderson GL, Prentice RL, LaCroix AZ, Kooperberg C, Stefanick ML, et al.: Risks and benefits of estrogen plus progestin in healthy postmenopausal women: Prinicipal results from the Women's Health Initiative randomized controlled trial. *JAMA* 2002; 288:321–33.

Teofilo JM, Azevedo AC, Petenusci SO, Mazaro R, Lamano-Carvalho TL: Comparison between two experimental protocols to promote osteoporosis in the maxilla and proximal tibia of female rats. *Brazilian Oral Res* 2003; 17(4):302–6.

U.S. Department of Health and Human Services: *Bone Health and Osteoporosis: A Report of the Surgeon General*. Rockville, MD: U.S. Department of Health and Human Services, Office of the Surgeon General, 2004.

Wactawski-Wende J, Grossi SG, Trevisan M, Genco RJ, Tezal M, Dunford RG, et al.: The role of osteopenia in oral bone loss and periodontal disease. *J Periodontol* 1996; 67(10 Suppl):1076–84.

Weaver CM, Peacock M, Johnston DD: Adolescent nutrition in the prevention of postmenopausal osteoporosis. *J Clin Endocrinol Metab* 1999; 84(6):1839–43.

White SC, Rudolph DJ: Alterations of trabecular pattern of the jaws in patients with osteoporosis. *Oral Surg Oral Med Oral Pathol Oral Radiol Endod* 1999; 88(5):628–35.

Immune System Disorders

American Cancer Society: *Cancer Facts & Figures—1995*. Atlanta: Author, 1995.

American Cancer Society: *Understanding Chemotherapy*. Atlanta: Author, 1999a.

American Cancer Society: *Understanding Surgery*. Atlanta: Author, 1999b.

Atkinson JC, Wu AJ: Salivary gland dysfunction: Causes, symptoms, treatment. *J Am Dent Assoc* 1994; 125:409–16.

Badger TM, Ronis MJ, Simmen RC, Simmen FA: Soy protein isolate and protection against cancer. *J Am Coll Nutr* 2005; 24(2):146S–49S.

Block G, Patterson B, Subar A: Fruit, vegetables, and cancer prevention: A review of the epidemiological evidence. *Nutr Cancer* 1992; 18(1):1–29.

Cassileth BR: Complementary therapies: The American experience [Review]. *Supportive Care in Cancer* 2000; 8(1):16–23.

Centers for Disease Control and Prevention: *HIV/AIDS Surveillance Supplemental Report*, 2003 (Vol. 15). Atlanta: Author, 2003.

Centers for Disease Control and Prevention: Preventing and controlling oral and pharyngeal cancer recommendations from a National Strategic Planning Conference. *MMWR* 1998; 47(RR14).

Centers for Disease Control and Prevention: Promoting oral health: Interventions for preventing dental caries, oral and pharyngeal cancers, and sports-related craniofacial injuries. *MMWR* 2001; 50(RR12):1–13.

Chandra RK: Nutrition and immunoregulation. Significance for host resistance to tumors and infectious disease in human and rodents. *J Nutr* 1992; 122: 754–57.

Chandra RK: Nutrition and the immune system: An introduction. *Am J Clin Nutr* 1997; 66:460S–63S.

Chandra RK: Impact of nutritional status and nutrient supplements on immune responses and incidence of infection in older adults. *Ageing Res Rev* 2004; 3(1):91–104.

Chao A, Thun MJ, Connell CJ, McCullogh ML, Jacobs EJ, Flanders WD, et al.: Meat consumption and risk of colorectal cancer. *JAMA* 2005; 293(2):172–82.

Charuhas PM: Drug and food interactions: nutrition support of the cancer patient. New York: Norwich Eaton Pharmaceuticals, 1990; 10(2):1–3.

Deapen D, Liu L, Perkins C, Bernstein L, Ross RK: Rapidly rising breast cancer incidence rates among Asian-American women. *Int J Cancer* 2002; 99:747–50.

Evans WJ, Roubenoff R, Snevitz A: Exercise and the treatment of wasting: Aging and human immunodeficiency virus infection. *Semin Oncol* 1998; 25(2 Suppl 6):112–22.

Ferlay J, Bray F, Pisani P, Parkin DM: *Cancer Incidence, Mortality and Prevalence Worldwide*. IARC CancerBase No.5, version 2.0. IARCPress, Lyon, 2004.

Greenwald P: Cancer risk factors for selecting cohorts for large-scale chemoprevention trials. *J Cell Biochem* 1996; 25(Suppl):29–36.

Hakim FT, Flomerfelt FA, Boyiadzis M, Gress RE: Aging, immunity and cancer. *Curr Opin Immunol* 2004; 16(2): 151–56.

Heald AE, Pieper CF, Schiffman SS: Taste and smell complaints in HIV-infected patients. *AIDS* 1998 Sep 10; 12(13):1667–74.

Hensel M, Haake K, Vogel S, Flugel W, Krausch D, Kox WJ: Management of swallowing disorders and chronic aspiration by glottic closure procedure. *J Neurosurg Anesthesiol* 1997; 9(3):273–76.

Hollister MC, Weintraub JA: The association of oral status with systemic health, quality of life, and economic productivity. *J Dent Ed* 1993; 75(12):901–12.

Hsu S: Research demonstrates cancer-fighting properties of green tea. February 15, 2001. Medical College of Georgia website. Retrieved from http://www.mcg.edu/2001newsrel/hsu.html.

Johns ME: The nutrition problem in head and neck cancer. *Otolaryngol Head Neck Surg* 1988; 88:691–94.

Key TJ, Schatzkin A, Willett WC, Allen NE, Spencer EA, Travis RC: Diet, nutrition and the prevention of cancer. *Public Health Nutr* 2004; 7(1A):187–200.

Khafif A, Schantz SP, al-Rawi M, Edelstein D, Sacks PG: Green tea regulates cell cycle progression in oral leukoplakia. *Head Neck* 1998; 20(6):528–34.

Levene MB, Harris JR (eds): *Overall Principles of Cancer Management: Radiation Therapy, Cancer Manual*. Boston: American Cancer Society, Massachusetts Division, 1982.

Linardaki G, Moutsopoulos HM: The uncertain role of immunosuppressive agents in Sjögren's syndrome. *Cleve Clinic J Med* 1997; 64(10):523–26.

Madeddu G, Spanu A, Solinas P, Calia GM, Lovigu D, Chessa F, et al.: Bone mass loss and vitamin D metabolism impairment in HIV patients receiving highly active antiretroviral therapy. *Q J Nucl Med Mol Imaging* 2004; 48(1):39–48.

Marques MA, Dib LL: Periodontal changes in patients undergoing radiotherapy. *J Periodontol* 2004; 75(9):1178–87.

Marti A, Marcos A, Martinez JA: Obesity and immune function relationships. *Obes Rev* 2001; 2(2):131–40.

Meguid MM, Muscaritoli M, Beverly JL, Yang ZJ, Cangiano C, Rossi-Fanelli F: The early cancer anorexia paradigm: Changes in plasma free tryptophan and feeding indexes. *J Parenter Enteral Nutr* 1992; 16(6 Suppl):56S–59S.

Molasssiotis A, Fernadez-Ortega P, Pud D, Ozden G, Scott JA, Panteli V, et al.: Use of complementary and alternative medicine in cancer patients: A European survey. *Ann Oncol* 2005; 16(4):655–63.

Moons P, DeGeest S, Abraham I, Cleemput JV, VanVanhaecke J: Symptom experience associated with maintenance immunosuppression after heart transplantation: patients' appraisal of side effects. *Heart Lung* 1998 Sep–Oct; 27(5):315–25.

National Cancer Institute: Nutrition in cancer (PDQ). Retrieved June 19, 2005, from http://www.nci.nih.gov/cancertopics/pdq/supportivecare/nutrition/healthprofessional/allpages#Section_298, 5/13/05.

National Institutes of Health: *Eating Hints for Cancer Patients Before, During, and After Treatment*. U.S. Department of Health and Human Services, Public Health Service, 1994. Retrieved from www.cancer.gov May 19, 2006.

National Screening Initiative: *Nutrition: Statement of principle*. 2002. Retrieved from http://www.eatright.org/Public/Files/nutrition(1).pdf.

Nutrition for Cancer Patients. American Cancer Society: www.cancer.org.

Palesty JA, Dudrick SJ: What we have learned about cachexia in gastrointestinal cancer. *Dig Dis* 2003; 21(3):198–213.

Pelucchi C, Talamini R, Negri E, Levi F, Conti E, Franceschi S, et al.: Folate intake and risk of oral and pharyngeal cancer [Review]. *Ann Oncol* 2003; 14(11):1677–81.

Ramaswamy G, Rao VR, Kumaraswamy SV, Anantha N, Serum vitamins' status in oral leucoplakias—a preliminary study. *Eur J Cancer B Oral Oncol* 1996; 32B(2):120–22.

Riboli E, Norat T: Epidemiologic evidence of the protective effect of fruits and vegetables on cancer risk. *Am J Clin Nutr* 2003; 78(Suppl):559S–69S.

Richardson MA, Masse LC, Nanny K, Sanders C: Discrepant views of oncologists and cancer patients on complementary/alternative medicine. *Supportive Care in Cancer* 2004; 12(11):797–804.

Rosenthal P, Griffin T, Hassey K, Lingos T, Maciewicz R, O'Connor L: Complications of cancer and cancer treatment. In Osteen R (ed): *Cancer Manual*, 8th ed. Boston: American Cancer Society, 1990.

Schwartz JL, Baker V, Larios E, Chung FL: Molecular and cellular effects of green tea on oral cells of smokers: A pilot study. *Mol Nutr Food Res* 2005; 49(1):43–51.

Scrimshaw NS, Sangiovanni JP: Synergism of nutrition, infection, and immunity: An overview. *Am J Clin Nutr* 1997: 66:464S–77S.

Scott JA, Kearney N, Hummerston S, Molassiotis A: Use of complementary and alternative medicine in patients with cancer: A UK survey. *Eur J Oncol Nurs* 9(2):131–37.

Shils ME, Olsen JA, Moshe S (eds): *Modern Nutrition in Health and Disease,* 8th ed. Malvern, PA: Lea & Febiger, 1994.

Spaulding-Albright N: A review of some herbal and related products commonly used in cancer patients. *J Am Diet Assoc* 1997; 97(10 Suppl 2):S208–S15.

Thomas DB: Alcohol as a cause of cancer. *Environ Health Persp* 1995; 103(Suppl 8):153–160.

U.S. Department of Health and Human Services, Panel on Clinical Practices for Treatment of HIV Infection: *Guidelines for the Use of Antiretorival Agents in HIV-1-Infected Adults and Adolescents.* Washington, DC: Author, 2005.

Williams EF, Meguid MM: Nutritional concepts and considerations in head and neck surgery. *Head Neck Surg* 1989; 11:393–99.

Wilson PR, Herman J, Chubon SJ: Eating strategies used by persons with head and neck cancer during and after radiotherapy. *Cancer Nurs,* 1991; 14(2):98–104.

Wood RM, Lander V, Mosby EL, Hiatt WR: Nutrition and the head and neck cancer patient. *Oral Surg Oral Med Oral Pathol* 1989; 68:391–95.

Yates JS, Mustian KM, Morrow GR, Gillies LJ, Padmanaban D, Atkins JN, et al.: Prevalence of complementary and alternative medicine use in cancer patients during treatment. *Support Care Cancer,* February 15, 2005.

Oral Lesions

American Academy of Periodontology: *Oral Features of Mucocutaneous Disorders (Position Paper).* Chicago: American Academy of Periodontology, 1994:1–5.

Boyd LD, Dwyer JT, Papas A: Nutritional implications of xerostomia and rampant caries caused by serotonin reuptake inhibitors: A case study. *Nutr Rev* 1997; 55(10):362–68.

Griffith RS, Walsh DE, Myrmel KH, Thompson RW, Behforooz A: Success of L-lysine therapy in frequently recurrent herpes simplex infection. Treatment and prophylaxis. *Dermatologica* 1987; 175(4):183–90.

Haisraeli-Shalish M, Livneh A, Katz J, Doolman R, Sela BA: Recurrent aphthous stomatitis and thiamine deficiency. *Oral Surg Oral Med Oral Pathol* 1996; 82(6):634–36.

Miller LS, Manwell MA, Newbold D, Reding ME: The relationship between reduction in periodontal inflammation and diabetes control: A report of 9 cases. *J Periodontal* 1992; 63:843–48.

National Cholesterol Education Program: *Third Report of the Expert Panel on Detection, Evaluation, and Treatment of High Blood Cholesterol in Adults.* Bethesda, MD: National Institutes of Health, National Heart, Lung, and Blood Institute, 2002.

Research and Therapy Committee of the American Academy of Periodontology: Position paper: Periodontal considerations in the management of the cancer patient. *J Periodontol* 1997; 68(8):791–801.

Rhodus NL, Michalowicz BS: Periodontal status and sulcular candida albicans colonization in patients with primary Sjogren's syndrome. *Quintessence Int* 2005; 36(3):228–33.

Taylor GW, Burt BA, Beeker MP, Genco RJ, Shlossman M: Glycemic control and alveolar bone loss progression in Type 2 diabetes. *Ann of Periodontol* 1998; 3(1):30–39

Thein DJ, Hurt WC: Lysine as a prophylactic agent in the treatment of recurrent herpes simplex labialis. *Oral Surg Oral Med Oral Pathol* 1984 Dec; 58(6):659–66.

U.S. Cancer Statistics Working Group: *United States Cancer Statistics: 2001 Incidence and Mortality.* Atlanta: Department of Health and Human Services, Centers for Disease Control and Prevention, National Cancer Institute, 2004.

U.S. Department of Health and Human Services: *Oral Health in America: A Report of the Surgeon General—Executive Summary.* Rockville, MD: US Department of Health and Human Services, National Institute of Dental and Craniofacial Research, National Institutes of Health, 2000.

Vissink A, Jasma J, Spijkervet FKL, Burlage FR, Coppes RP: Oral sequelae of head and neck radiotherapy. *Crit Rev Oral Biol Med* 2003; 14(3):199–212.

Weusten BL, van de Wiel A: Aphthous ulcers and vitamin B_{12} deficiency. *N Engl J Med* 1998; 53(4):172–75.

Wray D, Ferguson MM, Hutcheon WA, Dagg JH: Nutritional deficiencies in recurrent aphthae. *J Oral Pathol* 1978; 7:418–23.

Chapter 12

Nutrition in the Growth and Development of Oral Structures

Catherine Hayes and Kathryn Thornton

OBJECTIVES

The student will be able to:

- Discuss how general nutritional status can affect the growth and development of oral tissues and structures.
- Describe the role of specific nutrients in the development of oral tissues and structures.
- Describe how mastication, diet consistency, and texture relate to oral development.
- Describe the nutritional factors possibly associated with cleft palate and other oral deformities.

INTRODUCTION

Adequate nutrition provides the basis for development of all tissues and structures of the body including those in the oral cavity. Because it is unethical to cause malnutrition purposefully in humans to study developmental effects, most of the human research has been epidemiological in nature. The more definitive clinical studies have been conducted on animals, and the results have been used to suggest possible human effects as well.

This chapter highlights and summarizes the state of our knowledge about nutrition and oral development.

COMPOSITION OF ORAL TISSUES AND STRUCTURES

A variety of cells, tissues, and fluids compose the oral cavity (Figure 12–1). These include soft tissues (oral mucosa, salivary glands), mineralized tissues (alveolar bone, teeth), and fluid secretion (saliva, gingival sulcular fluid).

The *tooth* (including the enamel, dentin, cementum, and pulp) are unique among body tissues. Enamel is the most highly mineralized of the body's tissues. It is composed of about 96% mineral, 3% water, and 1% organic material (as compared to bone, which is only about 60% mineral) (Wefel, Dodds, 1999). *Enamel* is primarily composed of a crystalline structure, hydroxyapatite $Ca_{10}(PO_4)_6(OH)_2$. The major chemical constituents of enamel are calcium, phosphorus, magnesium, and carbonate. Enamel is much like bone in structure, but enamel crystals are larger and more densely packed than bone crystals; consequently teeth are harder than bone. Enamel is unique to mineralized tissues as it is relatively inert. Unlike bone, it does not remodel. Despite this fact, enamel is affected by topical demineralization and remineralization activity. (This becomes an important issue in dental caries susceptibility and prevention.) Enamel can be destroyed by organic acids, such as those involved in the production of dental caries and other types of demineralization. Ionic exchanges can take place between the

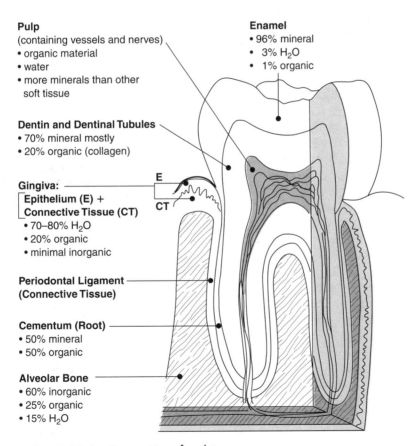

Pulp
(containing vessels and nerves)
• organic material
• water
• more minerals than other
  soft tissue

Dentin and Dentinal Tubules
• 70% mineral mostly
• 20% organic (collagen)

Gingiva:
Epithelium (E) +
Connective Tissue (CT)
• 70–80% H_2O
• 20% organic
• minimal inorganic

Periodontal Ligament
(Connective Tissue)

Cementum (Root)
• 50% mineral
• 50% organic

Alveolar Bone
• 60% inorganic
• 25% organic
• 15% H_2O

Enamel
• 96% mineral
• 3% H_2O
• 1% organic

E

CT

FIGURE 12-1 Composition of oral tissues.

environment and enamel crystal at the surface of the crystal, within the crystal body, or in the water spaces between crystals. Elements such as fluoride, zinc, lead, iron, silver, manganese, silicon, and tin can be found concentrated in external layers of enamel. Carbonate, sodium, and magnesium are in the subsurface. Other trace elements such as strontium can be evenly distributed in both. Only about 0.6% of enamel is organic and is made up of keratin, mucoprotein, collagen, peptide, citrate, phospholipid, and cholesterol. (See Chapter 8 for a discussion of the mineralization process of teeth and bone.)

Dentin is only about 70% mineralized, 20% organic (primarily collagen), and 10% water. Dentin is closer in composition to bone than enamel, and has less calcium and phosphorus and more magnesium, carbonate, and fluoride than enamel. Collagen accounts for about 18% of the organic matter in dentin. The remainder consists of lipids, mucopolysaccharides, and protein. *Cementum* is similar in composition to bone and dentin.

Pulp is primarily organic material and water, with much higher amounts of calcium, phosphorus, and fluoride than other soft tissues. The pulp is a vehicle for the physiological exchange of nutrients to and from the dentin to the rest of the body.

Periodontal tissues include gingiva (epithelium and connective tissue), periodontal ligament (connective tissue), and alveolar bone. The composition of these tissues is much the same as all other similar body tissues. The epithelium is made of about 70–80% water, 20% organic matter (protein-polysaccharide complexes), and a small amount of inorganic material. Gingival fluids are composed of water, proteins, and minerals.

Collagen is the major structural protein in connective tissue. Ground substance, which provides structure for collagen formation, is made of protein and structural polysaccharides such as hyaluronic acid and chondroitin sulfate.

Alveolar bone, similar to other bone throughout the body, is about 60% inorganic, 25% organic, and 15% water. The inorganic portion of the bone is primarily hydroxyapatite crystal as in enamel. There may be several apatite-type compounds in bone. The organic component is primarily collagen. Other constituents include mucopolysaccharides, lipids, and alkaline phosphatase enzymes.

The *salivary glands*, like other oral soft tissues, are composed primarily of collagen. Saliva is secreted from parotid, submaxillary, sublingual, and mucus glands. It is composed primarily of water and minerals such as sodium, chloride, potassium, magnesium, sulfate, and carbonate. It also contains a supersaturated solution of calcium phosphate, which is essential in promoting tooth remineralization. Saliva also contains small amounts of proteins and amino acids, as well as enzymes such as amylase (needed for the hydrolysis of starch), peroxidase, and decarboxylase (Wefel, Dodds, 1999) Saliva is an important buffer in the oral cavity. The normal pH of resting saliva is from 6.5 to 7.0 (a pH of 7.0 is neutral). When saliva is stimulated, the pH rises and becomes more alkaline. This allows saliva to neutralize the acids formed in the caries process and is a crucial factor in caries prevention. Conversely, when saliva production decreases (xerostomia or dry mouth) caries risk increases dramatically. Malnutrition can have a detrimental effect on saliva formation, primarily via effects on protein and mineral nutriture (Johnson, 1993).

Dental plaque is composed of approximately 80% water, with the remainder as salivary proteins, enzymes, bacteria, desquamated epithelial cells, and other oral debris. The plaque matrix is composed primarily of salivary mucins to which bacteria adhere, colonize, and proliferate. Enzymes such as glycosidases can hydrolyze dietary sucrose into monosaccharides, which can then be polymerized to dextrans and levans and stored in plaque. These products contribute significantly to plaque adhesion.

IMPORTANCE OF NUTRITION IN THE GROWTH AND DEVELOPMENT OF ORAL TISSUES AND STRUCTURES

Optimal nutrition is particularly important during early periods of growth and development (Table 12–1). Nutritional problems that occur during these critical periods of growth can have lifelong consequences. For example, deficiencies or toxicities that occur during oral tissue development may or may not be reversible depending on the timing of the insult. When a nutritional insult occurs during initial cell formation (hyperplasia), the results are usually permanent and not reversible. For example, malnutrition or nutrient toxicity during amelogenesis (enamel formation) may result in permanent enamel defects in the primary dentition (Boyle, 1934; Giunta, 1998; Pindborg, 1970). Conversely, problems that occur later during periods of cell growth and/or regeneration only (hypertrophy) are often reversible.

TABLE 12–1   Nutritional Considerations for Oral Growth and Development

Dietary Component	*Role in Oral Growth and Development*
Calcium/phosphorus/vitamin D/magnesium	Association with quantity of alveolar bone and bone density
Vitamin C	Association with bone density and soft tissue integrity via collagen formation
Diet consistency and texture	Firm diet aids proper growth of mandible and maxilla and proper tooth eruption
Malnutrition (animals)	Results in reduced mandible size and crowding of teeth
	Dental anomalies include wide pulp chambers and open apices, as a result of decreased osteogenic and osteoclastic activity
	Bone that is thin and not as radio-opaque as controls
Malnutrition (humans)	Delayed tooth development and eruption
	Enamel hypoplasia
	Increased risk for caries and periodontal disease
	Reduced collagen formation
Protein deficiency	Protein is needed for all cell replication
	Deficiency affects tooth size and eruption sequence
	Affects salivary gland formation and function

For example, scorbutic gingiva, resulting from vitamin C deficiency, is generally curable when adequate ascorbic acid is given (Figure 12–2).

Oral soft tissues have a more rapid turnover time (3 to 7 days) than other body tissues, which increases the susceptibility of these tissues to problems associated with nutrient variablility. Because of this rapid tissue turnover, nutrient requirements may be higher in the oral cavity than in the rest of the body, and when nutritional disturbances do exist, they may first manifest in the oral cavity. (DePaola, Faine, Palmer, 1999).

Effects of Nutrition on Oral Development and Caries Risk

Children's primary teeth are formed to a major degree before birth, with mineralization beginning around 3 to 4 months of embryogenesis. The primary teeth begin forming at 6 weeks in utero. At this point, the cells differentiate to form the dental lamina, the site of tooth bud development. Crown formation begins with a dentin matrix containing collagen fibrils. Minerals such as calcium and phosphorus enter the matrix and form small crystals on or between the collagen fibrils. After this first dentin layer is complete, enamel formation begins, and continues after the matrix is formed.

Mineralization begins as early as 4 months in utero and continues into late adolescence. At birth, the crowns of the primary incisors are almost completely formed, and the primary canines and primary first molars are one-third to one-half formed. Crown completion of the second primary molars occurs approximately 1 year after birth (Table 12–2). Once the tooth erupts into the oral cavity, mineralization continues throughout life topically from saliva, food, fluids, dentifrices, oral rinses, and so on. Table 12–3 shows how nutrition affects the developmental history of teeth.

There are two major distinctions between the mineralized tissues of the teeth and other body tissues:

1. Enamel does not contain any capillary or lymphatic vessels to transport nutrients. Therefore, chemical interchange in enamel occurs directly via external surface exchange. In contrast, dentinal tubules carry blood to the dentin systemically. Once the tooth erupts, the vascular supply of nutrients to enamel ceases, and further enamel effects become exclusively topical.
2. Consequently, mineralized dental tissues cannot repair themselves (other than some external re-mineralization). This is in contrast to bone, which is continually remodeling.

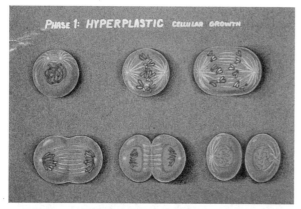

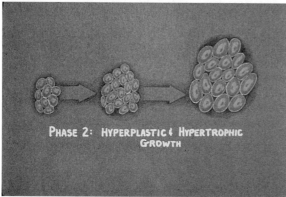

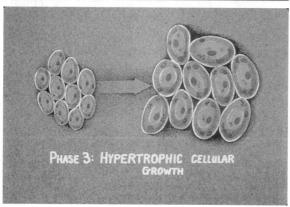

FIGURE 12–2 Cell hyperplasia versus hypertrophy.

Malnutrition has been related to decreased tooth size and a delayed eruption sequence in mice. In children, prenatal nutrition and the health of the pregnant mother may have an important impact on the child's developmental mineralization and the subsequent caries susceptibility of the child's teeth (Tinanoff, Palmer, 2000). Malnourished children may have delayed maxillary growth and general delays in tooth development and eruption in comparison to nutritionally normal children (Midda, Konig, 1994). Table 12–4 shows specific effects of malnutrition on oral development.

Malnutrition, although not the only cause, is one common contributor to linear enamel hypoplasia (Ismail, 1998). In human studies conducted in areas of the world where there is extreme malnutrition, developmental defects (enamel hypoplasia) of the primary teeth are common (Davies, 1988; Sweeney, Guzman, 1966). Surprisingly, a high prevalence (14%) of enamel hypoplasia also has been found in inner-city U.S. populations as well (Douglass, Wei, Zhang, Tinanoff, 1995). Several studies have shown strong associations between enamel hypoplasia and dental caries. Children with enamel hypoplasia reportedly have a 2.5 times greater risk of developing dental caries than children who do not have such defects (Davies, 1988; Seow, 1998). Children who are malnourished or have low birth weight (<2500 g), or both are more likely than well-nourished children to have hypomineralized primary teeth and increased risk of early childhood caries (ECC) (Ismail, 1998). A high incidence of enamel hypoplasia and subsequent dental caries in primary teeth has also been found in children born prematurely (Aine et al., 2000).

The eruption of primary teeth was found to be delayed in stunted and/or wasted infants in comparison with healthy infants. This delay in eruption persisted until age 2½ to 3. Furthermore, there was a significantly higher prevalence of dental caries in the primary and permanent dentitions of these nutritionally deprived children when compared with healthy children (Ismail, 1998). Indeed, even one mild or moderate episode of malnutrition during the first year of life is associated with increased caries in both deciduous and permanent teeth years later (Alvarez, 1995; Alvarez, Eguren, Caceda, Navia, 1990). This implies that if nutrient needs are not met in early life, the genetic potential of oral tissues and structures may also not be achieved, and permanent structural damage may result.

Effects of Specific Nutrient Deficiencies on Developing Dentition

Even moderate nutritional deficits can cause defects in tooth development. Nutritional factors can also affect tooth integrity, enamel solubility, and salivary flow and composition. In humans, deficiencies of protein,

TABLE 12–2 Calcification, Crown Completion, and Eruption Times of the Primary Teeth

		Tooth	*First Evidence of Calcification (Months in Utero)*	*Crown Completed (Months)*	*Eruption (Months)*
Primary dentition		Central incisor	3–4	4	$7\frac{1}{2}$
		Lateral incisor	$4\frac{1}{2}$	5	8
	Upper	Canine	$5\frac{1}{2}$	9	16–20
		First molar	5	6	12–16
		Second molar	6	10–12	20–30
		Central incisor	$4\frac{1}{2}$	4	$6\frac{1}{2}$
		Lateral incisor	$4\frac{1}{2}$	$4\frac{1}{4}$	7
	Lower	Canine	5	9	16–20
		First molar	5	6	12–16
		Second molar	6	10–12	20–30

Source: From Tinanoff, Palmer, 2000.

calories, vitamins A, C, and D, and iodine, and excesses of fluoride and vitamin D have all been shown to affect human dentition development (DePaola et al., 1999).

For example, protein-calorie malnutrition can result in enamel hypoplasia and dental caries. Low-protein diets can result in delayed tooth eruption. Vitamin A deficiency (usually associated with protein-calorie malnutrition) can affect epithelial tissue development, ameloblastic activity, odontogenic differentiation, and calcification (Boyle, 1933; Dreizen, 1989). Calcium, phosphorus, and vitamin D deficiencies can result in hypomineralization of developing teeth. This can decrease resistance to cariogenic challenges (Kisel'nikova et al., 1996; Leaver, 1971).

Vitamin D deficiency in children (rickets) is characterized by a widened layer of predentin and by hypoplastic defects in enamel. Vitamin D deficiency can also affect tooth structure in general and delay tooth eruption patterns and sequencing (Mellanby, 1918). Because the permanent incisors, cuspids, and first molars develop at the age in which rickets is most common, they are usually the teeth most affected (Dreizen, 1989) (Figure 12–3).

In vitamin C deficiency, the deciduous and permanent teeth have tiny pulpal hemorrhages. In older children, the pulp becomes hyperemic (engorged with blood), edematous, necrotic, and improperly calcified.

TABLE 12–3 Effects of Nutritional Problems on Tooth Development

Period	*Effects of Nutritional Problems*
Preeruptive period: Crown formation and mineralization within the jaw	• Developing enamel and dentin are susceptible to nutritional imbalances as any other developing tissues
Maturation period: Teeth are erupting into oral cavity and roots are forming	• Deficiencies affect secretory or maturation stages of enamel formation • Secretory stage deficiencies → hypoplastic lesions • Maturation stage deficiencies → hypomineralized defects
Maintenance: Teeth are functioning in the oral cavity	• Lack of constant mineralization from saliva, food, beverages, and oral care products results in decreased resistance to dental caries

Source: Adapted from DePaola D, Faine M, Palmer C: Nutrition in relation to dental medicine. In Shils M, Olsen JA, Shike M, Ross AC (eds): *Modern Nutrition in Health Disease*, 9th ed. Baltimore: Williams & Wilkins, 1999: 1099–1124. Reprinted with permission of Lippincott Williams & Wilkins, © 1999.

TABLE 12–4 Effects of Specific Nutrients on Developing Dentition

Nutrient	Deficiency or Excess
Vitamins	
Vitamin C	**Deficiency:**
	Mild: Exaggerated tissue response to and increased risk of infection; blood vessel fragility; increased periodontal signs and symptoms; delayed wound healing
	Severe: Scurvy red, swollen gingival; gingival friability and bleeding on provocation; interdental papillary infusions; petechiae; sore, burning mouth; increased risk of candidiasis; subperiosteal hemorrhages; periodontal destruction; increased tooth mobility and exfoliation; soft tissue ulceration; teeth malformation with normal enamel but inadequate dentin that can easily fracture
	Excess: Chronic overdosing can increase metabolism of vitamin C as an adaptation; rebound scurvy may occur after dose normalization
Vitamin D	**Deficiency:** Abnormal bone regeneration; osteoporosis; osteomalacia; incomplete calcification of teeth and alveolar bone; rickets
	Excess: Pulp calcification; enamel hypoplasia
Vitamin K	**Deficiency:** Increased risk of bleeding and candidiasis
Vitamin A	**Deficiency:** Inadequate differentiation of cells leading to impaired healing and tissue regeneration; desquamation of oral mucosa; early keratinization of mucosa (keratosis); increased risk of candidiasis, gingival hypertrophy, and inflammation; leukoplakia, decreased taste sensitivity, xerostomia, disturbed or arrested enamel development leading to poor or absent calcification and hypoplasia in mature teeth
	Severe: May lead to irregular tubular dentin formation and increased caries risk
	Excess: Impairs cell differentiation and epithelialization, resulting in delayed and impaired healing of oral tissues mimicking signs and symptoms of deficiency
B-complex in general	**Deficiency:** Angular cheilosis of lips; leukoplakia; burning tongue; papillary atrophy; magenta tongue; fissuring; glossitis
B_2 (riboflavin)	**Deficiency:** Angular cheilosis; atrophy of filiform papillae; enlarged fungiform papillae; shiny red lips; magenta tongue; sore tongue
B_3 (niacin)	**Deficiency:** Angular cheilosis; mucositis; stomatitis; oral pain; ulceration; denuded tongue; glossitis; glossodynia (tongue: tips are red, swollen, beefy, dorsum is smooth and dry); ulcerative gingivitis
Folic acid	**Deficiency:** Angular cheilosis; mucositis; stomatitis; sore or burning mouth; increased risk of candidiasis; inflamed gingiva glossitis (tongue: red, swollen tip or borders, slick bald pale dorsum); apthous-type ulcers
B_6 (pyridoxine)	**Deficiency:** Angular cheilosis; sore, burning mouth; glossitis; glossodynia
B_{12} (cynocobalamin)	**Deficiency:** Angular cheilosis; sore, burning mouth; mucositis/stomatitis; hemorrhagic gingival; halitosis; epithelial dysplasia of oral mucosa; oral paresthesia (numbness, tingling); detachment of periodontal fibers; loss or distortion of taste; glossitis; glossodynia (tongue: beefy red, smooth, glossy); delayed wound healing; xerostomia; bone loss; apthous-type ulcers
Minerals	
Fluoride	**Deficiency:** Decreased resistance to dental caries
	Excess: Fluorosis leading to enamel hypoplasia: *mild* = mottled enamel (white spots)/high caries resistance; milder signs of toxicity are esthetically unpleasant but increase caries resistance; *moderate* = unsightly brown stain/high caries resistance; *severe* = hypoplasia of enamel, with decreased caries resistance; more severe toxicity results in interference with amelogenesis and decreased caries resistance

Iron	*Deficiency:* Angular cheilosis; pallor of lips and oral mucosa; sore, burning tongue; atrophy/denudation of filiform papillae; glossitis; increased risk of candidiasis
Calcium	*Deficiency:* Incomplete calcification of teeth; rickets; osteomalacia; excessive bone resorption and bone fragility; osetoporosis; increased tendency to hemorrhage; increased tooth mobility and premature loss
Copper	*Deficiency:* Decreased trabeculae of alveolar bone; decreased tissue vascularity; increased tissue fragility
Zinc	*Deficiency:* Loss or distortion of taste and smell acuity; loss of tongue sensation; delayed wound healing; impaired keratinization of epithelial cells; eptithelial thickening; atrophic oral mucosa; increased susceptibility to periodontal disease and candidiasis; xerostomia; increased susceptibility to caries if present during tooth formation
Magnesium	*Deficiency:* Alveolar bone fragility; gingival hypertrophy
Phosphorus	*Deficiency:* Incomplete calcification of teeth; increased susceptibility to caries if present during tooth development; increased susceptibility to periodontal disease via effects on alveolar bone
Other nutrients	
Carbohydrates	*Deficiency:* Caries rate generally decreases when carbohydrate intake decreases in populations and individuals *Excess:* Increased frequency of any carbohydrates (other than fiber) is a causative risk factor for dental caries; cariogenic characteristics include physical form of foods, constancy of intake, total oral contact time with caries-susceptible dentition
Fats	*Deficiency:* No direct effect; difficult to get deficiency *Excess:* No direct effect, but fats may coat teeth and protect them against cariogenic challenges
Proteins	*Deficiency:* Defects in composition, eruption pattern, and resistance to decay during periods of tooth development; increased susceptibility to infection in soft tissues; poor healing and tissue regeneration
Water	*Deficiency:* Dehydration and fragility of epithelial tissue; decreased muscle strength for chewing; xerostomia; burning tongue

Source: DePaola D, Faine M, Palmer C: Nutrition in relation to dental medicine. In Shils M, Olsen JA, Shike M, Ross AC (eds): *Modern Nutrition in Health Disease*, 9th ed. Baltimore: Williams & Wilkins, 1999: 1099–1124. Reprinted with permission of Lippincott Williams & Wilkins, © 1999.

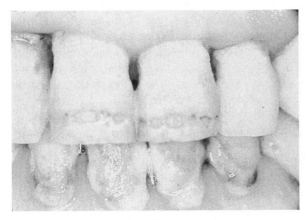

FIGURE 12-3 Dental malformations due to malnutrition.

The dentin is irregularly formed and has odontoblastic degeneration (Boyle, 1934).

Children born to mothers with severe goiter (iodine deficiency) have greatly delayed eruption of primary and secondary teeth. Altered patterns of craniofacial growth and development result in malocclusions (Dreizen, 1989).

In summary, malnutrition can result in abnormal and delayed development of teeth and surrounding structures and contribute to increased caries risk in primary teeth in children (Alvarez et al., 1990). The effects of malnutrition on caries risk are mediated by changes in salivary composition and volume (Johnson, 1993) and enamel defects (decreased resistance or increased enamel solubility) (Aponte-Merced, Navia, 1980; Seow, 1998).

Effects of Specific Nutrients on Mandible Formation

Specific nutrients also have been studied for their association with mandible development. One cross-sectional human study found a significant positive correlation between vitamin C intake and bone density, with higher intake resulting in denser bone (Clark, Navia, Manson-Hing, Duncan, 1990).

Controlled animal studies have also shown associations between nutrition and mandible formation. An early study of malnourished pigs reported reduced mandible size but normal tooth size, resulting in crowding of teeth, marked attrition of masticatory surfaces, and delayed dental development due to wide pulp chambers and open root apices. The pigs also had decreased osteogenic and osteoclastic acti, and the bone was thinner than with the well-nourished pigs (Guerrero et al., 1973).

Many studies have shown that rats fed high-calcium diets had greater alveolar bone density than did calcium-deficient rats (Ericsson, Ekberg, 1975), and that low-calcium diets resulted in a decreased quantity of alveolar bone which was reversible with calcium supplementation (Messer, Goebel, Wilcox, 1981).

Role of Mastication, Diet Consistency, and Texture in Oral Development

Many animal studies have concluded that a firm diet enhances proper growth and development when compared with a soft diet. Specifically, diet consistency has been shown to affect growth of the mandible and maxilla, and proper tooth eruption in animals. However, the implications for these findings in humans are unknown due to the unethical nature of conducting such studies in people.

For example, rats fed soft diets had smaller body mass and smaller mandibles and condyle, which were less radiographically dense than those fed hard food diets (Barber, Green, Cox, 1963). The group fed the soft diets also had significantly decreased width of the maxillary arch, in comparison to the group fed the hard food diet (Beecher, Corruccini, 1981). A study evaluating the effects of diet consistency and mechanical force on growth and development of alveolar bone in rats concluded that a softer diet resulted in decreased bone mineral density, trabecular bone volume, and thickness (Mavropoulos, Kiliaridis, Bresin, Ammann, 2004).

A related study in monkeys looked at diet consistency in relationship to craniofacial and occlusal development, and concluded that the developing craniofacial region (especially the dentition), needs a certain amount of mechanical stress to attain its proper configuration. The growth of various aspects of the oral cavity (maxillary length, width, palatal height) was greater for monkeys fed the hard diet, the intra-arch tooth displacement was less, and the maxillary and mandibular arch widths and lengths were larger (Beecher, Corruccini, Freeman, 1983).

Role of Nutrition and Hydration in Salivary Gland Development and Function

Malnutrition can affect salivary gland development, as well as salivary flow and composition. Because saliva is an important protective factor in the oral cavity, defects in salivary function may be a contributing factor in dental caries in all age groups (Johnson, 1993).

Again, animal studies have elucidated relationships between nutrition and salivary development and function. Protein is necessary in cell replication and thus is important in the growth of glands such as the salivary gland. Protein deficiencies in mice resulted in smaller salivary glands with less protein in the glandular tissue than in well-nourished mice (Humphreys-Behert, Hollis, Carlson, 1982; Jacobs, 1983).

Food consistency may also affect salivary function. In a study comparing solid and liquid diets in rats, solid food elicited a significantly higher parotid salivary flow (Ito, Morikawa, Inenaga, 2001). Another study ligated the submandibular and sublingual ducts of rats to observe parotid gland function under partial desalivation. Parotid gland weight and amylase activity were greatest in rats fed a powdered diet and least in those fed a liquid diet when comparing powdered, solid pellet, and liquid diets. The authors concluded that contact of dry food with the oral mucosa more likely caused functional changes in the parotid glands of these rats than the masticatory movement of the jaw used to eat dry food (Kurahashi, 2002). Dietary changes may contribute to differences in submandibular gland enzyme activity during maturation as well (Kuntsal, Firat, Sirin, 2003; Przybylo, Litynska, Hoja-Lukowicz, Kremser, 2004). Dehydration-induced xerostomia can also affect parotid salivary gland function in rats (Ito et al., 2001).

Effects of Nutritional Excesses on Oral Growth and Development

Although nutritional excesses have not been studied as extensively as deficiencies, nutrient excesses can have harmful oral effects on oral development as well. Harmful effects of hypervitaminosis D have been reported in the teeth of animals (Becks, Collins, Axelrod, 1946) and humans (Blank, Scanlon, Sinks, Lett, Falk, 1995; Giunta, 1998; Pindborg, 1970). Excess vitamin D results in hypercalcemia (due to acceleration of intestinal calcium absorption) and bone resorption. This leads to disturbances in tooth matrix formation and calcification and can result in either hypoplasia or hypocalcification, depending on the timing of the insult. Because enamel does not remodel, disturbances occurring during development remain as a permanent record. Two specific cases detailed in the vitamin D section of Chapter 8 report developmental defects resulting from excessive vitamin D consumption (overuse of vitamin supplements in one case, overfortification of milk with vitamin D by a local dairy in the other). Defects included linear hypoplastic defects on several deciduous and permanent teeth, and abnormal changes in pulp chambers.

NUTRITIONAL IMPLICATIONS IN ORAL CLEFT FORMATION

Cleft lip/palate is one of the most common birth defects and is estimated to affect 1 in 600 live births for whites and 1 in 1,850 live births for African Americans (*Oral Health in America*, 2000; van der Put et al., 1999). Oral clefts, which consist of cleft lip, cleft palate, and the combined defect, occur as a result of the failure of the normal fusion of the palatal or labial processes during embryogenesis.

There is a large body of research evaluating the effects of diet and/or specific nutrients on the formation of oral clefts. These studies include animal, human, and in vitro designs and have focused primarily on the role of multivitamins, folic acid, and vitamin A (Tables 12–5 and 12–6).

The results of studies evaluating the effect of multivitamin use (multivitamins, vitamin A, and folic acid) on decreased risk of oral cleft development have been equivocal. Some studies (Shaw, Schaffer, Velie, Morland, Harris, 1995; Tolarova, 1982, 1987; Werler, Shapiro, Mitchell, 1993) have shown a protective effect, whereas others have not (Czeizel, 1993; Czeizel, Dudas, 1992). It is possible that if an effect does exist, it may not

TABLE 12–5 Summary on Nutrition and Birth Defects

Nutrient	Type of Study	Findings
Vitamins with folic acid	Humans	Taking supplements with folic acid reduced subsequent clefts in women who had had babies with clefts previously. Other studies found no effect.
Folic acid	Humans	Women who took folic acid antagonists had children with clefts. Folic acid prevents neural tube defects, which are embryologically related to clefts.
Vitamin A excesses	Animals	Vitamin A in large doses decreased DNA synthesis. Vitamin A infusions in amniotic fluid resulted in increased clefts. Timing and length of supplementations has a major effect on development of clefts. Genetics may play a role in that some strains of rats are more susceptible than others. Incidence of clefts and maxillary bone development may be linked.
Vitamin A excesses	Humans	Teratogenic (causes birth defects). Inconclusive on oral clefts. Some increase in neural crest abnormalities.
Alcohol	Animals	Enhances the effect of vitamin A in cleft formation. Alcohol causes clefts at vitamin A levels that did not cause clefts alone.

TABLE 12–6 Possible Effects of Folic Acid on Oral Cleft Development

- Insufficient folic acid intake may be related to cleft etiology.
- Clefts have been seen in offspring of women taking folate antagonists during pregnancy.
- Folic acid supplementation periconceptionally results in reduction of neural tube defects that may be related to oral clefts.
- Neural tube defects and oral clefts are both considered midline defects and occur together more often than by chance.
- Folic acid protects against cleft development.

be very strong and may be mediated by other factors (e.g., gene–environment interactions).

Oral clefts may be embryologically related to neural tube defects (e.g., spina bifida) because facial and tooth tissue develop from neural crest cells that originate from the dorsolateral aspect of the forming neural tube (Bhaskar, 1990). Neural tube defects and oral clefts are both considered midline defects and occur together more frequently than would be expected by chance (Khoury, Cordero, Mulinare, Optiz, 1989). For oral clefts several areas of research suggest that folic acid deficiency may be related to cleft development. For example:

- Folic acid antagonists during pregnancy (methotrexate, aminopterin [4-pteroylglutamic acid], and anticonvulsants) were associated with oral clefts in the offspring (Friis, 1979; Hecht, Annegers, Kutland, 1989; Janz, 1975; Milunsky, Graef, Gaynor, l968; Nakane et al., 1980; Thiersch, 1952).
- Folic acid supplementation during the periconceptional period (around the time of conception) has been well documented to result in a substantial reduction in the occurrence of neural tube defects (NTDs) (Czeizel, Dudas, l992; Milunsky et al., 1989; MMWR, 1993; Shaw, Schaffer, et al., 1995; Werler et al., 1993).
- A number of human studies have shown a protective association between use of folic acid and/or multivitamins and the risk of oral clefts (Briggs, 1976; Conway, 1958; Peer, Gordon, Bernhard, 1964; Shaw, Lammer, Wasserman, O'Malky,

Tolarova, 1995; Tolarova, 1982, 1987; Werler, Hayes, Loiuk, Mitchell, 1999).
- Studies of several animal models have demonstrated a protective effect of folic acid on the risk of oral clefts (DePaola, Mandell, 1981; Evans, Nelson, Aslinq, 1951; Jordan, Wilson, Schumacher, 1977).

This protective effect has not been observed in all studies, however (Czeizel, Dudas, 1992; Hayes, Werler, Willett, Mitchell, 1996). Most of the earlier studies did not report information on timing of supplement use, compliance, or possible confounding factors.

A case control study by Hayes et al. (1996) found that vitamins containing folic acid had no protective effect on oral cleft formation. In this study, the controls were mothers of infants with other congenital malformations excluding NTDs and midline defects. In a subsequent study, however, when controls were infants without any type of malformation, a protective effect for multivitamin use was observed for cleft palate only (Werler et al., 1999). It may be that if folic acid has a protective effect against many malformations, the study that used controls with other malformations would not observe a protective effect for clefts alone.

Numerous animal studies have shown relationships between excess vitamin A consumption and the risk of developing oral clefts. The dosages and timing of the supplementation and genetic factors seem to be critical factors. Alcohol in combination with vitamin A greatly enhances the risk of clefting.

Maxillary bone development and the incidence of cleft palate may be linked, as hypervitaminosis A causes both clefting and heterotopic cartilage in the maxillary region. One hypothesis is that the cartilage does not exhibit the same pressures on the palate noted in bone growth. This growth is thought to help push the palatal shelves down from their vertical to horizontal positions, thus aiding in fusion (Nanda, 1970).

Although vitamin A toxicity is well known to be teratogenic (causing birth defects) in humans, there are fewer human studies than animal studies evaluating the role of vitamin A in oral cleft etiology. The few studies that have been conducted have been inconclusive. One study showed an increase in neural crest anomalies in women taking vitamin A supplements (Rothman et al., 1995), whereas another study found no increased risk of oral clefts among women taking vitamin A supplements (Shaw et al., 1996).

SUMMARY AND IMPLICATIONS FOR DENTISTRY

Adequate nutrition is essential from the earliest periods of development. Nutrient deficiencies or toxicities in early oral development can result in permanent damage to the developing oral structures. Other aspects of the diet, such as diet consistency, have been shown to affect growth of the mandible and maxilla, as well as tooth eruption in animals, but have not been studied in humans.

Ongoing research on harmful effects of nutrition on oral growth indicate that excess vitamin A can be a potent teratogen that can cause oral defects in animals. Protective effects of folic acid have also been shown in animal studies but not in humans as yet, probably owing to the complexity of factors involved.

To promote optimal growth and development of the oral cavity the dental health care team needs to emphasize to patients the importance of:

- An adequate diet throughout pregnancy
- Adequate intake of folic acid throughout the childbearing years
- Avoiding doses of vitamin A that exceed the recommended daily allowances
- Avoiding excessive doses of all vitamins (especially when pregnant)
- Optimum infant and child nutrition from birth

QUESTIONS PATIENTS MIGHT ASK

Q. Do I need to eat differently for good oral health than I do for general health during my pregnancy?

A. No, a good diet, which includes appropriate servings from the food pyramid (MyPyramid) will support your oral and overall health and that of your baby.

Q. Shouldn't I take supplements as a margin of safety to make sure my baby gets enough vitamins and minerals?

A. Your physician may recommend a daily multivitamin/mineral supplement for you. However, it is important to avoid taking large doses of vitamins, especially vitamin A, as it can cause irreversible harm to your baby.

Q. I've heard that folic acid supplements will help prevent birth defects in my baby. Should I be taking them after I get pregnant?

A. Actually, you should be sure to get enough folic acid *before* you get pregnant because the major effects of this vitamin occur in the first few weeks of pregnancy, before you may realize you're pregnant. A multivitamin/mineral supplement with folic acid will do the trick. In addition, nowadays many grain products like bread are fortified with folic acid for this very purpose.

CASE STUDY

History: Martha is a 27-year-old woman who works as a sales representative for an international cosmetics company. She travels frequently due to the nature of her job. She married 3 years ago, and is looking forward to having a child. She comes to the dental office twice a year for a checkup.

Medical history: Martha has mild hypertension, but no other medical problems. She is not taking any medication. Her last physical examination revealed blood pressure 140/90. Her total cholesterol, LDL cholesterol, and HDL cholesterol levels were within normal range. She has a BMI of 26 which places her within normal limits. Diabetes runs on her mother's side of the family; her grandfather and aunt both have Type 2 diabetes.

Dental history and examination: Martha has all her teeth. She had a plaque score of only 40% plaque free and had extensive calculus, especially on the lingual aspects of mandibular incisors. She has four new caries lesions. She brushes her teeth twice daily and uses dental floss once a week. She reports bleeding when she brushes her teeth and uses dental floss. She uses a fluoridated dentifrice but does not use any mouthwash.

Diet history: Martha eats most of her meals away from home and on the run. She does not usually eat breakfast. She just grabs items at the local store such as a candy bar, popcorn, and crackers. As she tries to meet as many customers as she can, she always gets takeout from a fast-food store, and rarely has a sit-down

(*continued*)

CASE STUDY (CONTINUED)

meal during the day. During weekends, she prefers eating TV dinners or calling for pizza delivery because she is "too tired to cook." Neither she nor her husband like fruits, so they never buy them.

24-Hour Recall

Breakfast:
Nothing or crackers/
    candy bar/popcorn
Mid-morning:
    1 cup of coffee with
    2 sugars and cream

Lunch:
Tuna salad sandwich
1 can of soda
1 small pack of chips
Afternoon:
    1 cup of coffee with
    2 sugars and cream

Dinner:
2 slices of pepperoni
    pizza
1 can of soda

Evening:
1/2 cup ice cream

Questions:

1. Is Martha's diet nutritionally adequate? Why or why not?
2. Are there any diet-related dental or oral problems?
3. Are there any risks to Martha or her baby if she becomes pregnant?
4. What would be appropriate nutritional and dental suggestions for Martha?

REFERENCES

Aine L, Backstrom MC, Maki R, Kuusela AL, Koivisto AM, Ikonen RS, Maki M: Enamel defects in primary and permanent teeth of children born prematurely. *J Oral Pathol Med* 2000 Sep; 29(8): 403–9.

Alvarez JO, Eguren JC, Caceda J, Navia JM: The effect of nutritional status on the age distribution of dental caries in the primary teeth. *J Dent Res* 1990; 69(9):1564–66.

Alvarez JO: Nutrition, tooth development, and dental caries. *Am J Clin Nutr* 1995; 61(2):410S–16S.

Aponte-Merced L, Navia JMM: Pre-eruptive protein-energy malnutrition and acid solubility of rat molar enamel surfaces. *Arch Oral Biol* 1980; 25:701–5.

Barber CG, Green LJ, Cox, GJ: Effects of the physical consistency of diet on the condylar growth of the rat mandible. *J Dent Res* 1963; 42(3):848–51.

Becks H, Collins D, Axelrod H: The effects of a single massive dose of vitamin D2 (D-stoss therapy) on oral and other tissues of young dogs. *Am J Orthodont Oral Surg (Orthodontic)* 1946; 32:452–62.

Beecher RM, Corruccini, RS: Effects of dietary consistency on craniofacial and occlusal development in the rat angle. *Orthodontist* 1981; 51(1):61–69.

Beecher RM, Corruccini RS, Freeman M: Craniofacial correlates of dietary consistency in a nonhuman primate. *J Craniofac Genet Dev Biol* 1983; 3:193–202.

Bhaskar, SN (ed): *Orban's Oral Histology and Embryology*, 11th ed. St. Louis: Mosby, 1990.

Blank S, Scanlon KS, Sinks TH, Lett S, Falk H: An outbreak of hypervitaminosis D associated with the overfortification of milk from a home-delivery dairy. *Am J Public Health* 1995; 85:656–59.

Boyle PE: Manifestations of vitamin-A deficiency in a human tooth-germ. *J Dent Res* 1933; 13:39–50.

Boyle PE: The tooth germ in acute scurvy. *J Dent Res* 1934; 14:172.

Briggs RM: Vitamin supplementation as a possible factor in the incidence of cleft lip/palate deformities in humans. *Clin Plast Surg* 1976; 3:647–52.

Clark DE, Navia JM, Manson-Hing LR, Duncan HE: Evaluation of alveolar bone in relation to nutritional status during pregnancy. *J Dent Res* 1990; 69(3):890–95.

Conway H: Effect of supplemental vitamin therapy on the limitation of incidence of cleft lip and cleft palate in humans. *Plast Reconstr Surg* 1958; 22:450–53.

Czeizel AE: Prevention of congenital abnormalities by periconceptional multivitamin supplementation. *Br Med J* 1993; 306:1645–48.

Czeizel AE, Dudas I: Prevention of the first occurrence of neural tube defects by periconceptional vitamin supplementation. *N Engl J Med* 1992; 327:1832–35.

Davies GN: Early childhood caries—a synopsis. *Commun Dent Oral Epidemiol* 1988; 26:(Suppl 1):106–16.

DePaola D, Faine M, Palmer C: Nutrition in relation to dental medicine. In Shils M, Olsen JA, Shike M, Ross AC (eds): *Modern Nutrition in Health and Disease*, 9th ed. Baltimore: Williams & Wilkins, 1999.

DePaola DP, Mandella RD: Folate deficiency and in vitro palatogenesis I: Effects of a folate-deficient culture on rabbit palate fusion and folate pools. *J Craniofac Gene Dev Biol* 1981; 1:5–13.

Douglass JM, Wei Y, Zhang BX, Tinanoff N: Caries prevalence and pattern in three- to six-year-old Beijing children. *Commun Dent Oral Epidemiol* 1995; 23:340–43.

Dreizen S: The mouth as an indicator of internal nutritional problems. *Pediatrician* 1989; 16:139–46.

Ericsson Y, Ekberg O: Dietetically provoked general and alveolar osteopenia in rats and its prevention or cure by calcium and fluoride. *J Periodont Res* 1975; 10:256–69.

Evans HM, Nelson MM, Asling CW: Multiple congenital abnormalities resulting from acute folic acid deficiency during gestation. *Science* 1951; 114:479.

Friis ML: Epilepsy among parents of children with facial clefts. *Epilepsia* 1979; 20:69–76.

Giunta JL: Dental changes in hypervitaminosis D. *Oral Surg Oral Med Oral Pathol Oral Radiol Endodont* 1998; 85(4):410–13.

Guerrero S, Otto B, Lacassie Y, Gattas V, Aquayo M, Hasbun J, et al.: The effect of nutrition on dental and craniofacial development. *J Dent Res* 1973; 55:345–52.

Hayes C, Werler MM, Willett WC, Mitchell AA: A case control study of periconceptional folic acid supplementation and oral clefts. *Am J Epidemiol* 1996; 143:1229–34.

Hecht JT, Annegers JF, Kutland LT: Epilepsy and clefting disorders: Lack of evidence of familial association. *Am J Med Genet* 1989; 33:244–47.

Humphreys-Behert M, Hollis D, Carlson D: Comparative developmental analysis of the parotid, submandibular and sublingual glands in the neonatal rat. *Biochem J* 1982; 204:673–79.

Ismail AI: The role of early dietary habits in dental caries development. *Special Care in Dent* 1998; 18(1):40–45.

Ito K, Morikawa M, Inenaga K: The effect of food consistency and dehydration on reflex parotid and submandibular salivary secretion in conscious rats. *Arch Oral Biol* 2001; 46:353–63.

Janz D: The teratogenic risk of antiepileptic drugs. *Epilepsia* 1975; 16:159–69.

Johnson DA: Effects of diet and nutrition on salivary composition. In Bowen WH, Tabak LA (eds): *Cariology for the Nineties*. Rochester, NY: University of Rochester Press, 1993.

Jordan RL, Wilson JG, Schumacher HJ: Embryotoxicity of the folate antagonist methotrexate in rats and rabbits. *Teratology* 1977; 15:73–80.

Khoury MJ, Cordero JF, Mulinare J, Opitz JM: Selected midline defect associations: A population study. *Pediatrics* 1989; 84:266–72.

Kisel'nikova LP, Leont'ev VK: The effect of the initial level of mineralization of the erupting molars on their caries susceptibility. *Stomatologiia (Mosk)* 1996; 75(2):55–8. Russian.

Kuntsal L, Firat D, Sirin Y: Prevention of liquid-diet-induced damages on submandibular glands by selenium supplementation in rats. *Tohoku J Exp Med* 2003; 210:191–99.

Kurahashi M: The effect of dietary consistency and water content on the parotid glands of submandibular and sublingual duct-ligated rats. *Arch Oral Biol* 2002; 47:369–74.

Leaver AG: Interrelationships of calcium, phosphorus, and Vitamin D in the bones and teeth of the rat. *Clin Orthop* 1971; 78:90–107.

Mavropoulos A, Kiliaridis S, Bresin A, Ammann P: Effect of different masticatory functional and mechanical demands on the structural adaptation of the mandibular alveolar bone in young growing rats. *Bone* 2004; 35:191–97.

Mellanby M: An experimental study of the influence of diet on teeth formation. *Lancet* 1918; 2:767.

Messer H, Goebel N, Wilcox A: Comparison of bone loss from different skeletal sites during acute calcium deficiency in mice. *Arch Oral Biol* 1981; 26:1001–4.

Midda M, Konig KG: Nutrition, diet, and oral health. *Int Dent J* 1994; 44:599–612.

Milunsky A, Graef JW, Gaynor MF: Methotrexate-induced congenital malformations. *J Pediat* 1968; 72:790–95.

Milunsky A, Jick H, Jick SS, Bruell CL, MacLaughlin DS, Rothman KJ, et al.: Multivitamin/folic acid supplementation in early pregnancy reduces the prevalence of neural tube defects. *JAMA* 1989; 262:2847–52.

MMWR: Recommendations for use of folic acid to reduce number of spina bifida cases and other neural tube defects. *JAMA* 1993; 269:1233–35.

Nakane Y, Okuma T, Takahashi R, Sato Y, Wada T, Sato T, et al.: Multi-institutional study on the teratogenicity and fetal toxicity of antiepileptic drugs: a collaborative study group in Japan. *Epilepsia* 1980; 21:663–80.

Nanda R: Maxillomandibular ankylosis and cleft palate in rat embryos. *J Dent Res* 1970; 49(5):1086–90.

Oral Health in America: A Report of the Surgeon General. Rockville, MD: U.S. Department of Health and Human Services, National Institute of Dental and Craniofacial Research, National Institutes of Health, 2000.

Peer LA, Gordon HW, Bernhard WG: Effect of vitamins on human teratology. *Plast Reconstr Surg* 1964; 34:358–62.

Pindborg JJ: *Pathology of the Dental Hard Tissues.* Philadelphia: WB Saunders, 1970.

Przybylo M, Litynska A, Hoja-Lukowicz D, Kremser E: Rat submandibular gland during the maturation process: Changes in enzyme activities, protein and lectin-binding profiles. *Physiol Res* 2004: 53:317–26.

Rothman KJ, Moore LL, Singer MR, Nquyen US, Mannino S, Milunsky A: Teratogenocity of high vitamin A intake. *JAMA* 1995; 333:1369–73.

Seow WK: Biological mechanisms of early childhood caries. *Commun Dent Oral Epidemiol* 1998; 26(Suppl 1):8–27.

Shaw GM, Lammer EJ, Wasserman CR, O'Malky CD, Tolarova MM: Risks of orofacial clefts in children born to women using multivitamins containing folic acid periconceptionally [see comments]. *Lancet* 1995; 346(8972):393–96.

Shaw GM, Schaffer D, Velie EM, Morlard K, Harris JA: Periconceptional vitamin use, dietary folate, and the occurrence of neural tube defects. *Epidemiology* 1995; 6:219–26.

Shaw GM, Wasserman CR, Block G, Lammer EJ: High material vitamin A intake and risk of anomalies of structures with a cranial neural crest cell contribution. *Lancet* 1996; 347:899–900.

Sweeney EA, Guzman M: Oral conditions in children from three highland villages in Guatemala. *Arch Oral Biol* 1966; 11:687–98.

Thiersch JB: Therapeutic abortions with a folic acid antagonist 4-aminopteroxyolutamic acid administered by the oral route. *Am J Obstet Gynecol* 1952; 63:1298–1304.

Tinanoff N, Palmer CA: Dietary determinants of dental caries and dietary recommendations for preschool children. *J Public Health Dent* 2000; 60(3):197–206.

Tolarova M: Orofacial clefts in Czechoslovakia. Incidence, genetics, and prevention of cleft lip and palate over a 19-year period. *Scand J Plast Reconst Surg* 1987; 21:19–25.

Tolarova M: Periconceptional supplementation with vitamins and folic acid to prevent recurrence of cleft lip. *Lancet* 1982; 2(8291):217.

van der Put NJM, Gabreels F, Stevens EMB, Smeitink JAM, Trijbels FJM, Eskes TKAB, et al.: A second common mutation in the methylenetetrahydrofolate reductase gene: an additional risk factor for neural-tube defects? *Am J Hum Genet* 1999; 62:1044–51.

Wefel JS, Dodds MWJ: Oral biologic defenses and the demineralization and remineralization of teeth. In Harris NO, Garcia-Godoy F (eds): *Primary Preventive Dentistry*, 5th ed. Stamford, CT: Appleton & Lange, 1999.

Werler M, Hayes C, Loiuk C, Mitchell A: Multivitamin use and multiple congenital anomalies. *Am J Epid* 1999; 150: 675–82.

Werler MM, Shapiro S, Mitchell AA: Periconceptional folic acid exposure and risk of occurrent neural tube defects. *JAMA* 1993; 269:1257–61.

Chapter **13**

Diet, Nutrition, and Teeth

Connie Mobley

OBJECTIVES

The student will be able to:

- Discuss the concept of enamel demineralization and remineralization.
- Explain how dental erosion differs from the demineralization of caries.
- Describe the caries process and the role of bacteria.
- Discuss the studies related to diet and caries.
- List the major risk factors for caries formation.
- List cariogenic and cariostatic food factors.
- Discuss the roles of saliva and oral hygiene in caries.

INTRODUCTION

Systemic nutrition affects the development, regeneration, and repair of both hard and soft oral tissues such as supporting bone, periodontal tissue, mucosal tissue, salivary glands, and dentinal, and pulpal tissues (DePaola, Faine, Palmer, 1999). Tooth enamel, however, is influenced by systemic nutrition only before eruption. After eruption, the effects of diet are exclusively topical and include enamel demineralization and dental caries. Food choices and dietary patterns are essential determinants of dental caries. In turn, the discomfort and possible tooth loss caused by dental caries can affect food choices and dietary patterns, and may lead to dietary inadequacies and compromised nutritional status.

This chapter focuses on:

- the interactions between diet and the oral environment that can harm or stabilize tooth enamel.
- the etiology and pathobiology of caries as related to dietary components and patterns.
- special considerations associated with the needs of special populations.

TOOTH ENAMEL INTEGRITY

As the hardest substance in the body, tooth enamel can be damaged only by trauma or by the effects of acid demineralization. Demineralization, or loss of the tooth's mineral structure, begins when the pH of the enamel surface drops to below 5.7 to 5.5 (Newbrun, 1989). The normal pH of the oral cavity is around 6, which is considered neutral. The dynamic process of tooth demineralization and remineralization is guided by the interaction of several factors: oral bacteria, salivary flow and composition, presence of fluoride, tooth integrity, and dietary habits. When the equilibrium of these factors shifts in the direction of demineralization, enamel dissolution occurs and caries is the end result. If the enamel demineralization has not reached the cementoenamel junction, calcium and phosphate (higher pH), as well as fluoride, can help remineralize previously demineralized areas. Tooth integrity (or stabilization) exists when these processes occur without any net loss of tooth mass. A tooth carious lesion results when the rate of demineralization exceeds the rate of remineralization over an extended time.

LOCAL EFFECTS OF DIET ON TEETH

Enamel Decalcification

Dental erosion is the loss of dental hard tissues (typically the enamel) caused by the local effect of acid on the teeth. The acid may come from dietary sources, such as citrus fruits (Asher, Read, 1987; Grobler, Senekal, Laubscher, 1990; Lussi, Jaeggi, Zero, 2004), acidogenic sports drinks (Milosevic, Kelly, McLean, 1997), snacks containing citrus acid (Dodds, Gragg, Rodriguez, 1997), carbonated beverages (Parry, Shaw, Arnaud, Smith, 2001), lemon-flavored iced tea (von Fraunhofer, Rogers, 2004), chewable vitamin C tablets, or excessive regurgitation of gastric contents into the mouth. Excessive consumption of acidic foods or beverages over time can cause enamel dissolution, especially when xerostomia (dry mouth) robs the teeth of the natural protection of saliva. It is important to differentiate this type of erosion from the caries process in which acid produced from plaque bacteria causes the enamel demineralization.

Dental Caries: The Caries Process

Dental caries is a dynamic process that involves demineralization of enamel and dentin by the products of bacterial metabolism (organic acids), with alternate periods of remineralization (Table 13–1). This pathological process occurs on a continuum, from early enamel microscopic demineralization, to gross macroscopic tissue destruction, to overt cavitation. Dental caries is considered a multifactorial disease, traditionally represented by Figure 13–1. This process requires a susceptible tooth, cariogenic bacteria in dental plaque, and a food source for the bacteria (fermentable carbohydrates). Protective factors, particularly saliva and its components, play an important role.

Soon after the teeth are cleaned, proteins from the saliva adsorb to the cleaned tooth and form the acquired enamel pellicle. This proteinaceous coating allows certain bacteria to start to colonize the tooth through protein interactions between the bacterial cell wall and the pellicle. The plaque thickens as it matures and contains many species of oral bacteria in a matrix of extracellular material. This material binds the bacteria together into an ecosystem. More than 500 species of bacteria are present in the mouth. A small proportion of these are acidogenic bacteria that use dietary sugars as an energy

TABLE 13–1   Terminology to Describe Foods and Their Specific Role
in the Progression of Caries

Term	Description
Acidogenic	Foods or beverages that readily cause a drop in plaque pH to <5.5 within 30 minutes.
Cariogenic	Foods or beverages that contain fermentable carbohydrates that can be metabolized by oral bacteria to cause a decrease in plaque pH to <5.5 and result in demineralization of tooth enamel and ultimately caries in animals and/or humans.
Anticariogenic	Foods or beverages that can prevent cariogenic activity when eaten before an acidogenic product.
Cariostatic	Foods or beverages that cannot be metabolized by dental plaque bacteria within 30 minutes and do not cause a drop in salivary pH to the critical level of <5.5.

source, produce acid, and are associated with the caries development (not all acidogenic bacteria are cariogenic). In the human population, the two species of interest are *Streptococcus mutans* and *Streptococcus sobrinus* (Loesche, 1986). *S. mutans* is now considered the major pathogenic bacterial species involved in the caries process. Evidence suggests that children are most likely to develop caries if *S. mutans* is acquired at an early age, although good oral hygiene and a noncariogenic diet may control the impact (Harris, Nicoll, Adair, Pine, 2004).

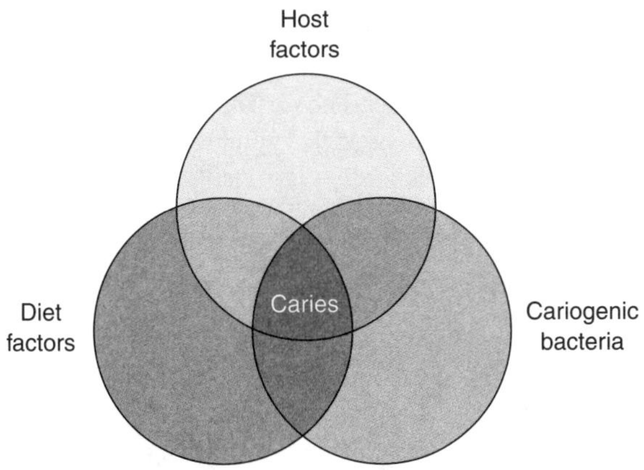

FIGURE 13–1   An etiologic model of dental caries: Caries occurs through the interaction of host factors (tooth, saliva flow, and composition), dietary factors, and bacterial factors.

The physiologic characteristics of the *S. mutans* that make them prime etiological agent in caries include their ability to:

1. adhere to tooth surfaces.
2. produce abundant insoluble extracellular polysaccharides from sucrose.
3. rapidly produce lactic acid from a number of sugar substrates.
4. be tolerant to acid.
5. produce intracellular polysaccharide stores. (Carlsson, 1984)

As a general rule, the cariogenic bacteria metabolize sugars to produce energy required for their growth and reproduction. The energy sources may be exogenous (from immediate food sources) or endogenous (from stored polysaccharide). Cariogenic bacteria can metabolize any monosaccharides or disaccharides for energy. Once within the cell, the end product, glucose, enters the Embden-Meyerhof glycolytic pathway, resulting in the formation of two 3-carbon pyruvate molecules from each 6-carbon glucose molecule, along with the generation of two molecules of adenosine triphosphate (ATP). Pyruvate can be converted to lactic acid (homofermentation) or other end products (heterofermentation), depending on a number of factors, including substrate concentrations. The result of this sugar catabolism is the production of organic acids in the dental plaque fluid, which lowers the plaque pH. As the pH decreases to around 5.2 to 5.5, the immediate tooth environment (interface between tooth and plaque) is no longer saturated with calcium and phosphate ions, and the tooth starts to demineralize (Figure 13–2). Once the decalcification reaches the dentinoenamel junction, acid decalcification of the dentin can progress, and the bacteria themselves can invade the protein of the dentin and destroy it through a process called proteolysis (Figure 13–3).

Carious lesions can occur in areas where plaque can sufficiently colonize such as:

- pit and fissure caries, found mainly on the occlusal surfaces of posterior teeth, and in lingual pits of the maxillary incisors.
- smooth surface caries that arises on intact enamel surfaces other than pits and fissures. Smooth surface caries can be further divided into free smooth surface caries (i.e., caries affecting the buccal and lingual tooth surfaces) and approximal caries, affecting the contact area(s) of adjoining tooth surfaces (i.e., mesial or distal surfaces).
- root surface caries, which might involve any exposed surface of the root.
- secondary, or recurrent, caries, which occurs on the tooth surface adjacent to an existing restoration.

The earliest clinically detectable stage of caries in the enamel is the incipient lesion. This is characterized by an opaque, white appearance. Although a certain amount of mineral loss has occurred, it is predominantly in the subsurface area of the enamel with the surface of the enamel essentially intact and amenable to

Chemistry of Dental Caries

Step 1
Sucrose ⟶ Dextrose ⟶ Lactic Acid

Step 2
Lactic Acid + Hydroxyapatite ⟶ Calcium Phosphate + Calcium Lactate + Water

Step 3
Tooth Organic Material + Proteolytic Bacteria ⟶ Decay

FIGURE 13–2 The caries process.

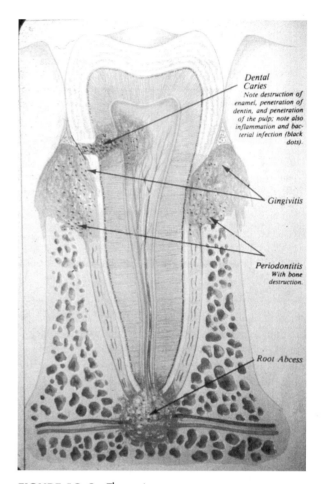

Dental Caries
Note destruction of enamel, penetration of dentin, and penetration of the pulp; note also inflammation and bacterial infection (black dots).

Gingivitis

Periodontitis
With bone destruction.

Root Abcess

FIGURE 13–3 The caries process.

remineralization. If the lesion progresses, demineralization continues to exceed remineralization. Further mineral loss eventually causes sufficient structural weakening of the enamel. The surface then breaks down, causing frank cavitation. At this point the only treatment option in most cases is the placement of a restoration (i.e., an amalgam filling or crown).

Trends in Caries Prevalence

Dental caries is traditionally viewed as a disease associated with sugar consumption, but dental caries may be more a disease of civilization. Prevalence is high in developed countries such as the United States, and low in developing countries, affecting 60 to 90% of school children (Blinkhorn, Davies, 1996; Petersen, 2003). Anthropological evidence suggests that as ancient populations increased sucrose consumption, their prevalence of caries increased (Moore, Corbett, 1978). Similarly, populations undergoing "Westernization" of their diets that includes higher sugar consumption have shown increased caries incidence. Conversely, caries rates declined in Europe (Sognnaes, 1948) and Japan (Takeuchi, 1961) during the sugar limitation of wartime.

There has been a decline in the number of decayed-missing-filled-surface (DMFS) rate in children, but an increase in adults, with fewer than 5% of persons over the age of 50 being free of caries (Bowen, 1994; DePaola et al., 1999). Data from the late 1980s indicate that 50% of 12-year-olds but only 20% of 17-year-olds were caries free (Kaste et al., 1996). Likewise only 2–3% of the elderly population were caries free, 41% were edentulous, and 57% had caries, missing teeth, or both (Miller, Brunelle, Carlos, Brown, Löe, 1987).

Caries rates also vary greatly within and between populations. Children of low socioeconomic groups and from certain ethnic minorities have higher levels of this disease (Blinkhorn, Davies, 1996; Petersen, 2003). When 3,000 Hispanic preschool children in South Texas were examined in the early 1990s, 28% presented with caries (Garcia-Godoy, Mobley, Jones, 1995). Black adults have not shown the same reductions in the number of decayed-missing-filled teeth (DMFT) noted in whites (Brown, Swango, 1993). Furthermore, medically compromised persons with chronic diseases, receiving pharmaceutical and medical therapies, or with physical disabilities are at increased risk for caries (Position of the American Dietetic Association, 1996).

Root Caries

Root caries is defined as caries occurring on the exposed root surfaces. Because gingival recession is a prerequisite for this pattern of disease, root caries is common in more than half of the dentate elderly (Saunders, Meyerowitz, 2005) Individuals approaching their 30s experience about 1 out of 100 surfaces with recession and root caries; when they leave their 50s, about 1 out of 5 exposed surfaces are involved (Katz, Hazen, Chilton, Mumma, 1982). By age 72, approximately 52% of these surfaces have been affected (*Oral Health of United States Adults,* 1987). Risk factors for root caries development include age, gender, fluoride exposure, systemic illness, medications, oral hygiene, salivary function, and diet (Banting, 1986). Although the clinical and histological appearance of root caries differ from coronal caries

(Mellberg, 1986), the etiology is fundamentally similar. The role of diet is at least as important in root caries as in coronal caries.

DIET AND DENTAL CARIES
Classic Studies Related to Diet and Caries Prevalence

A number of classic studies in specific human populations have shown a clear relationship between sucrose consumption and caries prevalence and incidence. These include the Vipeholm study from the 1940s (Gustafsson et al., 1954), the Hopewood House study from the 1960s (Harris, 1963), and the Turku Sugar study from the early 1970s (Scheinin, Mäkinen, 1976). The Vipeholm study remains the most influential study of diet and dental caries to date. This prospective study was conducted in Sweden between 1945 and 1953 with 436 patients at the Vipeholm Hospital (an institute for persons with mental illness), to determine the effect on caries activity of the consumption of either a retentive or nonretentive carbohydrate with or between meals. To summarize a complicated protocol, six major experimental groups received carbohydrate supplements in different forms. All subjects received the same nutritionally adequate basal diet. They also received the same total daily amount of supplemental carbohydrate, but in different forms and varying frequencies. A number of dietary changes and two separate study periods confounded interpretation of the data, but the conclusions were as follows:

- Increased frequency of sugar consumption results in increased caries incidence.
- The increase is greater when sugar is consumed in a retentive form, particularly between meals.
- The total amount of sugar consumed is not critical when consumed at mealtimes.
- Even under uniform experimental conditions, caries activity shows wide interpersonal variation.
- Withdrawal of a caries-promoting agent from the diet causes caries activity to drop, although new lesions may continue to develop despite severe dietary restriction of carbohydrate (Figure 13–4).

This study showed "not only the quantity of sugar consumed . . . but also the form in that it is served and whether it is consumed at meals or between meals" are

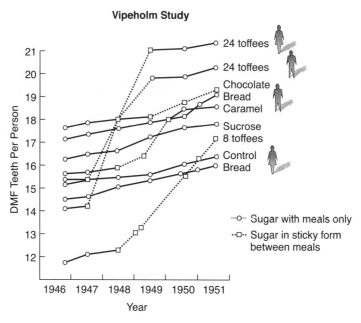

FIGURE 13-4 Vipeholm study results.

important factors in caries development. In fact, a reduction in the total daily sugar intake could be associated with increased caries if the sugar is consumed between meals, especially if in a retentive form that adheres to the teeth and provides fermentable carbohydrates for a prolonged period.

The Hopewood House study conducted in New South Wales over a 15-year period compared 52 children who followed a regimented lactovegetarian diet devoid of refined carbohydrate and rich in uncooked vegetables (Hopewood group) with children who followed a more refined diet (Harris, 1963). Neither group practiced adequate oral hygiene nor had significant dental care, but the Hopewood group had significantly lower caries incidence. These findings concur with the Vipeholm study conclusion that caries incidence is related to the form of carbohydrate consumed.

The Turku Sugar study (Scheinin, Mäkinen, 1976) was conducted in Finland in the early 1970s. A total of 125 subjects, divided into three groups, received all sweetened food items with sucrose, fructose, or xylitol. After 1 year, caries development in the xylitol group was insignificant compared with the other two groups. There was no difference between the sucrose and fructose groups in caries development initially, but the

sucrose group had significantly more caries than the fructose group after 2 years.

Two more recent investigations have shown only weak correlations between sucrose intake and caries. British (Rugg-Gunn, Hackett, Appleton, Jenkins, Eastoe, 1984) and American studies (Burt et al., 1988) in the 1980s involved children who consumed over 100 grams of sucrose per day, or a minimum of 20% of total kilocalories. The results showed that sucrose was an etiological factor but not the sole determinant of caries prevalence. Oral hygiene, fluoride, and dental health care were variables in these more recent studies and may account for the differences in results between them and earlier investigations.

It takes repeated cariogenic attacks to produce the cumulative mineral loss that characterizes caries. This factor is important when considering cariogenic eating patterns. As found in the Vipeholm study, the amount of sugar in the diet was not as important in caries progression as the *frequency* and *form* of consumption. For example, foods such as raisins, cooked starches, and candies that adhere to the teeth for some time will continue to slowly leach sugars. The local bacteria will use these sugars and extend the decrease in the plaque pH. Similarly, any food or beverage that contains fermentable carbohydrates and is consumed over a prolonged period or with increased frequency will have the same effect. Encouragement of remineralization by appropriate dietary strategies could prevent the progression of an incipient to a frank lesion.

Sugars and Sugar-Containing Foods

Over the years, the role of diet in dental health has been associated with "sugar." However, the term *sugar* warrants definition and clarification. To some, the term *sugar* is synonymous with the term *sucrose*. However, the term actually encompasses all mono-, di-, and polysaccharides. In relating sugar to dental health, it is more appropriate to refer to "fermentable carbohydrates," which include all sugars or cooked starches metabolized by oral bacteria to produce acids (Kandelman, 1997). Table 13–2 lists carbohydrates and sweeteners and their known caries-promoting potential.

In addition to the classic studies of sugar consumption patterns (Gustafsson et al., 1954; Harris, 1963; Scheinin, Mäkinen, 1976), others have examined the role of total sugars in dental health. Only a weak relationship was found between the *amount* of sugar consumed and caries occurrence in 12-year-old children in 90 countries (Woodward, Walker, 1994). However, other studies that assessed actual sugar intake provide contradictory findings (Rugg-Gunn, 1994; Sreebny, 1982). Dietary data from 141 elderly adults showed a higher incidence of root caries in those who consumed twice as much liquid sugar in coffee or tea (Papas, Joshi, Palmer, Giunta, Dwyer, 1995).

Sucrose continues to receive the greatest attention of all the fermentable carbohydrates. Among dental researchers, foods with 15% sugar by weight are considered high-sugar foods and therefore considered to have cariogenic properties (Huxley, 1977; Kandelman, 1997). However, categorizing foods as cariogenic is confusing and problematic because they have multiple properties. For example, fruits in general tend to have low cariogenic potential, with the exception of dried fruits (Mundorff et al., 1990) and certain fresh fruits. Apples, bananas, and grapes contain 10–15% sucrose, citrus fruit 8%, and berries and pears only 2% (DePaola et al., 1999). Although citrus fruits are high in water, stimulate saliva production, and provide an excellent source of vitamin C, they can potentially erode tooth enamel if consumed in large quantities over an extended period. Honey is often touted as a "healthy" food, yet it is

composed primarily of a variety of simple sugars along with some vitamins and minerals. In some studies, honey has been shown to be even more cariogenic than plain sucrose. Molasses and brown sugar are also less processed versions of sucrose. Molasses contains a little iron, but not enough to be considered a nutritious food.

In the United States, nonmilk sugars contributed to 18% of total energy intake in individuals between the ages of 11 and 50 years (Gibney, Sigman-Grant, Stanton Jr, Keast, 1995). Carbonated beverages were the major contributors to sugar intake, whereas chewing gum and candy were minor sources. Dairy foods were the primary source of total sugars in the diets of young children.

Glucan (bacterial storage form of carbohydrate) specifically requires sucrose for its production. Examples of the importance of glucan are seen in several clinical situations. For example, children who consume little or no sucrose because of sucrase or fructase enzyme deficiencies have a less cariogenic plaque. Similarly, individuals receiving long-term nourishment via a stomach tube have less plaque and fewer *S. mutans* (Littleton, McCabe, Carter, 1967). Individuals restricting their sucrose intake have a decreased proportion of *S. mutans* in their plaque that increases when sucrose is reintroduced into the diet (Dodds, Edgar, 1986; Sgan-Cohen, Newbrun, Huber, Tenebaum, Sela, 1988).

Hereditary Fructose Intolerance

Another example of the importance of sucrose as a cariogenic agent in the diet can be seen in the inborn error of metabolism known as hereditary fructose intolerance (HFI). People with HFI are unable to metabolize fructose. As a result, they are also unable to metabolize sucrose (since sucrose, a disaccharide, is composed of glucose and fructose) and must obtain all of their carbohydrate from starches, dairy products (lactose), and glucose. People with HFI have a much *lower caries incidence* than people who do not have HFI (Table 13–3).

In summary, frequent consumption of sugars (fermentable carbohydrates) is a major cariogenic risk factor because:

- Excessive sugar consumption will increase the number of occasions, as well as the total time, that the plaque pH is in the acidic range.
- This frequent exposure will cause the plaque to become more bulky, through formation of

TABLE 13-2 Caries-Promoting Activity and Food Sources of Carbohydrates and Sweeteners

Category	Chemical Structure	Examples	Caries-Promoting Potential	Food Sources
Sugars	Monosaccharide	Glucose, dextrose	Yes	Most foods
		Fructose, high fructose corn syrup	Yes	Fruits, honey
		Galactose	No	Milk
	Disaccharide	Sucrose, granulated or powdered or brown sugar, turbinado, molasses	Yes	Fruit, vegetables, table sugar
		Lactose	Yes	Milk
		Maltose	Yes	Beer
Other carbohydrates	Polysaccharide	Starch	Yes	Potatoes, grains, rice, legumes, bananas, cornstarch
	Fiber	Cellulose, pectin, gums, beta-glucans, fructans	No	Grains, fruits, vegetables
	Polyol-Monosaccharide	Sorbitol, mannitol, xylitol, erythritol	No	Fruit, seaweed, exudate of plants or trees
	Polyol-Disaccharide	Lactitol, isomalt, maltitol	No	Derived from lactose, maltose, or starch
	Polyol-Polysaccharide	Hydrogenated starch hydrolysates (HSH) or maltitol syrup	No	Derived from monosaccharides
High-intensity sweeteners	Saccharin	Sweet and Low	No	
	Aspartame	Nutrasweet, Equal	No	
	Aceulfame-K	Sunett	No	
	Sucralose	Splenda	No	
Fat replacers made from carbohydrates		Carrageenan, cellulose gel/gum, corn syrup solids, dextrin, maltodextrin, guar gum, hydrolyzed corn starch, modified food starch, pectin, polydextrose, sugar beet fiber, xanthan gum	Unknown	Baked goods, cheese, chewing gum, salad dressing, candy, frozen desserts, pudding, sauces, sour cream, yogurt, meat-based products

TABLE 13–3   Hereditary Fructose Intolerance

	HFI Subjects (n = 17)	*Control subjects* (n = 14)
DMFT score	2.1	14.3
DFMS score	3.3	36.1
Plaque index	1.2	1.2
Oral hygiene index	1.7	1.8
Mean daily sucrose consumption index	0.83	4.32
Average daily index of sucrose (g)	2.5	48.2
Percent caries free	59%	0%
Mean age (years)	29.1	26.5

Source: From Newbrun, E: *Cariology.* Chicago: Quintessence, 1989.

extracellular polysaccharides. This will also be used as a bacterial energy source between snacking events.

- There is likely to be a higher proportion of mutans streptococci bacteria in the plaque that forms during this period (especially *S. sobrinus*). The acidogenic bacteria in general are metabolically primed by this frequent exposure to use sugars and other carbohydrates very efficiently, thus becoming more acidogenic. Limiting the number of times during the day that sugars are consumed is an important factor controlling overall rates of demineralization.

Starch

Starch must first be split into simpler sugars by amylase from saliva and plaque to be used as a food source for cariogenic bacteria. Processed high-starch snacks, whether gelatinized, baked, or fried, produce as much acid in plaque as sucrose alone but at a slower rate (Grenby, 1990; Mörmann, Mühlemann, 1981). The addition of sucrose increases the cariogenicity of cooked starchy foods because the starch brings the sucrose into close contact with the tooth surface (Sgan-Cohan et al., 1988). An increased prevalence of dental caries was found in children with a high intake of sugar-starch foods (e.g., sweetened baked goods and others), but not with the intake of foods rich in sugar alone (Garcia-Closas, Garcia-Closas, Serra-Majem, 1997). Rugg-Gunn (1994) concluded that foods containing both cooked starch and a substantial amount of sucrose may be as cariogenic as an equal amount of sucrose. Also, cariogenicity was

enhanced in animal studies, when foods (e.g., bread, chocolate, graham crackers, potato chips) containing approximately 1% or more of hydrolyzable starch in combination with sugars were tested (Mundorff et al., 1990).

Raw and uncooked starches have low caries-promoting activity (Havenaar et al., 1984). Cooked staple starchy foods such as rice, potatoes, and bread have low cariogenicity potential in humans, but their cariogenicity increases when sugars are added (Rugg-Gunn, 1994). Finally, less refined starchy grains and cereals contain phytate or phytic acid and/or fiber that may protect teeth, but few studies have investigated their role (Rugg-Gunn, 1994). At best, fibrous foods, including fruits and vegetables, require more chewing and may produce the benefit of increased salivary flow and oral clearance.

Alternative Sweeteners

Alternative sweeteners may include any products used as a sweetening alternative to the natural sugars (monosaccharides and disaccharides) and their combinations. These include nutritive sweeteners (e.g., Aspartame and the sugar-alcohols sorbitol, mannitol, and xylitol) and nonnutritive sweeteners such as saccharine. For a detailed discussion of these alternative sweeteners see Chapter 4. Based on an extensive review of the dental literature on foods and acidogenicity/cariogenicity testing, the FDA has concluded that the sugar alcohols xylitol, sorbitol, mannitol, maltitol, isomalt, lactitol, erythritol, hydrogenated starch hydrolysates, and hydrogenated glucose syrups have a low potential for caries production. Since 1998, products containing less than 0.5 gram of a sugar and a sugar alcohol can be labeled "reducing" or "not promoting" tooth decay (FDA, 1996). Xylitol is actually cariostatic as shown in the Turku Finland study (Scheinin, Mäkinen, 1976). Sweeteners not derived from carbohydrates, such as Aspartame and saccharine, are also not cariogenic.

Physical Properties of Foods

Sugars are rarely found alone in the diet. More often they are combined with a variety of other food components that can affect their ultimate cariogenic potential. The consistency, temperature, and textural properties of food all affect mastication and oral clearance (Christense, 1984). Likewise, oral health status can impact biting, chewing, and swallowing. Whether a food is liquid or solid, hard or soft, fresh or cooked, retentive or cohesive, viscous or moisture absorbent, these physical properties influence caries risk by determining the salivary flow rate and oral clearance. Although beverages clear the mouth quickly, they can actually sustain a low pH level for as long a period as a more retentive food (Ismail, Burt, Eklund, 1984; Rugg-Gunn, 1994). The role of texture in dental health has been limited to oral functional studies.

Recommendations to avoid sticky foods have been somewhat misleading. A food like a caramel or jellybean may have high initial retention or "stickiness" but be followed by rapid oral clearance (Grenby, 1990). Conversely, a food like white bread, pretzels, chips, or cereal may be retentive and clear slowly from the mouth. In a study of perceived stickiness versus actual retention of 21 commercially available foods, Kashket, Van Houte, Lopez, and Stocks (1991) showed that cookies, crackers, and potato chips were the most retentive, whereas caramels, jelly beans, raisins, and milk chocolate bars were among those poorly retained in the oral cavity. Slowly dissolving items such as hard candies and breath mints tend to be highly cariogenic, because they are usually consumed frequently and are dissolved slowly in the mouth (Papas et al., 1995) (Table 13–4).

Dietary Patterns: Frequency of Eating

All people have varied dietary habits and patterns. It is the cariogenicity of dietary patterns rather than the extent of bacterial infection that has been identified as a primary determinant in caries severity (van Palenstein, Helderman, Matee, van der Hoeven, Mikx, 1996). The frequency of food consumption, food combinations, and nutrient adequacy of the diet greatly influence the risk for caries (König and Navia, 1995).

Reports on the frequency of meals and snacks have been difficult to analyze and interpret because of varying operational definitions of "meal," "snack," and "eating occasion." More consistent approaches are necessary before definitive interpretations can be made. Nonetheless, most people eat five to six times daily. A higher frequency, especially if it involves constant

TABLE 13–4 Physical Form Alone May Be Misleading

Toffee	vs.	Soda
1 piece		6 cans
consumed fast		sipped
once/week		daily

nibbling or sipping of foods and beverages, is caries promoting (Firestone, Schmid, Mühlemann, 1984; Gatenby, 1997; Kandelman, 1997). Eating fermentable carbohydrates at bedtime is discouraged because saliva production diminishes during sleep (Edgar, O'Mullane, 1996). The Vipeholm study (Gustaffson et al., 1954) clearly demonstrated that frequent sugar intake between meals as opposed to with meals was associated with increased caries incidence. Ismail and colleagues (1984) showed a significant positive association between the frequency of sucrose intake both with meals and between meals and caries activity. Other animal and human studies have reported contradictory findings (Firestone, Imfeld, Schiffer, Lutz, 1987; Rugg-Gunn, 1994), even though the continued introduction of substrate to oral bacteria will sustain a decreased plaque pH.

Food Combinations

There is evidence that combining foods has potential anticaries efficacy. For example, eating occasions that incorporate sweets as part of the meal, in combination with proteins and fats, can decrease caries potential. When fermentable carbohydrates are eaten alone, acid production is rapid and plaque pH falls. But the pH will rise if a nonsugary item that stimulates saliva, is eaten immediately before, during, or after the challenge (Geddes, 1994). Additionally, the remineralization potential is enhanced if the food contains calcium or fluoride. For example, inclusion of dairy products (e.g., nonfat yogurt, milk) with a meal or snack will enhance cariostatic effects and enhance enamel remineralization. In one study, subjects who ate more cheese had fewer root caries (Papas et al., 1995).

Even the sequence of eating foods within an eating occasion can affect the magnitude of change in plaque pH. Eating acidogenic foods between other foods and eating combinations of chewy foods with those that have minimal effect on saliva production can reduce tooth demineralization. However, fermentable carbohydrates eaten sequentially, one after another, over time can enhance the potential for demineralization of tooth enamel (Geddes, 1994).

Nutrient and Caloric Adequacy in Relation to Caries

Animal studies have suggested a possible association between total food consumption and caries (Lewis, Park, Dexter, Yetley, 1992; Mundorff et al., 1990). However, statistically significant associations between total calories and caries have not been shown in human studies (Mackeown, Cleaton-Jones, Hargreaves, 1995). One study of Greek children reported that higher intakes of vegetables and milk products were associated with lower caries indices, even though sugary foods were widely used (Petridou, Athanassouli, Panagopoulos, Revinthi, 1996). In an older population, the caries-free elderly group had diets higher in crude fiber, calcium, magnesium, phosphorus, and protein (Rugg-Gunn, 1994).

These studies reinforce the need to consume nutritionally adequate diets that follow the principles of the food guide pyramid (1992) and follow dietary patterns that promote oral health.

HOW FOODS ARE TESTED FOR CARIOGENIC POTENTIAL

Specific foods, their forms, combinations, and frequency of intake impact the caries process. For example, frequent exposure to sucrose increases the number of *S. mutans* and other oral bacteria in the plaque (Staat, Gawronski, Cressey, Harris, Folke, 1975). This increases the acidogenic potential of the plaque to other foods, including starch (Dodds, Edgar, 1986; Sgan-Cohen et al., 1988).

The absolute cariogenicity of a food or beverage can be determined by administering that food (in isolation) to human volunteers for a period long enough for caries to develop (usually at least 2 years). However, since this is impractical as well as unethical (caries could result), there are other experimental strategies to estimate the potential cariogenicity of foods and beverages.

Plaque pH Studies in Humans

Measuring the fall in dental plaque pH after exposure to fermentable carbohydrates is the basis of plaque pH studies (Harper, Abelson, Jensen, 1986). Since Stephan (1940) first described this methodology, the typical plaque pH response to fermentable carbohydrate is termed the *Stephan curve* (Figure 13–5). The Stephan curve shows plaque pH response to a 10% sucrose rinse. The plaque pH is normally around neutral at resting, decreases within 5 minutes after a sugar challenge to a minimum value, and then returns to the resting value within 40 minutes. The different techniques used to measure the plaque pH, the absolute values of the resting pH, minimum pH, and time to return to resting value, are termed *acidogenicity tests*. Acidogenicity tests measure plaque acid responses

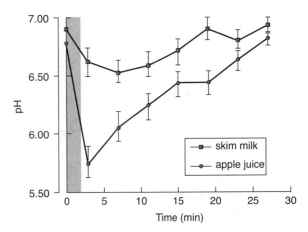

FIGURE 13–5   Stephan curves. Each point is the mean (± SE) of 12 measurements in different subjects. The hatched area represents the period of rinsing with either a reconstituted skim milk powder or a reconstituted dried apple juice powder.

and are only indirect tests of cariogenicity. In general, plaque pH studies have excellent reproducibility and are simple, inexpensive, and rapid means to determine food acidogenicity and potential cariogenicity.

Animal Studies

The rat model has been commonly used for food cariogenicity testing since it has relatively similar caries patterns to humans, requires reasonably short experimental periods, and is relatively inexpensive. Test foods can be administered in varying frequencies and forms while essential nutrition is given by gastric intubation or as a nutritive gel supplement (Shaw, 1986). Germ-free rats, even fed a highly cariogenic diet, do not develop caries. Caries patterns in rats are described as sulcal (analogous to fissure caries in humans) and buccal (smooth surface); sulcal caries is the better predictor of cariogenic potential for humans.

Other techniques for assessing the potential cariogenicity of foods include in vitro demineralization tests that use various combinations of bacteria, enamel, and test solutions (Clarkson, 1986; Ten Cate, 1986).

APPLICATION OF CARIOGENICITY TESTS IN FOOD RESEARCH

The scientific consensus was that foods with no or low cariogenic potential could be identified using combinations of these test techniques (Burt, Ismail, 1986;

Clarkson, 1986; Curzon, 1986; Edgar, Dodds, Higham, 1986; Stookey, 1986; Tanzer, 1986; Ten Cate, 1986). The 2nd European Conference on Diet, Nutrition and Dental Caries (Food Composition, 1990) recommended that dental researchers develop lists of foods with no cariogenic potential, and offered suggestions for the study of cariostatic/anticariogenic substances in food.

Despite the scientific integrity of conference findings (Edgar, 1993; Edmondson, 1990), the recommendations have not been followed extensively by either the food industry or caries research community. Reasons for this noncompliance may be that these testing programs are complicated and expensive to follow, particularly for food manufacturers who frequently reformulate products (Imfeld, 1994).

LABELING INITIATIVES FOR CARIOGENIC POTENTIAL

The ultimate goal of cariogenicity testing would be food labeling for consumers. The Swiss may label any food as "zahnschonend" (safe for teeth) if it is shown by plaque pH telemetry not to cause plaque pH to fall below a value of 5.7 (Imfeld, 1983).

The FDA (Health Claims, 1996) authorized the use of the terms "does not promote," "useful in not promoting," or "expressly for not promoting" dental caries on the packaging of foods containing sugar alcohols such as xylitol, sorbitol, mannitol, maltitol, isomalt, lactitol, erythritol, hydrogenated starch hydrolysates, and hydrogenated glucose syrups. The foods thus labeled must be sugar (i.e., sucrose) free, sweetened with one or a combination of the aforementioned sugar alcohols, and must not lower plaque pH below 5.7 if a fermentable carbohydrate is present.

CARIES PROTECTIVE FACTORS

Cariostatic Food Factors: Phytates, Proteins, Cheeses, Fats

Factors in addition to phytate and fiber have been identified in foods that may protect against or reduce the rate of demineralization of tooth enamel. Proteins act as neutral agents with buffering capacity and are adsorbed well onto surfaces of tooth enamel. Casein in milk plays a protective role by inhibiting adhesion of plaque to the tooth surface (Rugg-Gunn, 1994). Although milk contains sufficient lactose to be classified as cariogenic,

its high concentration of calcium and phosphorus also helps protect tooth enamel. Investigations using an artificial mouth test system found that foods containing sugars (e.g., cookies) had reduced cariogenicity when consumed with milk (Bibby, Huang, Zero, Mundorff, Little, 1980). Also, young adults who were caries free in one study consumed significantly more milk on a daily basis than those with caries (Dodds, Johnson, Mobley, Hattaway, 1997).

Cheeses such as cheddar and mozzarella, which also contain casein, have strong anticariogenic properties. As an additional benefit, the tyramine content of cheese stimulates saliva composition and flow (Bowen, 1994). The calcium and phosphate content of plaque rises after eating cheese, but this effect is lost when the cheese is eaten on a biscuit or is followed by an acidic beverage (Jenkins, Hargreaves, 1989). Other dietary sources of protein, such as meat, nuts and legumes, are metabolized by bacterial enzymes to alkaline products that raise plaque pH (Bowen, 1994). Daily food choices from the newly revised food guide pyramid (MyPyramid), especially from the dairy and meat groups, will promote anticariogenic activity.

Dietary fat accelerates oral clearance, but this action varies based on the type of fat and the cooking procedure (Brudevold, Kashket, Kent, 1990). Low concentrations of linoleic and oleic acids inhibit the growth of oral bacteria (Bowen, 1994). Promoting high-fat diets is contrary to dietary guidelines and therefore should not be routinely recommended for caries prevention. However, small amounts of high-fat foods, such as cheese, can be part of a low-fat diet. Tannins in cocoa, milk chocolate (that contains tannins, protein, and fat), glycyrrhizinic acid in licorice, a factor in rhubarb, and other food constituents have all been investigated for their roles as anticariogenic agents (Kashket, Paolino, Lewis, van Houte, 1985; Ten Cate, 1986). In the future, the addition of anticariogenic compounds to the food supply may be more effective in the dietary control of dental caries than the creation of "good" and "bad" foods lists for dental health promotion.

Fluoride and Other Micronutrients

The role of fluoride as a cariostatic agent both preeruptively and posteruptively has been well established (IOM, 1997). However, even optimum fluoride exposure will not fully protect the teeth from bad dietary practices, although it may limit the effects.

Other trace minerals, including molybdenum, vanadium, and strontium, also protect against caries. Conversely, selenium and lead may promote caries (Rugg-Gunn, 1994; Speirs and Beeley, 1992). Recent studies with animals fed iron-fortified sucrose identified iron as a cariostatic agent (Miguel, Bowen, Pearson, 1997). Food sources of these trace elements, their roles, and both optimal and toxic effects in humans must be examined carefully before recommendations can be made. Chapter 8 reviews fluoride in detail.

Water and Saliva

Water is an essential nutrient often overlooked in discussions of diet and caries, yet it is a significant component of saliva. The clearance of fermentable substrates can be enhanced by adequate intake at the time of fluid and food intake. This fact becomes paramount in the presence of conditions contributing to xerostomia (dry mouth).

Saliva contains supersaturated concentrations of calcium and phosphate relative to hydroxyapatite, the tooth mineral. Therefore, saliva can promote remineralization of the early carious lesion. Saliva has a number of other properties and functions that protect against caries. It contains antimicrobial proteins, such as lysozyme, lactoferrin, and secretory IgA. By virtue of its constant flow, saliva physically clears cariogenic materials from the mouth, buffers acid formation in the plaque, contains floruide, and forms a protective coating on the teeth (Dodds, Johnson, Yeh, 2005). Rapid caries development is often a problem in individuals who have little or no salivary flow due to disease (e.g., Sjögren's syndrome); radiation therapy to the head and neck, which damages salivary gland cells; or medications (see Chapter 11) (Figure 13–6).

Many medications cause xerostomia, increasing the risk for caries (Boyd, Dwyer, Papas, 1997; Edgar, O'Mullane, 1996). Dietary supplements such as vitamin A, when taken in toxic doses, can also cause oral dryness (Meyers, Maloley, 1996). Herbal preparations that include *ma huang* or ephedra act as diuretics and could potentially cause dry mouth, whereas ginger root is thought to stimulate saliva flow ("about Herbs" www.mskcc.org). It is important to identify patient use of these and similar products in determining caries risks.

Chewing and the taste of food (sweet, sour, bitter) can increase salivary flow. The gustatory response to food can increase salivary flow rate from 0.3 to 4.0 mL/min. During sleep, salivary flow rate drops to 0.1 mL/min, which reduces oral clearance of plaque acids and available

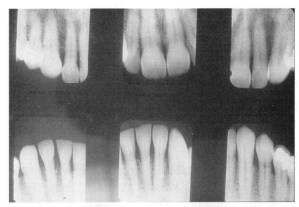
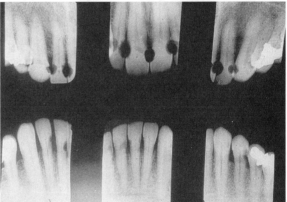

FIGURE 13–6   *Top:* Healthy teeth before xerostomia and use of candies. *Bottom:* Interproximal caries resulting from xerostomia and excessive use of slowly dissolving mint candies.

bacterial substrates (Edgar, O'Mullane, 1996; Kandelman, 1997). Stimulated saliva has a higher pH and buffer capacity than unstimulated saliva, and therefore impacts the removal of food and the neutralization and buffering of plaque acids. Stimulated saliva also helps repair early demineralization episodes by the redeposition of calcium and phosphate ions. This property of saliva has been promoted by the use of chewing gum to remineralize early decay. Sugar-free gum is usually sweetened with a mixture of sugar alcohols and intense sweeteners, such as Aspartame. The combination of chewing and the sweetness of the gum stimulates salivary flow. Thus, chewing sugar-free gum helps return the plaque pH to neutral or higher values (Jensen, Wefel, 1989).

Frequent use of sugar-free gums may increase basal salivary flow rates and reduce the acidogenicity of the dental plaque (Dodds, Hsieh, Johnson, 1991; Jenkins, Edgar, 1989). Long-term use of sugar-free gum has been shown to slow down, if not prevent, caries in prospective population-based studies (Kandelman, Gagnon, 1990; Mäkinen et al., 1995, 1996). Xylitol-sweetened gums appear better at promoting remineralization than sorbitol-sweetened gums (Edgar, 1998). Sugar-free gums may be especially useful to chew after meals or snacks, by those individuals with low salivary flow rates (Abelson, Barton, Mandel, 1990). Similarly, sugar-free candies and mints may have the same effect.

Even sucrose-sweetened gum also may help minimize plaque pH falls after food consumption, thereby promoting remineralization (Manning, Edgar, 1992, 1993). The effect of sucrose-sweetened gum is not as clear as with sugar-free gums and probably depends on how long and how frequently the gum is chewed. For example, it may be beneficial to chew one piece of gum for a prolonged period so that the sugar is dissipated and the salivary stimulation is effective. Conversely, constantly chewing a new piece of gum as soon as the sweet flavor is gone may have the same cariogenic effect as the frequent use of any other cariogenic item.

Oral Hygiene

Although plaque is a prerequisite for caries development, the literature shows poor correlation between home oral hygiene efforts and caries (Axelsson, Paulander, Svardstrom, Tollskog, Nordensten, 1993). Advising patients they can eat with impunity "just so long as you brush your teeth afterward" is inappropriate and possibly negligent. Better advice would be to monitor food choices and the frequency of eating, and to follow a sugary snack with an anticariogenic one such as sugar-free gum, or a cariostatic food such as milk, to raise the plaque pH (Higham, Edgar, 1989). These dietary practices can enhance the oral health benefits of brushing with a fluoride toothpaste.

DIET AND CARIES IMPLICATIONS FOR SPECIFIC POPULATIONS

Infants and Young Children

The Centers for Disease Control and Prevention has described patterns of tooth decay in infants and young children as early childhood caries (ECC) (Duperon, 1995) (Figure 13–7). Factors most implicated in this rampant disease process are:

- prolonged use of baby bottles containing highly fermentable sugars (e.g., fruit juice, soda, and other sweetened drinks).
- pacifiers dipped in sweet agents such as sugar, honey, or syrups.
- other high-frequency sugar exposures (Fitzsimons, Dwyer, Palmer, Boyd, 1998; Mobley, 1998). (ECC is detailed in Chapter 17.)

Older children's diets will include foods that contain fermentable carbohydrates. However, having them at mealtimes rather than between meals will reduce their cariogenic potential. Avoid allowing children to develop especially cariogenic habits such as snacking on sugared cereals while watching television, or sipping constantly on sweet beverages.

Athletes

Because tooth erosion is associated with prolonged use of sports drinks by athletes, oral health screening should address this behavior (Milosevic et al., 1997). The combined effect of the acidogenic medium with sucrose accelerates not only erosion but also caries. Athletes should rely on a variety of food and water for their energy and hydration needs. When long-term, sustained athletic performance is desired, the combined use of sugar-free gum and periodic sports drinks may be appropriate.

Vegetarians

Vegetarians consume diets primarily derived from plant sources, which tend to be fibrous and possibly more abrasive than nonvegetarian diets. However, the contribution

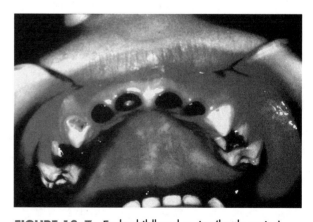

FIGURE 13–7 Early childhood caries (bottle caries).

of this type of diet to dental abrasion has not been consistently shown (Sherfudhin, Abdullah, Shaik, Johansson, 1998). Although the vegetarian diet tends to be higher in carbohydrates, the prevalence of caries is relatively low among traditional vegetarian populations when compared with nonvegetarian groups. This is especially true when frequency of eating is not excessive.

Elderly People

Root caries is common in elderly people due to exposed dentin from gingival recession and associated changes in the oral mucosa and periodontium (Papas et al., 1995). Likewise, changes in teeth and masticatory function can affect dietary intake that in turn can alter the risk for caries. For those with tooth loss, changes in the texture and consistency of foods may be necessary (Mobley, Saunders, 1997). Nutrition needs of older persons are detailed in Chapter 19.

SUMMARY AND IMPLICATIONS FOR DENTISTRY

Fermentable carbohydrates initiate the process of dental caries, but they do not operate in a vacuum. They interact dynamically with other variables such as oral bacteria

and saliva. Eating patterns are greater determinants of cariogenic risk than diet composition. Foods containing fermentable carbohydrates will continue to be a major component of a healthful diet and can be combined with other foods to enhance oral health. Health professionals can serve the public well by promoting basic dietary messages that are consistent with both good oral health and general health. Dietary advice should take into account social circumstances and dietary habits. Information should be based on foods as eaten, not solely on carbohydrate content. Most important, dental advice on diet should not contradict general nutritional principles (Nutrition and Your Health, 1995). Diet concepts of moderation, variety, and balance all support both good nutrition and good oral health.

Specific recommendations to reduce the cariogenic risk of the diet should include the following:

- Reduce the frequency of consumption of foods and drinks containing fermentable carbohydrate, especially between meals.
- Finish any eating or drinking occasion with a food or drink with no cariogenic potential or with cariostatic properties (Food Composition, 1990) (Table 13–5).

TABLE 13–5 Acidogenic Potential of Foods*

Non- or Low-Acidogenic	*Acidogenic (from lesser to greater)*
Raw vegetables (e.g., broccoli, cauliflower, cucumber, lettuce, dill pickle, carrot, peppers)	Cooked vegetables Fresh fruits (most)
Meat, fish, poultry	Sweetened canned or cooked fruits
Beans, peas	Fruit juices, fruit drinks
Nuts, natural peanut butter	Sweetened beverages
Milk, cheeses	Nondairy creamers
Flavored yogurts	Ice cream, sherbet, pudding, gelatin
Corn chips	Potato chips, pretzels, crackers
Peanuts	Marshmallows
Popcorn	Starches: bread, rice, pasta, sweetened cereals, french fries
Fats, oils, butter, margarine	Cookies, cakes, pies, pastry
Nonsugar sweeteners	Candy
	Bananas, dried fruits, fruit rolls
	Slowly dissolving sugar products: mints, cough drops, candies

* Independent items from rat studies, not related to usage patterns.
Source: From Palmer, C: Important Relationships Between Diet, Nutrition and Oral Health. *Nutr Clin Care* 2001: 4–14.

- Combine and sequence foods to enhance mastication, saliva production, and oral clearance. For example, follow an acidogenic food with one that promotes remineralization, such as xylitol chewing gum.
- Drink water to satisfy thirst and hydration needs.
- Consume sweetened and acidic beverages with meals and snacks that contain other foods that can buffer their cariogenic and acidogenic effects.

Finally, populations such as infants, children, older people, athletes, vegetarians, and those on certain medications or dietary supplements need to know how dietary choices can enhance their oral health. Health professionals should address dental health needs in the context of overall diet and provide nutrition messages that support health and decrease the risk for chronic diseases such as dental caries.

QUESTIONS PATIENTS MIGHT ASK

Q. I don't know why I'm getting so many cavities. I never eat candy and I don't eat a lot of sweets.

A. Sweets and candy are not the only foods that can contribute to dental caries. Any sugars, including those in juices, can promote caries. Additionally, although you say you don't eat a lot of sweets, you may be snacking frequently throughout the day. This is a more dentally risky pattern than just eating three normal-sized meals.

Q. If I use only "diet" sodas and eliminate sugar-containing beverages from my diet will I be protected against dental decay?

A. Not necessarily. Although diet sodas don't contribute to decay directly, they contain acids that can erode tooth enamel and make teeth more susceptible to developing decay. Also, if you are eating lots of other types of carbohydrates, especially between meals, these habits may pose a greater dental risk than the sodas.

Q. I was using a lot of sugar in my daily coffees. If I cut down on the sugar will that help reduce my risk of developing cavities?

A. Again, not necessarily. Cutting down from 3 teaspoons of sugar in your coffee to 1 teaspoon will have little dental impact, especially if you are having several cups of coffee daily. The frequency of sugar contacts with teeth is much more important than the amount of sugar in any one contact. Also, if you are using "creamer" in your coffee as well, the creamer has sugar in it. The best approach would be to try to eliminate the sugar totally *and* cut down on the total amount of coffee you drink.

CASE STUDY

Julia is a 24-year-old Hispanic woman who attends a community college part time and works part time as a convenience store clerk. She lives with a roommate who is a single parent with a 3-year-old child. At her recent dental visit, Julia was diagnosed with four incipient lesions and two frank caries. Previous to this time she had never needed dental treatment. She had received routine preventive care until 3 years ago when her parents' dental plan no longer provided coverage. Her periodontal health was good, but she did complain of dry mouth, which she blamed for her recent habit of constantly sipping on colas or sports drinks. Because she works late in the evening at least three nights a week, she frequently relies on sugary/starchy snack foods to supplement the one meal, breakfast, that she consistently eats every day. She is 62 inches tall and weighs 173 pounds. Recent concern with weight gain has led to skipping meals, attempting to restrict her intake of beverages, and avoiding breads, cereals, fruits, and vegetables because they are restricted on most weight-loss programs. Time constraints and "eating on the run" describe her eating patterns.

Questions:
1. What characteristics of Julia's diet are possibly contributing to her oral disease?
2. List and explain the key issues to consider in how these dietary variables are interacting with the infectious agents responsible for caries activity.
3. What changes can Julia make in her diet to alter the course of her future risk for caries and at the same time improve her general health status?

REFERENCES

Abelson DC, Barton J, Mandel ID: The effect of chewing sorbitol-sweetened gum on salivary flow and cemental plaque pH in subjects with low salivary flow. *J Clin Dent* 1990; 2:3–5.

"About Herbs" Memorial Sloan-Kettering Cancer Center. Retrieved from www.mskcc.org May 19, 2006.

Asher C, Read MJ: Early enamel erosion in children associated with the excessive consumption of citric acid. *Br Dent J* 1987; 162:384–87.

Axelsson P, Paulander J, Svardstrom G, Tollskog G, Nordensten S: Integrated caries prevention: effect of a needs-related preventive program on dental caries in children. *Caries Res* 1993; 27(Suppl 1):83–94.

Banting DW: Epidemiology of root caries. *Gerodontology* 1986; 5:5–11.

Bibby BG, Huang CT, Zero D, Mundorff SA, Little MF: Protective effect of milk against "in vitro" caries. *J Dent Res* 1980; 59:1565–70.

Blinkhorn AS, Davies RM: Caries prevention. A continued need worldwide. *Int Dent J* 1996; 46:119–25.

Bowen BH: Food components and caries. *Adv Dent Res* 1994; 8:215–20.

Boyd LD, Dwyer JT, Papas A: Nutritional implications of xerostomia and rampant caries caused by serotonin reuptake inhibitors: A case study. *Nutr Rev* 1997; 55:362–68.

Brown LJ, Swango PA: Trends in caries experience in US employed adults from 1971–74 to 1985: Cross-sectional comparisons. *Adv Dent Res* 1993; 7:52–60.

Brudevold F, Kashket S, Kent RL: The effect of sucrose and fat in cookies. *J Dent Res* 1990; 64:1278–82.

Burt BA, Eklund SA, Morgan KJ, Larkin FE, Guire KE, Brown LO, et al.: The effects of sugars intake and frequency of ingestion on dental caries increment in a three-year longitudinal study. *J Dent Res* 1988; 67:1422–29.

Burt BA, Ismail AI: Diet, nutrition, and food cariogenicity. *J Dent Res* 1986; 65:1475–84.

Carlsson J: Regulation of sugar metabolism in relation to the feast-and-famine existence of plaque. In Guggenheim B (ed): *Cariology Today*. Basel: Karger, 1984.

Christense CM: Food texture perception. *Adv Food Res* 1984; 29:159–99.

Clarkson BH: In vitro methods for testing the cariogenic potential of foods. *J Dent Res* 1986; 65:1516–19.

Curzon MEJ: Integration of methods for determining the cariogenic potential of foods: Is this possible with present technologies? *J Dent Res* 1986; 65:1520–24.

DePaola DP, Faine MP, Palmer CA: Nutrition in relation to dental medicine. In Shils ME, Olson JA, Shike M (eds): *Modern Nutrition in Health and Disease*, 9th ed. Baltimore: Williams & Wilkins, 1999.

Dodds MWJ, Edgar WM: Effects of dietary sucrose levels on pH fall and acid-anion profile in human dental plaque after a starch mouthrinse. *Arch Oral Biol* 1986; 31:509–12.

Dodds MWJ, Gragg PP, Rodriguez D: The effect of some Mexican citric acid snacks on *in vitro* tooth enamel erosion. *Pediatr Dent* 1997; 19:339–40.

Dodds MWJ, Hsieh SC, Johnson DA: The effect of increased mastication by daily gum-chewing on salivary gland output and dental plaque acidogenicity. *J Dent Res* 1991; 70:1474–78.

Dodds MWJ, Johnson DA, Mobley CC, Hattaway K: Parotid saliva protein profiles in caries-free and caries-active adults. *Oral Surg Oral Med Oral Pathol Oral Radiol Endodont* 1997; 83:244–51.

Dodds MWJ, Johnson DA, Yeh C: Health benefits of saliva: A review. *J Dent* 2005; 33:223–33.

Duperon DF: Early childhood caries: A continuing dilemma. *J Calif Dent Assoc* 1995; 23:15–23.

Edgar WM: Extrinsic and intrinsic sugars: A review of recent UK recommendations on diet and caries. *Caries Res* 1993; 27:64–67.

Edgar WM: Sugar substitutes, chewing gum, and dental caries: A review. *Br Dent J* 1998; 184:29–32.

Edgar WM, Dodds MWJ, Higham SM: The control of plaque pH and its significance in relation to the evaluation of food cariogenicity. In Leach SA (ed): *Factors Relating to Demineralisation and Remineralisation of the Teeth*. Washington, DC: IRL Press, 1986.

Edgar WM, O'Mullane DM: *Saliva and Oral Health*. London: British Dental Association, 1996.

Edmondson EMS: Food composition and food cariogenicity factors affecting the cariogenic potential of foods. *Caries Res* 1990; 24:60–71.

Firestone AR, Imfeld T, Schiffer S, Lutz F: Measurement of interdental plaque pH in humans with an indwelling glass pH electrode following a sucrose rinse: A long-term retrospective study. *Caries Res* 1987; 21:555–58.

Firestone AR, Schmid R, Mühlemann HR: Effect of the length and number of intervals between meals on caries in rats. *Caries Res* 1984; 18:128–33.

Fitzsimons D, Dwyer JT, Palmer C, Boyd LD: Nutrition and oral health guidelines for pregnant women, infants, and children. *J Am Diet Assoc* 1998; 98:182–89.

Food composition and food cariogenicity factors affecting the cariogenic potential of foods. *Caries Res* 1990; 24:75–76.

Food Guide Pyramid: A Guide to Daily Food Choices. Washington, DC: U.S. Dept of Agriculture, Human Nutrition Services, 1992.

Garcia-Closas R, Garcia-Closas M, Serra-Majem L: A cross-sectional study of dental caries, intake of confectionery and foods rich in starch and sugars, and salivary counts of *Streptococcus mutans* in children in Spain. *Am J Clin Nutr* 1997; 66:1257–63.

Garcia-Godoy F, Mobley CC, Jones DL: *Caries and Feeding Patterns in South Texas Preschool Children.* San Antonio: University of Texas Health Science Center at San Antonio, 1995.

Gatenby SJ: Eating frequency: Methodological and dietary aspects. *Br J Nutr* 1997; 77:S7–S10.

Geddes DAM: Diet patterns and caries. *Adv Dent Res* 1994; 8:221–24.

Gibney M, Sigman-Grant M, Stanton JL Jr, Keast DR: Consumption of sugars. *Am J Clin Nutr* 1995; 62:178S–94S.

Grenby TH: Snack foods and dental caries. Investigations using laboratory animals. *Br Dent J* 1990:353–61.

Grobler SR, Senekal PJ, Laubscher JA: In vitro demineralization of enamel by orange juice, apple juice, Pepsi Cola, and diet Pepsi Cola. *Clin Prev Dent* 1990; 12:5–9.

Gustafsson BE, Quensel CE, Lanke SL, Lundqvist C, Grahnen H, Bonow BE, et al.: The Vipeholm dental caries study. *Acta Odont Scand* 1954; 11:232–364.

Harper DS, Abelson DC, Jensen ME: Human plaque acidity models. *J Dent Res* 1986; 65:1503–10.

Harris R: Biology of the children of Hopewood House, Bowral, Australia. 4. Observations on dental caries experience extending over five years (1957–61). *J Dent Res* 1963; 42:1387–99.

Harris R, Nicoll AD, Adair PM, Pine CM: Risk factors for dental caries in young children: A systematic review of the literature. *Community Dent Health* 2004; 21:71–85.

Havenaar R, Drost JS, de Stoppelaar JD, Huis in 't Veld JH, Dirks OB: Potential cariogenicity of Lycasin® 80/55 in comparison to starch, sucrose, xylitol, sorbitol, and L-sorbose in rats. *Caries Res* 1984; 18:375–84.

Health claims: Dietary sugar alcohols and dental caries. United States Food and Drug Administration. *Fed Register*, August 23, 1996:43433–447.

Higham SM, Edgar WM: Effects of parafilm® and cheese chewing on human dental plaque pH and metabolism. *Caries Res* 1989; 23:42–48.

Huxley HG: The cariogenicity of dietary sucrose at various levels in two strains of rat under unrestricted and controlled-frequency feeding conditions. *Caries Res* 1977; 11: 237–42.

Imfeld T: Cariogenicity tests. *Adv Dent Res* 1994; 8:225–28.

Imfeld T: *Identification of Low Caries Risk Dietary Components.* Basel: Karger, 1983.

Institute of Medicine, National Academy of Science: *Dietary Reference Intakes for Calcium, Phosphorus, Magnesium, Vitamin D, and Fluoride.* Washington, DC: National Academies Press, 1997.

Ismail AI, Burt BA, Eklund SA: The cariogenicity of soft drinks in the United States. *J Am Dent Assoc* 1984; 109:241–45.

Jenkins GN, Edgar WM: The effect of daily gum-chewing on salivary flow rates in man. *J Dent Res* 1989; 68:786–90.

Jenkins GN, Hargreaves JA: Effect of eating cheese on Ca and P concentrations of whole mouth saliva and plaque. *Caries Res* 1989; 23:159–64.

Jensen ME, Wefel JS: Human plaque pH responses to meals and the effects of chewing gum. *Br Dent J* 1989; 167: 204–8.

Kandelman D: Sugar, alternative sweeteners and meal frequency in relation to caries prevention: New perspectives. *Br J Nutr* 1997; 77:S121–S28.

Kandelman D, Gagnon G: A 24-month clinical study of the incidence and progression of dental caries in relation to consumption of chewing gum containing xylitol in school preventive programs. *J Dent Res* 1990; 69:1771–75.

Kashket S, Paolino VJ, Lewis DA, van Houte J: In vitro inhibition of glycosyltransferase from the dental plaque bacterium *Streptococcus mutans* by common beverages and food extracts. *Arch Oral Biol* 1985; 30:821–26.

Kashket S, Van Houte J, Lopez LR, Stocks S: Lack of correlation between food retention on the human dentition and consumer perception of food stickiness. *J Dent Res* 1991; 70:1314–19.

Kaste LM, Selwitz RH, Oldakowski RJ, Brunelle JA, Winn DM, Brown LJ: Coronal caries in the primary and permanent dentition of children and adolescents 1–17 years of age: United States 1988–1991. *J Dent Res* 1996; 75: 631–41.

Katz RV, Hazen SP, Chilton NW, Mumma JDJ: Prevalence and intraoral distribution of root caries in an adult population. *Caries Res* 1982; 16:265–71.

König KG, Navia JM: Nutritional role of sugars in oral health. *Am J Clin Nutr* 1995; 62:275S–83S.

Lewis CJ, Park YK, Dexter PB, Yetley EA: Nutrient intakes and body weight of persons consuming high and moderate levels of added sugar. *J Am Diet Assoc* 1992; 92:708–13.

Littleton NW, McCabe RM, Carter CH: Studies of oral health in persons nourished by stomach tube. II. Acidogenic properties and selected bacterial components of plaque material. *Arch Oral Biol* 1967; 12:601–9.

Loesche WJ: Role of *Streptococcus mutans* in human dental decay. *Microbiol Rev* 1986; 50:353–80.

Lussi A, Jaeggi T, Zero D: The role of diet in the aetiology of dental erosion. *Caries Res* 2004; 38:34–44.

Mackeown JM, Cleaton-Jones PE, Hargreaves JA: Energy intake, dental caries and periodontal disease in 11-year-old black children in two regions of Southern Africa: Kwazulu and Nambia. *Community Dent Oral Epidemiol* 1995; 23: 182–86.

Mäkinen KK, Mäkinen PL, Pape HR Jr, Allen P, Bennett CA, Isokangas PJ, et al.: Stabilisation of rampant caries: Polyol gums and arrest of dentine caries in two long-term cohort studies in young subjects. *Int Dent J* 1995; 45:93–107.

Mäkinen KK, Mäkinen PL, Pape HR Jr, Peldyak J, Hujoel P, Isotupa KP, et al.: Conclusion and review of the Michigan Xylitol Programme (1986–1995) for the prevention of dental caries. *Int Dent J* 1996; 46: 22–34.

Manning RH, Edgar WM: pH changes in plaque after eating snacks and meals, and their modification by chewing sugared- or sugar-free gum. *Br Dent J* 1993; 174:241–44.

Manning RH, Edgar WM: Salivary stimulation by chewing gum and its role in the remineralization of caries-like lesions in human enamel in situ. *J Clin Dent* 1992; 3: 71–74.

Mellberg JR: Demineralization and remineralization of root surface caries. *Gerodontology* 1986; 5:25–31.

Meyers DG, Maloley PA, Weeks D: Safety of antioxidant vitamins. *Arch Intern Med* 1996; 156:925–35.

Miguel JC, Bowen WH, Pearson SK: Effects of frequency of exposure to iron-sucrose on the incidence of dental caries in desalivated rats. *Caries Res* 1997; 31:238–43.

Miller AJ, Brunelle JA, Carlos JP, Brown LJ, Löe H: *Oral Health in United States Adults.* Bethesda, MD: U.S. Department of Health and Human Services, NIH Pub No. 87-2868, 1987.

Milosevic A, Kelly MJ, McLean AN: Sports supplement drinks and dental health in competitive swimmers and cyclists. *Br Dent J* 1997; 182:303–8.

Mobley C: Spreading the message of good oral health care for children. *J Am Diet Assoc* 1998; 98:189.

Mobley C, Saunders M: Oral health screening guidelines for non-dental health care providers. *J Am Diet Assoc* 1997; 97(Suppl 2):S123–S26.

Moore WJ, Corbett ME: Dental caries experience in man: Historical, anthropological and cultural diet—caries relationships, the English experience. In Rowe NH (ed): *Diet, Nutrition and Dental Caries.* Ann Arbor: University of Michigan, 1978.

Mörmann JE, Mühlemann HR: Oral starch degradation and its influence on acid production in human dental plaque. *Caries Res* 1981; 15:166–75.

Mundorff SA, Featherstone JDB, Bibby BG, Curzon ME, Eisenberg AD, Espeland MA: Cariogenic potential of foods. 1. Caries in the rat model. *Caries Res* 1990; 24:344–55.

Newbrun E: *Cariology.* Chicago: Quintessence, 1989.

Nutrition and Your Health: *Dietary Guidelines for Americans,* 4th ed. Washington, DC: U.S. Department of Agriculture and U.S. Department of Health and Human Services, 1995. Home and Garden Bulletin No. 232.

Oral Health of United States Adults. U. S. Department of Health and Human Services. Bethesda, MD: NIH Publication 87-2868, 1987.

Papas AS, Joshi A, Palmer CA, Giunta JL, Dwyer JT: Relationship of diet to root caries. *Am J Clin Nutr* 1995; 61:423S–29S.

Parry J, Shaw L, Arnaud MJ, Smith AJ: Investigation of mineral waters and soft drinks in relation to dental erosion. *J Oral Rehabil* 2001; 28:766–72.

Petersen PE: The world oral health report 2003: Continuous improvement in oral health in the 21st century—the approach of the WHO global health programme. *Community Dent Oral Epidemiol* 2003; 31:3–24.

Petridou E, Athanassouli T, Panagopoulos H, Revinthi K: Sociodemographic and dietary factors in relation to dental health among Greek adolescents. *Community Dent Oral Epidemiol* 1996; 24:307–11.

Position of the American Dietetic Association: Oral health and nutrition. *J Am Diet Assoc* 1996; 96:184–88.

Rugg-Gunn AJ: *Nutrition and Dental Health.* Oxford: Oxford University Press, 1994.

Rugg-Gunn AJ, Hackett AF, Appleton DR, Jenkins GN, Eastoe JE: Relationship between dietary habits and caries increment assessed over two years in 405 English adolescent school children. *Arch Oral Biol* 1984; 29: 983–92.

Saunders RH Jr, Meyerowitz C: Dental caries in older adults. *Dent Clin North Am* 2005; 49(2): 293–308.

Scheinin A, Mäkinen KK: Turku sugar studies: an overview. *Acta Odont Scand* 1976; 34(6):405–8.

Sgan-Cohen HD, Newbrun E, Huber R, Tenebaum G, Sela MN: The effect of previous diet on plaque pH response to different foods. *J Dent Res* 1988; 67:1434–37.

Shaw JH: Animal caries models: resource paper. *J Dent Res* 1986; 65:1485–90.

Sherfudhin H, Abdullah A, Shaik H, Johansson A: Some aspects of dental health in young adult Indian vegetarians. A pilot study. *Acta Odont Scand* 1998; 54: 44–48.

Sognnaes RF: Analysis of war-time experience in dental caries in European children. *Am J Dis Child* 1948; 75:792–821.

Speirs RL, Beeley JA: Food and oral health: 1. Dental caries. *Dent Update* 1992; 19:100–6.

Sreebny LM: Sugar and human dental caries. *World Rev Nutr Diet* 1982; 40:19–65.

Staat RH, Gawronski TH, Cressey DE, Harris RS, Folke LE: Effects of dietary sucrose levels on the quantity and microbial composition of human dental plaque. *J Dent Res* 1975; 54:872–80.

Stephan RM: Changes in hydrogen-ion concentration on tooth surfaces and in carious lesions. *J Am Dent Assoc* 1940; 27:718–23.

Stookey GK: Considerations in determining the cariogenic potential of foods: How should existing knowledge be combined? *J Dent Res* 1986; 65:1525–27.

Takeuchi M: Epidemiological study on dental caries in Japanese children before, during and after World War II. *Int Dent J* 1961; 11:443–57.

Tanzer JM: Testing food cariogenicity with experimental animals. *J Dent Res* 1986; 65:1491–97.

Ten Cate JM: Demineralization models: mechanistic aspects of the caries process with special emphasis on the possible role of foods. *J Dent Res* 1986; 65:1511–15.

van Palenstein, Helderman WH, Matee MIN, van der Hoeven JS, Mikx FHM: Cariogenicity depends more on diet than the prevailing mutans streptococcal species. *J Dent Res* 1996; 75:535–45.

von Fraunhofer JA, Rogers MM: Dissolution of dental enamel in beverages. *Gen Dent* 2004; 52(6):308–12.

Woodward M, Walker ARP: Sugar consumption and dental caries: evidence from 90 countries. *Br Dent J* 1994; 176: 297–302.

Chapter 14

Nutrition and the Periodontium

Linda Boyd

OBJECTIVES

The student will be able to:
- Describe how nutrition affects the oral mucosa.
- Be familiar with the state of current research on nutrition in periodontal disease.
- List groups at high nutritional risk and recognize when consultation is required.
- Provide appropriate diet recommendations for patients with periodontal conditions.

INTRODUCTION

Nutritional status affects the development, growth, and maintenance of the periodontal tissues (gingiva, periodontal ligament, alveolar bone, cementum, and oral mucosa), and is important in immunity and resistance to infection. It is the balance between host resistance and the virulence of the infective process that determines the extent of periodontal health and disease (Figure 14–1). Periodontal health requires preventing and/or managing the host, environmental, and bacterial factors that may cause or exacerbate periodontal disease (Page, 1998), including nutritional factors.

Some systemic disease and conditions such as diabetes mellitus and acquired immunodeficiency syndrome (AIDS) may also place patients at high risk for periodontal disease and have nutritional implications. This chapter focuses on the role of nutrition in the maintenance and repair of the periodontium on host immune response. Practical dietary recommendations will also be provided for patients with periodontal conditions.

Maintenance of Host Immune Response

Decreased immunity increases the risk and extent of infectious diseases such as periodontal disease. Nutritional status is a critical determinant of immune response (Chandra, 1997). Nutritional deficiencies can alter immunocompetence and increase the risk and extent of oral infection. Because many nutrients play essential roles in immune cell function and proliferation, alterations in function are seen early in the course of reduced nutrient intakes (Chandra, 1997).

For example, mild protein malnutrition may impair the acute phase response to infection, resulting in reduced

host ability to mount an effective inflammatory response to the invading pathogens (Sherman, 1992). White blood cell (especially neutrophil) function is reduced in protein malnutrition (Enwonwu, 1995). High-risk groups with altered neutrophil function include poorly controlled diabetics, cancer patients, and people with AIDS (Chandra, 1997). These patients may exhibit severe periodontal disease and/or refractory periodontitis. In animal models, the volume and antimicrobial properties of saliva are also severely compromised when protein intake drops to 5–8% of calories (Johnson, Lopez, Navia, 1995). An overgrowth of pathogenic microorganisms, particularly the anaerobic microflora, results from the loss of saliva's antimicrobial properties (Enwonwu, 1994).

Vitamin C is present in high amounts in neutrophils (Washko, Rotrosen, Levine, 1991). Functions of vitamin C in immunity include (Enwonwu, 1994):

- Enhancing the migration of neutrophils to the site of infection.
- Preserving the integrity of neutrophil cell structure.
- Facilitating the oxidative destruction of microorganisms.
- Aiding the host by neutralizing the toxic bacterial products produced by neutrophils during phagocytosis.

Studies on periodontal disease in monkeys showed increased gingival inflammation, cellular permeability, and gingival exudate in those animals even marginally deficient in vitamin C (Alvares, Siegel, 1981).

The average selenium intake in the United Kingdom has declined over the last 20 years and is now about half of the recommended intake (Jackson et al., 2004). Epidemiologic studies suggest that this reduction in selenium intake may contribute to an increased risk of infection and some types of cancer (Jackson et al., 2004). Studies also indicate that selenium supplementation to the recommended levels improves immune function (Broome et al., 2004; Jackson et al., 2004). Other nutrients that play a major role in immune function include B-complex vitamins, vitamin A, vitamin E, copper, zinc, and iron.

EFFECTS OF FOOD ON SUPRAGINGIVAL PLAQUE

Food not only nourishes the individual but also serves as the source of nutrients for bacterial plaque. Sucrose intake is needed for the synthesis of glucan, which is

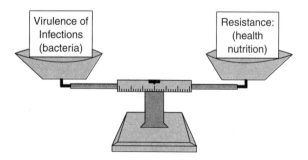

FIGURE 14–1   Periodontal health: A balancing act.

used to facilitate bacterial adherence to the dental pellicle (Carlsson, 1965; Mikkelsen, 1996; Schilling, Blitzer, Bowen, 1989). In addition an excess glucose intake in the early stages of biofilm formation results in an increased rate of bacterial growth (Bowden, 1997). However, there is little information at this time about how dietary carbohydrates may influence the gram-negative anaerobic pathogens involved in periodontal diseases.

In animal studies, consumption of hard, fibrous foods provides some physical cleansing of plaque from the teeth. These findings have not been replicated in human studies. Thus, the concept of apples as "nature's toothbrush" is somewhat misleading. It is true that fibrous foods such as apples stimulate saliva and are not particularly retentive in the oral cavity, both beneficial characteristics for oral health. However, the mere biting and chewing of such foods does not remove plaque to any significant degree. In humans, eating fibrous foods:

- *does not* remove plaque from areas adjacent to the gingiva.
- *does* increase food clearance via increasing salivary flow.
- *may* help maintain supporting tissues of teeth (bone and periodontal ligament).
- *is* a good alternative to more cariogenic foods. (Rugg-Gunn, 1993).

ROLE OF NUTRITION IN PERIODONTAL DISEASE

Poor nutrition does not initiate periodontal disease. However, nutritional status may be an important conditioning or modifying factor in the progression of the disease and the healing of the periodontal tissues. Most of the studies investigating the potential effect of nutrition on periodontal diseases are limited to protein-calorie malnutrition and vitamin C status, but there may be other nutrients that have, as yet, unidentified effects. Infections, even mild ones, have adverse effects on nutritional status. Ascorbic acid (vitamin C) is a cofactor in the formation of hydroxyproline and stimulates collagen expression by fibroblasts (Tajima, Pinnell, 1996). Deficiencies of vitamin C result in underhydroxylation of collagen, leading to an increase in intracellular permeability of blood vessels and sulcular epithelium (Alvares, Siegel, 1981; Nakamoto,

McCroskey, Mallek, 1984). For this reason, the symptoms of vitamin C deficiency appear first in the oral cavity. The classic symptoms of scurvy include swollen and inflamed gingiva, loosening of the teeth, follicular hyperkeratosis, perifollicular hemorrhage, weakness, malaise, sore joints, ecchymosis (bruising), and weight loss (Nakamoto et al., 1984).

Although frank scurvy is rare, even marginal deficiencies may result in alterations in collagen synthesis. Thus deficient or marginal ascorbic acid intakes may be a conditioning factor in the development of gingivitis and one of the early manifestations of vitamin C deficiency (Nakamoto et al., 1984). A recent animal study demonstrated that the need for ascorbic acid increased in the first 7 days of wound healing, although the optimal intake of ascorbic acid to aid wound healing remains uncertain (Kaplan, Gonul, Dincer, Kaya, Babul, 2004). This suggests that if a patient has marginal or inadequate intakes of vitamin C, supplementation at the RDA level prior to or at the beginning of the healing period following periodontal therapy will enhance the healing process (Kaplan et al., 2004).

The epidemiologic data from NHANES (National Health and Nutrition Examination Survey) suggests the odds of having periodontal disease were 20% greater with low intakes of vitamin C (Nishida et al., 2000b).

People with marginal vitamin C deficiency, when supplemented with ascorbic acid at the level of 100 mg/day, have a statistically significant increase in hydroxyproline in periodontal tissues (Buzina, Aurer-Kozelu, Srkak-Jorgic, Buhler, Gey, 1986). Smokers tend to have a higher metabolic turnover of vitamin C and require a higher daily intake than nonsmokers to reach normal plasma levels (Kallner, Hartmann, Hornig, 1981). Megadoses of vitamin C (1000 mg/day) have not been shown to have a strong effect on the gingival response to initial periodontal therapy and should not be recommended to patients without further research (Woolfe, Kenney, Hume, Carranza, 1984). Patients can easily obtain their daily vitamin C requirement from dietary sources such as citrus fruits or juice without the need for supplementation. One orange or 1/2 cup of orange juice contains approximately 60 mg of vitamin C.

A comprehensive study of vitamin C and periodontal disease was conducted on a representative sample of U.S. adults (20 to 90 years old), using nutritional and dental data from the Third National Health and Nutrition Examination Survey (NHANES III). Results showed a 20% increased risk for periodontal disease for those with low intakes of vitamin C (Nishida et al., 2000b). Current and former smokers with the lowest vitamin C intake had the greatest risk for periodontal disease (Nishida et al., 2000).

Evaluation of NHANES III data also suggests an increased risk of periodontal disease may be associated with low calcium intakes. A calcium intake of 500 mg/day resulted in a 56% greater risk for periodontal disease, and an intake of 500 to 800 mg/day of calcium resulted in a 27% greater risk (Nishida et al., 2000a).

Another epidemiological study using NHANES III data from over 12,000 participants suggests that vitamin D intake may be associated with loss of periodontal attachment independent of calcium intake (Dietrich, Joshipura, Dawson-Hughes, Bischoff-Ferrari, 2004). The study found that this association was stronger in men and women aged 50 years and older. Those at the lowest levels of intake lost 27% more attachment than those at the highest levels. Dietrich and colleagues hypothesized that the effect of vitamin D on attachment levels is due to its antiinflammatory effects, which inhibit cytokine production and C-reactive proteins.

Gingivitis

Vitamin C may influence the early stages of gingivitis, in particular crevicular bleeding. In one study, bleeding scores decreased during supplementation with 600 mg/day of vitamin C and increased during the depletion phase (Leggott et al., 1991). This may be related to the influence of vitamin C in maintaining the integrity of the microvasculature of the sulcus. However, limited effects on periodontal probing depths were shown (Leggott et al., 1991).

Periodontitis

Because of the myriad predisposing factors for periodontal disease and the difficulty in determining the individual effect of each on the actual initiation and progression of disease, little is known about the specific effects of suboptimal nutrition on periodontitis. A healthy, balanced diet (see Chapter 2) promotes periodontal health.

Necrotizing Ulcerative Gingivitis/Periodontitis

Significant predisposing factors to necrotizing ulcerative gingivitis/necrotizing ulcerative periodontitis (NUG/NUP) include poor oral hygiene, a preexisting gingivitis, mental

stress, smoking, physical stress (compromised immune system), and Caucasian race (Horning, Cohen, 1995; Wade, Kerns, 1998). Poor nutrition is usually included in the list of predisposing factors, but there is little literature to support this finding. Studies suggesting that poor nutrition is a predisposing factor are mainly among young people in developing countries with protein-calorie malnutrition and may have limited application to the populations seen in the United States (Bermejo-Fennoll, Sanchez-Perez, 2004; Enwonwu, 1972; Osujii, 1990). More studies are needed to determine the significance of overall nutritional status in NUG/NUP.

Some data from animal and human studies suggest an association between vitamin C deficiency and the risk for developing NUG/NUP. Animal studies show that ascorbic acid may be involved in both the pathogenesis and severity of period NUG through its effect on collagen synthesis and its effect on neutrophils of the immune system (Alvares et al., 1981). In a case-control study, subjects with ascorbate levels below normal had a sevenfold increase in NUG when compared with subjects with normal ascorbic acid levels (Melnick, Alvarez, Navia, Cogen, Roseman, 1988). Approximately 67% of the control group met the RDA for vitamin C compared with 48% of the study group. Thus data suggest that meeting RDA levels will decrease the risk for NUG.

Oral Bone and Tooth Loss

Osteoporosis is a complex condition that results in a reduction in bone mass as a result of imbalances in bone metabolism that favor bone resorption (Wactawski-Wende et al., 1996). Low lifetime calcium intakes along with other risk factors including smoking, genetics, medications, physical inactivity, and low estrogen status all contribute to accelerated rates of systemic bone loss eventually resulting in osteoporosis.

Evidence is accumulating to indicate a correlation between systemic osteoporosis, alveolar bone, and ultimately tooth loss in postmenopausal women (Jeffcoat, 1998; Krall, Dawson-Hughes, Papas, Garcia, 1994; Krall, Garcia, Dawson-Hughes, 1996; Wactawski-Wende et al., 1996). Reduction in total skeletal mass is directly related to reduction in mandibular bone density in women with osteoporosis (Wactawski-Wende et al., 1996). In one prospective study, postmenopausal women who lost teeth were also losing bone mineral of the whole body and femoral neck at greater rates than those who retained their teeth. The rates of change in bone mineral density were significant predictors of tooth loss (Krall et al., 1996). Thus, systemic bone loss appears to be related to generalized osteoporosis and a predictor of tooth loss in dentate postmenopausal women (Krall et al., 1996). (See Chapter 19 for more details on osteoporosis in aging.)

NUTRITION RECOMMENDATIONS TO MAINTAIN PERIODONTAL HEALTH

Nutrition recommendations for periodontal health are the same as those for promoting overall health: follow the USDA food guide pyramid and the dietary guidelines. The average American and Canadian diet contains more than adequate amounts of protein and calories. Nuts and legumes can help increase intakes of copper and boron. The average American eats approximately three and a half servings of fruit and vegetables daily (Serdula et al., 2004). This is significantly below the current recommendations. The 2005 version of the dietary guidelines and food guide pyramid recommend four servings of fruit and five servings of vegetables per day for a 2000 calorie diet (USDHHS, USDA, 2005). Fruits and vegetables are excellent sources of vitamins A, C, and K; beta-carotene; and magnesium. Low-fat dairy products should also be encouraged as excellent sources of protein, calcium, vitamin A, and vitamin D. For anyone with marginal nutrient intakes, extra portions of the USDA food guide pyramid food groups can help replete nutrient levels. Although research seems to indicate that low intake of vitamin C is a risk factor for periodontal disease, this does not imply that supplementation of vitamin C at levels above the RDA can be recommended for control of periodontal disease. A registered dietitian may need to be consulted for individualized nutritional advice.

NUTRITIONAL CONSIDERATIONS IN PERIODONTAL THERAPY

Screening and Presurgical Nutrition Recommendations

Patients should be screened before beginning treatment to determine if they are at nutritional risk, which may adversely affect healing. Those at nutritional risk may need diet guidance to assist them in attaining optimal nutritional status. The previous nutritional status of the individual, the nature and duration of the infection, and dietary intake during recovery are all important aspects of nutrition that must be considered to ensure optimal outcomes to periodontal treatment (Schrimshaw, SanGiovanni, 1997). Screening tools such as the Nutrition Screening Initiative designed to assess nutritional risk in elderly people (see Chapter 19) or the general diet screening scorecard may be useful. (see Chapter 22 and the Appendix).

Some groups such as patients with poor nutritional status before surgery (chronic alcoholics or patients who are medically compromised) and the diabetic patient cannot tolerate this short period of fasting. Before treatment for these nutritionally compromised patients, the physician and registered dietitian should be consulted and an attempt made to replete any nutrient deficiencies. Postoperative nutrient requirements increase because of blood loss, increased catabolism, tissue regeneration, and host defense activities. Thus it is helpful to provide the patient with a list of nutrient-dense foods and beverages before treatment so that these foods can be available during recovery. Dental professionals can also recommend a multivitamin supplement with nutrients at 100% of RDA levels.

Nutrition Recommendations after Periodontal Therapy

Patients undergoing initial periodontal therapy, which includes scaling and root planing, usually experience only mild, brief tissue discomfort after treatment, and no special dietary recommendations are necessary. Those undergoing periodontal surgery may have inadequate nutrient intakes for a short time, but most healthy people have adequate postoperative nutrient stores for 3 to 5 days, as long as fluid intake remains sufficient.

A liquid diet may be required for the first 1 to 3 days posttherapy if tissue discomfort makes it difficult to eat solid foods. Good sources of calories and protein needed in wound healing include milk-based foods such as pudding, milk shakes, custards, ice cream, and commercial complete liquid supplements (Ensure, Boost). The patient should be encouraged to continue taking the multivitamin supplement to help with other nutrient needs until eating returns to normal. During postoperative days 3 to 7, the diet can progress from a liquid diet to a soft diet until the patient tolerates a normal diet. A liquid diet generally should be of very short duration, as it is not nutritionally adequate (unless liquid supplements are used). For a soft diet, fruit nectars, soft fruits, scrambled eggs, yogurt, cottage cheese, and the like can be added to the nutrient-dense liquid diet.

Diabetic patients can also consume these nutrient-dense foods. It is recommended that they spread their carbohydrate intake evenly throughout the day to control blood glucose. There are also sugar-free and "no sugar added" products available for diabetics concerned about sugar intake. However, during this period of reduced dietary intake, diabetic patients may need the carbohydrate contained in liquid supplements.

The American Academy of Periodontology (American Academy of Periodontology, 1996) recommends that patients with NUG/NUP be instructed on proper nutrition and appropriate fluid intake. The acute nature of NUG/NUP may make eating difficult because of oral discomfort, so instructions for a high-calorie, high-protein soft or liquid diet should be provided to the patient. The patient is also at risk for dehydration because of the reduced oral intake, so fluids must be encouraged.

Nutrition tips for patients after periodontal surgery or when they have ulcerated oral lesions and cannot eat a normal diet are shown in Table 14–1.

SUMMARY AND IMPLICATIONS FOR DENTISTRY

Nutritional factors do not cause periodontal diseases directly, but can play an important role in immune function and in healing. In turn, periodontal conditions and their treatment may impair the desire and ability to eat and contribute to poor nutrition. Dental professionals should:

- screen patients for dietary risk before periodontal therapy.
- offer soft and liquid diet suggestions for the few days after surgery.
- offer palliative diet suggestions if there are oral lesions.
- inform patients that firm foods cannot substitute for toothbrushing and flossing to remove plaque.
- enlist the assistance of a registered dietitian when indicated.

QUESTIONS PATIENTS MIGHT ASK

Q. I was told that my diet has nothing to do with my gums because gum disease is caused by germs. Is this true?

A. It is true that gum disease is caused by bacteria in the mouth, but the effect that the bacteria have on the oral tissues is related to the health of the tissues and the ability to resist infection. Your nutrition affects both of these.

Q. Is it true that apples and other firm foods help clean my teeth?

A. Apples and other fruits and vegetables are important for the nutrients they provide to keep the oral tissues healthy. The effect of chewing also helps stimulate saliva which helps wash away food debris. However, foods do not remove the dental plaque that causes oral disease, so they cannot be considered nature's toothbrush.

TABLE 14–1   Nutrition Tips after Periodontal Surgery

- Have small, frequent high-calorie, high-protein meals and snacks primarily consisting of liquid or soft, moist foods such as:
  - Puddings, cream soups, and milkshakes
  - Custard
  - Scrambled eggs
  - Macaroni and cheese (add melted or grated cheese to foods)
  - Mashed potatoes
  - Fruit nectars and soft canned fruit (e.g., applesauce)
  - Yogurt
  - Cottage cheese
  - Instant Breakfast with milk for snacks
  - Commercial liquid nutrition supplements such as Ensure or Boost
- Attempt to eat all solid (soft foods) before consuming liquids at meals to prevent early fullness
- To avoid excessive irritation to oral tissues avoid:
  - Citrus fruit or juices, such as orange and grapefruit
  - Rough, coarse, or dry foods such as raw vegetables, granola, toast, and crackers
  - Spicy or salty foods
  - Textured or granular foods
  - Extremely hot or cold foods
- Take one multivitamin and mineral supplement daily with 100% of RDA for nutrients
- Consume adequate fluids, 8–10 glasses per day (not counting caffeine-containing fluids which may act as diuretics)

Q. I am concerned that my diet may not be good enough to protect my gums. Should I take extra doses of some diet supplements?

A. A well-balanced diet that follows the food guide pyramid should provide you with the nutrition you need for a healthy periodontium. If you feel you need a "diet boost," a multivitamin/mineral supplement at the level of the Dietary Reference Intakes is fine. You should *not* take larger doses of any of these supplements unless prescribed by a doctor or nutritionist for a specific reason, as there can be potentially harmful effects.

CASE STUDY

A 65-year-old white woman presents for an initial periodontal examination with a periodontist.

Dental history: She has seen her dentist infrequently over the years and has recently become concerned about her gums bleeding when she brushes her teeth. Her general dentist is concerned that she has "gum disease" and has referred her to the periodontist for an evaluation. She is quite upset at hearing that she has gum disease and wants to know what to do to "cure" it.

Medical history: Postmenopausal and not taking any hormone replacement therapy, she is also taking Fosamax due to a recent diagnosis of osteoporosis. She takes antacids (Tums) seven or eight times a day because of heartburn and as a calcium supplement.

Social history: Her husband died about 6 months ago and she is very fragile emotionally. Now that she is alone, she is not eating regular meals because she "just doesn't feel hungry."

Nutritional status: She reports having lost 15 pounds without trying in the last couple of months. The patient appears quite thin and frail. She says her doctor wants her to gain some weight. She eats mainly broth and crackers because she doesn't feel like cooking. She has never consumed many dairy products because she thought that only children needed them.

Clinical findings: She has generalized moderate chronic adult periodontitis with localized severe periodontitis affecting her maxillary molars. Home care is fair with a plaque index of 60%. Her therapy will include home care instruction, scaling, and root planing followed by a reevaluation to determine if localized periodontal surgery is indicated.

Questions:
1. What are the nutritional concerns with this patient? How might they affect her periodontal treatment?
2. Do you feel a consultation with her physician is indicated? Why or why not?
3. What dietary recommendations would you make for this patient?

REFERENCES

Alvares O, Altamn LC, Springmayer S, Ensign W, Jacobsen K: The effect of subclinical ascorbate deficiency on periodontal health in nonhuman primates. *J Periodont Res* 1981; 16(6):628–36.

Alvares O, Siegel I: Permeability of gingival sulcular epithelium in the development of gingivitis. *J Oral Pathol* 1981; 10(1):40–48.

American Academy of Periodontology: *Parameters of Care* (Position Paper). Chicago: Author, 1996:36.

Bermejo-Fenoll A, Sanchez-Perez A: Necrotising periodontal diseases. *Med Oral Patol Oral Cir Bucal* 2004; 9(Suppl): 114–19.

Bowden GH, Li H: Nutritional influences on biofilm development. *Adv Dent Res* 1997; 11:81–89.

Broome CS, McArdle F, Kyle JA, Andrews F, Lowe NM, Hart CA, et al.: An increase in selenium intake improves immune function and poliovirus handling in adults with marginal selenium status. *Am J Clin Nutr* 2004; 80(1): 154–62.

Buzina R, Aurer-Kozelu J, Srkak-Jorgic D, Buhler E, Gey KF: Increase of gingival hydroxyproline and proline by improvement of ascorbic acid status in man. *Int J Vitam Nutr Res* 1986; 56(4):367–72.

Carlsson J: Effect of diet on early plaque formation in man. *Odont Rev* 1965; 16:112–25.

Chandra RK: Nutrition and the immune system: An introduction. *Am J Clin Nutr* 1997; 66:440S–43S.

Dietrich T, Joshipura KJ, Dawson-Hughes B, Bischoff-Ferrari HA: Association between serum concentrations of 25-hydroxyvitamin D3 and periodontal disease in the US population. *Am J Clin Nutr* 2004; 80(1):108–13.

Ellis CN, Vanderveen EE, Rasmussen JE: Scurvy. A case caused by peculiar dietary habits. *Arch Dermatol* 1984; 120(9):1212–14.

Enwonwu CO: Cellular and molecular effects of malnutrition and their relevance to periodontal diseases. *J Clin Periodontol* 1994; 21:643–57.

Enwonwu CO: Epidemiological and biochemical studies of necrotizing ulcerative gingivitis and noma (cancrum oris) in Nigerian children. *Arch Oral Biol* 1972; 17:1357–71.

Enwonwu CO: Interface of malnutrition and periodontal disease. *Am J Clin Nutr* 1995; 61:430S–36S.

Horning GM, Cohen ME: Necrotizing ulcerative gingivitis, periodontitis, and stomatitis: Clinical staging and predisposing factors. *J Periodontol* 1995; 66:990–98.

Jackson MJ, Dillon SA, Broome CS, McArdle A, Hart CA, McArdle F: Are there functional consequences of a reduction in selenium intake in UK subjects? *Proc Nutr Soc* 2004; 63(4):513–17.

Jeffcoat MK: Osteoporosis: A possible modifying factor in oral bone loss. *Ann Periodontol* 1998; 3(1):312–21.

Johnson DA, Lopez H, Navia JM: Effects of protein deficiency and diet consistency on the parotid gland and parotid saliva of rats. *J Dent Res* 1995; 74(8):1444–52.

Kallner AB, Hartmann D, Hornig DH: On the requirements of ascorbic acid in man: Steady-state turnover and body pool in smokers. *Am J Clin Nutr* 1981; 34(7):1347–55.

Kaplan B, Gonul B, Dincer S, Kaya FN, Babul A: Relationship between tensile strength, ascorbic acid, hydroxyproline, and zinc levels of rabbit full-thickness incision wound healing. *Surg Today* 2004; 34:747–51.

Krall EA, Dawson-Hughes B, Papas A, Garcia RI: Tooth loss and skeletal bone density in healthy postmenopausal women. *Osteoporos Int* 1994; 4(2):104–9.

Krall EA, Garcia RI, Dawson-Hughes B: Increased risk of tooth loss is related to bone loss at the whole body, hip, and spine. *Calcif Tissue Int* 1996; 59(6):433–37.

Leggott PJ, Robertson PB, Jacob RA, Zambon JJ, Walsh M, Armitage GC: Effects of ascorbic acid depletion and supplementation on periodontal health and subgingival microflora in humans. *J Dent Res* 1991; 70(12):1531–36.

Melnick SL, Alvarez JO, Navia JM, Cogen RB, Roseman JM: A case-control study of plasma ascorbate and acute necrotizing ulcerative gingivitis. *J Dent Res* 1988; 67(5):855–60.

Mikkelsen L: Effect of sucrose intake on numbers of plaque expressing extracellular carbohydrate metabolizing enzymes. *Caries Res* 1996; 30:65–70.

Nakamoto T, McCroskey M, Mallek HM: The role of ascorbic acid deficiency in human gingivitis—a new hypothesis. *J Theor Biol* 1984; 108(2):163–71.

Nishida M, Grossi SG, Dunford RG, Ho AW, Trevisan M, Genco RJ: Calcium and the risk for periodontal disease. *J Periodontol* 2000a; 71:1057–66.

Nishida M, Grossi SG, Dunford RG, Ho AW, Trevisan M, Genco RJ: Dietary vitamin C and the risk for periodontal disease. *J Periodontol* 2000b; 71(8):1215–23.

Osujii OO: Necrotizing gingivitis and cancrum oris (noma) in Ibadan, Nigeria. *J Periodontol* 1990; 61:769–72.

Page RC: The pathobiology of periodontal diseases may affect systemic diseases: Inversion of a paradigm. *Ann Periodontol* 1998; 3(1):108–20.

Rugg-Gunn AJ: *Nutrition and Dental Health*. Oxford: Oxford University Press, 1993.

Schilling KM, Blitzer MH, Bowen WH: Adherence of *Streptococcus mutans* to glucans formed *in situ* in salivary pellicle. *J Dent Res* 1989; 68:1678–80.

Schrimshaw NS, SanGiovanni JP: Synergism of nutrition, infection, and immunity: An overview. *Am J Clin Nutr* 1997; 66(Suppl):464S–77S.

Serdula MK, Gillespie C, Kettel-Khan L, Farris R, Seymour J, Denny C: Trends in fruit and vegetable consumption among adults in the United States: Behavioral Risk Factor Surveillance System, 1994–2000. *Am J Public Health* 2004; 94(6):1014–18.

Sherman AR: Zinc, copper, and iron nutriture and immunity. *J Nutr* 1992; 122:604–9.

Tajima S, Pinnell SR: Ascorbic acid preferentially enhances type I and III collagen gene transcription in human skin fibroblasts. *J Dermatol* 1996; 11(3):250–53.

U.S. Department of Health and Human Services, U.S. Department of Agriculture. *Dietary Guidelines for Americans 2005*. Retrieved January 12, 2005, from http://www.nal.usda.gov

Wactawski-Wende J, Grossi SG, Trevisan M, Genco RJ, Tezal M, Dunford RG, et al.: The role of osteopenia in oral bone loss and periodontal disease. *J Periodontol* 1996; 67(10): 1076–84.

Wade DN, Kerns DG: Acute necrotizing ulcerative gingivitis-periodontitis: A literature review. *Military Med* 1998; 163 (5):337–42.

Washko P, Rotrosen D, Levine M: Ascorbic acid in human neutrophils. *Am J Clin Nutr* 1991; 54(Suppl): 1221S–27S.

Woolfe SN, Kenney EB, Hume WR, Carranza FA Jr: Relationship of ascorbic acid levels of blood and gingival tissue with response to periodontal therapy. *J Clin Periodontol* 1984; 11(3):159–65.

Nutritional Concerns for the Dentally Compromised Patient: Oral Surgery, Orthodontics, Dentures, Dysphagia, Temporomandibular Disorders

Lisa F. Harper and Mary P. Faine

OUTLINE

OBJECTIVES

The student will be able to:

- Discuss the nutritional implications of oral conditions such as orthodontia, extractions and orthognathic surgery, dentures, dysphagia, and temporomandibular disorders.
- Provide dietary suggestions for managing the nutritional issues associated with each of these conditions.
- Discuss the appropriate use of liquid dietary supplements.
- Develop a nutritionally adequate soft and liquid diet plan for patients who are functionally impaired or dentally compromised.

INTRODUCTION

Changes in oral health status can have a profound impact on nutritional status and ultimate health status. For example, the number of oral problems, including limited chewing ability, was found to be the most important predictor of weight loss in a study of older, frail adults (Sullivan, Martin, Flaxman, Hagen, 1993). Temporomandibular disorders or other oral facial structure dysfunctions may alter food choices drastically. Dysphagia (difficulty in swallowing) can cause a reduction in caloric intake and decreased consumption of important food components such as fiber. Oral surgery and maxillomandibular fixation can temporarily alter food intake and may contribute to weight loss. Orthodontic treatment may also result in dietary changes that can be detrimental to oral health. Poor oral function has also been associated with decreased self-esteem and a decline in general quality of life (Gift, Redford, 1992). As an example, adults with missing teeth or unstable dentures may avoid social activities because they are embarrassed to speak, smile, or eat in the presence of others. This chapter discusses the nutritional implications of these common oral conditions.

NUTRITIONAL CONSIDERATIONS IN ORTHODONTICS

Role of Systemic Nutrition

The nutritional status and the eating habits of those undergoing orthodontic care can affect the treatment outcomes. Healthy bones and tissues are required for the periodontal ligament and bone to respond positively to orthodontic tooth movement (Hickory, Nanda, 1981), so the well-nourished individual will be best able to respond to this stress. On the other hand, nutritional imbalances may interfere with tissue synthesis. For example, with ascorbic acid deficiency, collagen breakdown and synthesis during tooth movement are slowed. Guinea pigs deficient in ascorbic acid receiving orthodontic forces also showed histological alterations in the periodontal ligament and supporting alveolar bone (Litton, 1974). Calcium and vitamin D deficiencies undermine bone mineralization and remodeling, so positive calcium balance (especially during rapid growth periods) will promote a high peak bone mass and optimally mineralized alveolar process.

Role of Local Food Factors

Orthodontic bands and brackets can cause food retention as well as irritating the gingiva. Orthodontic appliances also provide a nidus for plaque growth in normally caries-free tooth surfaces (e.g., facial surfaces), thus increasing caries risk in these areas. Since fermentable carbohydrates provide the substrate for cariogenic bacteria, the frequency of exposure to sugars, sugar–starch combinations, and retentive carbohydrate foods is an important caries risk factor for people with orthodontic appliances. (Chapter 13 details the role of diet in dental caries.)

The risk of developing dental caries is greater for those who snack most often. Some of the most frequently chosen snacks by children aged 6 to 18 years are soft drinks, ready-to-eat cereals, and sweetened, baked products, all of which are cariogenic (Position of the American Dietetic Association, 1999; Subar, Krebs-Smith, Cook, Kahle, 1998). Because 100% juice, juice drinks, and sweetened beverages such as sodas all contain fermentable carbohydrates, all have similar cariogenic potential (Marshall et al., 2003).

Soft drinks are the biggest source of added sugars in the diet (Borrud, Wilkinson, Mickle, 1997), and are the most likely item to be chosen from vending machines (Kubik, Lytle, Hannan, Perry, Story, 2003). Soft drink consumption has increased by almost 500% in the past 50 years (Ludwig, 2004). About 27% of all drinks are soda. This is a 38% increase in soft drinks from 1989 to 1995 in 2- to 17-year-olds. Over 40% of preschoolers have up to 8.9 oz of soft drinks/day; 11.7% have 9+ oz/day. Adolescent boys average 21.7 oz/day (Grimm, Harnack, Story, 2004).

Independent of the sugar content, soft drinks and juices also contain acids, such as phosphoric or citric acid, that can demineralize dental enamel when consumed frequently (von Fraunhofer, Rogers, 2004).

Carbonated beverages have replaced milk as a snack beverage for some children and adults. This can make it difficult to meet calcium needs. Sipping soft drinks slowly between meals increases the risk of caries. Soda companies negotiate lucrative contracts with many school systems (called "pouring rights"), which provide the schools with needed financial and in-kind resources in return for allowing free usage of sodas throughout the day in classes. This means increased access to and consumption of sodas throughout the school day. Recently, in response to

TABLE 15-1 Foods to Avoid for People with Orthodontic Appliances

Food Group	Avoid
Grains	Corn chips, crisp tacos, large pieces of hard breads such as bagels, French bread, pizza crust.
Fruits and vegetables	Lemons (cut fresh corn-off-the-cob, and raw fruits and vegetables such as apples and carrots into thin slices so little biting force is required).
Proteins	Nuts (cut meat off the bone; and cut foods like steak, pizza, and submarine sandwiches into pieces).
Snacks	Hard candy; popcorn; nuts; peanut brittle; highly retentive, sticky foods such as caramels, taffy, jelly beans, and bubble gum; sipping on soft drinks or sweetened beverages.

criticism from health professionals and consumers, some major soda producers have vowed to reduce access to sodas in schools (Makers of Soft Drinks, 2006).

To prevent dislodging orthodontic bands and brackets, patients should avoid excessively hard foods that may loosen bands, and those foods that can become stuck in the bands and gingival sulcus (Table 15–1) Dietary guidance should be provided to individuals with orthodontic appliances to help them make wise food choices that will promote, rather than undermine, oral health (Riordan, 1997).

ORAL SURGERY

Oral surgery may include extractions, orthognathic surgery, osseous-integrated implants, fracture repair, or periodontal surgery (discussed in Chapter 14). Nutritional status is important prior to surgery, and maintaining good nutriture is important after surgery to facilitate healing and recuperation.

Preoperative Nutrition Considerations

The well-nourished oral surgery patient will experience fewer complications and a shorter healing time after oral surgery. The malnourished patient is at increased risk of postoperative infection (Badwal, Bennett, 2003) and may have diminished recuperation and healing. This does not mean that nutritional supplementation prior to surgery is indicated (unless the patient is severely malnourished prior to surgery) (Olejko, Fonseca, 1984). Rather, individuals need to

have an adequate supply of carbohydrates, protein, and vitamins A, C, D, and K to promote optimum healing (Badwal, Bennett, 2003). Some oral surgery patients who may be at nutritional risk (those severely underweight or having recent loss of 10% or more of body weight, alcohol or substance abusers, or those taking steroids, immunosuppressants, or antitumor agents that have catabolic properties) should be referred to a registered dietitian for nutrition therapy (Patten, 1995).

Postoperative Nutrition Considerations

Maintaining good nutrition during recovery from oral surgery enhances the host immune response, facilitates wound healing, and lowers the risk of infection. The challenge is that nutritional requirements increase (due to the stress of surgery) at the same time that eating well becomes the most difficult. Thus, it is important to educate and motivate patients to consume adequate calories in the early stages of recovery. Carbohydrates, fats, protein, vitamins, and minerals all play key roles in different phases of the tissue healing process. After surgery, minimally stressed patients require 25 to 30 kcal/kg of body weight and 1 g of protein/kg of body weight.

Guidelines for the first 12 to 24 hours:

- The patient should have a high-calorie liquid diet (Table 15–2).
- For optimal tissue healing response, a high-carbohydrate intake is important to spare tissue

TABLE 15–2 Suggestions for Liquid, Soft, and Normal Diets

Food Group/Daily Amount	Liquid Choices	Soft Choices	Normal Diet
Dairy products and other calcium sources At least 3 servings/day (a serving is 1 cup)	All forms of milk: milkshakes, Instant Breakfast type drinks, soft custards, ice cream, yogurt, pudding	All forms of milk: milkshakes, Instant Breakfast type drinks, soft custards, ice cream, yogurt, pudding; soft cheeses like cottage cheese	Low-fat or skim milk, milkshakes, Instant Breakfast type drinks, soft custards, ice cream, yogurt; cheeses collard greens, kale, broccoli
Proteins At least 5 ounces/day (1 slice of meat is about 1 oz, a usual serving of protein is 4–5 oz)	Broth, strained creamed soups, eggs in custard, strained or pureed meat or poultry in soups, plain yogurt, pudding	Eggs, cheese, milk and milkshakes, pea and bean soups, soups with tender meat, fish, poultry, chowders, tender meat in gravy	Meat, fish, poultry, eggs, milk products, dried peas, beans Avoid nuts and tough meats
Fruits At least 3 servings/day (a serving is 1/2 cup)	Fruit juices, nectars, ices, Popsicles, applesauce, strained fruits	Fruit juices, ices, nectars, Popsicles, applesauce, pureed or strained cooked fruits, canned fruits, fruit gelatins	All fruit juices, raw or cooked fruits as tolerated, especially vitamin C-rich citrus fruits Avoid berry seeds as in jams and canned berries Slice raw fruits into small pieces to facilitate chewing
Vegetables At least 4 servings/day (a serving is 1/2 cup)	Vegetable juices, strained or pureed vegetables mixed with broth	Vegetable juices, strained or pureed vegetables mixed with broth; Pureed, soft, canned, cooked vegetables	All vegetables, especially dark green (spinach, broccoli, peppers) and red/orange (peppers, tomato, sweet potato, carrots, squash) Slice raw vegetables into small pieces to facilitate chewing
Grains At least 3 servings/day (a serving is 1 slice)	Soft bread with crusts removed softened in soup or milk, diluted cereals	Cooked cereals, soft breads, mashed potatoes, pasta, rice, crackers in soup	Whole grain breads, bagels, crackers, enriched noodles, pasta, rice, fortified cereals, potatoes, wheat germ, pancakes/waffles Avoid grains with seeds

proteins (amino acids provided by dietary protein are used in tissue repair).

- Powdered skim milk, an excellent protein source, can be used to fortify fluid milk, soups, cereals, and puddings.
- Some patients will avoid eating because of the local pain or fear that eating will cause pain.

- Cool or cold foods (ice cream, milkshakes, eggnog, and chilled puddings) will help keep the local area comfortable and may be more soothing during the first 12 hours after surgery.
- Patients should be urged to consume eight glasses of fluids (water, fruit juices, or milk) every 24 hours.

TABLE 15–3 Soft Diet Meal Plan

Morning	*Noon*	*Evening*
Fruit juice	Cream soup	Vegetable juice
Cooked cereal w/milk	Flaked fish	Casserole (meat, fish, egg, cheese)
Canned fruit	Mashed potato w/gravy	Mashed, cooked vegetables
Milk	Cooked vegetable	Canned fruit
Coffee or tea	Pudding	Frozen dessert
	Milk	Milk
	Coffee or tea	Coffee or tea
Snack	**Snack**	**Snack**
Banana milkshake	Frozen yogurt	Eggnog

Guidelines for the second or third day after surgery:

- The patient should be able to consume a soft diet (Table 15–3).
- Because the volume of food a patient can consume is limited, foods of high-nutrient density (e.g., whole milk, omelets, soft casseroles topped with cheese, fortified cooked cereals, mashed vegetables, finely diced moist meats) should be recommended. Bread products with hard crusts may not be well tolerated.

The typical oral surgery patient should be able to return to a normal diet within a week, but people with multiple extractions throughout the mouth may need to maintain a soft diet for a longer time. If the patient reports losing weight, calorie intake may be inadequate. Fatigue is a common patient complaint and may lead to skipping meals. Adding snacks of fruit juice, Popsicles, milkshakes, or liquid supplements provides additional calories. Using more sauces, margarine, whole milk, regular yogurt, peanut butter, egg-based custards, and puddings will boost the calorie and protein intake.

Intermaxillary Fixation

Intermaxillary fixation (wiring the maxilla and mandible together) may be necessary for major reconstructive jaw surgery or to immobilize a fractured jaw. Intermaxillary fixation is no longer considered an appropriate treatment for morbidly obese adults.

Jaw fixation may last for several weeks. During this period, patients may be at increased nutritional risk from impaired eating ability. If the jaw wiring is prolonged, food intake may decrease dramatically. Weight loss is common after jaw fixation owing to the limited volume of food eaten. If patients have suffered injury, they may be in negative nitrogen balance as well. Diet recommendations during intermaxillary fixation include:

- A smooth liquid diet is recommended (Nelson, Moxness, Jensen, Gastineau, 1994).
- Generally, six to eight small meals a day may be required to obtain adequate calories.
- Dairy foods such as yogurt, milkshakes, soups, and pureed cooked meats, vegetables, and fruits that can pass through a straw are well tolerated (Soliah, 1987).
- Broth, milk, and juices can be used to thin foods.

Because of limited jaw opening, eating can be a tedious, fatigue-inducing process, and weight status needs to be monitored. Liquid meals give a feeling of fullness and become monotonous because of the limited variety of flavors, so patients often tend to prefer the variety of flavors in blenderized foods over the monotony of liquids.

However, if patients are unable to consume adequate food to maintain weight, a liquid nutritional supplement may be needed. High-protein liquid supplements may also be used as snacks between meals to promote nitrogen retention and tissue repair. In one study, Liquid supplements given to healthy orthognathic surgery patients for 6 weeks after surgery aided patients in maintaining nitrogen balance, body weight, and a balanced nutrient intake (Olejko, Fonseca, 1984). Various types of complete dietary supplements are listed in Chapter 3.

Because of the high sugar content of these supplements there is an increased risk for developing dental caries, so it is important to encourage patients to rinse with water after consuming a liquid drink, and brush frequently with a fluoridated dentifrice.

DENTATE STATUS AND NUTRITION

Despite the trend toward increased tooth retention throughout adult life in developed countries, 11% of adults aged 25 and older have lost all of their natural teeth. This number increases to 30% for people over age 65 and is even higher in those living in poverty (USD-HHS, 2000). In a 1996 study, half of all Americans aged 55 and older wore a partial or complete denture, and about 60% of denture wearers reported one or more problems with their denture (Redford, Drury, Kingman, Brown, 1996).

Loss of teeth is not a normal result of the aging process; the major cause of tooth loss is extractions resulting from dental caries and/or periodontal disease (Ship, Duffy, Jones, Longmore, 1996).

Chewing Ability

Masticatory ability is primarily a function of dentition status (Ship et al., 1996). Aging itself has little effect on chewing ability and efficiency. However, the associated reduction in muscle mass associated with aging may adversely affect oral motor function (Newton, Yemm, Abel, Menhinick, 1993). As adults age, they tend to use more chewing strokes and masticate longer to prepare food for swallowing (Wayler, Chauncey, 1983). One-fourth of older adults surveyed reported difficulty chewing one or more of the following foods: steaks, chops, fibrous meats, raw carrots, celery, fresh apple, lettuce or spinach salad, and cooked vegetables (Foerster, Gilbert, Duncan, 1998). Using the Swallowing Threshold Test Index (an objective measure of chewing ability, assessing the number of chewing strokes required to reduce a hard food such as a raw carrot to a small enough particle size for swallowing (Wayler, Chauncey, 1983)), individuals with intact dentitions chewed the best, followed in descending order by those with partially compromised dentitions (24 to 29 teeth) or compromised dentitions (20 to 26

teeth). People with one or two full dentures had the poorest chewing performance. Although dentures improve chewing ability, they do not restore full function. The measured chewing function of a person with complete dentures is only one-fifth that of a dentate person (Michael, Javid, Colaizzi, Gibbs, 1990; Moynihan, Bradbury, 2001). Individuals with altered dentate status often avoid hard foods such as fresh fruits and vegetables as well as those foods containing seeds or pits (Moynihan, Bradbury, 2001). Thus, the number of teeth affects both masticatory performance and food selection (Carlsson, 1984; Chauncey, Muench, Kapur, Wayler, 1984).

Other factors that affect masticatory function include tooth mobility, bone resorption, reduced sensory perceptions, and motor impairment. Adults who have chewing difficulties are more likely to have denture soreness, dry mouth, sore or bleeding gums, and toothache pain.

Dentate Status, Diet Quality, and General Health

The extent to which tooth loss can adversely affect nutritional status is not completely known (Ship et al., 1996). However, diet quality tends to decline as the degree of dental impairment increases (Gunne, 1985; Papas, Joshi, Giunta, Palmer, 1998; Krall, Hayes, Garcia, 1998). In a large group of free-living elders, three lifestyle factors were linked to inferior diets: low median family income, low educational attainment, and wearing dentures (McGandy et al., 1986). A subset of this group who were wearing one or two complete dentures had a 20% decline in the nutrient quality of their diets when compared with the dentate group (Papas et al., 1989). Intake of vitamin A, fiber, calcium, and other key nutrients declined as the number of teeth declined (Papas, Joshi, Giunta, Palmer, 1998). The Health Professionals study found that the edentulous subjects' diets contained fewer vegetables, less carotene and fiber, and more cholesterol, saturated fat, and calories than persons with 25 teeth or more (Joshipura, Willett, Douglass, 1996). A study of civilian, noninstitutionalized people found that intake of foods rich in dietary fiber, anticarciogenic nutrients, and other preventive health effects was lower in denture wearers than in the fully dentate group (Nowjack-Raymer, Sheiham, 2003). Also, a high number of smokers and former smokers are edentulous, and adults who smoke generally have poorer diets (Joshipura et al., 1996). Full-denture wearers also tend to eat fewer fruits and vegetables than dentate adults (Greska, Parraga, Clark, 1995; Ranta, Tuominen, Paunio, Seppänen, 1988).

Replacement of ill-fitting dentures does not necessarily result in significant improvements in dietary intake (Ettinger, 1998; Garret, Perez, Elbert, Kapur, 1996; Gunne, 1985; Gunne, Wall, 1985). Implant-supported mandibular dentures improve masticatory function, particularly biting force. However, no significant improvement in food selection or nutrient intake has been noted in patients exchanging optimal complete dentures for implant-supported dentures (Geertman et al., 1996; Sandström, Lindquist, 1987; Sebring, Guckes, Li, McCarthy, 1995).

Changes in food habits associated with denture wearing may also affect systemic health. These food choices may put the edentulous individual at greater risk for heart disease and cancer. Edentulous, middle-aged Swedish men and women were heavier and had lower high-density lipoprotein (HDL) cholesterol concentrations than dentate adults (Johannsson, Tidehag, Lundberg, Hallmans, 1999). Edentulous women had significantly higher plasma total cholesterol and triglycerides than dentate females. The prevalence of non-insulin-dependent diabetes mellitus (NIDDM) was significantly higher in older men who were edentulous than in dentate or partially edentulous men (Cleary, Hutton 1995). Among a healthy, well-educated group, denture wearers consumed more refined carbohydrates and sucrose than dentate adults (Papas, Palmer et al., 1998). In addition, a lower fiber intake by denture wearers may contribute to impaired functioning of the gastrointestinal tract. Indeed, the use of gastrointestinal drugs appears to be higher in adult edentulous subjects with poor masticatory ability (Laurin, Brodeur, Bourdages, Vallee, Lachapelle, 1994). It is important that the dental team provide dietary advice to those individuals who are becoming edentulous, and that they follow up with these recommendations at maintenance appointments (Walls, Steele, 2004). Table 15–4 lists the nutritional implications of dentures.

Effects of Dentures on Taste and Swallowing

Taste and swallowing ability may be impaired when wearing a full upper denture. The hard palate contains taste buds, so taste sensitivity may be reduced when the

TABLE 15–4 Nutritional Implications of Dentures

- Diet quality tends to decrease as number of missing teeth increases.
- Dentures do not necessarily improve diet quality.
- Dentures may be associated with health risks such as high cholesterol, high weight, non-insulin-dependent diabetes mellitus, and high sugar and carbohydrate intake.
- Upper denture can impair taste and swallowing function and increase risk of choking.
- Denture wearer may have accelerated alveolar bone resorption and lower calcium intake.

soft (upper) palate is covered with an upper denture. As a result, swallowing can be poorly coordinated and dentures can become a major contributing factor to deaths from choking (Anderson, 1977; Palmer, 2003).

Some adults with poorly fitting dentures may have experienced weight loss because of a low calorie intake or limited variety of foods.

Alveolar Bone Resorption

Resorption of the alveolar ridge (Figure 15–1) is common among complete denture patients, and it is difficult to construct a mandibular denture with good retention and stability in the presence of severe mandibular bone loss resorption. Loss of bone mass from the alveolar crest parallels osteoporosis of the long bones (Kribbs, Chestnut, Ott, Kilcoyne, 1990). With the loss of teeth, the occlusal forces on the mandible that occur during chewing are absent. Thus, the bone remodeling process is disturbed. During the first 6 months after tooth extractions, bone resorption accelerates and bone height is reduced. Resorption is greater in the mandible than in the maxilla, and reduction in height of the residual ridge is greater in women than in men.

Women appear to lose bone when their daily calcium intake is less than 425 mg/day (Dawson-Hughes et al., 1990), and there is some evidence that calcium intake is lower in denture wearers (Papas, Joshi et al., 1998). Some female denture wearers have calcium intakes below 425 mg, and the majority of female denture wearers have calcium intakes below 1200 mg/day

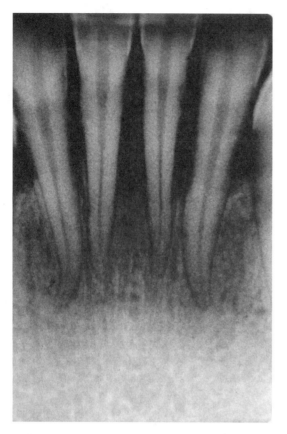

FIGURE 15–1   Bone resorption.

(Papas et al., 1989). Although a high calcium intake will not restore bone already lost, it may reduce the rate of future bone resorption.

Diet Suggestions for Denture Wearers

Despite their dental status, with nutritional guidance denture wearers can consume nutritionally adequate diets, so when patients present to the dental office for new prostheses, diet assessment and guidance is indicated (Knapp, 1989). Most patients receiving dentures for the first time will be able to obtain adequate nutrition by eating a soft diet while they become accustomed to the new denture. Tables 15–2 and 15–3 provide examples of nutritious foods that are easy to chew. Sometimes patients limit their food intake to liquids such as coffee, tea, juice, and broth due to the inflammation and pain they experience

during the first week after delivery of a new denture. In this case, use of a liquid nutritional supplement for 1 to 2 weeks will help promote tissue healing and provide needed calories while the patient adjusts to the new denture. Until comfortable-fitting dentures can be provided, consuming nutritional supplements between meals may also be helpful. For the lactose-intolerant person, low-lactose milk is readily available commercially.

Denture wearers can be advised to chew longer, eat more slowly, and cut fibrous foods such as apples and carrots to bite size. New denture wearers should begin adaptation to their new dentures by cutting up foods in small pieces and chewing them with the molars. They can then progress to biting and incising food.

Explaining the importance of adequate fiber, calcium, and vitamin D intakes, and reducing saturated fat intake for the prevention of chronic systemic diseases may also help motivate patients to improve their diets.

DYSPHAGIA

Adults swallow about 2,400 times a day, including during every meal, and regularly throughout the day and night to clear saliva from the mouth. Swallowing is so automatic that most people never think about it until it is impaired. Swallowing is, in fact, a complex series of movements involving five or six major central nervous system nerves and about 23 muscles (ALS Association [ALSA], 2005) (Figure 15–2).

Swallowing difficulty, called dysphagia, may result from stroke; head and neck radiation or other anticancer therapy; surgery involving the oral structures; severe trauma to the oral facial areas; multiple sclerosis; muscular dystrophy; or inflammation of the pharynx or esophagus. Swallowing difficulties may also be seen in older patients and those with neurological disorders (e.g., cerebral palsy), Parkinson's disease, or Alzheimer's disease (Ship et al., 1996).

The purpose of swallowing is to get food from the mouth, through the throat (pharynx), to the stomach without allowing it to come out the nose or go down the windpipe (trachea). The throat is a tube of muscle that is the common pathway for air, food, and drink. The throat (pharynx) divides into two sections near the top. The tube at the front is the windpipe

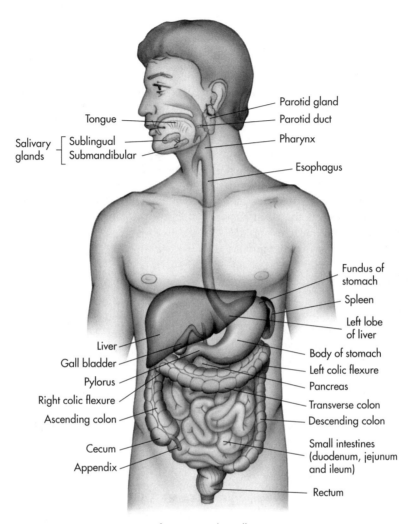

FIGURE 15–2 Anatomy of eating and swallowing.

(trachea) which goes to the lungs. At the top of the airway is the voice box, or larynx (Adam's apple). The larynx is behind the esophagus, the tube that takes food to the stomach. During swallowing, the muscular soft palate lifts to close off the nasal cavities and stop food from going upward. The muscular throat then squeezes the food down into the esophagus. To stop the food from going the wrong way, the larynx acts as a valve to close off the airway; then it tips forward, out of the way.

During swallowing, food is pushed into the throat, the windpipe closes off, and breathing is temporarily stopped. Once the food has passed through the throat, the windpipe opens up again and breathing can resume.

Any food or drink in the throat when the windpipe is open could move into the windpipe.

There are three different stages involved in swallowing:

1. **Oral preparation stage**—In the first phase of swallowing, food enters the mouth, it is chewed, and forms into a bolus. The food or liquid is then gathered into the center of the tongue by using a sucking movement of the tongue, lips, and cheeks. The tongue forms a cupped shape around the liquid and holds it ready for swallowing. The entire bite or sip (bolus) is then pushed by the tongue to the back of the

mouth, or oral cavity. Damage to cranial nerves may result in uncoordinated tongue movements making it difficult to form a bolus. If lip muscles are weak, it may also be difficult to form a seal around a glass or cup, and the result may be oral incontinence (Black, Matassarin-Jacobs, 1993).

2. **Pharyngeal stage**—The tongue then squeezes the food or liquid to the back of the mouth and the swallow reflex is triggered. As the food is being pushed to the back of the mouth, the larynx rises, the vocal folds close, and the soft palate rises to close off the nasal passage. The bolus is moved by muscles through the pharynx, past the closed larynx, and into the esophagus. Throat wall muscles facilitate the downward movement of food and drink through peristalsis.

3. **Oesophageal stage**—This is the movement of food from the lower part of the throat, through the gullet (oesophagus) to the stomach, assisted by a continuation of the peristaltic wave (ALSA, 2005).

Dysphagia can occur during any of the three phases of swallowing. People with dysphagia are at high risk for respiratory infections, malnutrition, and even death because food may be aspirated into the lungs when swallowing is impaired and/or the choking reflex is impaired (Elmstahl, Bulow, Ekberg, Petersson, Tegner, 1999; Smithard, O'Neill, Parks, Morris, 1996). Getting the adult with dysfunctional swallowing to consume adequate calories, protein, vitamins, minerals, and fluids to meet body needs is often a challenge. Patients with swallowing disorders often fear choking or aspirating food, and may resist eating by clenching the teeth or throat, pushing food away, regurgitating, or pushing food out of the mouth because of tongue thrust. Drooling also often embarrasses them. Inadequate nutrient intake is common and results in weight loss, dehydration, and vitamin and mineral deficiencies.

If the dental professional detects swallowing problems, the patient should be referred to the appropriate specialist. Nutrition therapy for dysphagia is a team effort, involving the physician, occupational or speech therapist, and registered dietitian. The nutrition goal is to nourish patients safely while they learn to compensate for the swallowing disorder (Nelson et al., 1994). Feeding by mouth is preferred, but if efforts to increase food intake are unsuccessful, more aggressive approaches may be necessary. Specialized dietary products, such as liquid nutritional supplements and food thickeners, are available to aid in swallowing disorders. Nursing home residents with swallowing disorders were able to maintain their weight better and lost less weight when using a daily oral liquid supplement (Kayser-Jones et al., 1998). As patients resume normal chewing and swallowing ability, they may be able to progress from thickened liquids to solid foods. Table 15-5 provides swallowing tips for people with dysphagia. Table 15-6 lists general diet suggestions for dysphagia. In 2002 the American Dietetic Association published the National Dysphagia Diet, which outlines four levels of food consistencies: dysphagia puree, dysphagia mechanically altered, dysphagia advanced, and regular. Table 15-7 describes the consistency of each stage and provides examples of foods acceptable for each stage. The National Dysphagia Diet also includes four levels of liquid consistencies: thin liquids (low viscosity), nectarlike liquids (medium viscosity), honeylike liquids (viscosity of honey), and spoon-thick liquids (viscosity of pudding) (National Dysphagia Diet Task Force, 2002).

TABLE 15–5 Swallowing Tips for People with Dysphagia

- Sit upright when eating or drinking.
- Maintain the head in a slightly chin-tucked position when eating or drinking to avoid opening the airway inadvertently.
- Concentrate on maintaining a slow, steady rate of feeding, and minimize distractions.
- Clear excessive saliva from the mouth prior to eating or drinking.
- Take small bites and small sips, drink slowly, place only one bite in the mouth before swallowing.
- Swallow two to three times to make sure all food has cleared the throat.
- Alternate swallowing food and liquids to help clear drier or more textured foods.
- Moisten food with sauces and gravy.
- Use a straw to drink liquids to keep the chin down.

Source: Adapted from ALSA, 2005.

TABLE 15–6   Diet Suggestions for the Patient with Dysphagia

Try	*Avoid*
• Soft, moist foods such as cooked cereals; chopped, ground, or pureed fruits, vegetables, and tender meats; yogurt, custards, and puddings; canned fruits or cooked vegetables; fish and chicken, complemented with gravies and sauces. • Thickened liquids that are easier to swallow and less likely to be aspirated into the lungs (may be life threatening). Thickening can be with cornstarch or flour, potato or banana flakes, or fruit purees. Commercial thickeners are also available such as Thick-It, Thicken-Up, etc. • Positioning the body correctly to reduce the risk of choking, the patient should be seated upright at a 90-degree angle with the head slightly forward (Nelson et al., 1994). • Cook food longer to soften (mash with the back of a fork or liquify in a blender). • Try nutritional supplements such as Ensure, or Instant Breakfast type drinks if necessary.	• Pureed diets that are not appetizing and do not encourage swallowing or stimulate the involuntary reflex. • Thin liquids, such as water. They require the most coordination and control to swallow. • Small, hard, or coarse textures such as peanuts, corn, raw fruits and vegetables, and whole grain breads that do not form a bolus easily. • Dry foods such as rice, pretzels, potato chips, crackers, and cookies. • Sticky foods such as peanut butter or mashed potatoes that may stick to the roof of the mouth. • Mixed consistencies or textures such as cold cereal and milk, chicken noodle or vegetable soups, and fruit cocktail (blend into one consistency). • Highly textured foods such as red meats and raw vegetables. • Stringy textures such as bacon, celery, and string beans. • Floppy textures such as lettuce and cabbage. • Dairy products if they seem to make secretions thicker.

TABLE 15–7   National Dysphagia Diet

Stage of Condition	*Food Consistency Required*	*Food Choice Examples*
Severe	**Puree** • Uniform • Pureed • Cohesive • Puddinglike texture	• Smooth, hot cereals • Mashed potatoes • Applesauce or pureed fruit • Pureed vegetables • Pureed meat • Pureed pasta • Rice porridge • Yogurt, custard, pudding
Moderate	**Mechanically Altered** • Moist • Soft textured • Easily forms a bolus	• Soft pancakes moistened with syrup • Cooked cereals • Dry cereals moistened with milk • Canned fruit (except pineapples) • Well-cooked, diced vegetables • Soft, moist cakes • Moist ground meat • Cottage cheese • Scrambled eggs • Tuna salad (without large chunks) • Potato salad • Well-cooked noodles in sauce or gravy

(continued)

TABLE 15–7 National Dysphagia Diet (Continued)

Stage of Condition	Food Consistency Required	Food Choice Examples
Mild	**Normal** • Regular foods (with the exception of very hard, sticky, or crunchy foods)	• Moist breads (using butter, jelly, spreads, etc.) • Well-moistened cereals • Peeled soft fruits (peach, plum, kiwi, mango) • Cooked vegetables • Shredded lettuce • Tender, thin-sliced meats • Eggs • Rice • Baked potato (without skin)

Source: Adapted from Kamer AR, Sirois DA, Huhmann M: Bidirectional impact of oral health and general health. In Touger-Decker R, Sirois DA, Mobley CC (eds): *Nutrition and Oral Medicine*. Totowa, NJ: Humana Press, 2005.

TEMPOROMANDIBULAR DYSFUNCTION

Dysfunction of the temporomandibular region, where the mandible joins the temporal bone, can result in pain and discomfort and impaired mandibular mobility. Inability to open the mouth wide can limit biting and chewing ability (Stegenga, Lambert, deLeeuw, Boering, 1993). Thus, jaw dysfunction may interfere with food intake and alter the types of foods chosen. Although the exact causes of many temporomandibular disorders (TMD) are not clear, the most commonly documented causes of TMD include injury to the joints or muscles of the jaw, occlusal disharmonies such as malocclusion or jaw misalignment, and parafunctional habits such as clenching, bruxing, or excessive gum chewing. These disorders are more common among postmenopausal women receiving hormone replacement therapy and young women using oral contraceptives (LeResche, Saunders, Von Korff, Barlow, Dworkin, 1997).

Dietary deficiencies have been proposed but not documented as factors in TMD. Treatment with large doses of vitamins A, C, E, B-complex, magnesium, calcium, iron, and zinc have also been proposed, but the effectiveness of vitamin or mineral supplementation has not been demonstrated in placebo-controlled trials (Dwyer, 1993). People with TMD may be told to eat soft foods and eliminate gum chewing to rest the jaw, but the effectiveness of these measures has not been demonstrated.

SUMMARY AND IMPLICATIONS FOR DENTISTRY

Impaired oral function can affect diet and nutritional status by altering patients' ability and desire to bite, chew, and swallow foods. Any decrease in eating ability increases the risk of malnutrition. The dental health care team should recognize the potentially detrimental effects of dental treatment on diet and provide counteractive dietary guidance. Problems vary with the individual patient and the specific dental condition, and recommendations should be appropriately tailored to meet the patient's specific needs.

The dental team should:

• determine if there are preexisting nutrition problems that may affect healing and recuperation before providing dental treatment. (This is especially important in nutritionally compromised patients.)
• provide dietary guidance before dental treatment to prepare patients for any potential changes in eating ability.
• provide diet suggestions after surgery, tailored to meet the patient's individual need.
• ensure diet adequacy by suggesting appropriate choices from each food group in the food guide pyramid (MyPyramid).
• consult with a registered dietitian if it appears that liquid nutritional supplements may be required to

provide adequate calories, protein, vitamins, and minerals for the dysphagic intermaxillary fixation patient.

QUESTIONS PATIENTS MIGHT ASK

Q. If I have dentures, do I still need to visit the dentist on a regular basis?

A. All patients should see a dentist on a regular basis, even if they have dentures. Dentures need to be monitored for proper fit, occlusion, wear, and the appearance of the oral mucosa. The complete denture patient should come in annually to have soft tissues checked for oral cancer and other problems; a biannual oral exam is recommended for those with implant-supported dentures (Wilkins, 2005).

Q. Is there a certain age limit for orthodontic treatment?

A. Children and adults can both benefit from orthodontics because healthy teeth can be moved at almost any age. Because monitoring growth and development is crucial to managing some orthodontic problems well, the American Association of Orthodontists recommends that all children have an orthodontic screening no later than age 7. Some orthodontic problems may be easier to correct if treated early. Waiting until all the permanent teeth have come in, or until facial growth is nearly complete, may make correction of some problems more difficult (American Orthodontic Association, 2005).

Q. Is it necessary to take out my dentures overnight to clean?

A. Dentures need to be removed once every 24 hours. The mucosa needs a rest from the pressure of the acrylic during occlusion, bruxism, and clenching. Daily cleaning of your denture is necessary to prevent buildup of plaque, food, calculus (tartar), and stain, which can cause problems with appearance or asthetics, mouth odor, irritation to the tissues under the denture, and infections in the mouth (Wilkins, 2005).

CASE STUDY

Hx: Margaret is a 78-year-old retired school teacher who comes to you for the first time complaining that her dentures don't fit properly. She is a widow with two grown children who live out of state. She spends most of her time working in her flower garden and reading.

Med. Hx: Margaret has rheumatoid arthritis. She sees her physician for regular checkups. At her annual visit in February her blood pressure was slightly elevated but her cholesterol levels were within normal limits. Her weight is slightly below normal. She takes medication for her rheumatoid arthritis, 1000 mg calcium carbonate, and a baby aspirin daily as a heart disease preventative. She can't remember the name of the arthritis medication. She also complains of frequent constipation.

Dental Hx and examination: Margaret has a full upper denture and a partial lower denture. The partial lower denture doesn't fit properly due to a broken clasp. She has heavy accumulation of plaque and supra and subgingival calculus on the linguals of her lower teeth. Margaret says she brushes her teeth with a medium-to-hard-bristle toothbrush and uses "whatever toothpaste is on sale." She brushes once daily in the mornings. She cleans her dentures with commercial denture cleaner. However, she is embarrassed to go without her dentures, so it is rare that she takes them out. She will often just quickly rinse them under tap water after eating. She uses toothpicks to clean in between her remaining natural teeth on the mandibular arch.

Diet history: Margaret eats most of her meals at home. Her husband died 6 years ago so she doesn't prepare large meals as she once did. She says it's too expensive to purchase fresh fruits and vegetables and they just go to waste since she lives alone. Plus, she has to cut things into bite-sized pieces because she has trouble chewing with her current dentures and because of her arthritis. She tries to stay away from anything that she might have to incise. She prefers soft foods that don't present a problem chewing or biting, and convenience foods that don't require much preparation.

(continued)

CASE STUDY (CONTINUED)

24-Hour Recall

Breakfast:
2–3 powdered doughnuts
1 cup orange juice
1 cup coffee with 2 T
  sugar and cream

1 cup coffee with 2T
  sugar and cream
Mid-day Snack:
3–4 Ritz crackers
2 T peanut butter

Lunch:
1 cup tomato soup
2 pieces of white bread
1 can potted meat
  prepared
2 T mayonnaise

Dinner:
Frozen dinner
1 cup coffee with
  2T cream and sugar

Questions:
1. Is Margaret's diet nutritionally adequate? Why or why not?
2. Might there be a relationship between Margaret's diet and any of her general health problems? If so, what?
3. How might her oral condition affect her diet?
4. How might her diet affect her oral condition?
5. What would be appropriate nutritional and preventive dental suggestions for Margaret?

REFERENCES

American Orthodontic Association: *Facts About Orthodontics.* Retrieved July 21, 2005, from http://www.braces.org

Anderson DL: Death from improper mastication. *Int Dent J* 1977; 27:349.

ALS Association of Oregon and SW Washington. 2005. alsa-or.org/treatment/Swallowing.htm.

Badwal RS, Bennett J: Nutritional considerations in the surgical patient. *Dent Clin North Am* 2003; 47(2):373–94.

Bjorvell H, Hadell K, Jonsson B, Molin C, Rossner S: Long-term effects of jaw fixation in severe obesity. *Int J Obesity* 1984; 8:79–86.

Black JM, Matassarin-Jacobs E (eds): *Luckmann and Sorenson's Medical Surgical Nursing. A Psychophysiologic Approach,* 4th ed. Philadelphia: WB Saunders, 1993.

Borrud L, Wilkinson EC, Mickle S: What we eat: USDA surveys food consumption changes. *Community Nutr Inst* 1997; 27:4–5.

Carlsson GE: Masticatory efficiency: Effect of age, the loss of teeth, and prosthetic rehabilitation. *Int Dent J* 1984; 34:93–97.

Chauncey HH, Muench ME, Kapur KK, Wayler AH: The effect of the loss of teeth on diet and nutrition. *Int Dent J* 1984; 34:98–104.

Cleary TJ, Hutton JE: An assessment of the association between functional edentulism, obesity, and NIDDM. *Diabetes Care* 1995; 18:1007–9.

Dawson-Hughes B, Dallal GE, Krall EA, Sadowski L, Sahyoun N, Tannenbaum S: A controlled trial of the effect of calcium supplementation on bone density in postmenopausal women. *N Engl J Med* 1990; 323:878–83.

Dwyer J: Fertile food for fads and fraud. Questionable nutritional therapies. *NY State J Med* 1993; 93:105–8.

Elmstahl S, Bulow M, Ekberg O, Petersson M, Tegner H: Treatment of dysphagia improves nutritional conditions in stroke patients. *Dysphagia* 1999; 14:61–66.

Ettinger RL: Changing dietary patterns with changing dentitions: How do people cope? *Spec Care Dent* 1998; 18:33–39.

Foerster U, Gilbert GH, Duncan P: Oral functional limitation among dentate adults. *J Public Health Dent* 1998; 58:202–9.

Garret NR, Perez P, Elbert C, Kapur KK: Effects of improvements of poorly fitting dentures and new dentures on masticatory performance. *J Prosthet Dent* 1996; 75:269–75.

Geertman ME, Boerrigter EM, Van't Hof MA, Van Waas MA, van Oort RP, Boering G, et al.: Two-center trial of implant-retained mandibular overdentures—chewing ability. *Community Dent Oral Epidemiol* 1996; 24:79–84.

Gift HC, Redford M: Oral health and quality of life. *Clin Geriatr Med* 1992; 8:673–83.

Greska LP, Parraga IM, Clark CA: The dietary adequacy of edentulous older adults. *J Prosthet Dent* 1995; 73:142–45.

Grimm GC, Harnack L, Story M: Factors associated with soft drink consumption in school aged children. *J A Diet Assoc* 2004; 104(8):1244–49.

Gunne HS, Wall AK: The effect of new complete dentures on mastication and dietary intake. *Acta Odontol Scand* 1985; 43:257–68.

Gunne HSJ: The effect of removable partial dentures on mastication and dietary intake. *Acta Odontol Scand* 1985; 43:269–78.

Hickory W, Nanda R: Nutritional considerations in orthodontics. *Dent Clin North Am* 1981; 25:195–210.

Johannsson I, Tidehag P, Lundberg V, Hallmans G: Dental status, diet, and cardiovascular risk factors in middle-aged people in northern Sweden. *Community Dent Oral Epidemiol* 1999; 22:431–36.

Joshipura KJ, Willett WC, Douglass CW: The impact of edentulousness on food and nutrient intake. *J Am Dent Assoc* 1996; 127:459–67.

Kapur KK, Soman SD: Masticatory performance and efficiency in denture wearers. *J Prosthet Dent* 1964; 14:687–94.

Kayser-Jones J, Schell ES, Porter C, Barbaccia JC, Steinbach C, Bird WF: A prospective study of the use of liquid oral dietary supplements in nursing homes. *J Am Geriatr Soc* 1998; 46:1378–86.

Knapp A: Nutrition and oral health in the elderly. *Dent Clin North Am* 1989; 33:109–25.

Krall E, Hayes C, Garcia R: How dentition status and masticatory function affect nutrient intake. *J Am Dent Assoc* 1998; 129:1261–69.

Kribbs PJ, Chestnut CH, Ott SM, Kilcoyne RF: Relationships between mandibular and skeletal bone in a population of normal women. *J Prosthet Dent* 1990; 63:86–89.

Kubik MY, Lytle LA, Hannan PH, Perry CI, Story M: The association of the school food environment with dietary behaviors of young adolescents. *Am J Public Health* 2003; 93:1168–73.

Laurin D, Brodeur JM, Bourdages J, Vallee R, Lachapelle D: Fibre intake in elderly individuals with poor masticatory performance. *J Can Dent Assoc* 1994; 60: 443–49.

LeResche L, Saunders K, Von Korff MR, Barlow W, Dwonkin SF: Use of exogenous hormones and risk of temporomandibular pain. *Pain* 1997; 69(1–2):153–60.

Litton ST: Orthodontic tooth movement during an ascorbic acid deficiency. *Am J Orthod* 1974; 65:290–302.

Ludwig DS: Hard facts about soft drinks. *Arch Pediatr Adolesc Med* 2004; 158(3):290.

Makers of soft drinks accept ban in schools. Retrieved from www.LATimes.com May 19, 2006.

Marshall TA, Levy, SM, Broffitt B, Warren JJ, Eichenberger-Gilmore JM, Burns TL, et al., Dental caries and beverage consumption in young children. *Pediatrics* 2003; 112(3):e184–91.

McGandy RB, Russell RM, Hartz SC, Jacob RA, Tannenbaum S, Peters H, et al.: Nutritional status survey of healthy noninstitutionalized elderly: Energy and nutrient intakes from three-day diet records and nutrient supplements. *Nutri Res* 1986; 6:785–98.

Michael CG, Javid NS, Colaizzi FA, Gibbs CH: Biting strength and chewing forces in complete denture wearers. *J Prosthet Dent* 1990; 63(5):549–53.

Moynihan P, Bradbury J: Compromised dental function and nutrition. *Nutrition* 2001; 17:177–78.

National Dysphagia Diet Task Force: *National Dysphagia Diet: Standardization for Optimal Care.* Chicago: American Dietetic Association, 2002.

National Institute on Deafness and Other Communication Disorders, http://www.nidcd.nih.gov/health/voice/dysph.asp.

Nelson JK, Moxness KE, Jensen MD, Gastineau CF: *Mayo Clinic Diet Manual: Handbook of Nutrition Practices,* 7th ed. St. Louis: Mosby, 1994.

Newton J, Yemm R, Abel RW, Menhinick S: Changes in human jaw muscles with age and dental state. *Gerodontology* 1993; 10:16–22.

Nowjack-Raymer RE, Sheiham A: Association of edentulism and diet and nutrition in US adults. *J Dent Res* 2003; 82(2):123–26.

Olejko RD, Fonseca RJ: Preoperative nutritional supplementation for the orthognathic surgery patient. *Oral Maxillofac Surg* 1984; 42:573–78.

Palmer CA: Gerodontic nutrition and dietary counseling for prosthodontic patients. *Dent Clin North Am* 2003; 47(2): 355–71.

Papas AS, Joshi A, Giunta JL, Palmer CA: Relationships among education, dentate status, and diet in adults. *Spec Care Dent* 1998; 18:26–32.

Papas AS, Palmer CA, Rounds MC, Herman J, McGandy RB, Hartz SC, et al.: Longitudinal relationships between nutrition and oral health. *Ann NY Acad Sci* 1989; 561:124–42.

Papas AS, Palmer CA, Rounds MC, Russell RM: The effects of denture status on nutrition. *Spec Care Dent* 1998; 18:17–25.

Patten JA: Nutrition and wound healing. *Compendium* 1995; 16:200–12.

Position of the American Dietetic Association: Dietary guidance for healthy children aged 2 to 11 years. *J Am Diet Assoc* 1999; 99:93–101.

Ranta K, Tuominen R, Paunio I, Seppänen R: Dental status and intake of food items among an adult Finnish population. *Gerodontics* 1988; 4:32–35.

Redford M, Drury TF, Kingman A, Brown LJ: Denture use and the technical quality of dental prostheses among persons 18–74 years of age: United States, 1988–1991. *J Dent Res* 1996; 75(Spec No):714–25.

Riordan DJ: Effects of orthodontic treatment on nutrient intake. *Am J Orthod Dentofac Orthop* 1997; 111:554–61.

Sandström B, Lindquist LW: The effect of different prosthetic restorations on the dietary selection in edentulous patients. *Acta Odontol Scand* 1987; 45:423–42.

Sebring NG, Guckes AD, Li S-H, McCarthy GR: Nutritional adequacy of reported intake of edentulous subjects treated with conventional or implant supported mandibular dentures. *J Prosthet Dent* 1995; 74:358–63.

Ship JA, Duffy V, Jones JA, Longmore S: Geriatric oral health and its impact on eating. *J Am Geriatr Soc* 1996; 44:456–64.

Smithard DG, O'Neill PA, Parks C, Morris J: Complication and outcome after acute stroke. Does dysphagia matter? *Stroke* 1996; 27:1200–4.

Soliah LA: Clinical effects of jaw surgery and wiring on body composition: A case study. *Diet Currents* 1987; 14:13–16.

Stark AL: *Liquid Diner.* Thousand Oaks, CA: Health Press, 1995.

Stegenga B, Lambert GM, deLeeuw R, Boering G: Assessment of mandibular function impairment associated with temporomandibular joint osteoarthritis and internal derangement. *J Orofacial Pain* 1993; 7:183–95.

Subar AF, Krebs-Smith SM, Cook A, Kahle LL: Dietary sources of nutrients among U.S. children 1989–1991. *Pediatrics* 1998; 102:913–23.

Sullivan DH, Martin W, Flaxman N, Hagen JE: Oral health problems and involuntary weight loss in a population of frail elderly. *J Am Geriatr Soc* 1993; 41:725–31.

U.S. Department of Health and Human Services: *Oral Health in America. A Report of the Surgeon General.* Rockville, MD: U.S. Department of Health and Human Services, National Institute of Dental and Craniofacial Research, National Institutes of Health, 2000.

von Fraunhofer JA, Rogers MM: *Dissolution of dental enamel in soft drinks. Gen Dent* 2004; 52(4):308–12.

Walls AWG, Steele JG: The relationship between oral health and nutrition in older people. *Mechanisms of Ageing and Development* 2004; 125:853–57.

Wayler AH, Chauncey HH: Impact of complete dentures and impaired natural dentition on masticatory performance and food choices in healthy aging men. *J Prosthet Dent* 1983; 49:427–33.

Wilkins E: *Clinical Practice of the Dental Hygienist*, 9th ed. Baltimore: Lippincott Williams & Wilkins, 2005.

Chapter **16**

How Medications Can Affect Nutrition, Diet, and Oral Health

R. Rebecca Couris and
William W. McCloskey

OBJECTIVES

The student will be able to:

- Explain how drugs and nutrients can interact.
- Explain how drug-induced nutritional problems can affect the oral condition.
- Discuss potential direct and indirect effects of various medications on the oral cavity.

INTRODUCTION

Medications, both prescription and over-the-counter (OTC), may have a variety of effects on oral health and nutrition. The importance of these effects and their potential impact on oral health become more significant when one considers the amount of money spent on medications in this country. In 2004, drug sales in the United States were approximately $235 billion, an increase of 8% over the previous year (Vaczek, 2005). Even though the nonprescription market was down slightly compared to 2003, 2004 OTC sales were $16 billion, and are projected increase by over 2% annually over the next few years (Kline and Company, 2005). Therefore, health care practitioners need to be aware of the oral and nutritional manifestations of medication use. This chapter reviews the most common medications that affect nutrition and oral health.

DRUG–NUTRIENT INTERACTIONS

Interactions between drugs and nutrients may occur through various mechanisms or processes and can have numerous biochemical and clinical consequences (Blumberg, Couris, 1999; Hottzapple, Schwartz, 1984; Roe, 1985).

Nutrient Effects on Drugs

Nutrients may alter the extent of drug absorption by alterations in gastrointestinal pH and motility, and by the formation of nonabsorbable precipitates and/or chelates. For example, the calcium found in dairy products may form nonabsorbable chelates with tetracycline antibiotics such that neither drug nor nutrient is bioavailable (Hottzapple, Schwartz, 1984). Nutrients may also affect drug metabolism (Edwards, Bellevue, Woster, 1996). The active components in grapefruit juice can increase the bioavailability and subsequent potency of calcium channel blockers (felodipine, nifedipine, and nisoldipine). The result can be elevated risk of serious side effects such as hypotension and tachycardia (Edwards et al., 1996).

Drug Effects on Nutrients

Drugs may alter food intake through changes in appetite or the senses of taste and smell, or through adverse gastrointestinal side effects (Pawan, 1974). For example, antineoplastic agents induce nausea, vomiting, and aversion to food, and oral hypoglycemic drugs stimulate appetite by pancreatic release of insulin (Morrison, 1978). In addition, drugs may alter nutrient status by their impact on absorption, metabolism/utilization, and excretion. The impact of drugs on nutrient absorption may be caused by direct injury to the intestinal mucosa, alterations in gastrointestinal pH and motility, modification of bacterial flora composition, formation of nonabsorbable precipitates, and/or chelates and solubilization (Blumberg, Couris, 1999; Hottzapple, Schwartz, 1984; Roe, 1985). For example, antacids impair the absorption of riboflavin, folic acid, copper, and iron by alkalinizing the intestinal lumen (Benn et al., 1971). Drugs may also affect the metabolism/utilization of nutrients by inhibiting essential intermediary metabolites or promoting their catabolism. For example, coumarin-based anticoagulants such as warfarin inhibit the synthesis of vitamin K (Roe, 1985). Drugs can affect nutrient excretion by displacing nutrients from binding sites, chelation, or reduced renal absorption. For example, diuretics enhance the renal excretion of calcium, chromium, magnesium, potassium, and zinc (Wester, 1975).

Indirect Effects of Drug-Induced Nutrient Deficiencies on Oral Health

Drug-induced nutrient deficiences can, in turn, affect oral health. These effects are particularly important because the oral mucosa is extremely susceptible to changes in nutrient status. Its susceptibility is due primarily to the rapid turnover rate of the oral mucosal cells, most of which turn over within 3 to 7 days and require sufficient availability of nutrients to sustain DNA replication, protein synthesis, and cell maturation (DePaola, Faine, Palmer, 1999).

The most important nutrients are those that affect tooth integrity and epithelial tissue development and health. These include all of the vitamins and minerals such as fluoride, iron, calcium, copper, zinc, magnesium, and phosphorus, which are essential for mineralization. An alteration of the status of any of these nutrients can affect the integrity of the oral cavity.

Table 16–1 lists common drugs that affect food intake via effects on taste or appetite. Table 16–2 summarizes some of the most common categories of medications (generic and trade names), and their interactions with nutrients and oral health.

TABLE 16–1   Drug-Induced Alteration of Food Intake

Undereating	*Overeating*	*Decreased/Lack of Taste*
Actinomycin D	Amitriptyline HCl	Amydricaine
Alcohol	Anabolic steroids	Amylocaine HCl
Amphetamine	Benzodiazepines	Captopril
Cisplatin	Buxclizine HCl	Clofibrate
Cocaine	Chlorpropamide	*d*-Penicillamine
Diethylopropion HCl	Chlortetracycline	Encainide
Fenfluramine HCl	Cyproheptadine HCl	5-Fluorouracil
Hydroxyurea	Glucocorticoids	Griseofulvin
Mazindol	Phenothiazines	Lincomycin
Methotrexate	Reserpine	Lithium carbonate
Phenethylbiguanide	Tolbutamide	Methimazole
Phenmetrazine		Methylthiouracil
Phenmetrazine HCl		Oxyfedrine

TABLE 16–2   Medications Affecting Nutrition and Oral Tissues

Drug Category/Medication	*Affected Nutrient(s)*	*Nutritional and Oral Effects*
Anticoagulants Warfarin (Coumadin)	Vitamin K	Creates partial deficiency of the active form of vitamin K involved in the posttranslational modification of vitamin K dependent coagulation factors Requires diet control of vitamin K intake No specific oral effects
Anticholinergics Benztropine (Cogentin) Dimenhydinate (Dramamine)		No specific nutritional effects Causes xerostomia (inhibition of salivary flow)—recommend administration of sugar-free candy or lozenges or artificial saliva
Anticonvulsants *Barbiturates* Phenobarbital	Vitamin D, calcium	Secondary impairment of calcium absorption with ↑ risk for osteomalacia or rickets No specific oral effects
	Folic acid	↑ risk for folic acid deficiency implicated in birth defects, cervical dysplasia and elevated homocysteine levels associated with cardiovascular disease No specific oral effects
Hydantoins Phenytoin (Dilantin)	Vitamin D, calcium	Secondary impairment of calcium absorption with ↑ risk for osteomalacia or rickets Gingival hyperplasia
	Folic acid	↑ risk for folic acid deficiency, cervical dysplasia, and elevated homocysteine levels associated with cardiovascular disease No specific oral effects
Antihistamines Terfenadine	Grapefruit juice increases drug effects	Consumption with grapefruit juice can increase the activity of the drug No specific oral effects but may contribute to xerostomia

(continued)

TABLE 16–2   Medications Affecting Nutrition and Oral Tissues (Continued)

Drug Category/Medication	Affected Nutrient(s)	Nutritional and Oral Effects
Antihyperlipidemics ***Bile Acid Sequestrants*** Cholestyramine (Questran) Colestipol HCl (Colestid)	Vitamins A, D, E, K, beta-carotene Vitamin B_{12}, folic acid Iron, zinc	↑ risk for malabsorption of fat-soluble vitamins involved in bone mineralization and antioxidant functions No specific oral effects ↑ risk for folic acid deficiency implicated in birth defects, cervical dysplasia, and elevated homocysteine levels associated with cardiovascular disease No specific oral effects ↑ risk for iron-deficiency anemia and immune function abnormalities No specific oral effects
Atorvastatin (Lipitor) Simvastatin (Zocor)	High niacin or grapefruit juice	May cause muscle aches and weakness
Antihypertensives ***Vasodilators*** Hydralazine (Apresoline)	Vitamin B_6	↑ risk for vitamin B_6 deficiency with clinical signs of peripheral neuropathy (numbness and tingling of extremities) No specific oral effects
Felodipine (Plendil, Renedil)	Grapefruit increases drug effects	Grapefruit, when taken with drug, increases blood levels of drug
Loop Diuretics Furosemide (Lasix) Ethacrynic acid (Edecrin) Bumetanide (Bumex)	Sodium, calcium, potassium, zinc, magnesium, vitamin B_1, B_6, chromium	↑ risk for altered electrolyte and mineral status and depletion of vitamins No specific oral effects
Thiazide Diuretics Hydrochlorothiazide (HydroDIURIL)	Sodium, potassium, zinc, magnesium	↑ risk for altered electrolyte and mineral status No specific oral effects
Antiinfectives Antibiotics (general)	Vitamins B_1, B_2, B_6, B_{12}, K, biotin	May cause temporary decrease in absorption due to vomiting, nausea, or diarrhea Causes loss of the beneficial intestinal bacterial flora—acidophilus and probiotics may help counteract loss No specific oral effects
Cephalosporins Ciprofloxacin (Cipro) Tetracyclines	Alcohol Calcium, iron, or zinc Calcium	May cause flushing, headache, rapid heartbeat Decrease cipro absorption ↑ risk for mineral depletion Can cause discoloration of teeth Should be avoided in pregnant women and children less than 8 years old
Isoniazid/INH	Vitamin B_6 Calcium	May affect vitamin B_6 absorption No specific oral effects Secondary impairment of calcium absorption with ↑ risk for osteomalacia or rickets No specific oral effects
Neomycin	Sodium, potassium, calcium, vitamins B_{12}, K	May impair absorption of several vitamins and minerals No specific oral effects

Trimethoprim/TMP	Folic acid	↑ risk for folic acid deficiency implicated in birth defects, cervical dysplasia, and elevated homocysteine levels associated with cardiovascular disease No specific oral effects
Antiinflammatories		
Prednisone (Deltasone)	Vitamin D, calcium	Secondary impairment of calcium absorption with ↑ risk for osteomalacia or rickets No specific oral effects
Colchicine	Vitamin B_{12}	
Indomethacin (Indocin)	Vitamin C, iron	↑ risk of gastrointestinal mucosa damage leading to iron deficiency, anemia, and ↓ absorption of vitamin C No specific oral effects
Nonsteroidal Antiinflammatories (NSAIDs)		
Sulindac (Clinoril) Naproxen (Naprosyn) Ibuprofen (Motrin/Advil)	Folic acid	↑ risk for folic acid deficiency implicated in birth defects, cervical dysplasia, and elevated homocysteine levels associated with cardiovascular disease No specific oral effects
Aspirin	Vitamin C, iron	↑ risk of gastrointestinal mucosa damage leading to iron deficiency, anemia, and ↓ absorption of vitamin C No specific oral effects
	Folic acid	↑ risk for folic acid deficiency implicated in birth defects, cervical dysplasia, and elevated homocysteine levels associated with cardiovascular disease No specific oral effects
Antineoplastics		
Methotrexate (Mexate)	Folic acid	↑ risk for folic acid deficiency implicated in birth defects, cervical dysplasia, and elevated homocysteine levels associated with cardiovascular disease Ulceration and mucositis—encourage proper oral hygiene and use of mouthwashes with local anesthetic
Antiulcer Agents		
H_2-Receptor Antagonists		
Cimetidine (Tagamet) Ranitidine (Zantac) Famotidine (Pepcid) Nizatidine (Axid)	Vitamin B_{12}, folic acid	↑ risk for folic acid deficiency implicated in birth defects, cervical dysplasia, and elevated homocysteine levels associated with cardiovascular disease No specific oral effects
	Iron, zinc	↑ risk for iron-deficiency anemia and immune function abnormalities No specific oral effects
	Vitamin D, calcium	Secondary impairment of calcium absorption with ↑ risk for osteomalacia or rickets No specific oral effects
Proton Pump Inhibitors		
Omeprazole (Prilosec) Lansoprazole (Prevacid) Esomeprazole (Nexium) Pantoprazole (Protonix) Rabeprazole (Aciphex)	Vitamin B_{12}, folic acid	↑ risk for folic acid deficiency implicated in birth defects, cervical dysplasia, and elevated homocysteine levels associated with cardiovascular disease No specific oral effects

(continued)

TABLE 16–2　Medications Affecting Nutrition and Oral Tissues (Continued)

Drug Category/Medication	*Affected Nutrient(s)*	*Nutritional and Oral Effects*
	Iron, zinc	↑ risk for iron-deficiency anemia and immune function abnormalities No specific oral effects
	Vitamin D, calcium	Secondary impairment of calcium absorption with ↑ risk for osteomalacia or rickets No specific oral effects
Antacids Aluminum (Amphogel)	Phosphorus	↑ risk for bone demineralization and induced hypophosphatemia with proximal limb muscle weakness No specific oral effects
	Vitamin B_{12}, folic acid	↑ risk for folic acid deficiency implicated in birth defects, cervical dysplasia, and elevated homocysteine levels associated with cardiovascular disease No specific oral effects
	Iron, zinc	↑ risk for iron-deficiency anemia and immune function abnormalities No specific oral effects
Aluminum and Magnesium (Maalox, Mylanta)	Vitamin B_{12}, folic acid	↑ risk for folic acid deficiency implicated in birth defects, cervical dysplasia, and elevated homocysteine levels associated with cardiovascular disease No specific oral effects
	Iron, zinc	↑ risk for iron-deficiency anemia and immune function abnormalities No specific oral effects
Sodium bicarbonate (Alka-Seltzer)	Vitamin B_{12}, folic acid	↑ risk for folic acid deficiency implicated in birth defects, cervical dysplasia, and elevated homocysteine levels associated with cardiovascular disease No specific oral effects
	Iron, zinc	↑ risk for iron-deficiency anemia and immune function abnormalities No specific oral effects
Blood Thinners Warfarin (Coumadin)	High vitamin K intake	Decreases drug effectiveness
Calcium Channel Antagonists Amlodipine (Norvasc) Diltiazem (Cardizem) Nifedipine (Procardia) Verapamil (Isoptin)	High vitamin C intake	Decreases drug absorption No specific nutritional effects Gingival hyperplasia—encourage proper oral hygiene
The Benzodiazepines: midazolam, triazolam	Interact with grapefruit juice	Consumption with grapefruit juice can increase the activity of the drug No specific oral effects
Corticosteroids (Inhaled) Beclomethasone (Beclovent) Flunisolide (Aerobid) Fluticasone (Flovent) Triamcinolone (Azmacort)		No specific nutritional effects Oral candidiasis—encourage rinsing after use

Cytotoxic Agents		No specific nutritional effects
Bleomycin (Blenoxane)		Ulceration and mucositis—encourage proper oral hygiene and
Doxorubicin (Adriamycin)		use of mouthwashes with local anesthetic
Fluorouracil (5-FU)		
Methotrexate (Mexate)		
Hormones		
Conjugated estrogens (Premarin)	Interacts with grapefruit	Can increase drug effects
Esterfied estrogens (Ogen)	juice	Gingivitis—encourage proper dental care
Ethinyl estradiol		
Immunosuppressants		
Cyclosporine (Sandosporin)		No specific nutritional effects
		Gingival hyperplasia—encourage proper oral hygiene
Laxatives		
Lubricants		
Mineral oil (Haley's M-O)	Vitamins A, D, E, K,	↑ risk for malabsorption of fat-soluble vitamins involved
	beta-carotene	in bone mineralization and antioxidant functions
		No specific oral effects
Stimulant Cathartics		
Phenolphthalein (Ex-Lax)	Potassium	↑ risk for hypokalemia
		No specific oral effects
Bisacodyl (Dulcolax)	Calcium, vitamin D,	↑ risk for osteomalacia
	potassium	No specific oral effects
Stool Softeners		
Dioctyl sulfosuccinate (Colace)	Potassium	↑ risk for hypokalemia
		No specific oral effects
Psychotherapeutic Agents		
Tricyclic Antidepressants		
Amitripyline (Elavil)	Vitamin B_2	↑ risk for riboflavin deficiency implicated in glossitis
Nortriptyline (Pamelor)		and dermatitis
Imipramine (Tofranil)		Inhibits salivary flow—recommend sugar-free lozenges
Desirpamine (Norparmin)		or artificial saliva
Doxepin (Sinequan)		
Antipsychotics		
Chlorpromazine (Thorazine)		No specific nutritional effects
Fluphenazine (Prolixin)		Inhibits salivary flow—recommend sugar-free lozenges
Thioridazine (Mellaril)		or artificial saliva
Trifluperazine (Stelazine)		
Thiothixene (Navane)		

Sources: Ameer, Weintraub, 1997; Frequently Asked Questions, http://www.powernetdesign.com/grapefruit/general/faq.html.

NUTRITIONAL IMPLICATIONS OF COMMON MEDICATIONS

Antiinfectives

Antiinfective agents in general alter bacterial flora, thus affecting absorption of the B-complex vitamins including riboflavin (B_2), niacin (B_3), pyridoxine (B_6), cyanocobalamin (B_{12}), and folic acid. In addition, tetracycline antibiotics form nonabsorbable chelates with calcium, dairy products, antacids, and iron, such that neither drug nor nutrient is bioavailable (Hottzapple, Schwartz, 1984).

Anticonvulsants

Anticonvulsant agents such as phenobarbital and phenytoin (Dilantin) promote the catabolism of vitamin D metabolites, thus causing deficiencies in vitamin D, which result in a secondary impairment in calcium absorption (Keith et al., 1983).

Antiinflammatory Agents

Antiinflammatory agents such as aspirin and indomethacin (Indocin) injure the intestinal mucosa by producing many small hemorrhages that may result in iron deficiency anemia and a decreased absorption of vitamin C (Leonards, Levy, 1973). Moreover, chronic use of aspirin in patients with low dietary folate intake may be associated with folate deficiencies and macrocytic anemia (Gough, McCarthy, Read, Mollin, Waters, 1964). In addition, prednisone (Deltasone) impairs the hydroxylation of vitamin D in the liver and kidney, thereby causing functional deficiencies in vitamin D and resulting in a secondary impairment of calcium absorption (Hottzapple, Schwartz, 1984).

Antihyperlipidemics

Antihyperlipidemic agents such as cholestyramine (Questran), an anion exchange resin, binds bile salts and impairs the absorption of the fat-soluble vitamins including vitamins A, D, E, and K; vitamins B_{12} and folate; and minerals including calcium, iron, and zinc (West, Lloyd, 1975). The statins, another group of cholesterol-lowering agents, lower plasma concentrations of endogenous ubiquinone, also known as CoQ10, a cellular antioxidant important in the maintenance of oral mucosa tissue (Blumberg, Couris, 1999).

Antiulcer Agents

Antacids formulated with aluminum or magnesium hydroxides, such as Maalox, form nonabsorbable phosphates in the gut lumen and may induce hypophosphatemia resulting in malaise, anorexia, and proximal limb muscle weakness (Insogna, Bordley, Caro, Lockwood, 1980; Lotz, Zisman, Bartter, 1968; Rude, Singer, 1981). Antacids also alkalinize the gastrointestinal pH, thus adversely affecting the optimal bioavailability of riboflavin (B_2), folic acid, copper, zinc, and iron, which depend on a low pH environment for absorption (Benn et al., 1971). Proton pump inhibitors, such as omeprazole (Prilosec), and H_2-receptor antagonists, such as cimetidine (Tagamet), also alkalinize the gastrointestinal pH and adversely affect the bioavailability of riboflavin (B_2), folic acid, copper, zinc, and iron. In addition, these agents also inhibit the hydroxylation of vitamin D in the liver and kidney, producing functional deficiencies in vitamin D, which result in secondary impairment of calcium absorption (Brodie et al., 1981; Hahn, Birge, Sharp, Avioli, 1972; Robbro, Christiansen, Lund, 1974).

Laxatives

The overuse or abuse of stimulant cathartic laxatives such as bisacodyl (Dulcolax) may damage intestinal epithelial cells and impair colonic reabsorption. This may result in steatorrhea, protein-losing enteropathy, and decreased absorption of glucose, potassium, calcium, and vitamin D (Fleming, Genuth, Gould, Kamionkowski, 1975). Laxative preparations containing mineral oil can solubilize and prevent the absorption of the fat-soluble vitamins A, D, E, and K (Hottzapple, Schwartz, 1984; Roe, 1985).

Antihypertensives

Antihypertensive therapy with diuretics such as furosemide (Lasix) and hydrochlorothiazide (Hydro DIURIL) effectively decreases the absorption of sodium. However, these agents concurrently enhance the renal excretion of potassium and minerals including calcium, magnesium, chromium, and zinc (Wester, 1975).

ORAL EFFECTS OF MEDICATIONS

Some medications affect oral health directly by causing side effects such as gingival hyperplasia, gingivitis, mucositis, tooth discoloration, xerostomia, oral candidiasis, and direct tooth damage. Some of these adverse effects can be relatively benign and transient in nature, whereas others may be permanent and severe. The changes in the oral cavity can, in turn, affect nutrition through changes in appetite, taste, and smell, and the ability to eat.

Children with chronic health conditions or special needs may take medications for prolonged periods. If these medications are consumed regularly, especially if the user has xerostomia, they may increase caries risk.

Gingival Hyperplasia

Overgrowth of gingival tissue is a common complication of chronic phenytoin (Dilantin) therapy, a frequently prescribed antiepileptic drug. The prevalence of gingival hyperplasia is reported to be approximately 50% of treated patients (Dongari-Bagtzoglou, 2004).

The risk of gingival hyperplasia may be related to the dose and serum concentration of phenytoin (Stinnett, Rodu, Grizzle, 1987). Although the exact mechanism of phenytoin-induced gingival hyperplasia has not been established, it has been suggested that low doses of phenytoin may act on craniofacial bone cells to stimulate cell proliferation, differentiation, and mature osteoblastic activities to stimulate bone formation (Nakade, Baylink, Lau, 1995). While chronic use of other anticonvulsants such as valproic acid, phenobarbital, and carbamazepine have been linked to gingival enlargement, the reports are rare or are poorly documented (Dongari-Bagtzoglou, 2004).

Because there is a relationship between inflammation and gingival hyperplasia, proper oral hygiene programs are recommended to reduce the degree and severity of gingival hyperplasia if practiced before therapy is initiated. Patients should be instructed of the importance of good oral hygiene in reducing this complication by flossing or stimulating gums when initiating phenytoin therapy. Treatment of existing gingival hyperplasia includes dosage reduction or discontinuation, especially if another antiepileptic agent could be substituted, thus resulting in partial or complete resolution of side effects (Stinnett et al., 1987). While gingivectomy is also an option, hyperplasia may recur.

Calcium channel blockers have also been associated with drug-induced gingival hyperplasia. Nifedipine has been reported to have the highest prevalence, although a recent study suggests that only 6% of patients taking nifedipine had clinically significant gingival enlargement (Ellis et al., 1999). Diltiazem has also been associated with an increased risk of gingival overgrowth (Miranda et al., 2005). Reports of gingival hyperplasia with other agents of this class such as verapamil, amlodipine, and felodipine are less common (Dongari-Bagtzoglou, 2004). Most cases of gingival enlargement with calcium channel blockers have been reported in patients over 50 years old, and may occur as early as 30 days after initiation of therapy or be delayed for upward of 3 years. Discontinuation of the drug appears to be the most effective treatment strategy. Proper oral hygiene alone may not prevent the degree of gingival hyperplasia caused by calcium channel blockers, and surgery may be required in severe cases (Bullon et al., 1996).

The incidence of gingival overgrowth has also been reported in 5 to 16% of transplant patients receiving the immunosupressant cyclosporine (Product Information,

2004). Cyclosporine-induced gingival hyperplasia usually occurs within 3 months of initiating therapy (Seymour, Jacobs, 1992) and may be associated with higher salivary concentrations of the drug (McGaw, Porter, 1988). Histologically, cyclosporine-induced gingival hyperplasia is characterized by cellular hyperplasia and collagen overgrowth. Although an aggressive program of oral hygiene may improve gum tissue, it may not prevent the occurrence of gingival hyperplasia (Seymour, Jacobs, 1992). Tacrolimus is an immunosuppressant that is less likely to be associated with gingival hyperplasia as compared to cyclosporine (Ellis et al., 2004). However, gingival overgrowth may persist when changing from cyclosporine to tacrolimus if patients are on medications that increase the risk of hyperplasia such as calcium channel blockers.

Gingivitis and Effects on Oral Mucosa

Hormone therapy, including corticosteroids, androgens, estrogens, and progestins, has been associated with tenderness, swelling, or minor bleeding of the gums, possibly leading to gingivitis. The clinical changes seen in plaque-induced gingivitis are intensified during elevated blood levels of these hormones, and may result from immune suppression, increased fluid exudation, stimulation of bone resorption, or stimulation of fibroblast synthetic activity (Sooriyamoorthy, Gower, 1989). A recent clinical study reported that women undergoing ovulation induction with agents such as clomiphene citrate, follicle-stimulating hormone, and human menopausal gonadotropin for more than three cycles had significantly more gingival inflammation and bleeding than a control group of patients receiving less than three cycles (Haytac, Cetin, Seydaoglu, 2004). Therefore, proper attention to oral care and regular dental visits should be encouraged in patients receiving hormone therapy.

Nearly 40% of patients treated with chemotherapeutic agents develop oral side effects such as mucositis, bleeding, and infection (Sonis, Sonis, Lieberman, 1978). Most chemotherapeutic agents target cells undergoing cell division, which makes the rapidly reproducing oral mucosal cells more susceptible to the effects of these drugs. Mucositis begins approximately 7 days after therapy is initiated and is evidenced by a decrease in surface thickness and keratinization of the mucous membrane in the mouth (Johnson, 1984). In addition to pain, it can lead to bleeding and infection, which may also compromise the patient's nutritional status (Lindley, Finley, LaCivita, 1995). Treatment is primarily palliative and includes mouthwashes that have local anesthetics such as lidocaine and dyclonine, or antihistamines such as diphenhydramine, corticosteroids such as hydrocortisone, and antifungals such as nystatin combinations (Johnson, 1984; Lindley et al., 1995). The mucositis generally resolves several days after the therapy is discontinued (Johnson, 1984).

Some agents can also cause erythematous or lichenoid lesions in the oral cavity. The lichenoid lesions generally appear as white striations on the tongue or buccal mucosa (Torpet, Kragelund, Reibel, Nauntofte, 2004). If these conditions are medication related, the onset of occurrence may vary from days to weeks, and they usually resolve when the drug is discontinued (Ciancio, 2004). Some medications that have been associated with these lesions are noted in Table 16–3.

Tooth Discoloration

Tetracycline discoloration of the teeth is a well-known complication of therapy in children. All tetracyclines can deposit in the dentin and enamel of developing teeth, thus causing permanent discoloration of yellow to gray-brown. The presence of tetracycline in mineralized tissue is thought to be the result of a calcium chelate and the antiobiotic (Moffitt, Cooley, Olsen, Hefferren, 1974). Discoloration of permanent teeth may occur in children less than 8 years old who receive

TABLE 16–3 Drug-Induced Lichenoid or Erythematous Lesions

Medication	Therapeutic Class
Clindamycin (Cleocin)	Antibiotic
Barbiturates	Sedatives/hypnotics
Captopril (Capoten)	Antihypertensive
Carbamazepine (Tegretol)	Anticonvulsant
Chlorpropamide (Diabinese)	Hypoglycemic
Diflusianl (Dolobid)	Nonsteroidal antiinflammatory agent
Flurbiprofan (Ansaid)	Nonsteroidal antiinflammatory agent
Furosemide (Lasix)	Diuretic
Ibuprofen (Motrin, Advil)	Nonsteroidal antiinflammatory agent
Methydopa (Aldomet)	Antihypertensive
Phenytoin (Dilantin)	Anticonvulsant
Sulfonamides (various)	Antibiotic

tetracyclines. Consequently, tetracycline antibiotics should be avoided in this age group. The drug should also be avoided during the third trimester of pregnancy because discoloration of deciduous teeth can occur (Scopp, Kazandjian, 1986).

There have been some case reports of tooth discoloration in children associated with the antibiotic combination of amoxicillin and clavulantic acid (Garcia-Lopez, Martinez-Blanco, Martinez-Mir, Palop, 2001). Unlike tetracycline-related irreversible damage, discoloration secondary to amoxicillin-clavulantic acid is cuased by deposits on the surface of the tooth and is not associated with internal alternations in the tooth. There was also a recent case report in an 11-year-old child of reversible tooth discoloration with linezolid, one of a new class of antibiotics, the oxazolidinones (Matson, Miller, 2003). The nature and significance of this adverse reaction has not been clearly established.

Some other agents also cause a superficial staining of the teeth. These include chlorhexidine, liquid iron products, and tobacco. Chlorhexidine oral rinse may cause tooth discoloration and staining of the dorsum of the tongue, dentures, and fillings with rough surfaces. Tooth staining appears to be dependent on the concentration of chlorhexidine and is estimated to occur in approximately 50% of patients after only a few days of use (Heyden, 1973). Chlorhexidine staining may be related to dietary factors (Rolla, Melsen, 1975). The discoloration is formed by precipitation of iron sulfide, produced by denatured proteins and dietary iron. This may explain the reason for the staining of teeth after smoking or the consumption of tannic acid containing beverages such as tea, coffee, and wine. Standard dental cleaning will remove staining from most tooth surfaces, while staining to tooth restorations may be permanent. Chewing sugar-free gum for 20 minutes after the use of chlorhexidine oral rinse may decrease the amount of staining without any effect on chlorhexidine's efficacy (Yankel, Emling, 1997).

Liquid dosage forms of iron salts may also produce a temporary discoloration of tooth enamel. Therefore, it is recommended that patients first dilute iron-containing products with a beverage such as water or fruit juice before consumption. The use of a straw for ingestion of liquid iron preparations is also recommended. These recommendations are based on in vitro studies that indicate the extent of staining is proportional to the concentration of iron (Nordbo, Eriksen, Rolla, Attramadal, Solheim, 1982).

Xerostomia

Drugs that cause xerostomia ("dry mouth") can increase dental caries risk (Kempe, Silver, O'Brien, 1982). Medications that have the greatest potential for reducing saliva production are those agents with anticholinergic side effects, including tricyclic antidepressants and certain phenothiazine antipsychotics. Other agents exhibiting anticholinergic properties include the anti-Parkinson drug cogentin, and the antihistamine diphenhydramine.

Artificial saliva products are available over-the-counter for patients experiencing xerostomia secondary to the anticholinergic effects of certain medications. Patients may also be counseled to suck on sugarless candies or lozenges to promote saliva production. If xerostomia becomes problematic, oral pilocarpine, which is a cholinergic agent, may be used to alleviate the condition (Winer, Bahn, 1967). Chapter 11 provides a detailed review of xerostomia.

Direct Tooth Damage

There is some evidence that certain drug treatments for asthma may cause tooth damage in children. Most drugs commonly used for the treatment of asthma in children have a pH of less than 5.5 in the powdered form. This is significant because tooth enamel begins to dissolve at a pH of 5.5. Aerosol dosage forms have a pH that is significantly higher, above 7.0. The pH of powdered or aerosol forms of corticosteroids (including fluticasone) and beta-agonists (including albuterol and terbutaline) differ significantly. These drugs may result in tooth erosion when used several times a day in the powdered form (O'Sullivan, Curzon, 1998). Recommendations may include rinsing the child's mouth after every inhalation and the use of spacer devices.

While there have been reports about the effects of aspirin on the oral mucosa (Dellinger, Livingston, 1998), chewing aspirin tablets can cause damage to tooth enamel and dentin (Grace, Sarlani, Kaplan, 2004). Patients should be advised about the risks of dental erosion caused by chewing aspirin products.

Oral Candidiasis

The use of inhaled corticosteroids is also associated with oral candidiasis resulting from corticosteroid-induced inhibition of normal host defenses. The development of thrush is related to the total daily dose of corticosteroid and dosing frequency. Patients who are also taking nasal steroids, systemic steroids, or antibiotics concurrently are more susceptible to oral candidiasis. Therefore, patients should be advised to use a spacer device or to rinse their mouth after every use of these products. Fortunately, most cases of candidiasis are self-limited and can be managed by a reduction in steroid dose. If treatment is required, however, nystatin suspension may be used (Hanania, Chapman, Kesten, 1995).

SUMMARY AND IMPLICATIONS FOR DENTISTRY

Interactions between drugs and nutrients may alter a patient's dental therapeutic outcome and nutritional status. The clinician must be aware of potential oral effects of medications to provide proper interventions to either prevent or reverse damage to teeth and gums and to safeguard the oral health of patients.

QUESTIONS PATIENTS MIGHT ASK

Q. Why is it so important that you know all of the drugs I am taking before you do dental work?

A. That is a very important question. Drugs can have major effects on dental treatment. For example, if you have a history of heart valve problems, your dentist will have you take an antibiotic before any dental treatment to avoid infection (bacteria from your mouth can get into your bloodstream). Some drugs, such as the blood thinner Coumadin, can affect blood clotting in the mouth, so your dentist needs to know that you're taking it.

Q. My child is taking a lot of medications prescribed by his doctor. Can they have any harmful effects on his nutrition?

A. They could affect his nutrition. Check with your doctor or pharmacist to see what the side effects of each medication can be. For example, some drugs can affect appetite or interfere with nutrient absorption. In these cases you will need to make sure that your child gets appropriate food or supplements to make up for the losses.

Q. Could these drugs have any effects in his mouth?

A. Possibly. Some drugs can affect teeth and gums. For example, Dilantin can cause gums to grow around the teeth. This makes it hard to brush the teeth, and allows food to get trapped easily, contributing to gum infection. Your dentist and hygienist can help you overcome any side effects of these medications.

REFERENCES

Ameer B, Weintraub RA: Drug interactions with grapefruit juice. *Clin Pharmacokinet* 1997; 33(2):103–21.

Benn A, Swan CJH, Cooke WT, Blair JA, Matty AJ, Smith ME: Effect of intraluminal pH on the absorption of pteroylmonoglutamic acid. *Br Med J* 1971; 16:148–50.

Blumberg JB, Couris RR: Pharmacology, nutrition, and the elderly: Interactions and implications. In Chernoff R (ed): *Geriatric Nutrition.* Rockville, MD: Aspen, 1999.

Brodie MJ, Boobis AR, Hillyard CJ, Abeyasekera G, MacIntyre I, Park BK: Effect of isoniazid on vitamin D metabolism and hepatic monooxygenase activity. *Clin Pharmacol Ther* 1981; 30:363–67.

Bullon P, Machuca G, Martincz-Sahuquillo A, Rios JV, Velasco E, Rojas J, et al.: Evaluation of gingival and periodontal conditions following causal periodontal treatment in patients treated with nifedipine and diltiazem. *J Clin Periodontal* 1996; 23:649–57.

Butler RT, Kaklwarf LL, Kaldahl WB: Drug-induced gingival hyperplasia: Phenytoin, cyclosporine, and nifedipine. *J Am Dent Assoc* 1987; 114:56.

Ciancio SG: Medications' impact on oral health. *JADA* 2004; 135(10):1440–48.

Dellinger TM, Livingston HM: Aspirin burn of the oral cavity. *Ann Pharmacother* 1998; 32(10):1107.

DePaola DP, Faine MP, Palmer CA: Nutrition in relation to dental medicine. In Shills M, Olsen JA, Ross AC (eds): *Modern Nutrition in Health and Disease*, 9th ed. Baltimore: Williams & Wilkins, 1999.

Dongari-Bagtzoglou A. Drug-associated gingival enlargement. *J Periodontol* 2004; 75:1424–31.

Edwards DJ, Bellevue FH, Woster PM: Identification of 6′, 7′-dihydroxy-bergamotten, a cytochrome P450 inhibitor, in grapefruit juice. *Drug Metab Disp* 1996; 24:1287–90.

Ellis JS, Seymour RA, Steele JG, Robertson P, Butler TJ, Thomason JM: Prevalance of gingival overgrowth induced by calcium channel blockers: A community based study. *J Peridontol* 1999; 70:63–67.

Ellis JS, Seymour RA, Taylor JJ, Thomason JM: Prevalence of gingival overgrowth in transplant patients immunosuppressed with tacrolimus. *J Clin Periodontol* 2004; 31: 126–31.

Fleming BJ, Genuth SM, Gould AB, Kamionkowski MD: Laxative-induced hypokalemia, sodium depletion and hypereninemia: Effects of potassium and sodium replacement on the renin angiotensin aldosterone system. *Ann Intern Med* 1975; 83:60–62.

Garcia-Lopez M, Martinez-Blanco M, Martinez-Mir I, Palop V: Amoxycillin-clavulanic acid-related tooth discoloration in children. *Pediatrics* 2001; 108:819–20.

Gough KR, McCarthy C, Read AE, Mollin DL, Waters AH: Folic acid deficiency in rheumatoid arthritis. *Br Med J* 1964; 1:212–16.

Grace EG, Sarlani E, Kaplan S: Tooth erosion caused by chewing aspirin. *JADA* 2004; 135:911–14.

Hahn TJ, Birge SJ, Sharp CR, Avioli LV: Phenobarbital-induced alterations in vitamin D metabolism. *J Clin Invest* 1972; 51:741–48.

Hanania NA, Chapman KR, Kesten S: Adverse effects of inhaled corticosteroids. *Am J Med* 1995; 98:196–208.

Haytec MC, Cetin T, Seydaoglu G: The effects of ovulation induction during infertility treatment on gingival inflammation. *J Periodontol* 2004; 75:805–10.

Heyden G: Relation between locally high concentration of chlorhexidine and staining as seen in the clinic. *J Periodontal Res* 1973; 12:76–80.

Hottzapple PC, Schwartz SE: Drug-induced maldigestion and malabsorption. In Roe DA, Campbell TC (eds): *Drugs and Nutrients: The Interactive Effects.* New York: Marcel Dekker; 1984:575–85.

Insogna KL, Bordley DR, Caro JF, Lockwood DH: Osteomalacia and weakness from excessive antacids. *JAMA* 1980; 244:2544–46.

Iwamoto Y, Nakamura R, Folkers K, Morrison RF: Study of periodontal disease and coenzyme Q. *Res Commun Chem Pathol Pharmacol* 1975; 11(2):265–71.

Johnson DH: Effects of medications on oral tissues. *Can Pharm J* 1984; 117:8–10.

Keith DA, Gundberg CM, Japour A, Aronoff J, Alvarez N, Gallop PM: Vitamin K-dependent proteins and anticonvulsant medication. *Clin Pharmacol Ther* 1983; 34:529–32.

Kempe CH, Silver HK, O'Brien D (eds): *Current Pediatric Diagnosis and Treatment*, 7th ed. Los Altos, CA: Lange Medical Publishers, 1982.

Kline and Company, Little Falls, NJ: Nonprescription drugs USA 2004. Retrieved November 2005 from http://www.klinegroup.com/brochures/cia6c/brochure.pdf

Leonards JH, Levy G: Gastrointestinal blood loss during prolonged aspirin administration. *N Engl J Med* 1973; 289:1020.

Lindley C, Finley RS, LaCivita CL: Adverse effects of chemotherapy. In Young LY, Koda-Kimble MA (eds): *Applied Therapeutics: The Clinical Use of Drugs*, 6th ed. Vancouver, WA: Applied Therapeutics, 1995.

Lotz M, Zisman E, Bartter C: Evidence for phosphorus depletion syndrome in man. *N Engl J Med* 1968; 278: 409–15.

Matson K L, Miller SE: Tooth discoloration after treatment with linezolid. *Pharmacotherapy* 2003; 23:882–85

McGaw WT, Porter H: Cyclosporine-induced gingival overgrowth: An ultrastructural stereologic study. *Oral Surg Oral Med Oral Med Oral Path* 1988; 65(2):186–90.

Miranda J, Brunet L, Roset P, Berini L, Farre M, Mendieta C: Prevalence and risk of gingival overgrowth in patients treated with diltiazem or verapamil. *J Clin Periodontol* 2005; 32:294–98.

Missouris GG, Kalaitzidis RG, Cappuccio FP, MacGregor GA: Gingival hyperplasia caused by calcium channel blockers. *J Hum Hypertens* 2000; 14:155–56.

Moffitt JM, Cooley RO, Olsen NH, Hefferren JJ: Prediction of tetracycline-induced tooth discoloration. *J Am Dent Assoc* 1974; 88:547–52.

Morrison SD: Origins of anorexia and neoplastic disease. *Am J Clin Nutr* 1978; 31:1104–7.

Nakade O, Baylink DJ, Lau KH: Pheytoin at micromolar concentrations is an osteogenic agent for human mandible derived bone cells in vitro. *J Dent Res* 1995; 74: 331–37.

Nordbo H, Eriksen HM, Rolla G, Attramadal A, Solheim H: Iron staining of the acquired enamel pellicle after exposure to tannic acid or chlorhexidine: preliminary report. *Scand J Dent Res* 1982; 90(2):117–23.

O'Sullivan EA, Curzon ME: Drug treatments for asthma may cause erosive tooth damage. *Br Med J* 1998; 317(7161):820.

Pawan GLS: Drugs and appetite. *Proc Nutr Soc* 1974; 33: 239–44.

Product Information: Neoral Oral Solution®, cyclosporine. Novartis Pharmaceuticals, East Hanover, NJ, 2004.

Robbro OT, Christiansen C, Lund M: Development of anti-convulsant osteomalacia in epileptic patients on phenytoin treatment. *Acta Neurol Scand* 1974; 50:527–32.

Roe DA: Nutrients and their interactions with drugs. In *Drug-Induced Nutritional Deficiencies*. Westport, CT: Avi Publishing, 1985.

Rolla G, Melsen B: On the mechanism of plaque inhibition by chlorhexidine. *J Dent Res* 1975; 54 (Spec B):B57–B62.

Rude RK, Singer FR: Magnesium deficiency and excess. *Ann Rev Med* 1981; 32:245–59.

Scopp IW, Kazandjian G: Tetracycline-induced staining of teeth. *Postgrad Med* 1986; 79:202–3.

Seymour RA, Jacobs DJ: Cyclosporine and gingival tissues. *J Clin Periodontal* 1992; 19:1–11.

Sonis ST, Sonis AL, Lieberman A: Oral complications in patients receiving treatment for malignancies other than of the head and neck. *J Am Dent Assoc* 1978: 97:468–72.

Sooriyamoorthy M, Gower DB: Hormonal influences on gingival tissue: Relationship to periodontal disease. *J Clin Periodont* 1989; 16:201–8.

Steele RM, Schuna AA, Schreiber RT: Calcium antagonist-induced gingival hyperplasia. *Ann Intern Med* 1994; 120:663–64.

Stinnett E, Rodu B, Grizzle WE: New developments in understanding phenytoin-induced gingival hyperplasia. *J Am Dent Assoc* 1987; 114:814.

Torpet LA, Kragelund C, Reibel J, Nauntofte B: Oral adverse reactions to cardiovascular drugs. *Crit Rev Oral Biol Med* 2004; 15(1):28–46.

Vaczek D: Top 200 prescription drugs of 2004. Pharmacy Times. Retrieved November 2005 from http://www.pharmacytimes.com/article.cfm?id=2534

West RJ, Lloyd JK: The effects of cholestyramine on intestinal absorption. *Gut* 1975; 16:93–98.

Wester PO: Zinc curing diuretic treatment. *Lancet* 1975; 1:578.

Winer JA, Bahn S: Loss of teeth with antidepressant drug therapy. *Arch Gen Psychiatry* 1967; 16:239–40.

Yankel SL, Emling RC: Efficacy of chewing gum in preventing extrinsic tooth staining. *J Clin Dent* 1997; 8:169–72.

Chapter **17**

Nutrition in Pregnancy, Infancy, and Childhood

Lisa F. Harper and Mary P. Faine

OBJECTIVES

The student will be able to:

- List the important nutrition issues for women of childbearing age.
- Discuss the roles of nutrition in conception, pregnancy, and lactation.
- Detail the nutritional needs of pregnant and lactating women.
- Describe the benefits of breastfeeding for the infant and the mother.
- List and describe the caloric and nutrient needs of infants, toddlers, and school-aged children.
- Identify and discuss the most common nutritional problems of children.
- Discuss the nutrition-related oral health issues of infants and children.
- Describe the role of snacks in the food pattern of toddlers and children, and identify snacks of low cariogenicity.

INTRODUCTION

A healthy baby needs a healthy mother. The mother's health before and during pregnancy (and the quality of her prenatal care) are crucial factors for the unborn baby. The birth of a healthy, biologically mature baby without complications is more likely to occur if the mother is well nourished before conception and during pregnancy. The ultimate goal is an infant whose gestational age is more than 37 weeks, and whose birth weight is greater than 2500 g (5.5 lb).

Maternal risk factors such as malnutrition, supplement abuse, smoking, alcohol, and controlled substance abuse can all cause significant problems in the developing fetus. Once the baby is born, appropriate feeding is essential to the baby's growth and development. Each stage of child growth and development presents new nutritional and behavioral challenges. This chapter details the important nutritional considerations for mother and baby from prepregnancy through childhood.

DIET NEEDS PRIOR TO PREGNANCY

Anticipatory guidance for women prior to conception is important to reduce modifiable risks and to reduce maternal and infant morbidity and mortality. Anticipatory guidance can help prevent disease during pregnancy and maternal habits harmful to a fetus, and improve the mother's nutrient stores and help prevent delivery of a preterm baby. The mortality rate of preterm babies is higher than with babies delivered at term (Jack, Culpepper, 1990).

Many factors can place a woman at risk for poor pregnancy outcome. These include low income, lack of education, lack of support, health issues (gynecological age, nutritional status, untreated diabetes, high blood pressure, infections, medication), and lifestyle factors (tobacco, alcohol, and recreational drug use).

For the health of both mother and infant, women need to have nutritious diets before becoming pregnant. This is sometimes a challenge, as about half of all pregnancies in the United States are unintended (CDC, 1999). Poor nutrition, especially low iron and folic acid intakes, is more common among women with unintended pregnancies.

Women who are optimally nourished at conception will have the nutrients needed for the growing fetus immediately available during the critical first few weeks of the pregnancy, before the mother even knows she is pregnant.

Folic acid is particularly important because it protects against the occurrence and recurrence of neural tube defects (NTDs) in newborns (Endres, Rockwell, Mense, 2004; MRC Vitamin Research Group, 1991). NTDs are among the most common major birth defects seen worldwide. NTDs include spina bifida (failure of the spinal cord to close properly resulting in permanent spinal cord and nerve damage), malformations of the brain and skull that cause death shortly after birth, anencephaly, and encephalocele. NTDs present enormous emotional and monetary costs to affected infants, families, and society.

Any woman of childbearing age should be sure to get at least 400 μg of folic acid daily. This is because the folic acid is essential during the first few weeks of pregnancy before many women even know they are pregnant. In folic acid deficient women, if the folid acid supplementation is begun when the pregnancy is diagnosed, it may be too late to prevent the fetal NTDs.

Folate intake can be in the form of synthetic folic acid from fortified foods or supplements, and from foods containing folic acid (e.g., leafy dark green vegetables, asparagus, broccoli, legumes, citrus fruits, and juices) (CDC, 1997). Due to the risk of folic acid deficiency in pregnant women and the need for folic acid for other groups of people, fortification of flour with folic acid began in 1998 (FDA, 1996). See Chapter 9 for more information on folic acid.

Prepregnancy weight is also an important determinent of pregnancy outcome, with either underweight and overweight preventing risks to the developing fetus.

NUTRITION DURING PREGNANCY

Pregnant women undergo several physiological changes designed to accommodate maternal metabolism and fetal growth and to prepare the mother for delivery and lactation (Worthington-Roberts, Williams, 2000). The pregnant woman's sense of taste is altered, appetite increases, and gastric motility is slowed to allow for absorption of nutrients. The breasts enlarge in preparation for lactation, and fat is deposited in the lower body during the third trimester to provide energy reserve for the fetus and to support lactation. Nausea, vomiting, and constipation are common.

Nutrient Needs

Eating healthy foods during pregnancy supplies the fetus with all the nutrients needed for growth and development. Although it is true that a pregnant woman needs to eat for two, this does not mean she needs to eat twice as much as normal. The average additional calories needed per trimester are 96 kcal/day in the first trimester, 265 kcal/day in the second trimester, and 430 kcal/day in the third trimester (IOM, 1990; Reifsnider, Gill, 2000). Pregnant teenagers, underweight women, and physically active women may have higher energy needs. An extra 10 to 15 g of protein, depending on the woman's age, is needed for tissue synthesis starting in the second month of pregnancy. This is the amount in $1\frac{1}{2}$ cups of milk or 2 oz of cheese. If protein comes exclusively from vegetable foods, a greater protein intake is needed (see Chapter 5). Special protein powders and formulated high-protein drinks are not recommended. Table 17–1 shows the daily food guide for pregnancy and lactation. Figure 17–1 compares the difference in nutrient requirements in pregnancy and lactation.

The need for B-complex vitamins and minerals is also increased. Food is the best source of these nutrients. Vitamin A requirements do not increase during pregnancy. In fact, high doses (>10,000 IU) of preformed vitamin A increase the risk of fetal malformations, so unless there is evidence of a vitamin A deficiency,

supplemental vitamin A is *not* advised during pregnancy (Worthington-Roberts, Williams, 2000). The use of a vitamin A analog, isotretinoin, in early pregnancy has also been associated with birth defects and spontaneous abortion.

Folic acid and iron are essential and may not be obtained in adequate amounts from food. So in addition to folate-rich foods, a 400 µg supplement of folic acid is recommended (IOM, 1998). The absorption of dietary iron increases during pregnancy, but iron-deficiency anemia is still common. Because the fetus draws on the mother's iron stores for synthesis of hemoglobin and to build up fetal stores, a 30 mg supplement of ferrous iron is recommended during the second and third trimesters of pregnancy for all women (McGanity, Dawson, Van Hook, 1999). Pregnant women may also need supplements of specific nutrients under some circumstances. A prenatal vitamin-mineral supplement that contains 100% of the Recommended Dietary Allowance (RDA), although not always necessary, may provide protection for some women.

Prenatal fluoride supplementation is not indicated or recommended in pregnancy because although fluoride does cross the placental barrier, there is no evidence that giving prenatal fluoride supplements to the pregnant woman prevents dental caries in children (Leverett et al., 1997).

Women who are lacto-ovovegetarians or lacto-vegetarians usually have little difficulty meeting their nutritional needs. They have similar requirements to nonvegetarian pregnant women (getting sufficient iron,

TABLE 17–1   Diet Recommendations during Pregnancy and Lactation

Food Group	Pregnancy (servings/day)	Lactation
Milk, yogurt, cheese	3+ servings/day	4–5 servings/day (one infant only)
Meat, poultry, fish, dry beans and peas, eggs, nuts	6 oz	7–8 oz/day
Fruit	3 servings/day	2–4 servings/day (at least one good source of vitamin C)
Vegetables	4 servings/day	3–5 servings/day
Breads, cereals, rice and pasta	9 servings/day	6–11 servings/day
Fats and oils	Sparingly	2–3 servings/day

Source: Adapted from the *Manual of Clinical Dietetics*, 5th ed. Chicago: American Dietetic Association, 1996.

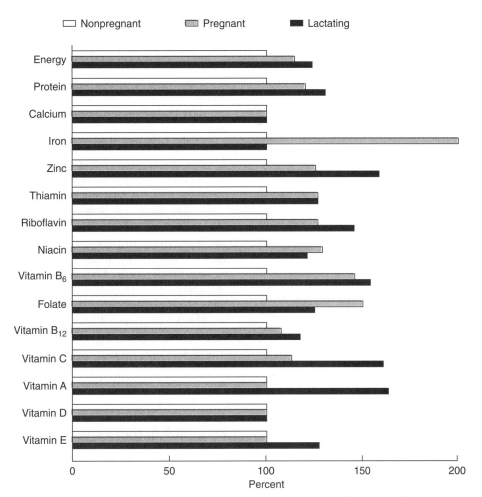

FIGURE 17-1   Percentage increase in nutrient recommendations for women during pregnancy and lactation (nonpregnant woman's goal set at 100%).

Source: Reprinted with permission from *Dietary Reference Intakes for Thiamin, Riboflavin, Niacin, Vitamin B$_6$, Folate, Vitamin B$_{12}$, Pantothenic Acid, Biotin, and Choline.* Copyright © 1998 by the National Academy of Sciences. Courtesy of the National Academy Press, Washington, D.C.

calcium, and folate). However, a strict vegan must carefully monitor her diet and if necessary work with a dietitian to ensure she is meeting her optimum nutrient needs (Schnuth, 1994). The Special Supplemental Food Program for Women, Infants, and Children (WIC) is a federal program to help improve the diets of low-income, pregnant, and lactating mothers, and children to age 5 who are at risk for poor nutrition. Monthly vouchers for a food package including dairy foods, protein sources, fruit and vegetable juices, formula, and iron-fortified cereals are provided. Food and nutrition education and referral to health services are also provided.

Maternal Weight Gain

The recommended total weight gain during pregnancy is related to prepregnancy body mass index (BMI) (Table 17–2). An ideal pregnancy would begin with a BMI of 20 to 26 (McGanity et al., 1999). Weight gain during pregnancy, especially during the second and third trimesters, is an important determinant of fetal growth and a strong predictor of infant birth weight (Brown, Berdan, Splett, Robinson, Harris, 1986). A steady rate of weight gain permits gradual buildup of muscle and fat in the mother and fetus. For the woman with a normal prepregnancy BMI, a weight gain of

TABLE 17–2   Recommended Total Weight Gain for Pregnant Women Based on Prepregnancy Body Mass Index (Weight/Height^2)*

Weight–Height Categories	Prepregnancy BMI	Recommended Total Weight Gain (lb)
Underweight	< 19.8	28–40
Normal weight	19.8–26.0	25–35
Overweight	>26.0–29.0	15–25
Obese	>29.0	≥15

*Body mass index is calculated in metric units.
Source: Reprinted with permission from *Nutrition During Pregnancy: Weight Gain, Nutrient Supplements.* Copyright © 1990 by the National Academy of Sciences. Courtesy of the National Academy Press, Washington, D.C.

2 to 4 pounds during the first trimester, and 1 pound per week in the second and third trimesters is recommended. A desirable range of weight gain for the healthy, normal weight woman over the 9-month period is 25 to 35 pounds (women carrying twins should gain 35 to 45 pounds). A rapid increase in weight, increased blood pressure, and generalized edema are symptoms of preeclampsia, a potentially dangerous condition that requires immediate medical attention. Table 17–3 shows where the weight gain goes in pregnancy.

Obese women and very lean women have worse prognoses for pregnancy outcome than normal weight

TABLE 17–3   Where Does the Weight Gain Go in Pregnancy?

Location	Average Weight Gain (lb)
Placenta	1–2
Amniotic fluid	2
Breasts	1
Uterus	2
Blood volume increase	3
Body fat	5+
More muscle and fluid	4–7
The baby itself	7–8
Total	25+lb

Source: Adapted from Duyff RL: *American Dietetic Association Complete Food and Nutrition Guide.* Hoboken, NJ: Willey & Sons, 2002.

women (Abrams, Parker, 1988). More late fetal deaths and fetal central nervous system congenital malformations occur in obese women than in normal weight women (Cnattingus, Bergstrom, Lipworth, Kramer, 1998). The obese woman is also more likely to have pregnancy-induced hypertension, gestational diabetes, preeclampsia, prolonged labor, and a cesarean section delivery. The recommended pregnancy weight gain for obese women is 15 to 25 pounds. Overweight women should strive to gain 0.66 pound per week during the second and third trimesters of pregnancy.

The underweight woman is more likely to develop iron-deficiency anemia, and anemic, underweight women are more likely to have a shorter gestational period, preterm delivery, and a small baby than women of normal weight (Edwards, Alton, Barrada, Kokanson, 1979). Weight gain by an underweight woman could lower her risk of preterm delivery and of having a low-birth-weight (LBW) infant. Low weight gain increases the risk of infant morbidity and mortality (McCormick, 1985). The total recommended weight gain for women with a prepregnancy BMI of less than 19.8 is 28 to 40 pounds.

Physical Activity during Pregnancy

Women who exercise during pregnancy may have less nausea, fatigue, leg cramps, round ligament pain, and backache than those who don't exercise (Sternfeld, 1997). Walking, low-impact aerobics, swimming, water exercises, stair climbing, and bicycling are appropriate exercises during pregnancy. The intensity and duration of exercise should be gauged so that a high internal body temperature does not develop. High-impact activities that involve jerky, jumping, or jarring motions, or rapid changes in direction should be avoided. A generous fluid intake before, during, and after exercise will prevent dehydration (American College of Obstetricians and Gynecologists [ACOG], 1994).

Adolescent Pregnancy

The United States has the highest frequency of teenage pregnancies among the industrialized countries of the world. Approximately 75% of pregnancies among women younger than 20 are unplanned (CDC, 1999). Babies born to adolescents are twice as likely to be preterm, of low birth weight (<2500 g), and the neonatal death rate is almost triple that of babies born to adult women (Committee on Adolescence, 1999; Hilgers, Douglass, Mathieu, 2003). The poor outcomes of teen pregnancies in the United States are thought to be due to immaturity, poor nutrition, lack of financial resources, and poor or nonexistent prenatal care.

The nutritional status of an adolescent prior to conception and during pregnancy can profoundly influence the outcome of pregnancy. It is a major challenge to provide nourishment to the growing fetus in addition to supporting the teenage girl's own physical growth. Teens often have low intakes of fruits, vegetables, and dairy foods, and they snack on foods high in fat and sugar. The result may be low intakes of many nutrients (e.g., calcium, iron, zinc) important for pregnancy (Neumark-Sztaner, Story, Resnick, Blum, 1998). Chronic dieting, binge eating, and eating disorders can also be a problem (Story, Alton, 1995). See Chapter 18 for information on eating disorders.

A weight gain of 26 to 35 pounds is recommended for girls who begin the pregnancy at a healthy body weight. Adolescents may need to gain more weight than adults to deliver infants with a favorable birth weight (Rees, 1997). Calcium requirements for the 14- to 18-year-old are high at 1300 mg/day, but can be met by consuming 4 glasses of milk per day. A 1000 mg calcium supplement is also indicated if intake of dairy foods is low. A 400 µg supplement of folic acid and supplemental iron are also usually prescribed for teens, especially those who may become pregnant. The WIC program can aid the low-income pregnant teen in obtaining adequate food to ensure a healthy weight gain. The most critical factor for the pregnant teen, however, is to receive early prenatal care.

Caffeine, Alcohol, Tobacco, and Drug Use

There is little evidence to warrant the prohibition of caffeine during pregnancy. In one study, women who drank up to three cups of coffee per day, (300 mg of caffeine) during pregnancy were not at greater risk of miscarriage or delivering LBW infants (Mills, Holmes, Aarons, Simpson, 1993); however, a prudent approach may be to limit caffeine intake by drinking decaffeinated coffee and caffeine-free soft drinks during pregnancy.

The leading cause of mental retardation and preventable birth defects in the United States today is alcohol use during pregnancy. Chronic alcohol intake by a woman during pregnancy can cause fetal alcohol syndrome (FAS). FAS is a pattern of congenital abnormalities in babies. The incidence of FAS in the general population is one to three cases per 1,000 live births (Worthington-Roberts, Williams, 1997). The child of a chronic alcoholic may exhibit a cluster of features: poor fetal and infant growth, mental retardation, physical deformities, minor facial malformations, and emotional and learning problems. The time of alcohol exposure during pregnancy determines the type of damage (Table 17-4). During the first trimester, the developing organs (brain, heart, and kidneys) may be malformed. During the second trimester, alcohol intake may cause spontaneous abortion. During the third trimester, body and brain growth may be retarded. More subtle effects that may occur when the mother is a moderate, social drinker include reduced birth weight, retarded growth, brain damage, and mild behavioral and learning disabilities. For every child born with FAS, there are 10 more children who suffer from alcohol-related problems.

Smokers have a reduced capacity to carry oxygen because smoking causes vasoconstriction resulting in lower blood flow to the placenta. Mothers who smoke any cigarettes during pregnancy have lower weight infants (Hellerstedt, Himes, Story, Alton, Edwards,

TABLE 17-4 Potential Alcohol Damage during Pregnancy

First trimester	Malformed developing organs (brain, heart, kidneys)
Second trimester	Spontaneous abortion
Third trimester	Retarded body and brain growth

1997). These high-risk women should take a low-dose vitamin-mineral preparation. To maintain serum vitamin C levels, smokers must consume twice as much vitamin C per day as nonsmokers.

Drugs are also of great concern during pregnancy. Many drugs can cause birth defects in the fetus, including over-the-counter and prescribed medications, and recreational drugs. Pregnant women should not take any drugs or nutritional supplements without physician supervision.

Oral Health Issues

A variety of oral complications can occur during pregnancy, so attention to oral health is important for the pregnant woman (Gulch, Giorgios, 1998; Loe and Silness, 1963). Untreated periodontal disease during pregnancy may increase the risk of a woman delivering a LBW baby (Offenbacher et al., 1996). Gram-negative anaerobic bacteria, linked to periodontal infections, are thought to influence the microflora of the genitourinary tract. These bacteria seem to increase the risk of preterm delivery and/or premature rupture of the membranes. Vomiting associated with morning sickness may result in decalcification of the anterior upper teeth. Pregnant women have an increased risk of developing dental caries if they have cravings for candy or snack on decay-promoting foods. Also, because oral bacteria are transmitted directly from mother to child, the mother needs to maintain good oral hygiene to protect her child (Berkowitz, Turner, Green, 1980). In addition, prenatal nutrition and the health of the pregnant mother may have an important impact on the child's tooth mineralization and subsequent caries susceptibility (Tirnanoff, Palmer 2001). Although highly interested and concerned about oral health, many expectant parents are not well informed about the subject (Shein, Tsamtsouris, Rovero, 1991; Tsamtsouris, Stack, Padamsee, 1986).

NUTRITION OF THE NEWBORN

The newborn grows rapidly both in length and weight. By the fourth month of life, an infant will have doubled his or her birth weight. By 1 year of age the baby will weigh three times his or her birth weight, and will increase in length by 50. Monitoring the infant's growth is the best way to determine if the child is receiving adequate nutrition.

The infant requires a high-calorie intake to support rapid growth and a high basal metabolic rate. The newborn's energy requirement is three to four times greater than that of an adult. Because of the newborn's small stomach capacity, frequent, small feedings are needed. Up to about 6 months of age, the child should be fed either breast milk or infant formula. Cow's milk should *not* be given to infants, as it varies in significant ways from breast milk and can be harmful to human babies. Table 17–5 compares the nutrients in breast milk, cow's milk, and infant formula.

Breastfeeding

Breast milk is the perfect food for all infants during the first year of life. Breastfeeding provides indisputable and significant benefits to both infants and mothers (American Academy of Pediatrics [AAP], 1997; American Dietetic Association, 1997). Nursing also promotes closeness and bonding between the mother and infant.

For the newborn, breastfeeding may significantly reduce infant morbidity and mortality during the early months of life. Breast milk provides immunity to viral and bacterial infections. Immune factors in human milk contribute to fewer respiratory infections, less otitis media, diarrhea, bacteremia, bacterial meningitis, botulism, urinary tract infections, and necrotizing enterocolitis in infants (AAP, 1997; Cushing et al., 1998). Human milk also reduces the chances of allergies developing in the allergy-prone newborn. Other benefits of breastfeeding include a lower risk of childhood obesity and healthy development of the jaws, teeth, and speech pattern. Breastfed children also appear to score higher on tests of cognitive function than do formula-fed children (Anderson, Johnstone, Remley, 1999).

For the mother, lactating women have less hemorrhaging, more rapid involution of the uterus, lower risk of developing premenopausal ovarian and breast cancer, delayed resumption of ovulation (which may delay another pregnancy), and improved bone remineralization.

Human milk has a unique composition. Colostrum, a thick, yellow fluid secreted the first few days

TABLE 17-5 Comparison of Human Milk, Cow's Milk, and Milk-Based Formula

Nutrient	Human Milk per 1000 mL*	Cow's Milk (Whole) per 1000 mL	Milk-Based Formula per 1000 mL
Fluid			
Water, mL	897	894	875
Energy and Macronutrients			
Energy, kcal	718	620	670
Protein, g	10.6	33.4	15–16
Fat, g	44.9	33.9	33–37
Carbohydrate, g	70.6	47.3	70–72
Vitamins			
Vitamin A, RE	656	315	340–500
Vitamin A, IU	2470	1279	1700–2500
Vitamin D, μg		10[†]	10
Vitamin E, mg TE	1.3–3.3	5.7	5.7–8.5
Vitamin C, mg	51	10	55
Thiamin, mg	0.14	0.39	0.4–0.7
Riboflavin, mg	0.37	1.65	0.6–1.0
Niacin, mg NE	2.0	0.85	7–9
Vitamin B_6, mg	0.11	0.43	0.3–0.4
Vitamin B_{12}, μg	0.46	3.63	1.5–2.0
Folate, μg	51	51	50–100
Minerals			
Calcium, mg	328	1208	550–600
Phosphorus, mg	144	945	440–460
Sodium, mg[†]	141	498	250–390
Potassium, mg[‡]	523	1544	620–1,000
Magnesium, mg	31	132	40–50
Iodine, μg	30–100		40–70
Iron, mg	0.3	0.5	1.4–12.5[§]
Zinc, mg	1.8	3.9	2.0–4.0

Source: From *Robinson's Basic Nutrition and Diet Therapy*: 8/E by Weigley/Mueller/Robinson, © 1997. Reprinted with permission.

*One liter of human milk = 1.025 g; 1 liter of cow's milk = 1.017 g.

[†]Assumes fortification of cow's milk with 10 μg vitamin D.

[‡]Allowances for sodium and potassium ranges are considered to be safe and adequate.

[§]Values for formula not fortified and fortified with iron.

after birth, contains many protective immune factors. Specific T- and B-cell lymphocytes and nonspecific macrophages and neutrophils convey passive immunity. Secretory immunoglobulin A and the presence of bifidus factors favor the establishment of friendly bacteria in the infant's intestinal tract (IOM, 1991).

The energy and nutrient composition of breast milk is uniquely designed to meet the needs of the human species (Jensen, 1995). The principal carbohydrate in breast milk, lactose, is easily digested and enhances absorption of calcium, phosphorus, and magnesium. The protein and mineral content is lower in breast milk than in cow's milk, resulting in a lower solute load for the immature kidney. The whey proteins found in large amounts in human milk form a soft, easily digestible curd; in contrast, casein, the predominant protein in cow's milk formula, forms a tough curd that is hard for the young child to digest. More than 50% of the calories in human milk come from fat, including generous amounts of the essential fatty acids (linoleic and linolenic). The long-chain polyunsaturated fatty acids, arachidonic and docosahexanoic acid, important for development of the central nervous system are found in human milk, but not modified cow's milk formula. Cholesterol, needed for myelin synthesis in the development of the central nervous system, is higher in human milk than in formula or cow's milk.

Breast milk contains adequate vitamins, with the possible exception of vitamin D. Deeply pigmented breastfed infants or those who have limited exposure to sunlight may be prescribed vitamin D before 6 months of age. Because of the high bioavailability of the iron in human milk, the breastfed infant receives adequate iron for the first 4 to 6 months (Butte, Garza, Smith, Wills, Nichols, 1987). By 6 months, iron-fortified cereals can provide additional iron. Cow's milk should not be introduced before 1 year of age. (see Table 17–5).

Nutritional Needs for Lactation (Breastfeeding)

During lactation, a nursing mother needs about an extra 500 kcal/day above prepregnancy calorie intake (Dewey, 1997; IOM, 1991). Body fat stored during pregnancy (about 4 to 9 lb) provides part of the additional energy used for lactation. An additional 15 g of protein is needed per day during the first 6 months and 12 g during the 17th through 12th months of lactation (IOM, 1991). If maternal dietary intake of water- and fat-soluble vitamins is inadequate, low amounts will be found in the milk. In contrast, the mineral content of human milk is not affected by maternal dietary intake because if intake is low, the mother's own mineral stores will be depleted to provide the missing nutrients (McGanity et al., 1999).

Regular aerobic activity by the nursing mother does not have adverse effects on lactation (Dewey, Lovelady, Nommsen-Rivers, McCrory, Lonnerdal, 1994). Generous fluid intake before and after workouts is important to prevent dehydration.

Effects of Caffeine, Alcohol, Tobacco, and Drugs

Most drugs and other substances ingested by the lactating woman will be transferred to her breast milk. Caffeine, alcohol, and smoking may also affect milk production. Although one to two cups of coffee per day appears to be acceptable, a high caffeine intake may make the infant irritable and less able to sleep. Alcohol passes from the mother's bloodstream into her milk, and may alter the flavor of milk, suppress feeding behavior, reduce a mother's milk production, and possibly contribute to delayed psychomotor development (Little, 1989). Cigarette smoking reduces the volume of milk produced and may be associated with sudden infant death syndrome (Cutz, Perrin, Hackman, Czegledy-Nagy, 1996).

Infant Formulas

Iron-fortified infant formula is an appropriate feeding approach for the full-term infant when it is not possible or practical for the mother to breastfeed. Infant formula is designed to imitate human milk, but is missing the mother's protective antibodies. Most infant formulas in the United States are nutritionally similar and follow standards set by the FDA. Lactose is usually the only sugar found in cow's milk formula. Lactose-free formulas and soy-based formulas are available for infants when cow's milk formula is contraindicated due to allergy or other reasons. Whole cow's milk, 1% fat, and 2% fat milk can be given to infants after 12 months of age. All formulas fed to infants should be fortified with iron because the infant's iron stores (received from the mother) are depleted by the fourth month and the bioavailability of iron in cow's milk formula is low (AAP, 1999).

An infant's hunger can vary from day to day and by time of day. The baby, not the clock, should regulate the feeding schedule. An infant should not be forced to finish the bottle. Propping the bottle should be discouraged because it can force the baby to consume more than necessary and may increase risk of choking. Table 17–6 discusses common bottle feeding practices to avoid.

Dental Issues in Infants

Nutritional deficiencies or excesses during periods of early oral development can have permanent deleterious effects. For example, developmental defects

TABLE 17–6   Top Common Bottle Feeding Practices to Avoid

Practice to Avoid	Rationale
Heating bottle in microwave	Possible burns
Using warm tap water	Possible lead exposure
Putting baby to bed with bottle	Increases caries risk
Not keeping filled bottles cold	Encourages bacterial growth
Overdiluting or overconcentrating formula	Inadequate nutrition
Not sterilizing bottles and nipples	Possible contamination
Adding cereal to bottle without doctor's approval	Ignores developmental needs
Adding sweeteners to the formula bottle	Can introduce harmful bacteria; increases caries risk
Not holding the infant during feeding	Increases choking risk, Prolongs feeding, leading to caries risk

Source: Adapted from *Food, Nutrition, and the Young Child* 5/E by Endres/Rockwell/Mense © 2004 by Pearson Education, Upper Saddle River, NJ.

TABLE 17–7   Determining Developmental Readiness for Solid Foods

Cues for Developmental Readiness for Solid Foods (approximately 6 months)

- Infant sits up with support in an upright chair, not an angled infant feeding chair
- Infant uses neck muscles to hold head up
- Infant doesn't slide down in the high chair
- Infant opens mouth to anticipate bites of food and closes mouth around the spoon
- Infant brings fingers and toys to mouth
- Infant doesn't push out food with tongue after it has been spooned in
- Infant can move food to the back of mouth
- Infant can turn head away from unwanted food
- Infant can "invite" food by opening mouth

Source: Adapted from *Food, Nutrition, and the Young Child* 5/E by Endres/Rockwell/Mense © 2004 by Pearson Education, Upper Saddle River, NJ.

(enamel hypoplasia) of the primary teeth are surprisingly common in malnourished children, who may have delays in tooth development and eruption compared to normal children. In turn, enamel hypoplasia is associated with increased risk of dental caries (Alvarez et al., 1993; Seow, 1991). Relationships between nutrition and oral development are detailed in Chapter 12.

No vitamin or mineral supplement is required for the formula-fed baby. However, infant formula is not manufactured with fluoridated water, so if the water used in preparing the formula contains less than optimal amounts of fluoride (0.3 ppm), and the infant gets no other source of fluoridated water, fluoride supplements may be indicated after 6 months of age (ADA, 1998). Chapter 8 includes a fluoride supplementation schedule.

Transition to Solid Foods

The transition to solid foods begins around 6 months of age and is determined by the infant's developmental readiness. Table 17–7 lists factors that determine readiness for solid foods. Feeding behavior develops sequentially (Table 17–8) (Satter, 1995). Iron-fortified rice cereal is usually the first solid food fed to infants because it is well tolerated. Pureed vegetables and fruits can be introduced in any order. Table 17–9 shows a typical sequence for food additions to an infant's diet. Honey should not be used to sweeten the foods of an infant less than 1 year old because it can contain spores of harmful *Clostridium botulinum* that are not destroyed when food is heated.

Transition to the cup should also begin at 6 months of age; infants should be weaned from the bottle to the cup by 12 months of age. Providing juices only in a cup also helps reduce the practice of putting juices in the bedtime bottle (a risk factor for early childhood caries). However, excessive use of fruit juices has become a health concern as well. Juices provide only limited essential nutrients (carbohydrate, vitamin C, and water), and high juice intake (>12 fl oz/day) has been linked to short stature and obesity (Dennison, 1996; Dennison, Rockwell, Baker, 1997). Juice sipped constantly in a "sippy cup" can also be a major contributor to dental caries. For these reasons, the young child should consume no more than 12 oz/day of 100% fruit juice.

TABLE 17–8 Sequence of Development of Feeding and Oral Behaviors

Stage	Nutritional Development	Oral Development
Fetal: Conception to Birth	Nourished via placenta	Embryological development of oral structures
Birth to 6 Months	Searches for nipple and suckles	Rooting reflex Gag reflex, sucking, and suckling Coordination of sucking, swallowing, breathing
5 to 7 Months	Begins to sit up and follow food with eyes Closes lips around spoon Begins to swallow solid foods	Cup drinking may begin Spoon feeding may begin Bite reflex develops
6 to 8 Months	Moves tongue laterally Controls position of food in mouth and swallows Chews food Spoon feeding begins Foods introduced as tolerated	Cup drinking continues More refined spoonfeeding and chewing
7 to 10 Months	Has more mature bite Rotary chewing: transfers food from side to side Curves lips around cup	Cup drinking improves More refined spoon feeding and chewing
12 Months	Sociability increases Interest in solid foods increases Cup drinking improves	Sucking, drinking, spoon feeding, chewing continue
Second Year and Beyond	Circular rotary chewing matures No pause in side-to-side food transfer Begins to use utensils	Masticatory reflexes more refined Self-feeding begins and continues

Sources: Adapted from *How to Get Your Kid to Eat: But Not Too Much* by Satter © 1987 by Bull Publishing, Palo Alto, CA; *Food, Nutrition, and the Young Child*: 5/E by Endres/Rockwell, © 2004 by Pearson Education, Upper Saddle River, NJ.

TABLE 17–9 Typical Sequence for Food Additions to Infants' Diets

Age	Food Additions

4–6 months
  (bottle fed)
5–6 months
  (breastfed)
	Iron-fortified rice cereal. Mix precooked cereal with formula for thin
	    consistency at first. Increase to 2 to 5 tablespoons by 7–8 months.
	Orange juice. Increase gradually to $\frac{1}{2}$ cup. May be diluted with water at
	    first. May be given from a cup.
	Mashed ripe banana, applesauce, strained pears, apricots, prunes, or
	    peaches. Start with 1 teaspoon and increase to 3 to 4 tablespoons by 1 year.
	Strained vegetables: asparagus, green beans, carrots, peas, spinach, squash, or tomatoes.
	    Start with 1 teaspoon and increase to 3 to 4 tablespoons by end of first year.

6–7 months	Strained meats and egg yolks. Mash hard-cooked egg yolk with a little formula, using $\frac{1}{4}$ teaspoon at first. Increase gradually. Plain yogurt. Avoid egg white until 10 months or so since it often causes allergic reactions.
5–8 months	Crisp toast, zwieback, teething biscuits, potato.
8–10 months	Chopped vegetables and fruits; pasta, rice.
10–12 months	Whole egg; plain puddings such as custard, junket; cooked and mashed dried beans or peas; cottage cheese or soft cheese.

Source: From *Robinson's Basic Nutrition and Diet Therapy*: 8/E by Weigley/Mueller/Robinson, © 1997. Reprinted with permission.

NUTRITION FOR TODDLERS AND SCHOOL-AGED CHILDREN

Children's dietary needs vary at different stages of development (Figures 17–2 and 17–3). Energy and nutrient requirements depend on body size and composition, rates of growth, and activity patterns. The growth rate slows after infancy into the preschool years, then increases into puberty.

In a national USDA survey, only 2% of children 2 to 19 years were receiving adequate servings from the 5 food groups outlined in the USDA food guide pyramid (Muñoz, Krebs-Smith, Bollard-Barash, Cleveland, 1997). Nearly 40–45% of children met none or only one of the food group recommendations. Table 17–7 provides some suggestions for making food easy for toddlers to eat. The chief nutrition-related health problems of children include obesity, high fat intakes, low calcium intakes, iron deficiency, and a low level of physical activity.

Bone health may be compromised by poor diet in early childhood. The new RDA for calcium, 1300 mg, can be met by consuming 4 servings of milk or dairy foods each day, but this goal may be difficult to meet because milk consumption has been declining among children. Table 17–10 offers some alternative ways of getting calcium into the diet.

Among U.S. children 1 to 3 years old, 9% suffer from iron deficiency (Looker, Dallman, Carroll, Gunter, Johnson, 1997). Iron stores are depleted in infants at about 6 months of age. Iron deficiency is partly attributed to use of cow's milk before 1 year of age, use of nonfortified formula, and use of foods lacking in iron. A high milk intake during the second year of life may also limit the number of iron-rich foods in the toddler's diet. Iron deficiency affects cognitive development, and children with iron-deficiency anemia in infancy have lower scores on mental and motor development tests. In one study, although iron therapy was provided to a group of anemic infants, the children had lower test scores on mental and motor development at age 5 (Lozoff, Jimenez, Wolf, 1991). The use of iron-fortified formula, infant cereals, and other foods is the best means of preventing iron deficiency in the young child.

During the second year, children learn to feed themselves independently. The 2- to 5-year-old is unable to eat large volumes of food; thus, snacks are important to ensure adequate calorie intake. Snack foods should be offered in small sizes so they can be finger-fed by the child. Table 17–11 provides some snack suggestions. Table 17–12 includes ideas for making toddler's foods easy to eat. Foods such as nuts, raw vegetables, grapes, hot dogs, snack chips, and popcorn should be avoided because they may cause choking or gagging.

CURRENT ISSUES REGARDING CHILD NUTRITION

Low-Fat Diets

The question of whether children should follow the dietary guidelines for fat intake (<30% of total calories from fat and <10% of calories from saturated fat) to prevent future cardiovascular disease has been a controversial issue in recent years. High blood cholesterol levels are seen among U.S. children over 2 years of age. On the other hand, restricting fat early in life may compromise growth, and protein and nutrient intake. It is currently recommended that when intake of calories, high-quality protein, and essential nutrients is adequate, dietary fat intake can be reduced to no more than 30% of calories between ages 2 and 5 without impairing growth and development (AAP, 1992; Williams, Bollela, Boccia, Spark, 1998). The fat intake should not be limited before age 2.

High Sugar Intake

Soft drinks are the single biggest source of refined sugars in the American diet (USDA, USDHHS, 2005).

Soft drink consumption is a contributing factor to the weight controversy surrounding toddlers and school-aged children as well as a major contributor to dental caries. Children that consume soft drinks, versus those children that do not, have higher energy intake. Overall diet quality is compromised as children are replacing nutrient-dense dairy products for calorie-dense soft drinks (Harnack, Stang, Story, 1999). The U.S. Surgeon General, in his 2001 report, *Overweight in Children and Adolescents*, proposed limitations in children's consumption of sugar-sweetened beverages—such as soft drinks, fruit juice drinks, and sports drinks—as an ongoing effort to promote health and reduce the risk of overweight and related chronic

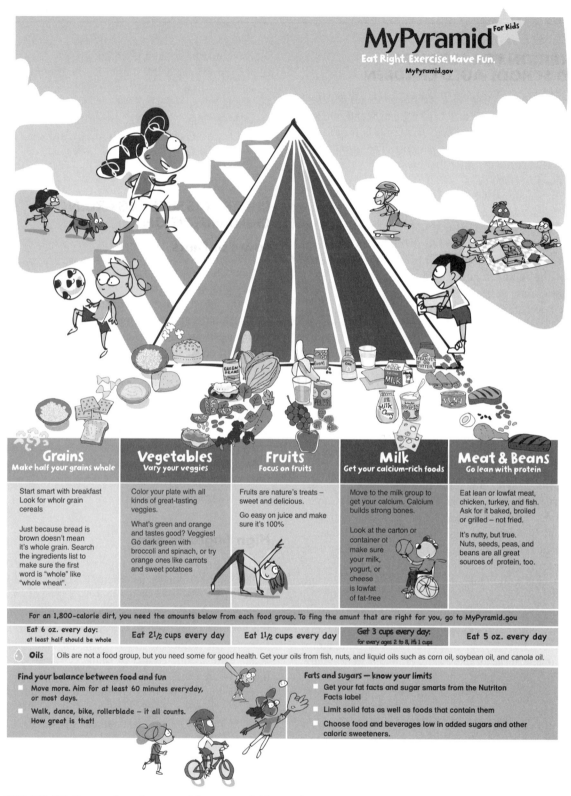

FIGURE 17-2 Food guide pyramid for young children with recommended serving sizes.

Source: U.S. Department of Agriculture, Food and Nutrition Service, 2005. MyPyramid.gov.

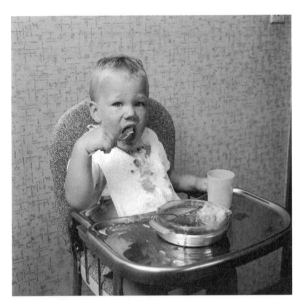

FIGURE 17–3 Child learning to self-feed.
Source: Getty Images, Hulton Archive Photos.

diseases among children (*Overweight in Children and Adolescents*, 2001). Table 17–13 shows sugars associated with specific health concerns in preschool-aged children.

TABLE 17–10 Ways to Increase Your Calcium Intake If You Avoid Most Milk Products

Foods equal to $\frac{1}{2}$ cup serving of milk:
3 oz of sardines (if the bones are eaten)
4 oz of tofu (if it has been processed with calcium sulfate)
4 oz of collards
1 waffle (7 inches in diameter)
4 corn tortillas (if processed with calcium salts)

Foods equal to about $\frac{1}{3}$ cup of milk:
1 cup of cooked dried beans
4 oz of bok choy or turnip greens or kale
1 medium square of cornbread
2 pancakes (4 inches in diameter)
7 to 9 oysters
3 oz of shrimp

Source: Reprinted with permission from *Nutrition During Pregnancy and Lactation: An Implementation Guide.* Copyright © 1992 by the National Academy of Sciences. Courtesy of the National Academy Press, Washington, D.C.

Obesity

Overweight is much more common than underweight or growth retardation among children. Intake of excess calories and physical inactivity are implicated in the rise in childhood obesity. Genetics also plays an important role in determining susceptibility to obesity, but interaction with environment may determine if obesity is expressed. If one or both parents are obese, the probability doubles that an obese or nonobese child will become an obese adult (Whitaker, Wright, Pepe, Seidel, Dietz, 1997). Because maintaining weight loss over a long time is so difficult, prevention of childhood obesity is an important public health goal (Dietz, 1998). The dental setting is an ideal place to implement recommendations for healthy eating not only for caries risk management but also for the overall health and well-being of the child. Children with complicated medical histories should be referred to a registered dietitian. However, for basic nutritional counseling a pediatric dental nutrition screening form (Figure 17–4) can be easily implemented in the dental setting.

Lack of Physical Activity

Physical activity provides many benefits for children, yet it is on the decline, both during and outside school. The percentage of children participating in physical education programs dropped from 21% in 1999, down from 42% in 1991. Fewer than 25% of children participate in even 20 minutes of daily aerobic activity (AAP, 2003). Poor eating habits coupled with inactivity are key factors in the increasing number of overweight children over the past decades (Carlson, Lino, Gerrior, Basiotis, 2001). One-fourth of all U.S. children watch 4 or more hours of television each day. Increased physical activity would help achieve healthy weights and promote optimum bone health.

Dental Issues

Dental team members should not recommend that children be prohibited from snacking as a caries preventive strategy, because this advice could deprive children of needed calories. One midmorning and one midafternoon snack composed of foods of low cariogenicity should not be harmful to oral health. Figure 17–4 is a useful tool that will provide nutritional insight and

TABLE 17–11 Nutritious Snack and Beverage Suggestions for Kids

Beverages	• Make cocoa with milk and cinnamon • Mix yogurt with fruit juice, add ice • Fruit shake: blend milk with fresh fruit and flavoring such as vanilla, cinnamon, or nutmeg • Fruit fizz: combine juice with club soda and ice
Deserts or snacks	• Frozen fruit: freeze fruit juice in ice cube trays with Popsicle sticks • Gelatin: add cottage cheese, cream cheese, fruits, nuts, vegetables for variety • Yogurt parfaits: add fruit, granola, coconut, nuts to flavored or plain yogurt
Grains	• Bagels: top with peanut butter, cream cheese, chopped pineapple, melted cheese, etc. • English muffins or pita bread: make mini pizzas with melted cheese, tomato sauce, chopped meats and vegetables • Muffins or quick breads: use whole wheat flour, add grated carrots, zucchini, bananas, nuts, dates, raisins, berries, squash, or pumpkin • Tortillas: fill with chili, refried beans, grated cheese, taco sauce • Crackers with peanut butter, cheese, hummus or other dips • Popcorn sprinkled with grated cheese
Fruits and vegetables	• Sliced apples with sliced cheese or peanut butter • Any fresh fruits and vegetables in bite-sized pieces used as "finger foods" • Celery stalks stuffed with cream cheese, hummus, peanut butter • Carrot sticks and celery stalks with cheese dips • Raw baby carrots • Fruit, cheese and meat kabobs (remove toothpicks before serving) • Grilled potato skins with shredded cheese and bacon bits
Protein	• Nuts (if children are old enough to avoid choking) • Tunafish as sandwiches or on crackers or pita bread • Ham or turkey rolls stuffed with cheese or pickle • Meat, cheese, and vegetable kabobs (remove toothpicks before serving)

TABLE 17–12 Making Toddlers' Food Easy to Eat

• Cut up meat finely (ground beef vs. steak) and cut other foods into bite-sized pieces.
• Serve foods close to room temperature.
• Soften and moisten foods that are too hard or dry.
• Serve salads as a finger food.
• Serve soups thin enough to drink or thick enough to spoon.
• Provide child-sized spoon and fork with dulled tines.
• Use unbreakable dishes with sides to push food against.
• Seat child at a comfortable height to the table with feet supported.
• Make food attractive and colorful.
• Don't bribe child to eat with promises or gimmicks.

Source: Adapted from *How to Get Your Kid to Eat: But Not Too Much* by Satter © 1987 by Bull Publishing, Palo Alto, CA.

guidance to the caregiver. Caregivers should be informed that the frequency of snacking and retentiveness of fermentable carbohydrates may be more critical than the total sugar intake. They should be advised to avoid caries-promoting snacks such as teething biscuits, raisins, sugarcoated cereals, and snack crackers. Soft fruits, lightly cooked vegetables, cheese sticks, small pieces of tender meats, and hard-cooked eggs are more appropriate snacks for the toddler. The American Academy of Pediatrics has identified dental caries and potential enamel erosion among the health risks associated with a high intake of sweetened drinks (AAP, 2004).

Many children's medications contain sucrose or other sugars as flavoring agents. This is of primary concern in children with specific health conditions

TABLE 17–13   Sugars Associated with Specific Health Concerns in Preschool Children

Sugar	Description	Reason for Concern	Comments
Sorbitol	Sugar alcohol present in pear, apple, and prune juices	Not absorbed from the gut and therefore may cause osmotic diarrhea at very high doses	Excessive amounts of sorbitol-containing juices should be limited, especially in children with gastrointestinal problems
Lactose	Sugar present in mammalian milks	Lactose deficiency and lactose intolerance cause gastrointestinal problems if lactose ferments in the colon	Lactose-intolerant individuals often digest enzyme-hydrolyzed lactose or yogurt with live cultures better than milk
Fructose	Commonly consumed monosaccharide	Fructose can cause problems in individuals with fructase deficiency, an autosomal recessive inborn error of metabolism	Rare genetic disorder
Honey	Contains a variety of fermentable carbohydrates: glucose, fructose, and sucrose	Infantile botulism from spores contaminating the honey has been reported	Honey should not be fed to infants under 1 year of age
Fermentable carbohydrates	Sugars fermented by *Steptococcus mutans* (sucrose, fructose, glucose, lactose, and cooked starch)	If sugars are retained in the mouth, dental caries may result	Pooling of milk or formula in the mouth or retention of other foods containing these sugars causes fermentation and acid production by *Streptococcus mutans*

Source: From Doucette RE, Dwyer JT: Is fruit juice a 'no-no' in children's diets? *Nutr Rev* 2000; 58(6):180–83.

(such as seizure disorders) whose carbohydrate intake must be carefully controlled. The use of these medications may also contribute to cariogenic risk in children who must use them frequently.

Behavioral Issues

The child's early experiences with food and eating help shape lifetime food preferences and diet (Birch, 1998). Caregivers are responsible for providing a variety of nutritious foods and a positive eating environment. The child should be allowed to decide independently which foods and how much will be eaten, based on signals of hunger and satiety. Feeding children is most successful when caregivers respect their children's internal feeding cues. Children have demonstrated that they can regulate their energy intake over a 24-hour period.

Conflict between parents and toddlers over food is common. It is common for preschool-aged children to insist on the same foods day after day. If a variety

of nutritious foods are available at mealtimes, eventually the child will experiment with them. Food should not be used for emotional purposes (e.g., reward good behavior, pacify or bribe, punish by withholding food). In one study, children whose mothers had restricted their access to snack foods and those whose mothers had not restricted their snacks, were provided with free access to snacks (Fisher, Birch, 1996). The group of toddlers with restrictive mothers ate the most snacks even if they weren't hungry. Thus, attempting to control a child's intake may actually promote eating of restricted foods. See Table 17–14 for common misconceptions about feeding children.

Food Allergies and Intolerances

Food allergies (also known as hypersensitivities) can be serious and even life threatening, and occur in up to 8% of the U.S. pediatric population, 25% of children in the United Kingdom and Japan, and 1–2% of U.S.

Dental Nutrition Risk Assessment

Questions for a child's parent/caregiver:

Has your child ever had any cavities or fillings?
  Enter 1 for yes
  Enter 0 for no

Have any of the child's brothers or sisters ever had cavities or fillings?
  Enter 1 for yes
  Enter 0 for no

How often does your child brush his/her teeth?
  Enter 0 for at least twice a day
  Enter 1 for once a day
  Enter 2 for never or less than once a day

Does your child use fluoride toothpaste?
  Enter 0 for yes
  Enter 1 for no

How often does your child floss?
  Enter 0 for every day or most days
  Enter 1 for at least once a week, but not daily
  Enter 2 for never/rarely (less than once a week)

Does your child take any sugar-containing medications or vitamins on a regular basis?
  Enter 1 for yes
  Enter 0 for no

How many snacks does your child eat per day?
  Enter 0 for 0, 1, or 2 snacks
  Enter 1 for 3 snacks
  Enter 2 for more than 3 snacks
  Enter 3 for constant snacking

Which best describes when your child eats sweets?
  Enter 0 for with meals
  Enter 1 for at the end of meals
  Enter 2 for with or as snacks
  Enter 0 for never

How often does your child snack before bedtime?
  Enter 0 for never
  Enter 1 for occasionally
  Enter 2 for often

How often does your child eat slowly dissolving candies and/or lozenges?
  Enter 0 for never/rarely
  Enter 1 for often
  Enter 2 for once a day
  Enter 3 for more than once a day

Does your child chew sugar-free gum?
  Enter 0 for yes
  Enter 1 for no

How often does your child drink fruit juice, soda, or other carbonated beverages?
  Enter 0 for never/rarely
  Enter 1 for often, but not every day
  Enter 2 for daily, one or more consumed fast
  Enter 3 for daily, one or more sipped slowly

If end score was:
  9 or higher: Very high risk and needs nutrition counseling.
  4–8: Moderate risk. Will probably benefit from instructions and handout.
  0–3: Low risk. Will probably benefit from review of basic instructions and handout.

FIGURE 17–4 Pediatric diet risk assessment.

---

adults (Asthma and Allergy Foundation of America). But people of any age can have sudden allergic reactions to a food that had previously not been a problem for them.

A food allergy is an immune system response to a food (usually protein referred to as an allergen) that the body mistakenly believes is harmful. The immune system then creates specific antibodies to the allergen. The next time the individual eats that food, the immune system releases massive amounts of chemicals, including histamine, to protect the body. These chemicals trigger a cascade of allergic symptoms that

TABLE 17–14   Misconceptions about Feeding Children

1. Children will automatically choose a nutritionally balanced diet when left to their own devices.
   Fact: This happens only when children's food choices are limited to a variety of healthy foods. Therefore, caregivers need to teach children early how to enjoy foods that promote health.
2. Delayed weaning onto solid foods can help prevent a child from becoming overweight.
   Fact: Late weaning can actually compound a tendency to gain too much weight.
3. Children who are gaining weight normally do not need vitamin supplements.
   Fact: More than 50% of American children under the age of 3 years do not get the RDAs for several essential nutrients without a daily multivitamin/mineral supplement.

Source: Adapted from *Feeding Your Child for Lifelong Health* by Roberts © 1999 by Bantam, New York, NY.

can affect the respiratory system, gastrointestinal tract, skin, or cardiovascular system.

Symptoms can range from a tingling sensation in the mouth, swelling of the tongue and the throat, difficulty breathing, hives, vomiting, abdominal cramps, diarrhea, drop in blood pressure, and loss of consciousness, to death. Symptoms typically appear within minutes to 2 hours after the person has eaten the food to which he or she is allergic.

Food allergies can have important nutritional implications if they result in the elimination of major food groups from the diet. Children can be allergic to any food, but 90% of all food allergies are to milk, eggs, peanuts and other tree nuts, fish, shellfish, soy, and wheat. Milk and egg allergies are usually outgrown, but nut and fish allergies can last a lifetime, and can cause fatal anaphylaxis (allergic reaction).

Food allergies are not the same as food intolerances. Food intolerances are commonly due to the lack of an enzyme (e.g., lactose intolerance) and are not life threatening. They also can cause nutrition problems, however, due to malabsorption and gastrointestinal discomfort.

With both food allergies and intolerances, diagnosis is based upon the relief of symptoms following the removal of the suspected food on several occasions. For people with food allergies, they must be acutely aware of the content of the foods they are eating, as even the tiniest amount of peanuts or shellfish may set off a potentially fatal reaction. They are usually cautioned to carry a source of quick epinephrine (e.g., Epi-pen) as a safeguard.

Helpful resources for more information on food allergies include the Food Allergy and Anaphylaxis Network (http://www.foodallergy.org); the American Academy of Allergy and Immunology (http://www.aaaai.org); the American College of Allergy, Asthma, and Immunology (http://www.acaai.org); and the Asthma and Allergy Foundation of America (http://www.aafa.org).

SUMMARY AND IMPLICATIONS FOR DENTISTRY

A healthy pregnancy is essential to the well-being of both mother and child. Pregnancy and the child's early years set the stage for lifelong health and health habits. Good nutrition during pregnancy fosters development of a healthy baby. Conversely, malnutrition during pregnancy can result in birth defects and can contribute to infant mortality. In the early years of life, growth is rapid and nutrient needs are great. Nutrient deficiencies during these years can have permanent effects on growth and development. Good nutrition and good oral health go hand in hand to help ensure a good start for mother and baby. The dental team needs to be aware of the major nutritional and oral health issues during these developmental periods, and promote and reinforce early development of good habits.

Dental professionals should:

- Reinforce the need for good dietary habits before pregnancy.
- Ensure that pregnant women are receiving good prenatal care.
- Educate women about the dental implications of pregnancy and provide appropriate oral care.
- Reinforce the principles of good infant care, including promoting breastfeeding.
- Prescribe appropriate fluoride modalities for mother and infant.

- Understand the need for children's frequent snacking and provide appropriate snack suggestions.
- Help parents deal with the common behavioral feeding issues of young children.
- Reinforce the importance of starting early with good dietary and dental practices.

QUESTIONS PATIENTS MIGHT ASK

Q. When should I start brushing my child's teeth?

A. When the first tooth erupts, you should brush it with water. After age 2 use a pea-sized amount of fluoride toothpaste daily (Soxman, 2005).

Q. My child is a picky eater. Are there any oral health precautions for children's chewable vitamins given to kids who are picky eaters?

A. Avoid vitamins with sugar listed as the first ingredient. Those sweetened with sorbitol would be a better alternative (Soxman, 2005).

Q. How does my child's diet affect his dental health?

A. A child must have a balanced diet for the teeth to develop properly. A balanced diet is also needed for healthy gum tissue around the teeth. A diet high in certain kinds of carbohydrates, such as sugar and starch, may place your child at increased risk of tooth decay (Soxman, 2005).

Q. How can I prevent tooth decay from a bottle or nursing?

A. Children should be encouraged to drink from a cup as they approach their first birthday. Children should not fall asleep with a bottle. Nighttime breastfeeding should be avoided after the first primary (baby) teeth begin to erupt. They should also avoid drinking juice from a bottle (Nainar, Mohummed, 2004).

Q. Won't children automatically choose a nutritionally balanced diet when left to their own devices?

A. This happens only when children's food choices are limited to a variety of healthy foods. Therefore, caregivers need to teach children early how to enjoy foods that promote health.

Q. Won't delayed weaning onto solid foods help prevent a child from becoming overweight?

A. No, actually late weaning can compound a tendency to gain too much weight.

Q. Is it true that children who are gaining weight normally do not need vitamin supplements?

A. Not necessarily true. More than 50% of American children under the age of 3 years do not get the RDAs for several essential nutrients without a daily multivitamin/mineral supplement.

CASE STUDY

Emily is 18 months old. Her mother Catherine is a strict vegetarian so she consumes no animal products. She still continues to breastfeed Emily because she would rather give Emily breast milk than cow's milk. Catherine works from home as a freelance writer. In order to keep Emily entertained while she writes, she often gives her a sippy cup filled with apple juice and a small container of honey-flavored toasted oats cereal and puts in an animated video for her to watch.

Questions:

1. What are the important differences between breast milk and cow's milk?

2. Is there a problem with letting Emily drink breast milk rather than weaning her to cow's milk?

3. What are the potential hazards of allowing Emily to sip on apple juice and eat honey-flavored toasted oats cereal over a long period? What alternatives could you offer?

4. What suggestions could you make to Catherine regarding Emily's diet?

REFERENCES

Abrams B, Parker J: Overweight and pregnancy complications. *Int J Obes* 1988; 12:293–303.

Alvarez JO, Caceda J, Woolley TW, Carley KW, Baiocchi N, Caravedo L, et al.: A longitudinal study of dental caries in the primary teeth of children who suffered from infant malnutrition. *J Dent Res* 1993; 72:1573–76.

American Academy of Pediatrics Committee on Nutrition: Statement on cholesterol. *Pediatrics* 1992; 90:469.

American Academy of Pediatrics Committee on Nutrition: Prevention of pediatric overweight and obesity. *Pediatrics.* 2003; 112:424–30.

American Academy of Pediatrics Committee on School Health Policy Statement: Soft drinks in schools. *Pediatrics.* 2004; 113:152–54.

American Academy of Pediatrics Work Group on Breastfeeding: Breastfeeding and the use of human milk. *Pediatrics* 1997; 100:1035–39.

American Academy of Pediatrics Work Group on Breastfeeding: Iron fortification of infant formulas. *Pediatrics* 1999; 104:119–21.

American College of Obstetricians & Gynecologists: *Exercise during Pregnancy and the Postpartum Period.* Washington, DC: Author, 1994.

American Dental Association: *ADA Guide to Dental Therapeutics.* Chicago: ADA Publishing, 1998.

American Dietetic Association: Position paper of the American Dietetic Association: position on breastfeeding. *J Am Diet Assoc* 1997; 97:662–66.

Anderson JW, Johnstone BM, Remley DT: Breastfeeding and cognitive development: A meta-analysis. *Am J Clin Nutr* 1999; 70:525–35.

Asthma and Allergy Foundation of America, http://www.aafa.org

Berkowitz RJ, Turner J, Green P: Primary oral infection of infants with *Streptococcus mutans. Arch Oral Biol* 1980; 25:221–24.

Birch LL: Psychological influences on the childhood diet. *J Nutr* 1998; 128:407S–10S.

Brown JE, Berdan KW, Splett P, Robinson M, Harris LJ: Prenatal weight gains related to birth of healthy sized infants to low-income women. *J Am Diet Assoc* 1986; 86:1679–83.

Butte NF, Garza C, Smith EO, Wills C, Nicholas BL: Macro trace-mineral intakes of exclusively breast-fed infants. *Am J Clin Nutr* 1987; 45(1):42–48.

Carlson A, Lino M, Gerrior S, Basiotis PP: Report card on the diet quality of children ages 2 to 9. *Fam Econ and Nutr Rev* 2001:52–54.

Centers for Disease Control and Prevention: Achievements in public health 1990–1999: Healthier mothers and babies. *MMWR* 1999; 48:849–58.

Centers for Disease Control and Prevention: Use of folic acid-containing supplements among women of childbearing age—United States—1997. *MMWR* 1998; 47:131–34.

Cnattingus S, Bergstrom R, Lipworth L, Kramer MS: Prepregnancy weight and the risk of adverse pregnancy outcomes. *N Eng J Med* 1998; 338:147–52.

Committee on Adolescence: Adolescent pregnancy—current trends and issues. *Pediatrics.* 1999; 103:516–20.

Cushing AH, Samet JM, Lambert WE, Skipper BJ, Hunt WC, Young SA: Breastfeeding reduces risk of respiratory illness in infants. *Am J Epidemiol* 1998; 147:863–70.

Cutz E, Perrin DG, Hackman R, Czegledy-Nagy EN: Maternal smoking and pulmonary neuroendocrine cells in sudden death syndromes. *Pediatrics* 1996; 98:668–72.

Dennison BA: Fruit juice consumption by infants and children: A review. *J Am Coll Nutr* 1996; 15:4S–11S.

Dennison BA, Rockwell HL, Baker SL: Excess fruit juice consumption by preschool children is associated with short stature and obesity. *Pediatrics* 1997; 99:15–22.

Dewey KG: Energy and protein requirements during lactation. *Annu Rev Nutr* 1997; 17:19–36.

Dewey KG, Lovelady CA, Nommsen-Rivers LA, McCrory MA, Lonnerdal B: A randomized study of the effects of aerobic exercise by lactating women on breast-milk volume and composition. *N Engl J Med* 1994; 330(7):449–53.

Dietz WH: Childhood weight affects adult morbidity and mortality. *J Nutr* 1998; 128:407S–10S.

Doucette RE, Dwyer JT: Is fruit juice a "no-no" in children's diets? *Nutr Rev* 2000; 58(6):180–83.

Edwards LE, Alton IR, Barrada MI, Kokanson EY: Pregnancy in the underweight woman: Cause, outcome, and growth patterns of the infant. *Am J Obstet Gynecol* 1979; 135:297–302.

Endres JB, Rockwell RE, Mense CG: *Food, Nutrition, and the Young Child,* 5th ed. Upper Saddle River, NJ: Pearson Education, 2004.

Fisher JO, Birch LL: Maternal restriction of young girls' food access is related to food intake of those foods in an unrestricted setting. *FASEB J* 1996; 10:A225(abs).

Food and Drug Administration: Food additives permitted for direct addition to food for human consumption; folic acid (folacin) final rule. *Fed Digest* 1996; 61:8797–807.

Gulch JI, Giorgios G: Risk factors related to periodontal disease before and during pregnancy. *Comp Cont Dent Educ Oral Hyg* 1998; 5:1–10.

Harnack L, Stang J, Story M: Soft drink consumption among US children and adolescents: Nutrititional consequences. *J Am Diet Assoc* 1999; 99:435–41.

Hellerstedt WL, Himes JH, Story M, Alton IR, Edwards LE: The effects of cigarette smoking and gestational weight change on birth outcomes in obese and normal-weight women. *Am J Public Health* 1997; 87:591–96.

Hilgers KK, Douglass J, Mathieu GP: Adolescent pregnancy: A review of dental treatment guidelines. *Pediatr Dent* 2003; 25(5):459–67.

Institute of Medicine, National Academy of Sciences: *Dietary Reference Intakes for Thiamin, Riboflavin, Niacin, Vitamin B_6, Folate, Vitamin B_{12}, Pantothenic Acid, Biotin, and Choline.* Washington, DC: National Academies Press, 1998.

Institute of Medicine, National Academy of Sciences: *Dietary Reference Intakes for Vitamin C, Vitamin E, Selenium, and Carotenoids.* Washington, DC: National Academies Press, 2000.

Institute of Medicine, National Academy of Sciences: *Nutrition During Lactation.* Washington, DC: National Academies Press, 1991.

Institute of Medicine, National Academy of Sciences: *Nutrition During Pregnancy and Lactation: An Implementation Guide.* Washington, DC: National Academies Press, 1992.

Institute of Medicine, National Academy of Sciences: *Nutrition During Pregnancy: Weight Gain, Nutrient Supplements.* Washington, DC: National Academies Press, 1990:1.

Jack BW, Culpepper JB: Preconception care, risk reduction, and health promotion. *JAMA* 1990; 264:1147–49.

Jensen RG: *Handbook of Milk Composition.* New York: Academic Press, 1995.

Leverett DH, Adair SM, Vaughan BW, Proskin HM, Moss ME: Randomized clinical trial of the effect of prenatal fluoride supplements in preventing dental caries. *Caries Res* 1997; 31(3):174–79.

Little RE: Maternal alcohol use during breastfeeding and infant mental and motor development. *N Engl J Med* 1989; 321:425–30.

Loe H, Silness J: Periodontal disease during pregnancy. 1. Prevalence and severity. *Acta Odontol Scand* 1963; 21: 533–51.

Looker AC, Dallman PR, Carroll MD, Gunter EW, Johnson CL: Prevalence of iron deficiency in the United States. *JAMA* 1997; 227:973–76.

Lozoff B, Jimenez E, Wolf AW: Long-term developmental outcome of infants with iron deficiency. *N Engl J Med* 1991; 325:687–94.

Manual of Clinical Dietetics, 5th ed. Chicago: American Dietetic Association, 1996.

McCormick MC: The contribution of low birthweight to infant mortality and childhood morbidity. *N Engl J Med* 1985; 312:81–89.

McGanity WJ, Dawson EB, Van Hook JW: Maternal nutrition. In Shils ME, Olson JA, Shike M, Ross AC (eds): *Modern Nutrition in Health and Disease,* 9th ed. Baltimore: Williams & Wilkins, 1999.

Mills JL, Holmes LB, Aarons JH, Simpson JL: Moderate caffeine use and the risk of spontaneous abortion and intrauterine growth retardation. *JAMA* 1993; 269:593.

MRC Vitamin Research Group: Presentation of neural tube defects: Results of the Medical Research Council Vitamin Study. *Lancet* 1991; 338:131–37.

Muñoz KA, Krebs-Smith SM, Bollard-Barash R, Cleveland LE: Food intakes of children and adolescents compared with recommendations. *Pediatrics* 1997; 100:323–29.

Nainar SM, Mohummed S: Diet counseling during the infant oral health visit. *Pediatr Dent* 2004; 6(5):459–62.

Neumark-Sztaner D, Story M, Resnick MD, Blum RW: Learned lessons about adolescent nutrition from the Minnesota Adolescent Health Survey. *J Am Diet Assoc* 1998; 98:1449–56.

Offenbacher S, Katz V, Fertik G, Collins J, Boyd D, Maynor G, et al.: Periodontal infection as a risk factor for preterm low birthweight. *J Periodontol* 1996; 67(10 suppl): 1103–13.

Overweight in Children and Adolescents. The Surgeon General's Call to Action to Prevent and Decrease Overweight and Obesity. Retrieved July 20, 2005, from http://www.surgeongeneral.gov/topics/obesity/calltoaction/fact_adolescents.htm.

Rees JM: Overview: Nutrition for pregnant and childrearing adolescents. *Ann NY Acad Sci* 1997; 817:241–50.

Reifsnider E, Gill S: Nutrition for the childbearing years. *J Obstet, Gynecol Neonatal Nurs* 2000; 29(1):43–55.

Roberts S: *Feeding Your Child for Lifelong Health.* New York: Bantam, 1999.

Satter E: *Child of Mine: Feeding with Love and Good Sense.* Palo Alto, CA: Bull Publishing, 1995.

Satter E: *How to Get Your Kid to Eat: But Not Too Much.* Palo Alto, CA: Bull Publishing, 1987.

Schnuth ML: You and your vegetarian patients. *RDH* 1994; 14(4):12–20.

Seow WK: Enamel hypoplasia in the primary dentition: A review. *J Dent Child* 1991; 58:441–52.

Shein B, Tsamtsouris A, Rovero J: Self-reported compliance and the effectiveness of prenatal dental education. *J Clin Pediat Dent* 1991; 15:102–8.

Soxman JA: Preventive guidelines for the preschool patient. *Gen Dent* 2005; 53(1):77–80.

Sternfeld B: Physical activity and pregnancy outcome. *Sports Med* 1997; 23:33–47.

Story M, Alton I: Nutrition issues and adolescent pregnancy. *Nutr Today* 1995; 30:142–51.

Tirnanoff N, Palmer CA: Dietary determinants of dental caries and dietary recommendations for preschool children. *J Public Health Dent* 2001; 60(3):197–206; discussion 207–9.

Tsamtsouris A, Stack A, Padamsee M: Dental education of expectant parents. *J Pedodont* 1986; 10:309–322.

U.S. Department of Agriculture, U.S. Department of Health and Human Services: *Dietary Guidelines for Americans 2005*. Washington, DC. Retrieved from http://www .healthierus.gov/dietaryguidelines.

Whitaker RC, Wright JA, Pepe MS, Seidel KD, Dietz WH: Predicting obesity in young adulthood from childhood and parental obesity. *N Engl J Med* 1997; 337:869–73.

Williams CL, Bollela M, Boccia L, Spark A: Dietary fat and children's health. *Nutr Today* 1998; 33:144–53.

Worthington-Roberts BS, Williams SR: *Nutrition in Pregnancy and Lactation*, 6th ed. Dubuque, IA:Brown & Benchmark, 1997.

Worthington-Roberts BS, Williams SR: *Nutrition throughout the Life Cycle*, 4th ed. Dubuque, IA: McGraw-Hill, 2000.

Chapter 18

Oral Health Nutrition and Dietary Considerations in Adolescence and Adulthood

Teresa Marshall

OBJECTIVES

The student will be able to:

- Identify key adolescent issues that affect dietary habits and oral health.
- Discuss the health and oral implications of eating disorders.
- Identify key adult issues that affect dietary habits and oral health.
- Discuss diet education strategies appropriate for adolescents and adults.

INTRODUCTION

The primary oral health issues in adolescence and adulthood are caries and periodontal disease prevention and treatment (see Chapters 13 and 14). This chapter discusses dietary practices common during adolescence and adulthood, identifies how these practices affect oral and systemic health, and reviews dietary practices that can promote optimal oral and systemic health.

Adolescence

Adolescence is defined as the period of physical and psychological development between childhood and adulthood (*American Heritage Dictionary*, 1994). This transition is progressive and rapid, although the different domains (physical, emotional, psychological, and cognitive) evolve independently (Lerner, Galambos, 1998). Good nutrition is important during adolescence for achieving growth potential and preventing chronic diseases. The rate of physical growth, metabolism, and activity determines nutrient and energy requirements, whereas emotional and psychological states influence food choices and meal patterns (Jacobson, Rees, Golden, Irwin, 1997; Miles, Eid, 1997; Miller, Maropis, 1998). During adolescence, adequate (but not excessive) intakes of energy-providing foods and nutrients are required for expected growth and physical maturity, metabolism, and activity. Insufficient energy or nutrient intakes can limit growth potential, delay or arrest puberty, impair tissue healing, and compromise immunity (Rickert, 1995). As the adolescent struggles to establish an identity and seeks autonomy, food issues can become part of the struggle and can affect current and future oral and systemic health and disease. For example, inadequate energy or nutrient intake can limit growth potential, excessive fat intake can predispose to cardiovascular disease, and frequent eating can increase caries risk.

Adolescence is a time when risk-taking behaviors are common, and unhealthy eating behaviors may be considered socially acceptable or even desirable. Frequent intake of food away from home, especially fast foods, can result in a high-fat, high-sugar, low-fiber dietary pattern. Cigarette and alcohol use and substance abuse are associated with a lower intake of fruits and vegetables (Adams, 1997). Greater access to healthy food choices at school and convenience food establishments could encourage youth to improve their diets.

Adulthood

Adulthood is defined as the state of being fully grown or mature (*American Heritage Dictionary*, 1994). Although physical growth and maturity have defined endpoints, emotional and psychological development may continue indefinitely (Bee, 1992). Life experiences continue to shape one's acceptance of new foods, willingness to change dietary habits, susceptibility to fad diets, and vulnerability to emotional eating. Previous experiences with food, often rooted in early childhood, are also strong determinants of food choices and dietary habits.

In adulthood, the primary role of good nutrition is to foster health promotion and chronic disease prevention, maintain oral tissue and supporting structures, and support a functional immune system.

OPTIMAL DIET FOR ADOLESCENTS AND ADULTS

The ideal diet for oral and systemic health during adolescence and adulthood provides adequate nutrients and energy to meet individual needs for growth or weight maintenance, metabolism, and activity. The dietary pattern should also limit exposure to fermentable carbohydrates. Dietary habits are deeply ingrained in tradition, culture, and religion; the ideal diet must work within and respect these variables. See Chapter 21 for a discussion of food habits.

The period of maximum linear growth in girls occurs between 10 and 13 years of age just prior to the onset of menarche. The period of maximum linear growth in boys occurs about 2 years later, between 12 and 15 years of age. Physiological age rather than chronological age should be used to establish nutrient requirements, because growth rates and body composition differ widely during adolescence (Heald, Gong, 1999). Nutritional requirements are greatest during the years of maximum growth. Energy needs peak during the growth spurt and then decline to adult levels. Estimated energy requirements range from 2071 to 2368 kcal/day for adolescent girls and 2403 kcal/day for adult females, with increased requirements for pregnancy and lactation (IOM, 2005). Estimated energy requirements are 2279 to 3152 kcal/day for adolescent boys and 3067 kcal/day for adult males (IOM, 2005). Protein intakes reported by both adolescents and adults typically are greater than requirements. Recommended Dietary Allowances for protein are estimated at 34–46 g/day and

34–42 g/day for adolescent girls and boys respectively, and at 46 g/day and 56 g/day for adult females and males, respectively (IOM, 2005).

Insufficient calcium and/or vitamin D intakes are associated with an increased risk of osteoporosis and, perhaps, periodontal disease in later life (Jeffcoat, 1998; Osteoporosis, 2000). A primary strategy for preventing osteoporosis is to maximize genetically predetermined bone mass during adolescence and early adulthood. A high calcium intake is required to support bone growth and to attain peak bone mass, yet teenage girls are less likely than boys to meet the Dietary Reference Intake (DRI) for calcium (1300 mg) (IOM, 1998). Foods of dairy origin, primarily milk, are the major source of calcium in Americans' diets. Analyses of national survey data suggests individuals in the highest quartile of dairy intake have greater calcium intakes (1353 mg) than those in the lowest quartile of dairy intakes (380 mg) (Weinberg, Berner, Groves, 2004). Women with low milk intakes during childhood and adolescence have less bone mass in adulthood and an increased risk of fractures (Kalkwarf, Khoury, Lanphear, 2003).

At the time of the pubertal growth spurt, additional iron is needed for synthesis of myoglobin and hemoglobin. Iron deficiency occurs in 9% of adolescent girls (Looker, Dallman, Carroll, 1997). Monthly blood loss is the main cause of poor iron status in females, and signs of iron deficiency often appear after the growth spurt at the initiation of menstruation. Thus, the iron recommendation for females exceeds that for males.

The major dietary sources of iron for adolescents are ready-to-eat cereals, fortified yeast breads, beef, bakery products, and pasta (Subar, Krebs-Smith, Cook, Kahle, 1998). Since the American diet provides about 6 mg iron per 1000 kcal, females with calorie intakes between 2000 and 2400 kcal often have difficulty obtaining the RDA for iron and may need to take an iron supplement.

Healthy adolescents and adults should easily be able to meet nutrient requirements for oral and systemic health by following the USDA's food pyramid (USDA, 2005). Active adolescents in a rapid growth phase have high-energy requirements, and structured snacks are often necessary to meet energy requirements. Efforts should be made to encourage teens to snack on foods that provide nutrients in addition to energy. Examples might be sandwiches, pizza, and milkshakes.

The rate, type, and quantity of food consumed influence satiation (the feeling of fullness that causes one to stop eating). Satiation usually occurs within 30 minutes following the onset of eating. Prolonging eating episodes or increasing the frequency of eating can result in excessive energy intake and increase the risk of caries and plaque development. Furthermore, energy consumed in liquid form is not compensated for as efficiently as that consumed in solid form; thus, liquid energy can increase overall energy intake.

ORAL RISKS OF THE ADOLESCENT OR ADULT DIET

Both dietary habits and nutrient intakes can affect oral disease at any life stage. Conversely, good dietary habits can help prevent the plaque diseases (caries and periodontitis). With advancing age, periodontal disease may cause gingival recession, newly exposing surfaces of teeth to the oral environment (Ravald, 1994). These root surfaces are less highly mineralized than crown surfaces, so they are at greater risk for caries, particularly if oral clearance is delayed due to xerostomia or declining oral motor skills. Eating habits can affect both caries risk and enamel demineralization (Harris, Garcia-Godoy, 1999; Middleman, Vazquez, Durant, 1998). Acid produced during fermentation of dietary carbohydrates demineralizes enamel and can result in site-specific caries development. The nature of the carbohydrate, length and frequency of consumption, and quantity consumed will determine the extent of acid exposure and subsequent demineralization. Prolonged exposure to acids contained within foods, beverages, medicines, or gastric contents can result in a generalized erosion of enamel surfaces. Table 18–1 shows some examples of foods that can increase risk of caries and/or erosion.

Nutrients and energy are necessary to support a functional immune system with the competent host defense mechanisms necessary to limit periodontal disease (see Chapter 14). Immune function can diminish with age, emphasizing the importance of the nutrition component (Patten, 1995).

The goal of dietary recommendations for caries risk reduction is to limit the contact time between teeth and fermentable carbohydrates to minimize plaque development and activity. This can be accomplished by limiting the frequency and length of meal and snack exposures (e.g., how long it takes to eat foods or drink beverages). Rinsing with water and brushing with fluoridated dentifrice after exposures will also reduce caries risk.

TABLE 18–1   Food Habits That May Increase Risk of Caries and/or Erosion

- Vitamin C supplements: ascorbic acid is acidic. When supplements are chewed, the risk of enamel erosion increases, particularly with multiple exposures throughout the day.
- Vitamin C lozenges: lozenges typically contain sugar, corn syrup, ascorbic acid, and citric acid. Frequent sucking on such lozenges increases risk of caries and enamel erosion.
- Hard candy: sucking on hard candy throughout the day, often as self-prescribed treatment for xerostomia, increases risk of caries.
- Breath mints: made with sugar and meant to be held in the mouth for prolonged periods. These are often the culprits in adult root caries.
- Sour candies: acidic candies; contain sugar, corn syrup, citric acid, and ascorbic acid. Marketing of these candies challenges consumers to see how long they can hold the candy in their mouth. Package labels contain the warning "eating multiple pieces within a short time period may cause a temporary irritation to sensitive tongues and mouths."* Consumption of such candies can increase risk of caries and enamel erosion in addition to producing lesions on the oral mucosa.
- Lemon wedges: holding or chewing acidic fruits in a specific location in the mouth increases risk of enamel demineralization.

*Mega Warheads, The Foreign Candy Company, Inc., 451 Black Forest Road, Hunt IA 51239-1499.

The presence of orthodontic appliances (braces) does not change nutrient requirements or appropriate dietary habits. However, food choices may be altered by dietary recommendations designed to protect brackets and minimize oral adherence (Riordan, 1997). Chapter 15 provides diet suggestions for persons undergoing orthodontia.

ADOLESCENT AND ADULT DIET-RELATED LIFESTYLE ISSUES

Nutrient intakes and dietary habits are influenced by multiple internal and external factors. A young teen is obviously different from a 50-year-old adult, physically, emotionally, cognitively, and psychologically. However, life is a continuum of growth subject to changing internal and external influences. Adolescents and adults occupy different positions along this continuum as a result of individual experiences. For this reason, the following issues are not categorized by lifecycle stage, although some issues prevail at each stage.

Environment

Environmental changes occur throughout the life span. During early adolescence, teens typically spend less time with their immediate family while they struggle to establish an identity and seek autonomy (Jacobson et al., 1997). As a result, peers have a greater influence than parents have in many areas, including food choices and dietary habits. Peer influences will continue throughout life concerning how, when, and where foods are consumed. Parents of young teens can minimize this influence by including peers within the family environment. Also, parents can participate in development of school policies to determine which foods and beverages should be available for purchase before, during, and after lunch.

Foods introduced and accepted during childhood continue to be accepted during adolescence and adulthood. Foods that were refused during childhood are not likely to be consumed during adolescence unless introduced by peers, but may be accepted during adulthood. As teens struggle for independence, parental guidance regarding food choices is often not well received. Caregivers have the right to determine what foods are purchased and available for consumption in the home (Satter, 2005). Teens should be active in the process of choosing foods and snacks and be allowed the autonomy to make their own dietary choices away from home.

Adulthood is generally thought to be a more stable state as a result of mature physical, emotional, and cognitive processes. However, adulthood continues to provide opportunities for growth, change, and stress associated with marriage and divorce, children, relocation, employment, hobbies, and activities (Barker, Thompson, McClean, 1996). All environmental changes, whether social, geographic, or financial, have the potential to influence diet by affecting access to food, resources for food, or time for food preparation, in addition to influencing food choices and dietary habits.

Adolescents and adults at school or work generally eat their midday meal away from home. Teens and adults have multiple commitments including school, work, and organized activities. Coordinating schedules to accommodate these responsibilities and leisure activities affects meal habits. Time conflicts may result in eating meals alone or separate from family, snacking instead of eating meals, having meals on the run, and skipping meals. When people skip meals, for whatever reason, the natural response is "bingeing" later due to severe hunger. Such bingeing may result in excessive calorie intake. Skipping breakfast can impair mental and physical performance. Skipping meals may also undermine weight control efforts, as this habit leads the body to conserve energy.

Weight Concerns

Weight management is a huge issue in today's world as people dissatisfied with their body size attempt to gain weight (bulk up) or to lose weight (Nowak, Speare, Crawford, 1996). The prevalence of obesity is increasing among children, adolescents, and adults. Obese adolescents are at an increased risk of becoming obese adults. Obesity and overweight during adolescence and adulthood increases the risk of atherosclerosis, hypertension, adult obesity, Type 2 diabetes, and eating disorders (Berenson, Srinivasan, 1998; Dietz, 1998; Rickert, 1995). In addition to the health risks, the stigma of obesity may lead to social isolation. Genetic factors, limited physical activity, and unstructured eating patterns are associated with adolescent and adult obesity. For example, eating while preoccupied with sedentary activities such as television viewing, computer use, or reading may result in a lack of awareness of what and how much is consumed.

During adolescence, many teens engage in some type of weight gain or loss program that they may pursue throughout adulthood (Jacobsen et al., 1997; Middleman et al., 1998). Diets that eliminate or minimize intake from specific food groups increase the risk of marginal nutrient intake. Thus, growth, tissue maintenance, healing, and immune function may be affected resulting in an increased susceptibility to oral and systemic disease, particularly those of infectious origin including periodontal disease. Rapid, extreme weight loss may also limit linear growth potential and delay the progression or completion of puberty in adolescents. (Chapter 3 details the characteristics of sound and unsound diets.)

Many adults select diets with a goal of preventing chronic diseases that can impair length and quality of life. Self-imposed, overly restrictive, or poorly understood diets may lead to unwarranted food restriction and can undermine good nutritional status. For example, individuals selecting foods high in simple sugars as part of the very-low-fat, high-carbohydrate craze increase

their risk of metabolic syndrome (i.e., hypertriglyceridemia, low high-density lipoprotein cholesterol, hypertension, and hyperinsulinemia). More recently, high-protein, high-fat, low-carbohydrate diets (i.e., ketogenic) have been associated with short-term safety, but long-term cardiovascular disease risk.

Eating Disorders

The media, food industry, and society influence dietary habits by fostering a preoccupation with thinness while promoting high-fat, low-nutrient foods. Such influences have contributed to a society of weight-conscious adolescents and adults, discrimination based on body size, and an increase in eating disorders (Kalodner, 1997). Eating disorders, in turn, have serious medical, oral, and psychological implications and can be life threatening. Eating disorders commonly present during adolescence and adulthood. The most well known are anorexia nervosa and bulimia nervosa; however, other eating disorders including female athlete triad, night-eating syndrome, binge eating disorder, compulsive overeating, and chronic dieting syndrome are increasingly recognized.

The statistics on disordered eating are staggering. In a study of 600 colleges, 75% of students and faculty interviewed had clinically significant symptoms of frequent bingeing or purging and obsessions with food and weight (Berg, 1998). Even more disturbing is a California-based study in which 81% of 10-year-old girls reported disordered eating (Berg, 1998). Most of those who suffer from eating disorders are 14 to 25 years old, white, and affluent, although the incidence of eating disorders is increasing among all racial and socioeconomic groups. The occurrence of eating disorders is more common in females; the female–male ratio is 10:1 (APA, 1994; Hartung, 1997).

Eating disorders are complex in origin, but underlying causes are thought to include sexual abuse, depression, early detachment from the mother (Garner, 1998), and media influences (Field et al., 1999). Table 18–2 provides a complete description of eating disorder characteristics.

Anorexia Nervosa
Anorexia nervosa, or self-induced starvation, is a psychiatric disorder characterized by an abnormal fear of being fat and manifested by significant body image distortions, refusal to eat, unusual eating habits, and

TABLE 18-2   Eating Disorder Characteristics

Disorder	General Characteristics	Physical Characteristics	Dental Implications
Anorexia nervosa	• Abnormal fear of being fat exhibited in body image distortions, refusal to eat, strange eating habits, excessive exercise • Typically affects adolescent females who are perfectionists, conscientious, and conforming	• Muscle wasting, amenorrhea, dry skin, thin and brittle hair, degradation of finger nails, dehydration, edema, constipation, sleep disturbance	• Diminished gum health
Bulimia nervosa	• Restriction of food intake, leading to physical and psychological urges to binge; food then purged by vomiting; use of laxatives • Afraid to gain weight, diminished self-worth, rebellious, emotional instability, extreme guilt	• Tooth enamel demineralization, gum damage, scratched and bruised knuckles, throat irritation, esophageal inflamation, cracked and damaged lips, broken facial blood vessels, rectal bleeding and calcium deficiency with laxative use, dehydration electrolyte imbalances, upper GI fistulas, kidney damage, reversible myopathies	• Tooth enamel demineralization and sensitivity, gingival recession, dental caries, orthodontic complications, angular cheilosis, xerostomia, decreased salivary flow, tooth erosion
Binge eating disorder	• Feeling of loss of control during bingeing episode • Duration of 2 hours to entire day • Volume of food more than most people would eat • Associated with psychiatric comorbidity, particularly depression	• Greater and earlier obesity than nonbingeing obese peers • Dental caries	• Dental caries

Sources: From Hubbard, O'Neill, Cheakalos, 1999; Jones, Jones, 1989; Rock, Curran-Celentano, 1994.

excessive exercise. It affects at least 5% of college women. Anorexia sufferers are often perfectionistic, conscientious, and conforming adolescents (Hubbard, O'Neill, Cheakalos, 1999). In acute anorexia, weight loss is often extreme.

Physical signs of possible anorexia nervosa include muscle wasting, amenorrhea, edema, dry skin, constipation, brittle nails, and thin brittle hair. Lack of estrogen associated with amenorrhea limits calcium deposition into bone and increases risk of osteoporosis. If the anorexia is accompanied by self-induced vomiting, lesions on the lingual side of the teeth resulting from acid reflux may be present (Faine, Mobley, 1999).

Bulimia Nervosa

Bulimia nervosa is more common than anorexia, and is a continuous cycle of fasting, bingeing, and purging that typically results in minor or no weight loss. Food intake is restricted, leading to physical and psychological urges to binge and ultimately the desire to purge the food, either by vomiting, excessive exercise, or laxative abuse (Wonderlich, Swift, Slotnick, Goodman: 1990).

Dentists can easily identify an eating disorder in their patients with bulimia because of significant tooth hypersensitivity from enamel erosion or gingival recession (Faine et al., 1999; Rytomaa, Jarvinen, Kanerva, Heinonen, 1998). A diagnosis of bulimia is likely if erosion occurs on the lingual surface of the maxillary anterior teeth as well as on the buccal surfaces of maxillary canines, premolars, and maxillary incisors. In one study, 69% of bulimics had significant perimylolysis (demineralization) of smooth maxillary lingual enamel surfaces resulting from regurgitation. In some cases the penetration extended into the pulp (Jones, Jones, 1989). Because many of the preferred foods for binge eating are laden with fat and sugar, these individuals may also suffer from dental caries (Garner, 1998).

Additionally, the soft palate may be traumatized by objects used to induce vomiting (e.g., pencils), and orthodontic complications can ensue from purging behavior (Jones, Jones, 1989). Bulimics often have xerostomia as a result of swollen glands, especially the parotid. They also tend to consume fruits or fruit juices to satisfy thirst after vomiting, which contributes to the risk of enamel erosion. Other signs of bulimia nervosa include scratched and bruised knuckles from inducing vomiting, esophageal inflammation, cracked and damaged lips, and throat irritation. In those who abuse laxatives, rectal bleeding, dehydration, and electrolyte imbalances also occur (Hubbard et al., 1999).

Female Athlete Triad

The term *female athlete triad* was coined to describe young female athletes with disordered eating (restrictive dieting, overexercising, weight loss, and a lack of body fat), osteoporosis, and amenorrhea (West, 1998). Again, dental risks include enamel decalcification, increased caries, and increased periodontal and soft tissue inflammation.

Binge Eating Disorder

Obese individuals with binge eating disorder typically have more severe obesity, an earlier onset of obesity, and greater psychopathology (i.e., depression, substance abuse, emotional problems) than obese peers (Stunkard, Allison, 2003). Binge eating episodes are characterized by a feeling of loss of control and consumption of more food than expected. The length of binges can range from 2 hours to entire days. Individuals who binge eat are at increased risk of dental caries and periodontal disease.

Night Eating Syndrome

Night eating syndrome is characterized by morning anorexia, evening hyperphagia, and insomnia (Stunkard, Allison, 2003). Subjects are typically obese and the majority of food is consumed during the evening and

night-time hours. The etiology is associated with a disorder of the biological rhythm. Individuals with night eating syndrome are conscious of their nocturnal eating. A similar disorder, nocturnal sleep-related eating disorder, is characterized by multiple waking and eating episodes during the night in which the individual is not conscious of his or her eating. Excessive energy consumed due to either condition increases risk of obesity; frequent eating, particularly of carbohydrate-containing foods, increases caries risk.

Diagnosis and Management of Eating Disorders

Anorexia nervosa and bulimia nervosa are considered psychiatric diseases with significant medical and nutritional complications (APA, 1994). Table 18–3 lists the diagnostic criteria used for eating disorders (DSM-IV, 1994). Successful intervention is more likely if disordered eating is detected early in the disease process and treatment is initiated promptly. Successful management of these disorders requires a team approach including psychiatrists, psychologists, physicians, nurses, dietitians, social workers, and dentists (Rock, Curran-Colentano, 1994). The road to recovery is often long and costly (Hubbard et al., 1999).

Dentists are often the first health care providers to diagnose an eating disorder (Mueller, 2001). In addition to providing palliative oral care, the dentist is obligated to assist the patient in obtaining psychotherapy and medical care. Table 18–4 shows the "red flags" of eating disorders. Dentists should provide palliation, restoration, preventive education, and proper referrals (Bedi, 1992; Bishop, Briggs, Schmidt, 1994).

The patient needs to understand that until the underlying problem is resolved, the oral problems will continue. Table 18–5 shows the dental considerations for treatment of the oral problems. The primary nutrition goals for individuals with eating disorders are restoration of weight and normalization of eating habits (Muscari, 1998; Powers, 1996). Table 18–6 shows the diet principles for managing eating disorders.

Beverage-Related Issues

Recent trends in the beverage consumption patterns of adolescents and adults have caused concern to health care providers. Children, adolescents, and adults have greatly increased juice and carbonated beverage intakes, and decreased milk and water intakes

TABLE 18–3 Eating Disorders—DSM-IV Criteria

Eating Disorder	Criteria
Anorexia nervosa	• Refusal to maintain weight at or above 85% ideal body weight • Intense fear of gaining weight • Distorted body image • Amenorrhea (absence of three menstrual cycles)
Bulimia nervosa	• Recurrent binge eating episodes followed by eating a large amount of food within a 2-hour time period, or a sense of lack of control during a binge episode • Recurrent inappropriate compensatory behavior to prevent weight gain (e.g., vomiting, laxatives, diuretics, excessive exercise, fasting) • Bingeing and compensatory behavior occurs at least two times/week for 3 months • Self-evaluation unduly influenced by body shape, weight • Disturbance doesn't occur exclusively during anorexia nervosa episodes
Binge eating disorder (BED)	• Recurrent episodes of binge eating characterized by eating within a 2-hour time period an amount of food larger than normal, and a sense of lack of control during binge episodes • Episodes associated with at least three of the following: eating more rapidly than normal, eating until uncomfortably full, or eating large amounts of food when not feeling physically hungry • Eating alone out of embarrassment over food intake • Feeling disgusted with self, depressed, or feeling guilty after eating • Marked distress regarding binge eating • Binge occurs at least 2 days a week for 6 months • Binge not associated with regular use of inappropriate compensatory behaviors (purging, fasting, excessive exercise) and does not occur exclusively during anorexia nervosa or bulimia nervosa

Source: Adapted from DSM-IV: Anorexia Nervosa, 1994.

TABLE 18–4 "Red Flags" for Eating Disorders

• Enamel demineralization
• Tooth hypersensitivity
• Mucosal trauma
• Xerostomia
• Swollen salivary glands

TABLE 18–5 Dental Treatment for Eating Disorders

• Oral prophylaxis
• Fluoride treatment
• Home care guidance
• Pain palliation
• Limited restoration

TABLE 18–6 Nutritional Treatment for Eating Disorders

• Evaluating average daily intake
• Examining weight for height
• Determining trigger and avoided foods
• Establishing a working eating plan
• Encouraging development of a healthy body image

(Harnack, Stang, Story, 1999; Nielsen, Popkin, 2004). A decrease in milk intake, particularly by adolescent females, is associated with decreased calcium and vitamin D intakes and an increased risk of osteoporosis (Gallo, l996) (Figure 18–1). Chapter 7 provides more information on dietary fluids. Of equal concern is the excess energy intake associated with increased regular carbonated beverage, juice, and juice drink consumption. These beverages contribute few nutrients to the diet and between 12 and 22 kcal/oz; all of the calories are from sugars. It is not unusual for individuals to consume 6 to 8 cups of juice or 6 to 8 12 oz cans of carbonated beverages daily, contributing 720 to 1,440 kcal to total energy intake. The individual may compensate by reducing food intake with a subsequent decrease in nutrient intake. Or, individuals may not compensate for the additional energy intake and gain weight as a result.

Battle Of The Beverages
Milk's nutrients compared to the competition.

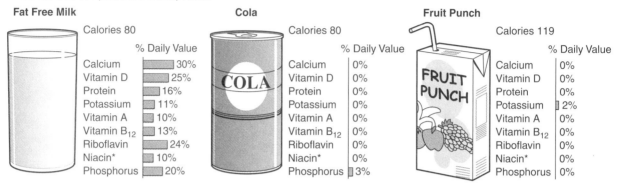

	Fat Free Milk		Cola		Fruit Punch	
Calories	80		80		119	
		% Daily Value		% Daily Value		% Daily Value
Calcium		30%		0%		0%
Vitamin D		25%		0%		0%
Protein		16%		0%		0%
Potassium		11%		0%		2%
Vitamin A		10%		0%		0%
Vitamin B_{12}		13%		0%		0%
Riboflavin		24%		0%		0%
Niacin*		10%		0%		0%
Phosphorus		20%		3%		0%

Serving size = 1 cup (8 fl. oz.). Fat free milk is fortified with vitamin D. The fruit punch is not fortified. Percent daily values are based on a 2,000 calorie diet. *Includes niacin equivalents.

FIGURE 18–1   Battle of the beverages.
Source: Developed by Milk Processor Education Program, 1999. U.S. Department of Agriculture nutrient analysis.

From an oral health perspective, beverages can be categorized as caloric (containing sugars) or noncaloric (containing no sugars). The frequency of consumption of soft drinks is positively associated with highly decayed, missing, and filled teeth scores (Ismail, Burt, Eklund, 1984). Consumption of regular carbonated beverages by young children was associated with greater caries risk than consumption of 100% juice (Marshall et al., 2003). Drinking sugared beverages as part of a meal has negligible caries risk. At the other extreme, a 64 oz carbonated beverage nursed throughout the day increases caries risk as the plaque pH rarely returns to normal. Reports of increased caries incidence, possibly associated with increased use of sugar-containing beverages, have caused recent concern among dentists (Meskin, 1999). Figure 18–2 shows rampant caries from excessive soda drinking.

Sports drinks contain 6 to 9 kcal/oz; all calories are from sugar. Originally designed to replenish electrolytes and glucose during intense workouts, sports drinks are often consumed as snack beverages. They also have the potential to increase caries risk (Milosevic, Kelly, McLean, 1997).

"Diet" carbonated beverages are not cariogenic because they do not contain a carbohydrate substrate for bacteria. However, diet carbonated beverages are acidic, and can cause enamel demineralization, particularly if used frequently by individuals with xerostomia (Al-Hiyasat, Saunders, Shardey, Smith, 1998; Larsen,

Nyvad, 1999; Nunn, 1996; von Frauhhofer, Rogers, 2004; Zero, 1996). For diet carbonated beverages, risk of enamel demineralization is dependent on the quantity and nature of consumption and the susceptibility of the individual. Sugar-containing carbonated beverages, juices, and sports drinks are also acidic, and the combination of acid and sugar may act synergistically to cause the severe caries associated with regular carbonated beverage consumption.

Absorption of pigments from coffee, tea, or similar dark beverages by plaque and enamel can lead to discoloration or staining of teeth (Harris, Garcia-Godoy, 1999).

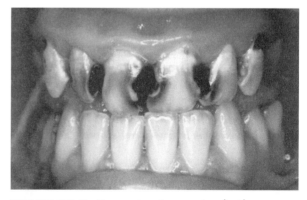

FIGURE 18–2   Rampant caries associated with consumption of 6 to 12 cans regular carbonated beverages daily.
Source: Courtesy of Teresa A. Marshall, University of Iowa.

Diet and Athletics

Participation in athletic or fitness programs increases energy requirements both to support the activity and to maintain lean body mass developed in response to the activity. Vitamins and minerals are required for metabolism of the energy-yielding nutrients. However, supplemental vitamins and minerals do not enhance performance and additional protein does not build muscle (Johnson, Landry, 1998). Muscle size or bulk is a reflection of genetic potential; strength training can increase muscle bulk. A number of ergogenic aids are marketed to facilitate this process, but the efficacy and safety of these products are not well established (Johnson, Landry, 1998). Chapter 10 reviews dietary supplements.

Females engaging in endurance sports are at an increased risk for iron deficiency from increased iron losses associated with sweating, red blood cell destruction, gastrointestinal losses, poor absorption, and inadequate iron intake. Water requirements are increased during activity because of increased sweating and breathing losses. Fluid requirements depend on length and intensity of activity, as well as on environmental conditions.

A variety of carbohydrate-loading regimens are often recommended to enhance glycogen storage and maximize performance. Other strategies include high-carbohydrate pre- and postgame meals. Long-distance runners and other endurance athletes often consume carbohydrate snacks and beverages during events. Sports drinks and gels that contain sugar and electrolytes may provide benefits to endurance athletes, but frequent intake of high-carbohydrate foods, beverages, and gels before, during, and after training or competition can increase caries risk.

Alcohol and Recreational Drugs

Although alcohol is not cariogenic or acidic, excessive consumption of alcohol has the potential to affect oral and systemic health. The direct effects of alcohol on the liver and other organs are well known. Alcohol provides energy when metabolized and may contribute to excessive energy intake. On the other hand, if increased energy intake from alcohol results in decreased food intake, then nutrient intake may decline. Low food intake and altered nutrient metabolism place individuals with frequent alcohol intake at risk for malnutrition. Many alcoholic beverages also contain fermentable carbohydrates, so frequent consumption increases caries risk, as do irregular dietary habits and poor oral hygiene. Marginal nutrient intake also increases susceptibility to periodontal disease.

Use of addictive drugs such as marijuana, cocaine, and nicotine alters food choices and dietary habits during both addiction and withdrawal (Asghar, 1986; Mohs, Watson, Leonard-Green, 1990). Depending on the nature of the food choices and the frequency of cariogenic exposures, the individual may be at increased risk of caries or malnutrition. Methamphetamine abuse by adolescents is increasing, particularly in the Midwest region of the country. Rampant caries is a hallmark of chronic abuse (i.e., meth mouth), and attributed to xerostomia, frequent sugared beverage consumption, and poor oral hygiene associated with methamphetamine use (Shaner, 2002).

SUMMARY AND IMPLICATIONS FOR DENTISTRY

Adolescence and adulthood present unique challenges to oral health and nutrition. Eating disorders occur primarily in young adults; root caries begin to appear in middle age. A host of lifestyle factors can contribute to increased oral risk in both groups. Nutritional risk factors tend to be problems of excess rather than deficiency. The dental team needs to understand the issues common to adolescents and adults and provide appropriate education and counseling. Tips for effective patient education include:

For Teens

- Counsel girls about the importance of achieving dense bones and make appropriate diet suggestions (see Chapter 8 on minerals).
- Respect teen struggles for independence and autonomy. Identify the oral or systemic health issue, discuss the risks of current dietary habits, and outline benefits of alternative dietary habits. Provide "how to" information. Encourage open dialogue to assess goals and willingness to change.
- Be realistic. Do not expect someone consuming 6 to 8 cans of regular carbonated beverages daily to stop doing so. One suggestion might be to substitute milk for some of the carbonated beverages.
- Be observant and watch for signs of eating disorders. Confront the patient with any suspicions in a caring and nonjudgmental manner, and provide referral to an eating disorders clinic.

For Adults

- Provide dietary recommendations within the family context. Although family members may have different nutritional requirements, it is rare that the same diet cannot meet these needs. Good eating habits may help prevent or delay chronic diseases.
- Keep recommendations simple for increased compliance. Food purchases and preparation techniques should be consistent with current resources, lifestyle, and cooking skills.

QUESTIONS PATIENTS MIGHT ASK

Q. I have heard that all the soda machines in schools are responsible for teenagers having many more cavities than in the past. Is this true?

A. Yes and no. It is true that there has been an increase in teen caries in recent years. However, it is important not to oversimplify the problem. Teen caries is likely due to a variety of lifestyle factors. Increased soda drinking could be one factor, but other factors may include increased snacking in general, xerostomia from tobacco and drug use, and undiagnosed eating disorders, just to name a few.

Q. Isn't it true that dental decay is a problem of young people, and that periodontal disease is the major cause of dental problems in adults?

A. Not anymore. In the past, most adults lost their teeth to periodontal disease relatively early, so there were no teeth left to decay. Today, however, people are taking better care of their teeth and adult dental caries as well as periodontal disease are common. The dental caries in adults tends to be recurrent caries around fillings, and root caries. Root caries occurs when the gums have receded due to periodontal disease, newly exposing the roots of teeth. These roots are not as "hard" as the tooth enamel, so they can "decay" faster, especially when there is a lack of protective saliva.

Q. My son is active in sports, and I have confidence in his coach, but I've heard that athletes don't necessarily get the best nutrition advice. Is this true? I would think that the sports world is so health conscious that nutrition advice would be sound.

A. It is true that athletes are health conscious. The majority of coaches make an effort to provide sound advice to their athletes. Unfortunately, the need to excel may lead athletes to follow unsafe dietary practices. For example, wrestlers or dancers may adopt severe calorie restrictions and even develop eating disorders to remain in certain weight classes. Weight lifters and athletes in other strength-related sports may try steroids and other muscle-enhancing nutritional supplements that can be dangerous. Today, coaches are aware of these problems and are making a greater effort to work with qualified nutritionists to provide sound, appropriate guidance to their athletes.

CASE STUDY

Andrew, a 30-year-old Caucasian male, alert and normally developed, presented to the Periodontics Department with this chief complaint: "I need to get my broken teeth fixed." Andrew was 6 feet 1 inch tall, weighed 190 lb (BMI = 25.8), and had a blood pressure of 129/88. He had a 12-pack per year smoking history, was on no medications, had no known drug allergies, and denied systemic disease. His most recent dental visit was 14 years ago at which time tooth #30 was extracted.

Extraoral examination was within normal limits. Intraoral examination revealed generalized gross caries (teeth #1–5, 7–10, 12–15, 17, 18, 10, 23, 24, 29, 31, and 32) and plaque-associated gingivitis with localized areas of early-onset periodontitis. His treatment plan included disease control and caries restoration. Disease control included removal of supragingival plaque and calculus, oral hygiene instruction, and dietary evaluation.

Evaluation of his 3-day diet record revealed that Andrew consumed 1 to 2 meals per day. Foods consumed included pizza, hamburgers, chicken strips, potatoes, and donuts. Daily beverage intake included 6 to 12 cans of soda consumed throughout the day, and occasional beer. Evaluated by food guide pyramid standards, the diet contained inadequate servings of foods from the milk, fruit, and vegetable groups, and excessive intake from the other group. Nutrient analysis of this diet showed 2300 kcal (68% CHO, 9% protein, 19% fat, and 4% alcohol), 350 g sugar, 3 g fiber, and deficient intakes of the following nutrients (percentages of RDAs in parentheses): vitamin A (37%), thiamin (51%), riboflavin (51%), pyridoxine (45%), folate (43%), vitamin E (14%), pantothenic acid (39%), vitamin C (23%), vitamin D (12%), calcium (30%), magnesium (30%), and zinc (38%).

Questions
1. What are the effects of Andrew's beverage consumption?
2. How appropriate is Andrew's calorie intake?
3. What would be appropriate dietary recommendations for Andrew?

REFERENCES

Adams LB: An overview of adolescent eating behaviors. Barriers to implementing dietary guidelines. *Ann NY Acad Sci* 1997; 817:36–48.

Al-Hiyasat AS, Saunders WP, Shardey SW, Smith GM: The effect of a carbonated beverage on the wear of human enamel and dental ceramics. *Prosthodont* 1998; 7:2–12.

American Heritage Dictionary: New York: Dell, 1994.

American Psychiatric Association: *Diagnostic and Statistical Manual of Mental Disorders*, 4th ed. Washington, DC: Author, 1994.

Asghar K: Role of dietary and environmental factors in drug use. *Alcohol Drug Res* 1986; 7:61–83.

Barker ME, Thompson KA, McClean SI: Do type As eat differently? A comparison of men and women. *Appetite* 1996; 26:277–86.

Bedi R: Dental management of a child with anorexia nervosa who presents with severe tooth erosion. *Eur J Prosthodont Restor Dent* 1992; 1(1):13–17.

Bee HL: *The Journey of Adulthood*, 2nd ed. New York: Macmillan, 1992.

Berenson GS, Srinivasan SR, Nicklas TA: Atherosclerosis: A nutritional disease of childhood. *Am J Cardiol* 1998; 82:22T–29T.

Berg F: Congress asked to take eating disorders seriously. *Healthy Weight J* 1998; 12:41–43.

Bishop K, Briggs P, Schmidt E: Identification and immediate management of the oral changes associated with eating disorders. *Br J Hosp Med* 1994; 52(7):326, 329–34.

Dietz WH: Childhood weight affects adult morbidity and mortality. *J Nutr* 1998; 128:407S–10S.

DSM-IV: Anorexia nervosa (Table 23.1), bulimia nervosa (Table 23.2), and binge eating disorder (Table 24.3). In *Diagnostic Criteria from the American Psychiatric Association's Diagnostic and Statistical Manual of Mental Disorders*, 4th ed. Portland, OR: Book News, Inc., 1994.

Faine M, Mobley C: Case problem: Balancing nutrition advice with dental care in patients with anorexia and bulimia. *J Am Diet Assoc* 1999; 99:1291–92.

Field AE, Cheung L, Wolf AM, Herzog DB, Gortmaker SL, Colditz GA: Exposure to mass media and weight concerns among girls. *Pediatrics* 1999; 103(3):36–44.

Gallo AM: Building strong bones in childhood and adolescence: reducing the risk of fractures in later life. *Pediatr Nurs* 1996; 22(5):369–74, 422.

Garner D: The effects of starvation on behavior: Implications for dieting and eating disorders. *Healthy Weight J* 1998; 12:68–72.

Harnack L, Stang J, Story M: Soft drink consumption among US children and adolescents: Nutritional consequences. *J Am Diet Assoc* 1999; 94(4):436–41.

Harris NO, Garcia-Godoy FL: *Primary Preventive Dentistry*, 5th ed. Stamford, CT: Appleton & Lange, 1999.

Hartung L: Disordered eating patterns in relation to gender in the college environment. *J Am Diet Assoc* 1997; 97(9): SA–60.

Heald FP, Gong EJ: Diet, nutrition, and adolescence. In Shils M, Olsen JA, Shike M, Ross AC (eds): *Modern Nutrition in Health and Disease*, 9th ed. Baltimore: Williams & Wilkins, 1999.

Hubbard K, O'Neill AM, Cheakalos C: Out of control. *People*, April 12, 1999:52–72.

Institute of Medicine, National Academy of Sciences: *Dietary Reference Intakes for Energy, Carbohydrate, Fiber, Fat, Fatty Acids, Cholesterol, Protein, and Amino Acids (Macronutrients)*. Washington, DC: National Academies Press, 2005.

Institute of Medicine, National Academy of Sciences: *Dietary Reference Intakes for Thiamin, Riboflavin, Niacin, Vitamin B_6, Folate, Vitamin B_{12}, Pantothenic Acid, Biotin, and Choline*. Washington, DC: National Academies Press, 1998.

Ismail AI, Burt BA, Eklund SA: The cariogenicity of soft drinks in the United States. *J Am Dent Assoc* 1984; 109:241–45.

Jacobson MS, Rees JM, Golden NH, Irwin CE: Adolescent nutritional disorders: Prevention and treatment. *Ann NY Acad Sci* 1997; 817:1–48.

Jeffcoat MK: Osteoporosis: A possible modifying factor in oral bone loss. *Ann Periodontol* 1998; 3:312–21.

Johnson WA, Landry GL: Nutritional supplements: Fact vs fiction. *Adolesc Med* 1998; 9(3):501–13.

Jones R, Jones P: Depth and area of dental erosions, and dental caries in bulimic women. *J Den Res* 1989; 68:1275–78.

Kalkwarf HJ, Khoury JC, Lanphear BP: Milk intake during childhood and adolescence, adult bone density, and osteoporotic fractures in US women. *Am J Clin Nutr* 2003; 77:257–65.

Kalodner C: Media influences on male and female non-eating disordered college students. *Eating Disorders* 1997; 5:47–57.

Larsen MJ, Nyvad B: Enamel erosion by some soft drinks and orange juices relative to their pH, buffering effect and contents of calcium phosphate. *Caries Res* 1999; 33:81–87.

Lerner RM, Galambos NL: Adolescent development: Challenges and opportunities for research, programs and policies. *Annu Rev Psychol* 1998; 49:413–46.

Looker AC, Dallman PR, Carroll MD, Gunter EW, Johnson CL: Prevalence of iron deficiency in the United States. *JAMA* 1997; 227(12):973–76.

Marshall TA, Levy SM, Broffitt B, Warren JJ, Eichenberger-Gilmore JM, Burns TL, et al.: Dental caries and beverage consumption in young children. *Pediatrics* 2003; 112: e184–91.

Meskin LH: Outrageous. *J Am Dent Assoc* 1999; 130(3): 308–10, 312.

Middleman AB, Vazquez I, Durant RH: Eating patterns, physical activity, and attempts to change weight among adolescents. *J Adolesc Health* 1998; 22(1):37–42.

Miles G, Eid S: The dietary habits of young people. *Nurs Times* 1997; 93(50):46–48.

Miller EC, Maropis CG: Nutrition and diet-related problems. *Primary Care* 1998; 25(1):193–210.

Milosevic A, Kelly MJ, McLean AN: Sports supplement drinks and dental health in competitive swimmers and cyclists. *Br Dent J* 1997; 182:303–8.

Mohs ME, Watson RR, Leonard-Green T: Nutritional effects of marijuana, heroin, cocaine, and nicotine. *J Am Diet Assoc* 1990; 90:1261–67.

Mueller JA: Eating disorders identification and intervention. *J Contemp Dent Prac* 2001; 2(2):98.

Muscari ME: Walking a thin line: Managing care for adolescents with anorexia and bulimia. MCN. *Am J Matern Child Nurs* 1998; 23(3):130–40.

Nielsen SJ, Popkin BM: Changes in beverage intake between 1977 and 2001. *Am J Prev Med* 2004; 27:205–10.

Nowak M, Speare R, Crawford D: Gender differences in adolescent weight and shape-related beliefs and behaviors. *J Paediatr Child Health* 1996; 32:148–52.

Nunn JH: Prevalence of dental erosion and the implications for oral health. *Eur J Oral Sci* 1996; 104:156–61.

Osteoporosis Prevention, Diagnosis, and Therapy. NIH Consensus Statement Online 2000 March 27–29; [cited 2005, 2, 23]; 17:1–36. http//consensus.NIH.Gov/2000/2000_osteoporosis111.html.htm.

Patten JA: Nutrition and wound healing. *Compendium* 1995; 16(2):200–14.

Powers PS: Initial assessment and early treatment options for anorexia nervosa and bulimia nervosa. *Psychiatr Clin North Am* 1996; 19(4):639–55.

Ravald N: Root surface caries. *Curr Opin Periodontol* 1994: 78–86.

Rickert VI: *Adolescent Nutrition: Assessment and Management*. New York: Chapman & Hill, 1995.

Riordan DJ: Effects of orthodontic treatment on nutrient intake. *Am J Orthod Dentofac Orthop* 1997; 111:554–61.

Rock C, Curran-Celentano A: Nutritional disorders of anorexia nervosa, a review. *Int J Eat Disord* 1994; 15:187.

Rytomaa I, Jarvinen V, Kanerva R, Heinonen OP: Bulimia and tooth erosion. *Acta Odontol Scand* 1998; 56(1):36–40.

Satter E: *Your Child's Weight: Helping Without Harming*. Madison, WI: Kelsey Press, 2005.

Shaner JW: Caries associated with methamphetamine abuse. *J Mich Dent Assoc* 2002; 84:42–47.

Stunkard AJ, Allison KC: Two forms of disordered eating in obesity: Binge eating and night eating. *Int J Obesity* 2003; 27:1–12.

Subar AF, Krebs-Smith SM, Cook A, Kahle LL: Dietary sources of nutrients among U.S. children, 1989–1991. *Pediatrics* 1998; 102:913–23.

USDA MyPyramid, 2005, http://www.mypyramid.gov.

Von Frauhhofer A, Rogers M: Dissolution of dental enamel in soft drinks. *Gen Dent* 2004; 52(4):308–12.

Weinberg LG, Berner LA, Groves JE: Nutrient contributions of dairy foods in the United States: Continuing Survey of Food Intakes by Individuals, 1994–96, 1998. *J Am Diet Assoc* 2004; 104:895–902.

West RV: The female athlete: the triad of disordered eating, amenorrhea, and osteoporosis. *Sports Med* 1998; 26(2): 63–71.

Wonderlich S, Swift WJ, Slotnick HB, Goodman S: DSM-III-R personality disorders in eating-disorder subjects. *Int J Eat Disord* 1990; 9:607–16.

Zero DT: Etiology of dental erosion—extrinsic factors. *Eur J Oral Sci* 1996; 104:162–77.

Chapter 19

The Older Dental Patient

Elizabeth A. Krall and Michelle Henshaw

OBJECTIVES

The student will be able to:

- List and discuss the factors that affect the nutritional requirements of older persons.
- Describe how nutritional requirements of elders may differ from those of younger persons.
- List and explain the oral health considerations for patients with conditions such as osteoporosis and impaired cognition.
- List the common oral conditions of elders and describe how they can affect nutritional status.
- List solutions to some of the common nutritional problems of older people.

INTRODUCTION

Improvements in health and subsequent longevity throughout the 20th century have resulted in tremendous growth in the size of the elderly population. In 1950 about 15 million people in the United States were over age 65 and few people were older than 85. By 2050 the number of adults over 65 is expected to reach 80 million, and the number over the age of 85 is expected to reach 20 million (Bahls, 2002). Indeed, in 2001 there were 48,999 people in the United States aged 100 or older (Administration on Aging, 2002).

Successful aging is defined as the ability to maintain three key behaviors:

1. low risk of disease-related disability
2. high mental and physical function
3. active engagement of life (Rowe, Kahn, 1998)

Nutrition is a major determinant of successful aging. Nutrition affects the aging process, and conversely, the aging process can have significant effects on nutrition. From the perspective of primary prevention, nutrition helps promote health and functionality. At secondary and tertiary preventive levels, nutrition interventions help lessen chronic disease risk, slow disease progression, reduce disease symptoms, and improve quality of life (Position of the American Deitetic Association, 2002). Good nutritional status is associated with a healthy immune function and reduced risk of chronic diseases such as cancer and heart disease. In elderly people, these factors help ensure a high quality of life. Yet, because they are often preoccupied with the many challenges of aging, people may relegate eating to a low priority, thereby contributing inadvertently to further nutritional risk.

The many changes that accompany aging can affect nutritional status and nutritional requirements (Blumberg, 1997). This chapter reviews the relationships between nutrition and aging, and provides strategies for helping optimize the nutritional status of older patients (Figure 19–1).

NUTRITIONAL CONCERNS OF OLDER PATIENTS

Although today's aging population is the most diverse and well educated ever seen, the average 75-year-old has three chronic conditions and uses five different

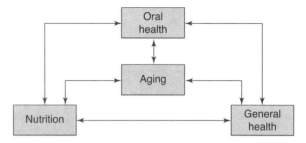

FIGURE 19–1 Multidirectional relationships between aging and nutrition.

prescription drugs (CDC, Merck Institute on Aging and Health, 2004). Obesity is the most common nutritional disorder in older persons, affecting three quarters of Americans over age 65; yet undernutrition is a pervasive problem as well (Watts, 2005). Both underweight and overweight contribute to increased morbidity and disability. Dietary excesses and poor food choices combined with decreased activity have resulted in an increased prevalence of overweight and obesity over the past two decades (Hedley et al., 2004). Overweight contributes to increased risk of heart disease, some cancers, hypertension, stroke, sleep apnea, diabetes mellitus, and osteoarthritis (Dewan, Wilding, 2003). Underweight contributes to poor immunity and healing, and associated high risk of early mortality (Position of the American Dietetic Association, 2005). Note that people can be overweight and still malnourished if their diet is high in calories but low in essential nutrients.

Diet quality decreases substantially with age. The consumption of poor-quality diets can result in inadequate nutrient intake, which can lead to malnutrition. Average energy (calorie) intakes decline by 1000–1200 calories in men and 600–800 calories in women from ages 20 to 80. Along with the decrease in calories comes a decline in nutrient intakes, especially calcium, zinc, iron, and B vitamins. As a result, with increasing age there is an increase in the prevalence of anemia. The primary contributor to the anemia is vitamin B_{12} deficiency. Deficiencies of vitamins B_6 and B_{12} also result in increased homocysteine, significant risk factors for heart disease (Guralnik, Eisenstaedt, Ferrucci, Klein, Woodman, 2004), and cognitive dysfunction (Malouf, Grimley, 2003). Deficiencies of vitamin D and calcium are also common. Older bodies are less efficient in synthesizing vitamin D from the sun's rays, and many older people limit their intake of dairy foods due to perceived intolerances.

In addition, frequently used medications can impair appetite and interfere with nutrient absorption and utilization (see Chapter 16). Ongoing research into the changes in nutritional requirements that accompany aging has led to revision of dietary guidelines for some nutrients for the elderly (IOM, 1997, 1998) (see the DRI tables in the Appendices). One significant change from previous Recommended Dietary Allowances (RDAs) is the recognition that the very old—that is, individuals aged 70 and above—may have different needs than adults between 51 and 70 years old. For example, the dietary reference value for vitamin D doubles from ages 31 to 50, to ages 51 to 70, and doubles again for individuals 70 and older.

Meeting dietary recommendations can be a challenge for older patients for a variety of reasons that are detailed below.

AGE-RELATED CHANGES AFFECTING NUTRITIONAL STATUS

Physiological Changes

Changes in body composition can be dramatic in elderly patients (Table 19–1). Lean body mass and associated basal metabolic rate decline with increasing age resulting

TABLE 19–1   Age-Related Changes Affecting Nutritional Status

Physiological Changes
Sensory
Cognitive
Functional
Social and Psychological Changes
Poverty
Food insecurity
Loneliness
Depression
Changes in living situation
Medications and alcohol
Oral Changes
Root caries
Periodontal disease and diabetes mellitus
Oral cancers
Osteoporosis and tooth loss
Dentition status
Xerostomia

in a decrease in calorie requirements. Lower physical activity also contributes to the reduced energy requirement. The prevalence of chronic diseases and infections increases with age, and may result from age-related declines in immune function. Both chronic and acute conditions can affect food intake and requirements.

Sarcopenia, the loss of muscle mass with aging, is a common problem in adults over age 65 and increases with age. Sarcopenia leads to functional disability, falling, decreased bone density, and intolerance to heat and cold. Malnutrition, decreased physical activity, oxidative stress, and changes in cytokine and hormone activities have been implicated as contributing factors to sarcopenia (Position of the American Dietetic Association, 2005).

The functioning of the gastrointestinal tract often declines with age, resulting in delayed gastric emptying, slowed digestion and absorption, and decreased appetite. Atrophic gastritis (chronic inflammation of the stomach lining, resulting in reduced secretion of hydrochloric acid) is common in the aging population, and can have a major impact on nutritional status. Reduction of hydrochloric acid in the stomach interferes with absorption of iron, calcium, vitamin B_6, and folate. Vitamin B_{12} deficiency associated with atrophic gastritis is a common problem in the elderly and contributes to anemia, weakness, and decreased appetite.

Changes in kidney function and total body water metabolism contribute to dehydration, a major concern in older people. Dehydration can be insidious and unrecognized until serious side effects occur. Because the thirst threshold may be impaired in elders, thirst is not an accurate monitor of hydration. Therefore, people should be encouraged to drink six to eight 8 oz glasses of fluid daily (not including caffeine-containing beverages, which are diuretics) (Ausman, Russell, 1999).

Dehydration can lead to constipation—often a major complaint in older people. Major contributors to constipation include decreased intestinal function and the adoption of low-fiber diets in response to chewing difficulties or dentures. Overuse of laxatives to relieve constipation may also contribute to malnutrition by contributing to nutrient malabsorption.

Sensory Changes

Changes in the oral cavity that occur with aging or disease may lead to alterations in food intake and dissatisfaction with eating ability. The senses of taste and smell decline with age. As people age, there is a decreased number of taste buds on the tongue and a decrease in nerve ending response to taste and smell (taste thresholds increase between 2 to 9 times with age). There are also changes in the threshold for salt and bitter tastes and smell (Morley, 2001; Winkler et al., 1999). Decreased smell acuity can make it harder to differentiate between food odors. Factors contributing to sensory changes include the aging process itself, medical conditions, drugs, and dentures. Taste is the strongest determinant of food choices, and the sense of smell is a major determinant of appetite. Compensation for the loss of these functions can result in either overconsumption or underconsumption and less enjoyment of food (Ship, Duffy, Jones, Langmore, 1996). Flavor-enhanced diets result in enhanced immune function and even enhanced grip strength (Position of the American Dietetic Association, 2005).

Cognitive Changes

Dementia is another major risk for nutritional deficiencies (Burns, Marsh, Berder, 1989; Gray, 1989). Almost half of nursing home residents have been diagnosed with some form of dementia or a chronic organic brain syndrome. Although the exact etiology is unclear, individuals with Alzheimer's disease and other forms of dementia often demonstrate inadequate nutritional status and weight loss. Contributing factors likely include memory loss, disorientation, and anxiety as well as biochemical and metabolic disturbances (Nordenram, Ryd-Kjellen, Johansson, Nordstrom, Winblad, 1996). Regardless of the cause, most individuals with Alzheimer's disease experience some changes in their eating habits. Most individuals reduce food intake. A shift in taste preference also occurs in one-third of individuals, most commonly an increased preference for sweet or spicy foods, and about 25% develop a tendency to eat inedible, inappropriate food (Cohen, 1994).

In one study, institutionalized Alzheimer's patients had a greater need for mashed food and support at mealtimes compared with a community dwelling control group. In this study, no association was found between dental status and nutritional status; however, dental status was correlated with the ability to eat unaided. It may be that having few or no natural teeth may impair the ability to eat unaided at an earlier stage of dementia than if the patient had natural teeth (Nordenram et al., 1996). These data suggest that individuals with poor oral health and Alzheimer's disease are at increased risk for nutritional inadequacies at an earlier stage of the disease.

Functional Changes

Any physical disability such as arthritis, stroke, or vision or hearing impairment can affect nutritional status indirectly. It may be difficult for an older person to get to and from grocery stores, reach food on shelves, carry groceries, open cans and packages, and prepare meals in general (Figure 19–2). Such barriers can impair ability to cook and eat and can dampen appetite considerably. Inability to handle eating utensils, see food clearly, or hear others' conversation may all lead to social isolation. This can lead to poor eating and subsequent malnutrition. Arthritis is the leading cause of disability, affecting approximately 60% of older adults (Position of the American Dietetic Association, 2005).

Social and Psychological Factors

Psychosocial factors may play even greater roles than physical, medical, and dental issues in determining the health and well-being of elders. Food habits are determined by lifetime food preferences, physiological changes, living arrangements, finances, transportation, disability, and social interaction, to name but a few relevant factors. Poverty is a major contributor to malnutrition. Hunger and food insecurity are real issues for a portion of community-residing older adults, thus

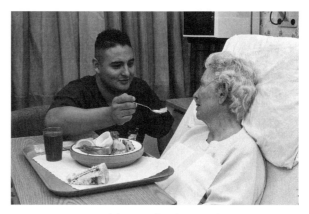

FIGURE 19–2 Older people often need assistance.

placing them at risk for poor nutritional status and deteriorating physical and mental function (Food Security Institute). Elders may see declines in economic status as a result of retirement, inflation, death of a wage earner, and increasing health care costs (Posner, Jette, Smigelski, Miller, Mitchell, 1994). When resources are low, rent and utilities may have to take precedence over food purchases (by now everyone has heard the horror stories about elders buying canned cat food for themselves). Food insecurity occurs whenever people are unable to acquire nutritionally adequate, safe food in socially accepted ways. Approximately 1.5% of elderly households experienced hunger, the most severe form of food insecurity. Elders who have food insecurity are at higher risk of being underweight (body mass index less than 19) and subsequently at higher risk of earlier mortality than elders who have sufficient food (Position of the American Dietetic Association, 2005).

There is also a strong social aspect to eating, and loneliness can be a contributing factor to malnutrition. Individuals who have a strong social network of family and friends are more likely to be physically and emotionally fulfilled and tend to have better nutrition. Those at highest nutrient risk from a social standpoint are individuals who have lost an eating companion, such as a spouse. This loss can affect the individual's desire to prepare and eat food and may lead to at least short-term malnutrition. Conversely, both women and men consume about 23% more food when dining with family and friends (Thomas, Morley, 2004).

Depression is also a common problem that can affect nutritional status. Depression is commonly associated with losses of loved ones, financial problems, medical conditions, and disruption in living arrangements. Depression, anxiety, and loneliness can undermine the desire to prepare and eat food, and have been associated with anorexia, weight loss, and increased morbidity and mortality.

Living Situation

Changes in living situations can also affect nutritional status indirectly. Living alone has a major impact on the nutritional status of elderly men (not elderly women). Elders may refuse to eat unfamiliar foods provided in nursing homes. Resident elder care facilities have all fostered communal dining because such environments foster appetite and eating.

Free-Living Homebound Elders. Homebound elders are at particularly high risk for malnutrition for the reasons previously mentioned (e.g., chronic illness, medication use, oral health problems, a physical inability to shop for or prepare food, the psychosocial effects of social isolation, and economic factors).

One study showed that whether rural or urban, 70% of homebound elders had intakes below 66% of the RDA for three or more nutrients, most commonly energy, vitamin B_6, calcium, magnesium, and zinc (Stevens, Grivetti, McDonald, 1992). In a physician-monitored population of homebound elders, results of a 24-hour diet history showed that these patients did not meet requirements for major energy sources and fiber (Lee, Novielli, 1996).

Little research has been done on oral health and nutrition in frail homebound elders. One comprehensive assessment of the nutritional status of urban, frail homebound elders found that undernutrition was common (29% of the women and 37% of the men were underweight), 19% of the subjects had low albumin levels, and 38% consumed insufficient protein and energy. Predictors of low body mass index were age, educational status, and oral symptoms (Ritchie et al., 1997). This study identified a relationship between oral problems and low body mass index in frail homebound elders, which is consistent with studies of other elderly populations such as nursing home residents (Blaum, Fries, Fiatarone, 1995), rehabilitation patients (Sullivan, Martin, Flaxman, Hagen, 1993), and healthy community-dwelling elders (Posner et al., 1994).

Nursing Home Residents. Elders over age 85, the fastest growing segment of the U.S. population, are at increased risk for functional impairment, with currently 22% of this group residing in nursing homes (U.S. Special Committee on Aging, 1991).

Nursing home residents commonly exhibit a loss in manual dexterity, which makes it difficult to self-feed and perform adequate oral hygiene. They often also suffer from impaired arm function and oral or pharyngeal neurogenic dysphagia (swallowing disorder) (Siebens et al., 1986).

Nursing home residents are at increased risk for nutritional inadequacies despite the adequate quantity and quality of foods provided. Calorie and protein intakes are frequently low, as are blood levels of water-soluble and fat-soluble vitamins. As a result,

30–50% of nursing home residents have substandard body weight, midarm muscle circumference, and serum albumin levels. Malnutrition makes this already frail and vulnerable population at increased risk for medical complications and delayed recovery from illness (Siebens et al., 1996).

The causes of undernutrition in a nursing home population are complex and include functional, behavioral, environmental, medical, and dental variables, complicated by problems with taste, smell, cognition, attention, manual dexterity, and impairments in the ability to chew and swallow.

Medications and Alcohol

The elderly use about one-third of all prescription drugs in the United States, and many elders living at home take three or more medications daily. In addition to prescription drugs, a high percentage of older people take over-the-counter drugs regularly. This "polypharmacy" increases the risk of drug–drug and drug–nutrient interactions. Drug–nutrient interactions are more common in elderly people because inefficient metabolization allows drugs to stay in the body for longer periods. Prescription drugs are the primary cause of anorexia, nausea, vomiting, gastrointestinal disturbances, xerostomia, taste loss, and interference with nutrient absorption and utilization. These conditions can lead to nutrient deficiencies, weight loss, and ultimate malnutrition. (Chapter 20 discusses drug–nutrition relationships.)

Alcohol abuse is a potential risk factor in elders as well. Abuse may be a response to stress, unwanted changes in the life situation, depression, and social isolation. Alcohol provides calories but is of little nutritional value and can undermine nutritional status by decreasing appetite and by substituting for more nutritious foods in the diet. A small alcoholic beverage before meals may enhance appetite, but greater amounts can suppress it.

PREVALENT ORAL CONDITIONS IN ELDERLY PEOPLE AND THEIR NUTRITIONAL IMPLICATIONS

An increasing number of people will keep more of their teeth into old age. Over the next three decades, the average number of teeth remaining among the elderly is predicted to rise to 26 teeth (Ettinger, 1997) from the current average of 20. Although the proportion of edentulous patients in the elderly population is declining, the number of persons with no teeth in the United States is likely to remain constant at 9 million over the next few decades. These individuals have unique dietary needs that must be acknowledged and treated. Moreover, recognition of the role of nutritional factors in the development and prevention of caries, periodontal disease, oral cancer, and tooth loss becomes increasingly important as the number of older individuals and number of teeth at risk continue to grow.

The maintenance of good oral health and efficient chewing ability enhance quality of life and help ensure adequate dietary intake. Many of the common oral problems seen in the dentate elderly have a similar etiology to those in younger adults; however, the lifelong cumulative effects of diet, lifestyle, and disease factors tend to make these problems more widespread and severe in older patients. The resulting diminished oral health may ultimately affect their nutritional status.

Common oral conditions in elderly patients include caries, periodontal disease, oral cancers, and xerostomia. Among dentate elders, more than 93% exhibit teeth with past or present coronal decay and nearly half of individuals show root decay. In addition, the majority of persons age 65 and older have one or more sites with mild or moderate signs of periodontal pocketing, attachment loss, and gingival bleeding. Severe attachment loss (≥ 5 mm) and gingival recession (≥ 3 mm) are found in fewer individuals but become more prevalent with increasing age.

The relationship between nutrition and oral health in the elderly is multidirectional. Nutritional factors may play a role in the etiology and prevention of the oral diseases and in tooth loss. The oral condition, especially the number of teeth remaining, affects the patient's ability and desire to eat and maintain adequate nutritional status. There is also increasing recognition of the link between oral and systemic disease (e.g., cardiovascular disease), in which nutritional factors can play an important role.

Root Caries

Caries on the root surfaces are becoming more prevalent with the increase in the elderly population and the greater number of teeth being retained into old age. In addition, because of cumulative gingival recession and loss of attachment, older people have more root surfaces exposed and at risk of decay. According to a national survey, 47% of this age group show evidence of root caries (Winn et al., 1996).

A less acidic environment is needed to initiate demineralization of the root cementum (pH of 6.7) compared with dental enamel (pH of 5.4), so root surfaces can develop caries more easily and progress more rapidly than coronal surfaces. The nutritional factors that lead to coronal or root caries in adults are similar to those in crown caries and are reviewed in Chapter 13. Major nutritional factors associated with root caries are frequent intake of fermentable carbohydrates (Griffin, Griffin, Swann, Zlobin, 2004; Steele, Sheiham, 2001) and limited exposure to fluoride. The current generation of elderly had little exposure to fluoridated water or toothpaste until they reached early adulthood.

Many nonnutritional factors also contribute to root decay in the elderly, including reduced salivary flow; limited ability to perform oral hygiene; and extent of plaque, calculus, and gingival recession. Presence of coronal caries and restorations, partial dentures, and fixed bridges are also associated with increased root caries. Institutionalized elders are at particularly high risk of root caries.

Periodontal Disease and Diabetes Mellitus

Most adults have mild to moderate signs of periodontal disease. Severe periodontal disease is seen in a relatively small subset of the population. Few nutritional factors have been related directly to the development or control of periodontal disease in older humans. Low intake of vitamin C, necessary for maintenance of healthy gums and connective tissues, is weakly associated with increased periodontal disease prevalence (Ismail, Burt, Eklund, 1983). Physiological roles of other nutrients include the maintenance of healthy mucosal, connective, and calcified tissues, and an adequate host response to inflammatory stimuli. For example, vitamin A is crucial for the differentiation of epithelial cells. Calcium and phosphorus constitute the major minerals in bone tissue. Low levels of zinc impair wound healing. Inadequate intake of these nutrients may provide a framework for increased susceptibility to periodontal infection and reduced ability to slow or reverse disease progression with periodontal treatment; however, there are little human data to confirm this. Periodontal disease is discussed in detail in Chapter 14.

Diabetes affects 10% of the U.S. population over 60 years old. The most common type, non-insulindependent diabetes mellitus (NIDDM), accounts for more than 90% of all cases of diabetes, and nearly all cases in the elderly. Features of diabetes include delayed wound healing and impaired immune response, which can increase susceptibility to periodontitis. Periodontal disease, as measured by attachment loss or radiographic alveolar bone loss, is more widespread among patients with diabetes and has an earlier age of onset than in nondiabetics. This relationship is independent of oral factors such as plaque, calculus, gingival bleeding, or numbers of caries and restorations. As with other common complications of diabetes, periodontal disease progression is more likely to occur in patients with poor glycemic control (Taylor, 2001; Taylor et al., 1996). Conversely, treatment of periodontal disease with systemic antibiotics may improve glycemic control but further studies are needed (Taylor et al., 2004).

Oral Cancers

The incidence and prevalence of oral cancers also increase with age. More than 90% of oral cancers occur in persons over 45 years old, with average ages at diagnosis of 57 to 64 depending on race. Oral cancers, which include the lip, mouth, tongue, and pharynx, account for 4% of total cancer cases. Oral cancer is discussed in detail in Chapter 11.

Osteoporosis and Tooth Loss

There are an estimated 1.5 million osteoporotic fractures in the United States annually. Of these, approximately 80% occur in postmenopausal women, and nearly a quarter million occur in older men. The adult skeleton begins to lose mineral mass around middle age, and by age 65, the average rate of bone loss can reach upward of 1% of total skeletal mass/year in women (Dawson-Hughes, Harris, Krall, Dallal, 1997).

The same process of age-related bone loss that occurs throughout the skeleton may also affect the alveolar bone that supports the teeth, resulting in increased risk of tooth loss and edentulism (Figure 19–3). Although inflammation due to periodontal disease is a primary cause of localized alveolar bone loss, systemic bone loss may contribute to loss of alveolar bone and teeth but to a lesser degree. Many studies have found associations between bone mineral density and tooth

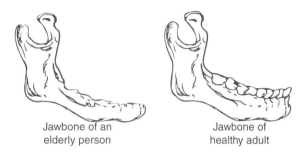

Jawbone of an   Jawbone of
elderly person   healthy adult

FIGURE 19–3 *Jawbone diminishes with age.*

loss or periodontal disease measures such that individuals with low bone mineral density (BMD) at skeletal sites such as the forearm, spine, hip, and whole body tend to have fewer teeth, deeper probing pockets, and more loss of clinical attachment (Krall, Dawson-Hughes, Papas, Garcia, 1994; May, Reader, Murphy, Khaw, 1995; Pilgram et al., 2002; Ronderos, Jacobs, Himes, Pihlstrom, 2000; Wactawski-Wende, 2001). The few prospective studies that exist to date suggest that alveolar bone loss is more extensive in women with osteoporosis (Payne, Reinhardt, Nummikoski, Patil, 1999), and greater rates of bone loss at systemic sites are related to risk of tooth loss (Krall, Garcia, Dawson-Hughes, 1996). But not all studies have detected significant relationships between systemic bone density and number of teeth remaining, radiographic alveolar bone height, or attachment loss (Elders, Habets, Netelenbos, van der Linden, van der Stelt, 1992; Weyant et al., 1999). Discrepant findings may reflect the different ages of the populations studied or lack of control for confounding factors such as smoking, level of periodontal disease, or oral hygiene.

Therapies that preserve skeletal bone appear to also improve periodontal status and tooth retention. Estrogen-deficient women lose alveolar bone more rapidly than estrogen-sufficient women (Payne, Zachs, Reinhardt, Nummikoski, Patil, 1997). Three large independent studies reported that women who ever used hormone replacement therapy (HRT) had more teeth remaining and less likelihood of being edentate than nonusers (Grodstein, Colditz, Stampfer, 1996; Krall, Dawson-Hughes, Hannan, Wilson, Keil, 1997; Paganini-Hill, 1995) even after controlling for measures of dental care (Grodstein et al., 1996). But the long-term use of HRT has significant adverse effects (Writing group for the Women's Health Initiative Investigators, 2002), and

other osteoporosis drugs are becoming widely prescribed. Although clinical studies are few, the bone antiresorptive drug bisphosphonate may increase alveolar bone density (Takaishi, Ikeo, Miki, Nishizawa, Morii, 2003).

The long-term success of dental implants depends in part on the amount of alveolar bone present to support the implant and the rate of bone remodeling. In osteoporosis or rapid systemic bone loss, bone remodeling rates are altered and may increase the implant failure rate, but studies on the effect of systemic bone status on implant failure rate are inconsistent (Becker, Hujoel, Becker, Willingham, 2000; Blomqvist, Alberius, Isaksson, Linde, Hansson, 1996).

Adequate calcium and vitamin D intake are major determinants of peak bone mass attainment before the onset of age-related bone loss. Increasing dietary intakes of calcium and vitamin D has been shown to reduce the rate of systemic bone loss in middle-aged and elderly men and women (Dawson-Hughes et al., 1997). Several studies suggested higher calcium intake, owing to its role in the prevention of systemic bone loss, may be associated with lower prevalence of periodontal disease (Nishida et al., 2000) and risk of tooth loss (Krall et al., 1996), but the findings need to be replicated. It remains to be determined whether dietary interventions with calcium, vitamin D, or other vitamins and minerals have a significant impact on the risk of tooth loss. See Chapter 11 for a more detailed discussion of osteoporosis.

Dentition Status

In the third U.S. Health and Nutrition Examination Survey conducted in 1988–1991, the proportion of persons with no teeth rose from 26% of men and women aged 65 to 69 years to 44% of those aged 75 and older (Marcus, Drury, Brown, Zion, 1996). Replacement with complete upper and lower dentures does not completely restore masticatory function and sensory ability. Individuals with full dentures have significantly poorer masticatory function and perceived ease of chewing (Wayler, Chauncey 1983; Wayler, Muench, Kapur, Chauncey, 1984), reduced intakes of many nutrients and food groups (Joshipura, Willett, Douglass, 1996; Krall, Hayes, Garcia, 1998; Lee et al., 2004; Sahyoun, Lin, Krall, 2003; Sheiham, Steele, 2001), and are at higher risk for weight loss (Ritchie, Joshipura, Hung, Douglass, 2000; Sheiham, Steele, Marcenes, Finch, Walls, 2002) than persons with intact dentition. Large cross-sectional studies of the relationship between dentate status and plasma nutritional levels in Great Britain and the United States also found that edentulous older adults had significantly lower mean blood levels of retinol, beta-carotene, ascorbate, tocopherol, and folate (Sahyoun et al., 2003; Sheiham, Steele, 2001) when compared to dentate elders.

Nutrient deficiencies are not inevitable, however. Some individuals compensate for decline in masticatory ability by choosing processed or cooked foods rather than fresh and by chewing longer before swallowing. Nutrient intakes of individuals with impaired dentition can fall below minimum requirements if an already marginal eating pattern is subjected to sudden insults such as illness, loss of taste, inability to chew, or changes in economic status and living situation (Ship et al., 1996). Chapter 15 provides details on nutrition and dentures.

Xerostomia

Although xerostomia was once considered a normal consequence of aging, it is now known that saliva levels remain unchanged in healthy elders (Baum, 1989). Instead, the hyposalivation observed in many older people is a side effect of certain diseases, medications, and radiation treatment. Medication use is the most common cause of xerostomia in the elderly, with more than 400 medications listing xerostomia as a minor or major side effect (Arky, 1997). These medications include antidepressants, antipsychotics, and certain antihypertensive agents commonly used by elders. Almost 50% of individuals over age 65 take medications that can diminish salivary flow (Beck, Hunt, 1985), and almost one in five older adults exhibit xerostomia (Rhodus, Brown, 1990).

When salivary levels are reduced, then teeth are more susceptible to carious attack. The soft cementum of exposed root surfaces is particularly at risk. The concurrent presence of gingival recession and xerostomia is an important risk factor in the formation of root caries, a serious problem in elders that can ultimately lead to tooth loss. Reduced salivary flow also decreases complete denture retention and is associated with increased periodontal disease, burning or soreness of the oral mucosa, and difficulties in chewing and swallowing, all of which can adversely affect food selection.

Xerostomic individuals have a significantly lower caloric intake than people without xerostomia, as well as inadequate fiber intake, potassium, vitamin B_6, iron, calcium, and zinc (Rhodus, Brown, 1990). This effect was seen regardless of the cause of xerostomia and held true for both community dwelling and institutionalized patients; however, the effect was more pronounced in institutionalized elders.

Saliva is also responsible for initiating carbohydrate digestion and for dissolving food intraorally. The influence of saliva in taste perception has been demonstrated in xerostomic individuals who reported alterations in taste and food perception (Dolan, Monopoli, Kaurich, Rubenstein, 1990). These alterations can result in a decreased interest in eating and resultant nutrient deficiencies. Xerostomia is discussed in detail in Chapter 11.

SCREENING OLDER PATIENTS FOR NUTRITIONAL RISK

Nutrition care is most effective when it is integrated into care management across all settings. Dental team members are important allies in screening older patients for health risks, including nutrition issues. To adequately determine the nutritional status of the older patient, an in-depth medical and psychosocial assessment must be conducted. However, the dental team can implement a quick patient screening to help pinpoint areas of possible nutritional risk. The Nutrition Screening Initiative (Table 19–2) has developed a risk assessment tool that targets issues of common concern with older patients (Nutrition Screening Initiative, 1992). Common oral complaints that affect nutritional status such as dry mouth, impaired taste, or difficulty chewing and swallowing, can be quickly identified with the use of oral health screening tools (Table 19–3).

IMPROVING THE NUTRITIONAL STATUS OF AGING PATIENTS
Dietary Guidance

The best way to ensure nutritional adequacy and balance is to consume a wide variety of foods. A key recommendation to lower risk for chronic diseases is to consume liberal amounts of fruits and vegetables. Nevertheless, only one-third of people aged 65 and older consume five or more fruits and vegetables a day.

TABLE 19–2 The Nutrition Screening Initiative Checklists for Nutritional and Oral Health

DETERMINE YOUR NUTRITIONAL HEALTH

The warning signs of poor nutritional health are often overlooked. Use this checklist to find out if you or someone you know is at nutritional risk.

Read the statements below. Circle the number in the Yes column for those that apply to you or someone you know. For each yes answer, score the number in the box. Total your nutritional score.

	YES
I have an illness or condition that made me change the kind and/or amount of food I eat.	2
I eat fewer than 2 meals per day.	3
I eat few fruits or vegetables or milk products.	2
I have 3 or more drinks of beer, liquor, or wine almost every day.	2
I have tooth or mouth problems that make it hard for me to eat.	2
I don't always have enough money to buy the food I need.	4
I eat alone most of the time.	1
I take 3 or more different prescribed or over-the-counter drugs a day.	1
Without wanting to, I have lost or gained 10 pounds in the last 6 months.	2
I am not always physically able to shop, cook, and/or feed myself.	2
TOTAL	

TOTAL YOUR NUTRITIONAL SCORE. IF IT'S:

0–2 **GOOD!** Recheck your nutritional score in 6 months.

3–5 **You are at moderate nutritional risk**. See what can be done to improve your eating habits and lifestyle. Your office on aging, senior nutrition program, senior citizens center, or health department can help. Recheck your nutritional score in 3 months.

6 or more **You are at high nutritional risk**. Bring this checklist the next time you see your doctor, dietitian, or other qualified health or social service professional. Talk with them about any problems you may have. Ask for help to improve your nutritional health.

Source: From *Nutrition Interventions Manual for Professionals Caring for Older Americans* by the Nutrition Screening Initiative © 1992 by Greer, Margolis, Mitchell, Grunwald & Associates, Washington, DC.

In addition, many of the fruits and vegetables consumed are not those most associated with reduced disease risk. The most beneficial fruits (citrus, melons, berries) make up less than half of fruit servings eaten. Only one-fourth of the vegetables consumed are those rich in protective phytochemicals (dark green, deep yellow/orange vegetables, tomato products) (CDC, 5 a day, 2005; Cooper, 2004; USDA, 2005).

The revised recommendations for the elderly are also reflected in a modified food pyramid guideline for age 70 and above (Russell, Rasmussen, Lichtenstein, 1999). This modified pyramid (Figure 19–4) remains fairly consistent with the 2005 *Dietary Guidelines for Americans* (USDHHS, USDA, 2005), which bases the

recommendations of daily or weekly servings from major food groups on an individual's caloric need (Table 19–4). However, the revised pyramid still highlights several age-specific needs in its recommendation of three servings of dairy foods, regardless of caloric intake, and eight glasses of water. It also recognizes that supplements may be necessary to supply adequate intakes of some nutrients that are consistently found at low intake levels in the elderly population.

When dietary problems are identified, they can sometimes be improved by making minor changes in food selection and cooking habits. Improving the intakes of fresh fruits and vegetables among patients with impaired dentition is a primary goal and has many

TABLE 19–3 The Nutrition Screening Initiative Checklists for Nutritional and Oral Health

DETERMINE YOUR ORAL HEALTH

Oral health can affect your nutritional health. A healthy mouth, teeth, and gums are needed to eat.

If you answered "yes" to "I have tooth or mouth problems that make it hard for me to eat" on the **Determine Your Nutritional Health** checklist, answer the questions below.

Check all that apply:

Do you have tooth or mouth problems that make it hard for you to eat, such as loose teeth, ill-fitting dentures, etc.? _____

Is your mouth dry? _____

Do you have problems with:
- Lips (soreness or cracks in corners of your mouth)? _____
- Tongue (pain/soreness)? _____
- Sores that do not heal? _____
- Bleeding or swollen gums? _____
- Toothaches or sensitivity to hot or cold? _____
- Pain or clicking in your jaw? _____

Have you visited a dentist:
- Within the past 12 months? _____
- In the past 2 years? _____
- Never been to a dentist. _____

If you have visited a dentist, was the main reason for your visit:
- Regular checkup? _____
- To have denture made? _____
- To have teeth cleaned? _____
- Bleeding or sore gums? _____
- To have tooth filled? _____
- Loose teeth/loose tooth? _____
- To have tooth pulled or other surgery? _____
- Oral or facial pain? _____
- To have a root canal? _____
- Adjustments or repair of denture? _____
- Other? _____

Source: From *Nutrition Interventions Manual for Professionals Caring for Older Americans* by the Nutrition Screening Initiative © 1992 by Greer, Margolis, Mitchell, Grunwald & Associates, Washington, DC.

potential benefits. Fruits and vegetables are important sources of antioxidants and fiber, and tend to be low in fat. High fiber intake is associated with reduced risk of chronic diseases such as cancer, diabetes, and cardiovascular disease in population studies. Table 19–5 lists a variety of suggestions for patients with specific oral problems. Table 19–6 provides suggestions for improving appetite through better flavor. Patients with complex nutritional concerns and underlying medical conditions should be referred to a registered dietitian. Chapter 23 provides helpful social service resources for the aging population.

It is also important to encourage older people to stay active whenever possible. Regular physical activity can help improve weight, blood pressure, diabetes mellitus, lipid profile, osteoarthritis, osteoporosis, cognitive and emotional functioning, and arthritis (Nied, Franklin, 2002; USDHHS, 2004).

Dietary Supplements

The percentage of elders using supplements has been higher than for any other age group in the United States, and senior supplement users tend to have healthier

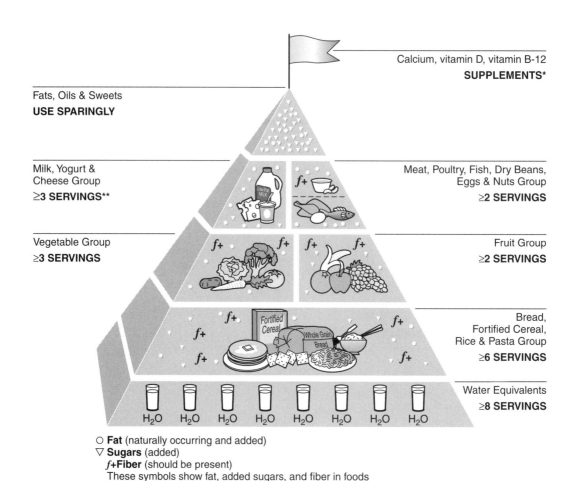

Calcium, vitamin D, vitamin B-12
SUPPLEMENTS*

Fats, Oils & Sweets
USE SPARINGLY

Milk, Yogurt & Cheese Group
≥3 SERVINGS**

Meat, Poultry, Fish, Dry Beans, Eggs & Nuts Group
≥2 SERVINGS

Vegetable Group
≥3 SERVINGS

Fruit Group
≥2 SERVINGS

Bread, Fortified Cereal, Rice & Pasta Group
≥6 SERVINGS

Fortified Cereal
Whole Grain Bread

H₂O H₂O H₂O H₂O H₂O H₂O H₂O H₂O

Water Equivalents
≥8 SERVINGS

○ **Fat** (naturally occurring and added)
▽ **Sugars** (added)
f+**Fiber** (should be present)
These symbols show fat, added sugars, and fiber in foods
*Not all individuals need supplements, consult your healthcare provider
** ≥ Greater than or equal to

FIGURE 19–4 Modified food pyramid for 70 + adults.
Source: © Tufts University with permission.

TABLE 19–4 Recommended Number of Daily or Weekly Servings of Food Groups by Caloric Needs

	Number of servings* by Daily Caloric Intake Level			
	1,600 Calories	*2,000 Calories*	*2,600 Calories*	*3,100 Calories*
Grains	6	7–8	10–11	12–13
Vegetables	3–4	4–5	5–6	6
Fruits	4	4–5	5–6	6
Low-fat or fat-free dairy foods	2–3	2–3	3	3–4
Meat, poultry, fish	1–2	2 or less	2	2–3
Nuts, seeds, legumes	3–4 /wk	4–5 /wk	1	1
Fat and oils	2 /wk	2–3 /wk	3	4
Sweets	0	5 /wk	2	2

* Servings per day unless indicated otherwise.
Source: Dietary Guidelines for Americans 2005, USDHHS, USDA, 2005.

TABLE 19–5   Dietary Suggestions for Common Oral Complaints in Elderly People

Food Group	Difficulty Chewing or Swallowing	Impaired Taste or Appetite	Xerostomia	Food Intolerance
Dairy	Cottage cheese, yogurt instead of hard cheeses.	Use flavored milk and yogurt. Add powdered milk to foods to increase protein and calorie intakes.	Add milk or yogurt to moisten dry foods.	Use milk in small amounts; use more cheese, yogurt, buttermilk, greens.
Meat	Substitute fish, eggs, peanut butter, tofu for hard-to-chew meats. Cut into small pieces.	Chew thoroughly. Add herbs and spices instead of salt.	Add broths, gravies, and sauces.	Use less fatty, fried meat; prepare by broiling, baking, stewing.
Fruits and Vegetables	Use cooked, canned fruits and vegetables. Cut into small pieces or puree foods.	Choose ripe fruits and raw vegetables with skins.	Use soups and stews with high water content.	Use cooked vegetables, fruit, sauces.
Grains	Avoid breads with hard crusts; use pasta, rice, cooked cereals.	Use whole grains such as rye and pumpernickel.	Moisten breads, cereals with milk or broths.	Choose plain breads and cereals, others as tolerated.
Other	Avoid seeds and nuts that tend to slip under dentures.	Wine before a meal may stimulate the appetite when used in moderation.	Use candy or gum with non-nutritive sweeteners instead of sucrose-containing products. Drink plenty of fluids.	

lifestyles and better diets than nonusers (Costello, Finkelstein, Saldanha, Dell'Orto, 2004). Older people who take supplements tend to want to maintain health, slow aging, and have more control over their health issues. Other factors leading to supplement use include dissatisfaction with conventional medical care, excessive dependency on prescription medications, and lack of social and spiritual support by traditional health care providers (Costello et al., 2004).

When there are indications that seniors may not be able to get an adequate diet, nutrient supplementation with Daily Value (DV)-appropriate levels of multivitamin/mineral combinations may be appropriate and useful (Barringer, Kirk, Santaniello, Foley, Michielutte, 2003; Costello et al., 2004). However, there is not yet strong evidence to support the value of supplements in reducing risk of chronic concerns such as heart disease, cataracts, osteoporosis, and immune deficiencies. Even more important, taking more than 100% of the Daily Value of some nutrients

like vitamin A, vitamin D, and iron (from supplement or fortified foods like some cereals and drinks) can be harmful. Too much folic acid can hide the symptoms of vitamin B_{12} deficiency, too much vitamin D can cause calcification of soft tissues like the heart and liver, too much vitamin A can destroy organs such as the liver, and too much iron can be harmful for men.

Supplements can interact with the medicine elders are taking as well. Some supplements can increase the effectiveness of drugs and lead to overdoses. Others can decrease drug effects. Some supplements also have unwanted effects before, during, and after surgery, so supplement use needs to be reported to apropriate health care professionals. See Chapter 16 for more details.

Elders should be encouraged to eat a balanced, nutritious diet and may take a daily multivitamin/mineral supplement that contains no more than 100–200% of the DRI for the nutrients contained.

TABLE 19–6   Tricks to Improve Flavor for Elders

Plan meals that include a wide palette of colors and shapes for eye appeal, and a variety of textures and temperatures for tongue appeal.

Perk up food flavors with small amounts of intense-flavored ingredients such as sharp cheese, toasted nuts, or fruity olive oil.

Try a spoonful of cheese sauce, a shaving of sweet butter, or a drizzle of creamy dressing to add luscious flavor to bitter vegetables and salad greens, and promote absorption of fat-soluble nutrients.

Enhance the natural flavor of foods with reduced, concentrated stocks, monosodium glutamate (MSG), flavored vinegars, zesty condiments, or an extra dash of herbs or spices.

Stave off taste fatigue. Encourage older adults to alternate between bites of food with different tastes, temperatures, and textures.

Try shakes made with coffee or chocolate extracts to mask bitter tastes from medications.

Be adventurous! Expand your tastes to enjoy a variety of foods. Your tastes buds will thank you.

Source: Food Insight, July/August 1999, with permission of the International Food Information Council Foundation.

CURRENT RESEARCH IN NUTRITION AND AGING

Relationships between nutrition and aging are undergoing active research. For example, research is currently under way on protein, vitamins A and K, magnesium, and phytoestrogens and their roles in bone health. The role of antioxidants in aging and disease risk reduction is also an important area of research. Researchers are studying how low dietary intakes of the antioxidant nutrients vitamins C, E, and carotenoids are associated with increased cataract risk, and how lycopene, lutein, and zeaxanthin (major carotenoids in human blood and tissue) in fruits and vegetables may help reduce the risk of developing age-related macular degeneration (Mozaffarieh, Sacu, Wedrich, 2003). In the future, biomarkers of oxidative stress may be used to determine relationships between antioxidant nutrients and chronic disease risk. These biomarkers also may be able to identify dietary patterns associated with reduced disease risk and to develop dietary recommendations.

SUMMARY AND IMPLICATIONS FOR DENTISTRY

Good oral health is essential for the maintenance of overall health. The well-being of the body is often reflected by changes in the oral cavity. As we learn more about the roles of nutrients in the aging and disease processes, findings can be applied to oral health as well. The elderly as a group tend to suffer from a wide range of oral problems that can have a negative impact on food selection, frequency of intake, and nutritional adequacy. To meet their needs, older adults should eat a diet that emphasizes nutrient-dense, high-fiber foods while controlling calories (Table 19–7). However, the elderly population is a heterogeneous group, and it must be recognized that whereas some individuals can obtain the recommended intake levels from foods, others will need to consider dietary supplements. The dental health professional is in an ideal position to identify nutritional problems and counsel the elderly patient on these points. The results will have a long-lasting effect on oral health.

Oral health professionals should:

- Be aware that elders may be at greater risk for nutritional problems than younger patients.
- Routinely screen older patients for nutritional risk factors.

TABLE 19–7   Better Nutrition for Mature Adults

Drink 6 to 8 glasses of water every day.

Eat calcium-rich foods such as milk, cheese, yogurt, fish with bones, and some dark green vegetables like broccoli. Calcium is important for strong bones.

Get plenty of vitamin A and vitamin C by eating fresh fruits and vegetables, such as carrots and oranges. Vitamin A is good for your eyes and skin. Vitamin C keeps gums healthy and prevents infection.

Eat foods high in iron, which helps the body use energy. Iron is abundant in red meat, poultry, fish, and dried beans.

Include meats, seafood, and poultry in your diet to protect against zinc deficiency. Zinc helps wounds heal faster.

Practice regular physical activity. Outdoor activity is best because your body can make vitamin D with the help of the sun.

Source: A joint project of the USDA Food and Consumer Service and Georgia State University. Also available in Spanish (404-651-2542).

- Recognize that oral conditions may contribute to nutritional problems and vice versa.
- Develop community resources to assist patients who are at nutritional risk (see Chapter 21).
- Provide dietary suggestions to help overcome common conditions such as xerostomia, lack of appetite, and problems with mastication.

QUESTIONS PATIENTS MIGHT ASK

Q. How can I eat a nutritious diet as you recommend when I can't chew properly due to my loose dentures?

A. We will help improve your dentures, but meanwhile, you can eat nutritious foods that don't require a lot of chewing such as soft meats and fish, cooked vegetables, canned fruits and juices, and dairy products (provide information from Table 19–2).

Q. Why should I worry about nutrition when I have so many more important problems to deal with like my fixed income, health problems, and loneliness?

A. You may not think that what you eat is so important, but poor diet can actually contribute to feeling poorly, tired, and depressed, and make it harder to fight infection and other health problems. If you make some simple wise food choices, at least you will know that something easy like good diet is not adding to your problems.

Q. Why can't I just take a dietary supplement instead of having to worry about the nutritional value of the foods I eat?

A. A multivitamin/mineral supplement is a good thing for added protection. However, supplements don't substitute for foods because foods contain a lot of important things that are not in supplements, such as fiber, calories, and protective phytochemicals.

Q. How can I get my calcium from dairy products when I am unable to tolerate milk products?

A. There are several solutions to milk intolerance (most often lactose intolerance). You can buy lactose-reduced milk products in the grocery store. You may also be able to tolerate yogurt (with active cultures) and hard cheeses. You can also buy pills in the pharmacy, such as LactAid and Dairy Ease, that you can add to the milk to break down the lactose.

CASE STUDY

Mrs. Murphy, an 82-year-old Caucasian woman, presents to your office with a chief complaint of an upper denture that keeps falling out. Her medical history includes hypertension, diabetes, asthma, and arthritis. She has no known drug allergies and currently takes Clonidine for hypertension, Atrovent for asthma, and was recently prescribed Prozac for depression. Mrs. Murphy denies any alcohol or tobacco intake. Mrs. Murphy was recently widowed and currently lives alone. She has three children, all of whom live in other states, and one sister who lives 5 minutes away.

Your extraoral examination is unremarkable. Intraorally, Mrs. Murphy has an edentulous maxilla and only teeth 22–28 on the mandible. There is generalized moderate gingival recession on all remaining teeth and 5 to 6 mm loss of attachment. Active root caries is present on the buccal of 22, 25, 26, and 27 and the distal of 22 and 28. The oral mucosa appears dry and the tongue is red and fissured.

Mrs. Murphy has a complete upper and partial lower denture that were made at Mrs. Murphy's last dental appointment 3 years ago. Both dentures appear in good condition; however, Mrs. Murphy has experienced some bone resorption and could benefit from relining both dentures.

Mrs. Murphy's dietary history includes two servings of meat and poultry, two servings of fruits and vegetables, and seven servings of breads and grains. Mrs. Murphy reports frequent sugar use, as she sucks on hard lemon candies almost continuously throughout the day. She also reports frequently missing meals, as she doesn't like to cook only for herself.

Questions:

1. What are Mrs. Murphy's oral problems?
2. What are her nutritional problems?
3. How would you manage Mrs. Murphy's oral and nutritional problems?

REFERENCES

Administration on Aging: *Profile of Older Americans: 2002*. Retrieved June 27, 2005, from http://www.aoa.gov/aoa/stats/profile/2002/2002profile.pdf.

Arky R: *Physicians' Desk Reference*, 51st ed. Montvale, NJ: Medical Economics, 1997.

Ausman L, Russell RM: Nutrition in the elderly. In Shils M, Olsen JA, Shike M, Ross AC (eds): *Modern Nutrition in Health and Disease*, 9th ed. Baltimore: Williams & Wilkins, l999.

Bahls C: Alzheimer research joins the mainstream. *The Scientist* 2002; 16:2.

Barringer TA, Kirk JK, Santaniello AC, Foley CL, Michielutte R: Effect of a multivitamin and mineral supplement on infection and quality of life. *Ann Int Med* 2003; 138(5):365–71.

Baum BJ: Salivary gland fluid secretion during aging. *J Am Geriatr Soc* 1989; 37:453–58.

Beck JD, Hunt RJ: Oral health status in the United States: Problems of special patients. *J Dent Ed* 1985; 49:407–25.

Becker W, Hujoel PP, Becker BE, Willingham H: Osteoporosis and implant failure: An exploratory case-control study. *J Periodontol* 2000; 71:625–31.

Blaum CS, Fries BE, Fiatarone MA: Factors associated with low body mass index and weight loss in nursing home residents. *J Gerontol Series A, Biol Sci Med Sci* 1995; 50:M162–68.

Blomqvist JE, Alberius P, Isaksson S, Linde A, Hansson BG: Factors in implant integration failure after bone grafting. *Int J Oral Maxillofacial Surg* 1996; 25(1):63–68.

Blumberg J: Nutritional needs of seniors. *J Am Coll Nutr* 1997; 16:519–23.

Burns A, Marsh A, Bender DA: Dietary intake and clinical, anthropometric and biochemical indices of malnutrition in elderly demented and non-demented subjects. *Psychol Med* 1989; 19:383–91.

Centers for Disease Control and Prevention: 5 a day. Retrieved June 29, 2005, from http://apps.nccd.cdc.gov/5AdaySurveillance/displayV.asp.

Centers for Disease Control and Prevention, Merck Institute on Aging and Health: *The State of Aging and Health in America 2004*. Retrieved June 27, 2005, from http://cdc.gov/aging/pdf/State_of_Aging_and_Health_in_America_2004.pdf.

Cohen D: Dementia, depression, and nutritional status. *Primary Care* 1994; 21:107–19.

Cooper DA: Carotenoids in health and disease prevention: Recent scientific evaluations, research recommendations and the consumer. *J Nutr* 2004; 134:

Costello R, Finkelstein J, Saldanha L, Dell'Orto M: Executive summary: Conference on Dietary Supplement Use in the Elderly—proceedings of the conference held January 14–15, 2003, Natcher Auditorium, National Institutes of Health, Bethesda, MD. *Nutr Rev* 2004; 62(4):160–75.

Dawson-Hughes B, Harris SS, Krall EA, Dallal GE: A controlled trial of calcium and vitamin D supplementation on bone density in men and women 65 years of age or older. *N Engl J Med* 1997; 337:670–76.

Dewan S, Wilding JP: Obesity and type 2 diabetes in the elderly. Gerontologist 2003; 49:137–45.

Dolan TA, Monopoli MP, Kaurich MJ, Rubenstein LZ: Geriatric grand rounds: Oral diseases in older adults. *J Am Geriatr Soc* 1990; 38:1239–50.

Elders PJ, Habets LL, Netelenbos JC, van der Linden LW, van der Stelt PF: The relation between periodontitis and systemic bone loss in women between 46 and 55 years of age. *J Clin Peridontol* 1992; 19(7):492–96.

Ettinger R: The unique oral health needs of an aging population. *Dent Clin North Am* 1997; 41:633–49.

Food Security Institute: Hunger and food insecurity among the elderly. Retrieved June 28, 2005, from http://www.centeronhunger.org.pdf/Elderly.pdf.

Gray CE: Nutrition and dementia. *J Am Diet Assoc* 1989; 89:1795–1802.

Griffin SO, Griffin PM, Swann JL, Zlobin N: Estimating rates of new root caries in older adults. *J Dent Res* 2004; 83:634–38.

Grodstein F, Colditz GA, Stampfer MJ: Post-menopausal hormone use and tooth loss: A prospective study. *J Am Dent Assoc* 1996; 127:370–77.

Guralnik JM, Eisenstaedt RS, Ferrucci L, Klein HG, Woodman RC: The prevalence of anemia in persons age 65 and older in the United States. Evidence for a high rate of unexplained anemia. *Blood* 2004; 104(8):2263–68.

Hedley AA, Ogden CL, Johnson CL, Carroll MD, Curtain LR, Foegal KM: Prevalence of overweight and obesity among US children, adolescents, and adults, 1999–2002. *JAMA* 2004; 291:2847–50.

Institute of Medicine, National Academy of Sciences: *Dietary Reference Intakes for Calcium, Phosphorus, Magnesium, Vitamin D, and Fluoride*. Washington, DC: National Academies Press, 1997.

Institute of Medicine, National Academy of Sciences: *Dietary Reference Intakes for Thiamin, Riboflavin, Niacin, Vitamin B_6, Folate, Vitamin B_{12}, Pantothenic Acid, Biotin, and Choline*. Washington, DC: National Academies Press, 1998.

Ismail AI, Burt BA, Eklund SA: Relation between ascorbic acid intake and periodontal disease in the United States. *J Am Dent Assoc* 1983; 107:927–31.

Joshipura KJ, Willett WC, Douglass CW: The impact of edentulousness on food and nutrient intake. *J Am Dent Assoc* 1996; 127:459–67.

Krall EA, Dawson-Hughes B, Hannan MT, Wilson PW, Kiel DP: Postmenopausal estrogen replacement and tooth retention. *Am J Med* 1997; 102(6):536–42.

Krall EA, Dawson-Hughes B, Papas A, Garcia RI: Tooth loss and skeletal bone density in healthy postmenopausal women. *Osteoporos Int* 1994; 4:104–9.

Krall EA, Garcia RI, Dawson-Hughes B: Increased risk of tooth loss is related to bone loss at the whole body, hip, and spine. *Calcif Tissue Int* 1996; 59:433–37.

Krall E, Hayes C, Garcia R: How dentition status and masticatory function affect nutrient intake. *J Am Dent Assoc* 1998; 129:1261–69.

Lee JS, Weyant RJ, Corby P, Kritchevsky SB, Harris TB, Rooks R, Rubin SM, et al.: Edentulism and nutritional status in a biracial sample of well-functioning, community-dwelling elderly: The health, aging, and body composition study. *Am J Clin Nutr* 2004; 80:1453–54.

Lee MY, Novielli KD: A nutritional assessment of home-bound elderly in a physician-monitored population. *J Nutr Elderly* 1996; 15:1–13.

Malouf R, Grimley EJ: The effect of vitamin B_6 on cognition. Cochrane Database Syst. Rev. 2003; 4:CD004393.

Marcus SE, Drury TF, Brown LJ, Zion GR: Tooth retention and tooth loss in the permanent dentition of adults: United States, 1988–1991. *J Dent Res* 1996; 75(Spec No):684–95.

May H, Reader R, Murphy S, Khaw K-T: Self-reported tooth loss and bone mineral density in older men and women. *Age Aging* 1995; 24:217–21.

Morley JE: Decreased food intake with aging. *J Gerontol Biol Sci Med Sci* 2001; 56A:81–88.

Mozaffarieh M, Sacu S, Wedrich A: The role of the carotenoids, lutein and zeaxanthin in protecting against age-related macular degeneration. A review based on controversial evidence. *Nutr J* 2003; 2:20.

Nied RJ, Franklin B: Promoting and prescribing exercise for the elderly. *Am Fam Physicians* 2002; 65:419–26.

Nishida M, Grossi SG, Dunford RG, Ho AW, Trevisan M, Genco RJ: Calcium and the risk for periodontal disease. *J Periodontol* 2000; 71(7):1057–66.

Nordenram G, Ryd-Kjellen E, Johansson G, Nordstrom G, Winblad B: Alzheimer's disease, oral function, and nutritional status. *Gerodontology* 1996; 13(1):9–16.

Nutrition Screening Initiative. *Nutrition Interventions Manual for Professionals Caring for Older Americans*. Washington, DC: Greer, Margolis, Mitchell, Grunwald & Associates, 1992.

Paganini-Hill A: The benefits of estrogen replacement therapy on oral health. *Arch Intern Med* 1995; 155:2325–29.

Payne JB, Reinhardt RA, Nummikoski PV, Patil KD: Longitudinal alveolar bone loss in postmenopausal osteoporotic/osteopenic women. *Osteoporosis Int* 1999; 10:34–40.

Payne JB, Zachs NR, Reinhardt RA, Nummikoski PV, Patil K: The association between estrogen status and alveolar bone density changes in postmenopausal women with a history of periodontitis. *J Periodontol* 1997; 68(1):24–31.

Pilgram TK, Hildebolt CF, Dotson M, Cohen SC, Hauser JF, Kardaris E, et al.: Relationships between clinical attachment level and spine and hip bone mineral density: Data from healthy postmenopausal women. *J Periodontol* 2002; 73(3):298–301.

Position of the American Dietetic Association: *Nutrition Across the Spectrum of Aging*. American Dietetic Association. Retrieved June 27, 2005, from http://www.eatright.org/Member/PolicyInitiatives/index_21992.cfm.

Posner BM, Jette A, Smigelski C, Miller D, Mitchell P: Nutritional risk in New England elders. *J Gerontol* 1994; 49(3):M123–32.

Rhodus NL, Brown JB: The association of xerostomia and inadequate intake in older adults. *J Am Diet Assoc* 1990; 90:1688–92.

Ritchie CS, Burgio KL, Locher JL, Cornwell A, Thomas D, Hardin M, et al.: Nutritional status of urban homebound older adults. *Am J Clin Nutr* 1997; 66(4):815–18.

Ritchie CS, Joshipura K, Hung HC, Douglass CW: Nutrition as a mediator in the relation between oral and systemic disease: Associations between specific measures of adult oral health and nutrition outcomes. *Crit Rev Oral Biol Med* 2002; 13:291–300.

Ronderos M, Jacobs DR, Himes JH, Pihlstrom BL: Associations of periodontal disease with femoral bone mineral density and estrogen replacement therapy: Cross-sectional evaluation of U.S. adults from NHANES III. *J Clin Periodontol* 2000; 27:778–86.

Rowe JW, Kahn RL: *Successful Aging*. New York: Pantheon Books, 1998.

Russell RM, Rasmussen H, Lichtenstein AH: Modified food guide pyramid for people over seventy years of age. *J Nutr* 1999; 129:751–53.

Sahyoun NR, Lin C-L, Krall E: Nutritional status of the older adult is associated with dentition status. *J Amer Diet Assoc* 2003; 103:61–66.

Saunders MJ: Incorporating the Nutrition Screening Initiative into the dental practice. *Spec Care Dent* 1995; 15:26–37.

Sheiham A, Steele J: Does the condition of the mouth and teeth affect the ability to eat certain foods, nutrient and dietary intake, and nutritional status amongst older people? *Public Health Nutr* 2001; 4:797–803.

Sheiham A, Steele JG, Marcenes W, Finch S, Walls AW: The relationship between oral health status and body mass index among older people: A national survey of older people in Great Britain. *Br Dent J* 2002; 192:703–06.

Ship JA, Duffy V, Jones JA, Langmore S: Geriatric oral health and its impact on eating. *J Am Geriatr Soc* 1996; 44:456–64.

Siebens H, Trupe E, Siebens A, Cook F, Anshen S, Hanauer R, Oster G: Correlates and consequences of eating dependency in institutionalized elderly. *J Am Geriatr Soc* 1986 Mar; 34(3):192–8.

Steele JG, Sheiham A: Clinical and behavioural risk indicators for root caries in older people. *Gerodontol* 2001; 18:95–101.

Stevens DA, Grivetti LE, McDonald RB: Nutrient intake of urban and rural elderly receiving home-delivered meals. *J Am Diet Assoc* 1992; 92:714–17.

Sullivan DH, Martin W, Flaxman N, Hagen JE: Oral health problems and involuntary weight loss in a population of frail elderly. *J Am Geriatr Soc* 1993; 41:725–31.

Takaishi Y, Ikeo T, Miki T, Nishizawa Y, Morii H: Suppression of alveolar bone resorption by etidronate treatment for periodontal disease: 4- to 5-year follow-up of four patients. *J Int Med Res* 2003; 31:575–84.

Taylor GW: Bidirectional interrelationships between diabetes and periodontal diseases: An epidemiologic perspective. *Ann Periodontol* 2001; 6:99–112.

Taylor GW, Burt BA, Becker MP, Genco RJ, Shlossman M, Knowler WC, et al.: Severe periodontitis and risk for poor glycemic control in patients with non-insulin dependent diabetes mellitus. *J Periodontol* 1996; 67(10suppl): 1085–93.

Taylor GW, Manz MC, Borgnakke WS: Diabetes, periodontal diseases, dental caries, and tooth loss: A review of the literature. *Compendium Cont Ed Dent* 2004; 25:179–84.

Thomas DR, Morley JE: Regulation of appetite in older adults. Retrieved October 13, 2004, from http://www .ltcnutrition.org/PDF/ApetiteRegulation.pdf.

U.S. Department of Agriculture: Diet and health. Food consumption and nutrient intakes. Retrieved June 27, 2005, from http://www.ers.usda.gov/briefing/DietAndHealth/data/foods/table1.htm.

U.S. Department of Health and Human Services, Office of the Surgeon General: *Bone Health and Osteoporosis: A Report of the Surgeon General*. Rockville, MD: Author, 2004.

U.S. Department of Health and Human Services and U.S. Department of Agriculture: *Dietary Guidelines for Americans 2005*, 6th ed. Washington, DC: U.S. Government Printing Office, January 2005.

U.S. Special Committee on Aging, United States Senate: *Developments in Aging: 1990*, Vol. 1, Res. 66, Sec. 19, February 28, 1990. Washington, DC: U.S. Government Printing Office, 1991.

Wactawski-Wende J: Periodontal diseases and osteoporosis: association and mechanisms. *Ann Periodontol* 2001; 6:197–208.

Watts ML: Improving nutrition for American seniors: A new look at the Older Americans Act. *J Am Diet Assoc* 2005; 105(4):527–29.

Wayler AH, Chauncey HH: Impact of complete dentures and impaired natural dentition on masticatory performance and food choice in healthy aging men. *J Prosthet Dent* 1983; 49:427–33.

Wayler AH, Muench MS, Kapur KK, Chauncey HH: Masticatory performance and food acceptability in persons with removable partial dentures, full dentures, and intact natural dentition. *J Gerontol* 1984; 39:284–89.

Weyant RJ, Pearlstein ME, Churak AP, Forrest K, Famili P, Cauley JA: The association between osteopenia and periodontal attachment loss in older women. *J Periodontol* 1999; 70(9):982–91.

Winkler S, Garg AK, Mekayarajjananonth T, Bakaeen LG, Khan E: Depressed taste and smell in geriatric patients. *J Am Dent Assoc* 1999 Dec; 130(12):1759–65.

Winn DM, Brunelle JA, Selwitz RH, Kaste LM, Oldakowski RJ, Kirgman A, et al.: Coronal and root caries in the dentition of adults in the United States, 1988–1991. *J Dent Res* 1996; 75(Spec No):642–51.

Writing Group for the Women's Health Initiative Investigators: Risks and benefits of estrogen plus progestin in healthy postmenopausal women. Principal results from the Women's Health Initiative randomized controlled trial. *JAMA* 2002; 288:321–33.

Chapter **20**

Oral and Nutritional Concerns for People with Special Health Care Needs

Katherine Kwon and Carole A. Palmer

OBJECTIVES

The student will be able to:

- Discuss why people with special health care needs in particular require nutrition and dental services.
- List and describe common oral dysfunctions seen in people with special health care needs and the nutritional implications of these problems.
- Describe common nutritional concerns for children with special health care needs.
- Discuss different feeding strategies to enhance food intake and overall health of this population.
- Identify ways to help minimize oral disease, which can lead to compromised nutritional status in people with special health care needs.

INTRODUCTION

Specific dental–nutritional relationships have been discussed thus far for people of all ages from infants to elders. However, people with special health care needs have unique oral health and nutrition issues that may be overlooked due to more pressing medical needs. This chapter discusses common oral and nutritional problems associated with specific special needs conditions and provides recommendations to help optimize the nutritional status of this population.

DEVELOPMENTAL DISABILITY AND SPECIAL HEALTH CARE NEEDS

Currently in the United States there are approximately 4.5 million individuals living with a developmental disability, the most common being mental retardation (USDHHS, 2005). (See Table 20–1 for the complete definition of *developmental disability*.) Children with special health care needs are defined as "those who have or are at an increased risk for a chronic physical, developmental, behavioral, or emotional condition and who also require health and related services of a type or amount beyond that required by children generally" (McPherson et al., 1998). As of 2001 approximately 9.4 million children in the United States under the age of 18 are estimated to have special health care needs (USDHHS, 2004b). Common special health care conditions include, but are not limited to, Down syndrome, epilepsy, cerebral palsy, muscular dystrophy, autism, and spina bifida.

Regardless of age, individuals with developmental disabilities or special health care needs have increased dental and nutritional risks as a result of many different factors related to their specific conditions. Maintaining optimal oral health and ensuring adequate nutrition are difficult challenges in children and adults of this particular population. This chapter will review the oral health–nutrition challenges faced by people with disabilities or special needs and provide some guidelines for managing these issues.

NEED FOR DENTAL AND NUTRITION SERVICES

Individuals with developmental disabilities and special health care needs may require an array of medical and support services such as specialized medical care and equipment; prescription medications; speech, physical, and occupational therapies; family and genetic counseling; and dental and nutritional care. According to a 2001 national survey, dental care was determined to be the second most needed service for approximately 78% of the special needs population, ranked only behind prescription medicine. More than 8% of children in this group needed but did not receive dental care (USDHHS, 2004b).

The landmark surgeon general's report (*Oral Health in America: A Report of the Surgeon General*) highlighted the relationship between compromised oral health and increased nutritional risk, and sent a clear message that oral health is critical to the general health and well-being of all Americans, including those with special needs (USDHHS, 2000b). *Healthy People 2010*, a government report published every decade, sets specific national objectives for disease prevention and public

TABLE 20–1   Definition of "Development Disability"

(A) IN GENERAL the term "developmental disability" means a severe chronic disability of an individual that—
  (i) is attributable to a mental or physical impairment or combination of mental and physical impairments;
  (ii) is manifested before the person attains age twenty-two;
  (iii) is likely to continue indefinitely;
  (iv) results in substantial functional limitations in three or more of the following areas of major life activity;
    (a) self-care,
    (b) receptive and expressive language,
    (c) learning,
    (d) mobility,
    (e) self-direction,
    (f) capacity for independent living,
    (g) economic sufficiency; and
  (v) reflects the person's need for combination and sequence of special, interdisciplinary, or generic services, individualized supports, or other forms of services that are of lifelong or extended duration and are individually planned and coordinated,
(B) INFANTS AND YOUNG CHILDREN—
  Individual from birth to age 9, inclusive, who has substantial developmental delay or specific congenital or acquired condition, may be considered to have a developmental disability without meeting 3 more of the criteria described in clauses (i) through (v) of subparagraph (A) if the individual, without services and supports, has a high probability of meeting those criteria later in life.

Source: Developmental Disabilities Assistance and Bill of Rights Act, PL 106-402; 2000.

TABLE 20–2 Oral Health in the Surgeon General's Report and *Healthy People 2010*

Oral Health in America: A Report of the Surgeon General:
- Oral health is related to well-being and quality of life as measured along functional, psychosocial, and economic dimensions. Diet, nutrition, sleep, psychological status, social interaction, school, and work are affected by impaired oral and craniofacial health.
- Oral and craniofacial diseases and conditions contribute to compromised ability to bite, chew, and swallow foods; limitations in food selection; and poor nutrition. These conditions include tooth loss, diminished salivary functions, oral-facial pain conditions such as temporomandibular disorders, alterations in taste, and functional limitations of prosthetic replacements.
- The burden of oral diseases and conditions is disproportionately borne by individuals with low socioeconomic status at each life stage and by those who are vulnerable because of poor general health.
- Many inherited and congenital conditions affect the craniofacial complex, often resulting in disfigurement and impairments that may involve many body organs and systems and affect millions of children worldwide.

Healthy People 2010
Maternal and Child Health
Objective 16–14: Reduce the occurrence of developmental disabilities.
Objective 16–23: Increase the proportion of territories and states that have service systems for children with special health care needs.
Nutrition
Objective 19–4: Reduce growth retardation among low-income children under age 5 years.
Objective 19–17: Increase the proportion of . . . counseling or education related to diet and nutrition.
Oral Health
Objective 21–2: Reduce the proportion of children, adolescents, and adults with untreated dental decay.
Objective 21–5: Reduce periodontal disease.

Sources: From *Healthy People 2010: Understanding and Improving Health*: 2E by U.S. Department of Health and Human Services © 2000 by U.S. Government Printing Office, Washington, DC; and *Oral Health in America: A Report of the Surgeon General—Executive Summary* by U.S. Department of Health and Human Services © 2000 by National Institutes of Health, Rockville, MD.

health promotion, and also targets the needs of special populations (USDHHS, 2000a). Summary guidelines from both documents are listed in Table 20–2.

In the face of often complex and extensive health issues in the special needs population, oral health and nutrition concerns may be unrecognized or overlooked. Therefore, it is important for the dental health professional to be knowledgeable of the common oral problems seen in individuals with special health care needs and their nutritional implications, and provide meaningful solutions and referral for further care. The common oral problems associated with common disabilities are summarized in Table 20–3.

WHAT ARE THE NUTRITION PROBLEMS OF PEOPLE WITH SPECIAL HEALTH CARE NEEDS?

Persons with developmental disabilities and special health care needs are at increased risk for nutritional problems. The most common issue is inadequate caloric intake, which can lead to slow growth and poor weight gain (USDHHS, 1991). Multiple factors increase the

nutritional risk for this population including poor growth and development, inadequate feeding skills, and side effects of medications (Position of the American Dietetic Association, 2004). In children, feeding development (age-appropriate foods, self-feeding skills) may be delayed due to motor dysfunctions and oral malformations (Cloud, 2004; McKinney, Palmer, Dwyer, Garcia, 1991). Additionally, extended feeding and mealtimes increases the exposure of teeth to cariogenic foods, increasing the risk of dental caries (Boyd, Palmer, Dwyer, 1998). Compromised oral health such as tooth or gum disease combined with oral motor dysfunctions may also affect feeding ability and desire, which further contributes to poor nutrition. This perpetuating cyclic relationship of poor oral health and nutrition is depicted in Figure 20–1.

Poor nutrition can increase mortality risk in children with special needs. Several studies of children with cerebral palsy have found relationships between feeding dysfunction, self-feeding skills, and nutritional status and increased risk of mortality or morbidity. One study of 12,000 children 6 months to 3.5 years of age with cerebral palsy found that lack of self-feeding skill was associated with a sixfold increased risk in

TABLE 20–3 Oral Motor Problems Often Associated with Common Special Needs Conditions

	Cerebral Palsy	Down Syndrome	Epilepsy/Seizure Disorder	Muscular Dystrophy	Autism	Cystic Fibrosis
Increased risk for periodontal disease	X	X	X	X	X	X
Increased caries risk	X		X	X	X	X
Poor sucking reflex	X				X	
Jaw clenching	X		X			
Excessive bleeding			X			
Drooling	X					
Gingival overgrowth	X		X			
	Due to Rx		Due to Rx			
Tongue and lip fissuring		X				
Malformed/ missing teeth		X				
Xerostomia	X	X			X	
Bruxism	X	X			X	
Hyperactive gag reflex	X	X				
Malocculsion	X	X		X		
Mouth breathing		X		X		
Inefficient chew	X	X		X		
Reduced motor tone	X	X		X		
Narrow/small oral cavity		X		X		
Tongue thrust	X	X		X		
Inability to cough/clear secretions				X		X
Taste sensitivity						X
Thick saliva			X			X

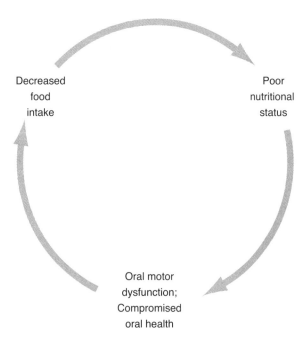

FIGURE 20–1 Cyclic relationship of oral health and nutrition.

mortality (Strauss, Shavelle, Anderson, 1998). Another study showed that those with mild feeding dysfunction had poor growth and inadequate fat stores (Fung et al., 2002). Therefore, detecting these feeding problems and treating or correcting them early on can significantly impact the health of this population.

HOW DOES ORAL DYSFUNCTION AFFECT NUTRITIONAL STATUS?

Problems in the oral cavity can affect ability and desire to eat, and ultimate nutritional status. Many oral conditions common in people with developmental disabilities and special health care needs have important nutritional implications, which are reviewed below and summarized in Table 20–4.

Mastication

Mastication and chewing problems are common among individuals with cerebral palsy, muscular dystrophy, autism, and Down syndrome. Impaired chewing ability

TABLE 20–4 Common Oral Problems and Their Dietary Implications

Oral Problem	Dietary Implication
Mastication difficulties	Decreased desire to eat Decreased eating ability Insufficient calories and/or nutrients and fiber
Abnormal muscle tone	Poor sucking, swallowing Impaired self-feeding ability Elongated mealtimes Inadequate calories and/or nutrients
Malocclusion	Difficulty chewing food Soft diet may be inadequate in calories and/or nutrients and fiber
Bruxism	Difficulty chewing food Soft diet may be inadequate in calories and/or nutrients and fiber
Gingival overgrowth	Sore mouth Difficulty chewing Diminished food intake Insufficient calories, nutrients, and fiber Increased caries risk due to drugs that cause xerostomia
Dysphagia	Food and beverage avoidance due to fear of aspiration Inadequate calories and/or nutrients
Prolonged feeding	Increased caries risk Possible inadequate calories and nutrients
Periodontal disease	Pain and discomfort Poor food intake Possible inadequate calories and nutrients

may be a result of poor occlusion, which can cause pain and difficulty during feeding. The result is a decreased desire and ability to eat, which ultimately increases nutritional risk for this population.

Abnormal Muscle Tone

Abnormal muscle tone (hypotonia or hypertonia) creates barriers to feeding development. Poor motor control and coordination often lead to problems with sucking,

chewing development, swallowing, and self-feeding skills. Feeding problems are intensified in children with a strong tongue thrust, which not only impedes normal feeding progression but also elongates mealtime and may result in decreased food intake.

Malocclusion

Malocclusion (resulting from muscle dysfunction) is commonly seen in persons with cerebral palsy. Poorly aligned teeth or crowded teeth can make mastication difficult (Figure 20–2). As a result, the person may avoid chewing, and may require a diet of soft consistency. It is important that this diet be as nutritionally adequate as a more traditional diet. Furthermore, because abnormally developed and aligned teeth are difficult to keep clean, the resulting food debris retention and poor oral hygiene may contribute to periodontal disease and dental caries.

Bruxism

Bruxism is commonly seen in children with cerebral palsy and Down syndrome (Figure 20–3). Long-term clenching and grinding of the teeth may erode and flatten dental crowns and cause difficulty when chewing. Teeth may also become loose leading to the inability to chew foods of tougher consistency (e.g., meats, raw vegetables). This may also lead to the need for a diet of softer consistency. The lack of dietary fiber can contribute to a problem of constipation.

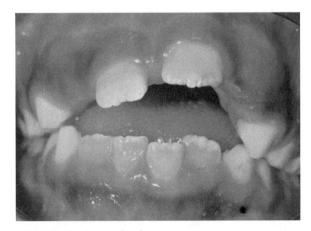

FIGURE 20–2 Malocclusion.
Source: U.S. Department of Health and Human Services, Health Resources and Services Administration. *Oral Conditions in Children With Special Needs.* Bethesda, MD: National Institutes of Health, 2004.

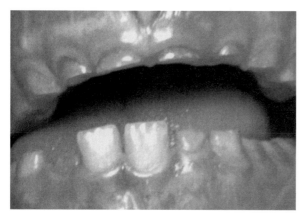

FIGURE 20–3   Bruxism.
Source: U.S. Department of Health and Human Services, Health Resources and Services Administration. *Oral Conditions in Children With Special Needs.* Bethesda, MD: National Institutes of Health, 2004.

Gingival Overgrowth

Gingival overgrowth (hyperplasia) may be a side effect in individuals who take the anticonvulsant medication Dilantin (phenytoin) and exhibit poor oral hygiene (Figure 20–4). It can also be a side effect of other medications including calcium channel blockers and cyclosporine. Severe gingival overgrowth may impede tooth eruption, chewing ability, cause discomfort while eating, and may result in an increased risk for gum infections. Furthermore, gingival overgrowth may negatively affect the child's self-esteem and self-image.

Again, it may be difficult for the individual to chew normal foods. A soft diet can and should be

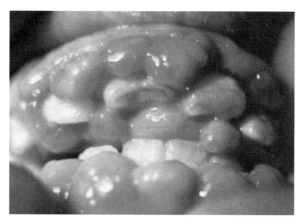

FIGURE 20–4   Gingival overgrowth.
Source: U.S. Department of Health and Human Services, Health Resources and Services Administration. *Oral Conditions in Children With Special Needs.* Bethesda, MD: National Institutes of Health, 2004.

nutritionally adequate if properly designed, but may be low in fiber.

Dysphagia

During the progression of feeding development, some children with special needs experience dysphagia (difficulty swallowing foods or liquids). This increases their risk of aspiration and may make the child afraid to eat or drink. Understandably, this increases the risk of nutritional deficiency.

Prolonged Feeding

Children with special health care needs are at high risk for dental caries because of multiple factors. Prolonged use of the bottle for infants and children with delayed feeding ability may lead to early childhood caries (ECC) due to the extended contact of dietary starches with the teeth. Frequent high-sugar snacks often given as behavioral rewards coupled with irregular tooth brushing increases the risk of dental caries in children with special needs. In addition, long-term consumption of certain medications in sucrose-based solutions or syrups can contribute to dental caries.

Periodontal Disease

Poor oral hygiene complicated by medications may lead to gingivitis and periodontal disease. Swollen gums that easily bleed upon contact can cause enough pain and discomfort to interfere with ability and desire to eat. If left untreated, periodontal disease can lead to premature tooth loss, which further compromises eating ability.

MANAGING DIETARY AND NUTRITIONAL NEEDS OF PEOPLE WITH SPECIAL HEALTH CARE NEEDS

Although many children and adults with developmental disabilities experience oral problems that may affect food intake, choosing healthful foods and engaging in physical activity are important lifestyle habits to adopt for long-term health. To the extent possible, children and adults with special needs should still practice healthful eating habits by following the food pyramid guidelines at the USDA's website: (http://www.mypyramid.gov) and the *Dietary Guidelines for Americans* summarized in Table 20–5.

Because of the different metabolic activity and growth rates of the special needs population, meeting

TABLE 20–5 Key Dietary Recommendations for Individuals Aged 2 Years or Older

- Balance dietary calories with physical activity to maintain normal growth.
- Engage in 60 minutes of moderate to vigorous play or physical activity daily.
- Eat vegetables and fruits daily; limit juice intake.
- Use vegetable oils and soft margarines low in saturated fat and trans fatty acids instead of butter or most other animal fats in the diet.
- Eat whole grain breads and cereals rather than refined grain products.
- Reduce the intake of sugar-sweetened beverages and foods.
- Use nonfat (skim) or low-fat milk and dairy products daily.
- Eat more fish, especially oily fish, broiled or baked.
- Reduce salt intake, including salt from processed foods.

Source: Adapted from Gidding et al., 2005; AHA Pediatric Dietary Strategies for Individuals Aged >2 Years.

the established DRIs for children and adults is not always applicable (Cloud, 2005). Diet and feeding recommendations should, therefore, be made on an individual basis depending on the individual's feeding ability, and growth should be carefully monitored. Due to the various oral motor and feeding problems that are seen in children and adults with developmental disabilities, it is important that the dental health professional and registered dietitian work together to help deliver appropriate oral health care and nutrition guidance. The dental professional can check with the state department of nutrition or the local dietetic association to locate registered dietitians who specialize in special needs. A registered dietitian with special needs experience will be able to provide nutrition strategies and instruction regarding appropriate food choices, feeding methods, and behavior modification skills to deal with specific feeding problems. Table 20–6 outlines strategies to

TABLE 20–6 Cincinnati Children's Hospital Medical Center Strategies for Identification and Intervention of Oral Motor Problems

Reflex	*Diagnosis*	*Stimulation-Mechanics*
Sucking	• Place pacifier or finger in mouth. Lips should close around it with strong suction applied.	• Use gloved finger to stimulate by pushing gently downward on tongue to encourage initiation of sucking. • Experiment with various nipple types. • Encourage use of straw; use cold liquids.
Swallowing	• Offer drink of water (observe for signs of gagging, coughing). • Check positioning; develop tongue control. • Modify barium swallow.	• Ensure good positions and alignment. • Keep head stable and in a downward position/chin tuck. • Position cup centrally; use other hand under chin to apply gentle upward pressure to minimize fluid loss. • Offer cold/sour items (e.g., lemon ice).
Tongue thrusting	• Place pretzel stick or small tongue blade in mouth and observe; tongue section will push out solid food.	• Place foods in corners of mouth between teeth. • When spoon feeding, use spoon with a shallow bowl (small amounts of food); when food is placed in mouth, produce a slight downward pressure on tongue with spoon.
Loosening jaw	• Place small pieces of cracker between molars. • Observe chewing action for rotary movement.	• Use hand to guide jaw up and inward while child chews. • Have child imitate adult while feeling adult's jaw.
Chewing	• Observe chewing for rotary motion, not loose vertical motion.	• Massage gums with index finger, gauze, or warm washcloth before feeding. • Have child imitate adult while feeling adult's jaw. • Slowly progress from soft, well-cooked foods to those of tougher consistencies.
Drooling	• Observe; accompanies poor swallowing reflex and/or jaw control.	• Use jaw control actions at feeding and nonfeeding times. • Stimulate swallowing reflex.

Source: Adapted from H. Cloud, "Feeding problems of the child with special health care needs," in *Pediatric Nutrition in Chronic Diseases and Developmental Disorders: Prevention, Assessment, and Treatment* 2/E by Ekvall/Ekvall (eds.) © 2005 by Oxford University Press, New York, NY.

identify and manage oral motor problems commonly seen in children and adults with special health care needs.

Improving Calorie Intake

Proper growth assessment of the child who has feeding problems is important because it may indicate whether his or her current food intake is adequate. Various oral motor problems may lead to limited food intake and severe nutritional risk. So modifying foods to increase caloric and protein intake may be necessary to meet the individual's needs. Table 20–7 lists foods that can be added to pureed foods for increased calories and protein.

Overcoming Oral Impairments

Children with special needs often have oral impairments such as problems chewing, abnormal oral muscle tone, malocclusion, bruxism, gingival overgrowth, and periodontal disease. Depending on the mastication abilities of the child, the texture, temperature, or caloric density of foods may need to be modified to improve nutritional status. Although these changes are important

to ensure adequate caloric intake, the dental health consequences of a modified diet must also be taken into consideration and properly managed. For example, foods may need to be pureed due to oral motor dysfunction. However, because pureed foods have a slower oral clearance time, they can increase the child or adult's risk for dental caries. Generally, firm-textured foods are recommended because they tend to promote salivary flow, which exerts a protective effect on teeth, and they also provide stimulation for oral–facial muscles. Table 20–8 provides diet suggestions for oral impairment.

Managing Dysphagia

Dysphagia, or swallowing dysfunction, may lead to increased aspiration risk in children and adults with special health care needs, as previously discussed. Because dysphagia usually leads to insufficient food intake, modifying the consistency and caloric content of the foods and liquids may be necessary for adequate nutrition. Children and adults with swallowing difficulties should be referred to an occupational or speech therapist for a feeding evaluation to determine the appropriate foods and liquids. Once the level of dysphagia is assessed, appropriate treatment to improve swallowing

TABLE 20–7   Soft Diet Suggestions for Chewing Impairments

Dairy Products and Other Calcium Sources	Proteins	Fruits	Vegetables	Grains
At least 3 servings/day (a serving is 1 cup)	At least 5 oz/day (1 slice of meat is about 1 oz, a usual serving of protein is 4–5 oz)	At least 3 servings/day (a serving is $\frac{1}{2}$ cup)	At least 4 servings/day (a serving is $\frac{1}{2}$ cup)	At least 3 servings/day (a serving is 1 slice of bread or $\frac{1}{2}$ cup cooked rice, pasta, cereal)
All forms of milk, milkshakes, Instant Breakfast type drinks	Eggs	Applesauce	Pureed or strained vegetables (mixed with broth)	Cooked cereals
	Cheese	Pureed or strained cooked fruits		Soft breads
Yogurt	Milk and milkshakes	Canned fruits	Steamed vegetables	Pasta
Soft cheeses like cottage cheese	Pea and bean soups	Fruit gelatins	Vegetable soups, curries	Mashed potatoes
Soft custards	Pureed meats	Fruit smoothies		Rice
Pudding	Tender meats (in soups or with gravy)	Popsicles	Vegetable juices	Rice porridge (with ground meat)
Ice cream	Fish	Fruit juices		Crackers in soup
	Tofu	Nectars		

Note: Applies to children aged 1 year or older.

TABLE 20–8 Foods That Can Be Added to Pureed Foods to Increase Calories and Protein

Food	Calories	Protein (g)
Infant cereal	9/Tbsp	0.25/Tbsp
Nonfat dry milk	25/Tbsp	1.3/Tbsp
Cheese	120/oz	5.0/oz
Margarine	101/Tbsp	Negligible
Evaporated milk	40/oz	1.1/oz
Vegetable oils	110/Tbsp	Negligible
Strained infant meals	100–150/jar	14.0/jar

Source: Adapted from H. Cloud, "Feeding problems of the child with special health care needs," in *Pediatric Nutrition in Chronic Diseases and Developmental Disorders: Prevention, Assessment, and Treatment* by Ekvall (ed.) © 1993 by Oxford University Press, New York, NY.

function should begin. This includes oral motor exercises, swallowing techniques, positioning during feeding, and diet modification (Kamer, Sirois, Huhmann, 2005). Strategies to minimize the risk of aspiration include having the child sit upright, supporting the trunk, and avoiding extension of the head and neck (Cloud, 2005). The consistency of foods and liquids may need to be altered for ease of swallowing.

In 2002 the American Dietetic Association published the National Dysphagia Diet, which outlines four levels of food consistencies: dysphagia puree, dysphagia mechanically altered, dysphagia advanced, and regular (National Dysphagia Diet Task Force, 2002). See Chapter 15 for details. Proper assessment and treatment of dysphagia will help optimize food and liquid intake of individuals with special health care needs. Treating dysphagia using an interdisciplinary approach is important to ensure adequate nutrition and good overall health.

DENTAL AND DIETARY PRACTICES TO PREVENT ORAL PROBLEMS

In addition to modifying foods and liquids to accommodate oral motor problems in people with developmental disabilities, maintaining good oral health in this population is imperative to help achieve optimal nutrition status. Periodontal disease is common in people with special health care needs mainly due to poor oral hygiene, in addition to other oral problems including malocclusion, bruxism, and gingival hyperplasia (USDHHS, 2004). Physical or cognitive impairments

TABLE 20–9 Recommendations to Help Minimize Oral Disease

- Encourage motivated patients to establish and maintain a daily oral care routine.
- Ensure that patients are practicing proper brushing and flossing techniques by asking them to demonstrate how they brush and floss.
- Discuss oral hygiene practices with the caretaker if the patient is unable to independently brush and floss; demonstrate basic brushing and flossing techniques to the caretaker.
- Recommend special devices to help make oral care easier including: electric/motor toothbrushes, dental floss holders, and special handles for toothbrush (for better grip).
- Suggest daily use of antimicrobial agent such as chlorhexidine. Depending on the patient's oral motor abilities, choose an appropriate method for delivery; rinsing, spraying, or brushing chlorhexidine are all equally efficacious.
- Encourage noncariogenic foods and beverages for snacks and rewards.
- Promote increased water consumption for patients taking medications that cause xerostomia.
- Suggest sugar-free medications if available; encourage water rinses after taking sugar-based medications.
- Recommend preventive measure including topical fluoride and sealants.

may result in improper brushing and flossing leading to inadequate plaque removal. Table 20–9 provides guidelines for preventing oral problems.

SUMMARY AND IMPLICATIONS FOR DENTISTRY

Unfortunately, oral health may be often overlooked in individuals with special health care needs due to other pressing medical issues. However, it is important for dental health professionals today to be aware of the oral problems commonly seen in children and adults with developmental disabilities and the negative consequences this may have on feeding and nutrition. Due to the complexity of medical, dental, and nutritional issues seen in this population, an interdisciplinary health care plan will likely be the most beneficial approach for treatment. Working together with a specialized registered dietitian will help the dental

TABLE 20–10 Additional Resources for Dental and Nutrition Services for Individuals with Special Health Care Needs

American Academy of Pediatric Dentistry
http://www.aapd.org
211 East Chicago Avenue, Suite 700
Chicago, IL 60611-2663
Phone: (312) 337-2169

American Dietetic Association
http://www.eatright.org
120 South Riverside Plaza, Suite 2000
Chicago, IL 60606-6995
Phone: (800) 877-1600

Family Voices, Inc.
http://www.familyvoices.org
2340 Alamo SE, Suite 102
Albuquerque, NM 87106
Phone: (505) 872-4774, (888) 835-5669
E-mail: kidshealth@familyvoices.org

Federation for Children with Special Needs
http://www.fcsn.org
1135 Tremont Street, Suite 420
Boston, MA 02120
Phone: (617) 236-7210, (800) 331-0688
E-mail: fcsninfo@fcsn.org

National Center on Birth Defects and Developmental Disabilities
Centers for Disease Control and Prevention
http://www.cdc.gov/ncbddd/

National Dissemination Center for Children with Disabilities
http://www.nichcy.org
P.O. Box 1492
Washington, DC 20013
Phone: (800) 695-0285
E-mail: nichcy@aed.org

National Foundation of Dentistry for the Handicapped (NFDH)
http://www.nfdh.org
1800 15th Street, Suite 100
Denver, CO 80202
Phone: (303) 534-5360
E-mail: fleviton@nfdh.org

National Maternal and Child Oral Health Resource Center (OHRC)
http://www.mchoralhealth.org
2115 Wisconsin Avenue N.W., Suite 601
Washington, DC 20007-2292
Phone: (202) 784-9771
E-mail: info@mchoralhealth.org

professional manage various oral and nutrition problems in individuals with special needs to optimize their nutritional status and overall health. Table 20–10 provides dental and nutrition services resources for this population.

QUESTIONS PATIENTS (OR CAREGIVERS) MIGHT ASK

Q. According to my dietitian, my child is not eating enough and is not growing properly. It's very difficult to feed her because every meal is such a battle. How can I make sure she gets enough calories and protein?

A. Inadequate caloric intake due to various oral motor problems puts individuals (especially children) with special health care needs at high nutritional risk. It may be necessary to modify foods to increase calorie and protein intake to meet the child's needs. For example, you can add margarine, oils, or cheese to pureed or soft foods. This way, the child can get more calories without having to eat more food.

Q. Why would a pureed diet increase my risk for cavities? What can I do to prevent this?

A. A pureed or soft diet is designed for people who have dysphagia (difficulty chewing or swallowing food). People with these feeding problems tend to hold the pureed food in their mouths longer, giving more time for bacteria to grow on their teeth.

Preventing cavities (or dental caries) or treating them early is very important for good oral health. Be sure to visit your dentist regularly. If you can't brush your teeth after every meal, try to rinse your mouth with water. Use fluoridated toothpaste (but don't swallow it) and drink tap water (usually contains some fluoride) because fluoride helps prevent tooth decay. Sealants may also protect the deep fissures and crevices of teeth from bacteria.

Q. My child has been grinding her teeth at night for several months. What should I do about this?

A. Grinding teeth, also known as bruxism, is common in children with special health care needs. Continuous bruxism may result in flattened teeth, which can lead to feeding difficulties. Bite guards are usually given to protect the child's teeth if treatment is indeed necessary and possible. Generally, bruxism is a habit that is outgrown.

CASE STUDY

Clark is an 18-month-old boy who has cerebral palsy. He is on a baby food/pureed diet and is slightly underweight for his height. His parents report that he likes to have a bottle at night to help him fall asleep and he will only drink diluted apple juice or milk. Many of his primary teeth have erupted but he hasn't visited a dentist yet due to other pressing medical needs. His medications include Dilantin, which he has just started taking recently.

Questions

1. Is a baby food/pureed diet appropriate for this child? Why or why not? What dental risks are associated with this type of diet?
2. Identify three common nutritional problems seen in individuals with special health care needs.
3. How does prolonged bottle feeding affect oral health?
4. Discuss the oral consequences of anticonvulsant medications such as Dilantin.

REFERENCES

Boyd LD, Palmer, C, Dwyer JT: Managing oral health related nutrition issues of high risk infants and children. *J Clin Pediatr Dent* 1998; 23(1):31–36.

Cloud H: Feeding problems of the child with special health care needs. In Ekvall SW (ed): *Pediatric Nutrition in Chronic Diseases and Developmental Disorders: Prevention, Assessment and Treatment*. New York: Oxford University Press, 1993.

Cloud H: Feeding problems of the child with special health care needs. In Ekvall SW, Ekvall V (eds): *Pediatric Nutrition in Chronic Diseases and Developmental Disorders: Prevention, Assessment, and Treatment*, 2nd ed. New York: Oxford University Press, 2005.

Cloud HH, Posthauer ME: Providing nutrition services for infants, children, and adults with developmental disabilities and special health care needs. *J Am Diet Assoc* 2004; 104:97–107.

Developmental Disabilities Assistance and Bill of Rights Act, PL 106–402; 2000.

Fung EB, Samson-Fang L, Stallings VA, Conaway M, Liptak G, Henderson RC, et al.: Feeding dysfunction is associated with poor growth and health status in children with cerebral palsy. *J Am Diet Assoc* 2002; 102:361–73.

Gidding SS, Dennison BA, Birch LL, Daniels SR, Gilman MW, Lichtenstein AH, et al.: American Heart Association scientific statement: Dietary recommendations for children and adolescents. *Circulation* 2005; 112(13):2061–75.

Institute of Medicine, National Academy of Sciences: *Dietary Reference Intakes for Energy, Carbohydrate, Fiber, Fat, Fatty Acids, Cholesterol, Protein, and Amino Acids (macronutrients)*. Washington DC: National Academies Press, 2002.

Kamer AR, Sirois DA, Huhmann M: Bidirectional impact of oral health and general health. In Touger-Decker R, Sirois DA,

Mobley CC (eds): *Nutrition and Oral Medicine*. Totowa, NJ: Humana Press, 2005.

McKinney LA, Palmer CA, Dwyer JT, Garcia R: Common dentally related nutrition concerns of children with special needs: Part 1 and Managing dentally related nutrition concerns of children with special needs: Part 2. *Top Clin Nutr* 1991; 6(2):70–85.

McPherson M, Arango P, Fox H, Lauver C, McManus M, Newacheck P, et al.: A new definition of children with special health care needs. *Pediatrics*. 1998; 102(1):137–40.

National Dysphagia Diet Task Force: *National Dysphagia Diet: Standardization for Optimal Care*. Chicago: American Dietetic Association, 2002.

Position of the American Dietetic Association: Providing nutrition services for infants, children, and adults with developmental disabilities and special health care needs. *J Am Diet Assoc* 2004; 104(1):97–107.

Strauss DJ, Shavelle RM, Anderson TW: Life expectancy of children with cerebral palsy. *Pediatr Neurol* 1998; 18:143–49.

U.S. Department of Health and Human Services: *Healthy People 2010: Understanding and Improving Health*, 2nd ed. Washington, DC: U.S. Government Printing Office, 2000a.

U.S. Department of Health and Human Services: *Oral Health in America: A Report of the Surgeon General—Executive Summary*. Rockville, MD: U.S. Department of Health and Human Services, National Institute of Dental and Craniofacial Research, National Institutes of Health, 2000b.

U.S. Department of Health and Human Services: *Project SPOON: Special Program of Oral Nutrition for Children with Special Needs*. Madison, WI: Office of University Publications, 1991.

U.S. Department of Health and Human Services, Administration for Children of Families: Administration on Developmental Disabilities Fact Sheet. Retrieved August 20, 2005, from: http://www.acf.dhhs.gov/programs/add.

U.S. Department of Health and Human Services, Health Resources and Services Administration, Maternal and Child Health Bureau: *The National Survey of Children with Special Health Care Needs Chartbook 2001*. Rockville, MD: Author, 2004a. Retrieved August 20, 2005, from http://mchb.hrsa.gov/chscn/pages/needs.htm.

U.S. Department of Health and Human Services, National Institutes of Health, National Institute of Dental and Craniofacial Research: *Practical Oral Care for People With Developmental Disabilities*. Bethesda, MD: National Institutes of Health, 2004b.

Chapter **21**

Effective Communication in Dental Practice

Carole A. Palmer and Glenda Butt

OBJECTIVES

The student will be able to:

- Explain why understanding food habits is essential to effective guidance.
- List the common factors that influence the food habits of individuals and groups.
- Discuss the factors that determine clients' readiness to change their habits.
- List aspects of oral health professional behavior that can undermine rapport with clients.
- Discuss the factors that can facilitate or impede the interview process.
- Discuss factors that can facilitate or impede efforts at effective client education.
- Describe oral health professional behaviors that may increase or decrease the likelihood that clients will be willing to change.
- List the major barriers to change.
- Describe strategies to assist clients to maintain change over time.

INTRODUCTION

Good patient communication skills are essential for success in clinical practice. The ability to listen to patients' concerns and problems, explain treatments and procedures effectively, and guide patients to institute better health habits are fundamental practitioner skills. Indeed, the word "doctor" evolved from the Greek word for teacher. It is often *more* difficult and challenging to communicate effectively with others than it is to provide technical services that are completely under one's own control. Many of the formal complaints lodged against dental health personnel are a result of miscommunication rather than clinical deficits.

Traditionally communication skills have been learned informally through "osmosis," by observation of mentors. However, consumer complaints to state dental boards and the lack of apparent effectiveness of informal mentoring have led to the recognition that effective communications skills can and must be learned and practiced. Dental team members need to feel that their communications skills are as important as their restorative, surgical, or prophylaxis skills. This chapter provides an overview of the important underlying principles of effective communications and provides specific strategies to foster effective patient communications. Although the communications concepts detailed here are targeted toward effective communication for diet assessment and guidance, these are foundation skills necessary for and applicable to *all* interpersonal interactions, professional and personal.

FOUNDATIONS OF EFFECTIVE NUTRITION COMMUNICATION

Types of Communication

Effective client communication involves skills in interviewing, teaching, and guiding.

Interviewing

Interviewing is a process designed to elicit needed information from the client. However, it is not a one-way street from patient to interviewer. Interviewing is a dynamic process whereby the interviewer instills trust in the client, gets the client to talk freely, and elicits important information through appropriate questioning.

Teaching

Teaching requires the use of appropriate approaches to facilitate client learning. It also requires a dynamic interchange between teacher and learner to ensure that information is correctly understood. The teacher provides information and monitors learning by obtaining constant feedback from the learner. Figure 21–1 shows this feedback system.

Guidance

Guidance involves both interviewing and teaching, with one important distinction: There is always an issue or problem to be resolved. Guidance involves identifying patient concerns and goals, problem solving, and helping implement change (Holli, Calabrese, 1998). The dental team member helps the client understand the

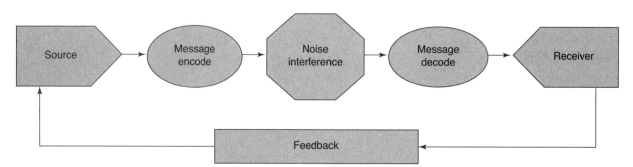

FIGURE 21-1 The process of communication.
Source: Adapted from the Shannon-Weaver model of communication, http://www.cultsock.ndirect.co.uk/MUHome/cshtml/introductory/sw.html.

issues and develop appropriate solutions to his or her unique situation.

Having a Philosophy of Communication

Most health professionals have not thought much about their "philosophy" of communication, yet the attitude and approach of the professional are crucial to the success of communication efforts. To be effective with dental clients, the oral health professional needs to adopt the approaches that have been proven most successful and adapt them to the dental setting. The most common approaches to communication are summarized as follows:

Directiveness: An Inappropriate Clinician-Centered Approach

The directive approach values the more knowing (counselor) over the less knowing (client). This approach *is* appropriate in certain situations, such as when asked for specific information, or when telling a child to "get out of the street." Unfortunately, this approach is also often used in the dental office, with undesirable results: We are being directive every time we tell someone what we think they should do. For example:

> Counselor: Now, I want you to floss every day for at least 5 minutes to reduce that gum inflammation.
> Client: Whatever you say, doctor.

When told what to do, most clients will merely nod and say okay rather than argue or speak up, but often they will not carry out the recommendations.

This directive approach is usually ineffective because:

- It does not respect the client's value and importance in making his or her own decisions.
- Directions are coming from an oral health professional who knows little about the situation of the person who has to follow them.
- It may result in suggestions that are totally inappropriate (e.g., saying "you should eat apples instead of candy" to a person who is allergic to apples).
- People who are being told what to do find many reasons for not doing it (perhaps a throwback to childhood).

Nondirectiveness: An Appropriate Client-Centered Approach

Nondirectiveness is a more appropriate approach for health promotion guidance. Nondirectiveness, commonly called client-centeredness, focuses on the client, with the health professional functioning as a facilitator (Rogers, 1965). Nondirectiveness acknowledges that the client is the only one in a position to solve his or her problem, and the professional's role is to guide the client to make the best decisions for himself or herself. The oral health professional provides information and direction to assist in the process, but clients make their own decisions. When clients make their own decisions, they are much more likely to remain committed to the changes. For example:

> Counselor: Given what you now know about the probable causes of your new dental caries, is there anything you can do about the problem?
> Client: Now I see that I haven't been brushing as well as I should be, and I've been using breath mints that I didn't realize were harmful. I am going to spend more time brushing in the evening, and switch to sugar-free mints.

Understanding Clients' Food Habits

In order to provide appropriate guidance and assistance to patients in areas that will require client follow-through, it is essential to understand as much as possible about what makes the client "tick," so to speak. This means getting to understand the factors driving current behavior so that they can be harnessed effectively to facilitate new behavior. These factors include food habits, motivation, and readiness to change.

Factors That Contribute to Food Habits

Nothing symbolizes the essence of life more than food. Food can mean love, happiness, danger, passion, identity, hospitality, romance, and security. Feeding is instinct-driven consumption, but human eating is social and encompasses learning, motivation, attitudes, values, social factors, and emotions as well as physiological needs (Curry et al., 2004).

Therefore, more important than understanding "what" people eat is the need to understand "why" they eat as they do. What are the driving factors underlying their eating habits? Food habits are intensely personal, steeped in culture, and difficult to change. No two people have the same food habits. People eat for many reasons other than hunger or appetite. Hunger is the need for fuel to feed the body. Appetite is the psychological and sensory reaction to foods that look and smell good. Appetite may also be a conditioned response—such as eating because it is noon rather than because we are hungry. Appetite, on the other hand, can be affected by many other factors such as health status and personal responses to specific foods.

A major barrier to effective dietary guidance is the failure to understand the underlying reasons for food habits, thereby making inappropriate suggestions for changes that may conflict with the client's values or lifestyle. The factors that influence food habits are discussed here and summarized in Table 21–1.

Biological and Health Factors. People differ in their ability to taste varying sensations such as sweet, sour, and bitter. These taste changes are genetically determined and can help explain differences among individuals such as why some people like artificially sweetened beverages and others find them "leaving an unpleasant aftertaste." With age and changes in the oral cavity, taste senses can become blunted, contributing to decreased desire to eat or preferences for highly flavored foods. Health conditions such as gastrointestinal disorders and lactose intolerance can help determine what foods can and cannot be eaten without negative side effects.

Social, Lifestyle, and Environmental Factors. Eating is very much a social activity. All major and most minor social occasions include food. Attitudes toward food are formed and become deeply embedded in the early childhood years, and continue to influence food choices throughout life (Curry, 1998).

Lifestyle and social interactions play an important role in determining food habits. People who are not "morning people" may arise late and grab a snack as they are running out the door in the morning (or eat nothing at all). Morning people may rise early and enjoy a leisurely big breakfast before continuing on in the day. The availability of food on the way to work or school may explain the usual morning donut and coffee. After work or school, people may go out for a drink with friends or stop by the local store for a snack before or after sports practice. In the office, a handy soda machine may explain the frequency of sodas consumed through the work day. If people live with others, and especially if others do the meal preparation, the family eating patterns usually dictate the individual habits. On the other hand, if people live alone, they may be totally responsible for what, when, and where they eat. Some people have a very structured life with well-defined eating periods. Others eat on the run and are hostage to whatever happens to be available.

TABLE 21–1 Factors Influencing Food Habits

Factors	Examples
Cultural Factors	
Ethnicity, symbolism, tradition	• Ethnic groups have strong cultural identities in which food often plays an integral role; for example, Italian emphasis on pasta and antipastos, and Hispanic staples such as plantain and cassava.
	• If changes are to be acceptable, they must be consistent with cultural food habits.
	• Foods serve as cultural symbols. For example, the turkey dinner with all of the "fixins" is the traditional Thanksgiving dinner in the United States. Birthdays are celebrated with birthday cake, candles, and ice cream. Champagne toasts are traditional at celebrations honoring individuals or groups.
	• Foods considered delicacies in some cultures are considered inedible in others. Raw fish (as sushi) is a delicacy in Asia, but may be considered worthy only as fish bait by others.
Religion	• Religious groups have retained their food practices for generations. For example, orthodox Jews do not eat dairy foods with or after meat dishes and do not eat pork or shellfish. Muslims also eschew pork and alcohol. Seventh-day Adventists are lacto-ovovegetarians.

Family	• Parents pass on their food likes and dislikes to their children whether they mean to or not. Some families always have dinnertime without outside distractions. In other families people eat in shifts due to conflicting schedules.
	• Family traditions surrounding food stay with people for a lifetime. When families merge as through marriage, for example, the composition of the traditional Thanksgiving dinner may incite conflict ("We always had baked sweet potatoes, not candied!").
Social status	• Food has social connotations. For example, caviar and paté de fois gras are considered status foods; meatloaf and macaroni and cheese are not. Candy and liquor are hostess gifts.
Geographics	• People tend to eat indigenous foods. For example, in the United States, Canada, and Europe the nucleus of the diet is often considered to be protein sources (meat, poultry, fish, beans), which are in abundant supply. In Asia, where meat is scarcer and rice is plentiful, rice is the mainstay and meat is used more as a garnish or for flavor. As improved transportation brings the world closer together, food nationalism decreases.
	• Seasonal variations also affect eating habits; when a particular food is in season, it is more available, less expensive, and eaten more often.
	• There are many regional food habit patterns. For example, in New England people eat baked beans (with molasses), brown bread, and clam chowder. Southerners eat collard greens, black-eyed peas, biscuits with country gravy, grits, and country fried steak.
	• Names of foods can differ by region: Cola in one part of the United States is called soda in another, pop in yet another, and tonic in New England.
Educational Factors	• Eating habits are strongly influenced by peer groups, friends, relatives, and mass communication (television, radio, magazines, newspapers, the Internet).
Economic Factors	• Food prices and financial considerations can greatly influence types and amounts of foods purchased.
Current trends	• Eating away from home in school, from street vendors, at food courts, or in fast-food restaurants is a current trend.
	• Reliance on prepared packaged meals and other convenience foods has increased.
Psychological Factors	
Emotional	• Food may be a way to soothe distress or discomfort. An unhappy person may "drown his pain" in food by eating excessively or gravitating to "comfort foods." Conversely, a person may develop anorexia nervosa and refuse to eat at all.
Associations with past experiences	• People avoid foods associated with former unpleasant incidents (e.g., becoming ill after eating a certain food) and gravitate toward those associated with pleasant memories (e.g., Grandma's delectable fried chicken).
Reward and punishment	• Foods can be used as manipulators of behavior ("If you eat all your vegetables, you can have ice cream for dessert"). Or favorite foods may be withheld as a method of punishment. In turn, at a young age children learn to use food to get attention and control parents (the louder they cry, the quicker they get the lollipop).
Physiological Factors	
Medical conditions	• Medical conditions such as diabetes or heart disease can cause people to change their eating habits. Some people have allergic reactions to certain foods (e.g., nuts, eggs) and must avoid them. Others have food intolerances such as lactose intolerance, which cause them to limit their consumption of milk products.
The senses	• People react positively or negatively to foods' appearance, color, consistency, or odor. Some people dislike the consistency of liver, whereas others object to the slimy sensation of custard and gelatins. Blue food is popular with children and unpopular with adults (with the exception of blueberries).

Source: Adapted from "Cultural factors in nutritional care," in *Applications in Medical Nutrition Therapy* 2/E by Zeman/Ney © 1988 by Merrill, Upper Saddle River, NJ.

Cultural, Experiential, and Religious Factors.
Cultural preferences may strongly influence what people eat. Ethnic diversity leads to many cultural dietary habits, as immigrants bring the food habits from their home country with them. The prevalence of ethnic restaurants is testament to the variety of ethnic foods available and desired by the populace. As people emigrate to different areas, they adopt the food habits of their new home, but usually maintain their homeland diet patterns as well. These patterns are held dear to them and must be considered when adaptations are needed.

People tend to retain the food habits that they become accustomed to in early family life. Such factors may include timing and content of meals (large meal at noon rather than evening), cooking practices, preferences for mother's method of cooking over others, the use of seasonings, acceptable versus unacceptable foods, to name but a few. For example, some foods that are considered delicacies in some families are considered inedible in others.

Most religions also have special dietary customs that are central to their practice. Many religions have specific foods that are prohibited, or foods that are eaten at specific times (holy days). The counselor must be aware that the client may be following specific religious dietary practices, and should determine what they are by asking the client about them. This shows respect of the client and will help the counselor avoid making any inappropriate suggestions.

Socioeconomic Factors. Some people have limited economic resources and may not be able to purchase a variety of fresh foods. Instead they may need to use processed or canned foods that will last longer. They may not have adequate transportation to grocery stores or may have to shop in nearby neighborhood stores with limited selections. Some people may not have the facilities to cook or freeze foods properly. In families where both parents work or there is only a single parent, there may not be time to prepare traditional meals and the family may rely heavily on fast foods and prepared convenience foods.

It is important not to take these conveniences of today's life for granted and assume that everyone has the same resources.

Psychological, Personal, and Emotional Factors.
Food can be highly symbolic of personal and family values. Some of these connections become prevalent in societies as well. For example, chicken soup is associated with caring, candy with love, red meat with manliness, and so on. The more entrenched these values are, the more difficult it is to change the related food habit.

Emotions can have a great impact on the food choices made from day to day. Most people at some point have turned to food for solace, relaxation, comfort or to relieve boredom or loneliness. Eating is a way to cope with emotion. Eating can also be a way to exert control. Food is often a first tool for young children in the battle for self-control and independence. Young children may refuse to eat when they realize that this is a way to get Mother to give them what they want. Young adults may develop eating disorders as one way to exert control over their lives.

Parents or other role models often pass on to children their concepts about foods and dieting, as well as their likes, dislikes, attitudes, and beliefs about food.

Understanding Clients' Attitudes and Values

Values are closely held personal feelings and attitudes. Values are all powerful because they determine the way people perceive what they hear, and they are the underpinnings of behavior. A major error of counselors is to provide clients with *information* and expect that this will result in *changed behavior*. (Figure 21–2). Increased knowledge and information of healthy food choices alone are unsuccessful in altering behavior toward choosing healthy diets (Contento et al., 1995; Lytle-Trenkner, Kelder, 1991). People filter what they hear through their personal perceptions, experiences, attitudes, and current habits. They then decide whether the information or

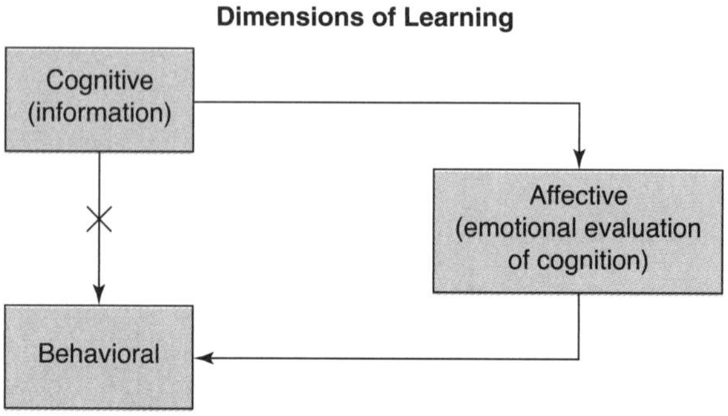

Dimensions of Learning

FIGURE 21–2 Dimensions of learning.

guidance is relevant, desirable for them, and actionable. If the clinician's approach is perceived by the client as inappropriate, the session is likely to be unsuccessful. Human values are slow to form and slow to change. Success in attaining change is determined partly by the degree of "fit" between potential change and the individual's value system. A major goal of patient communications (especially client-centered interviewing) is to help determine client values. A good counselor can then pursue an approach that will be consistent with these values (Christen, Katz, 2003).

Understanding Clients' Motivation and Readiness to Change

Motivation is the inner drive that pushes the person to satisfy a need. It cannot be produced in others; it can only be determined, fostered, and reinforced. Human motivations are extremely complex and spring from feelings, expectations, desires, attitudes, values, past experience, self-image, socioeconomic factors, and more.

Internal motivation is self-generated and usually produces long-lasting learning or action. External motivation comes from outside the individual. For example, in persuasion, reinforcement such as rewards, approval, or encouragement, or punishment, fear, and

threats are often used. Changes made under these conditions are manipulative and usually short lived, and last only as long as the reinforcer has control. Another risk inherent in threats is that clients will associate the expected action with the unpleasant threat and avoid the action entirely. Factors that can affect external motivation are numerous and, again, are best determined by skillful interviewing.

Many hours of clinicians' time (and frustration) have been wasted trying to get unwilling clients to make changes. A basic principle of behavioral change is that people will change only if they are ready and willing to do so. For this reason, the clinician must assess client readiness as part of the initial assessment. If clients aren't ready to make changes, basic information can be provided, and this reluctance should be documented in their record. The following models are useful because they provide ways for clinicians to assess client readiness to change. The dental professional can then use this information to be more effective in the counseling process.

Maslow's Hierarchy of Needs

Maslow's approach (Figure 21–3) to understanding human needs can be a useful and effective tool in the dental office (Christen, Katz, 1999). Basic human needs are physiological (e.g., food, water, sleep) and include

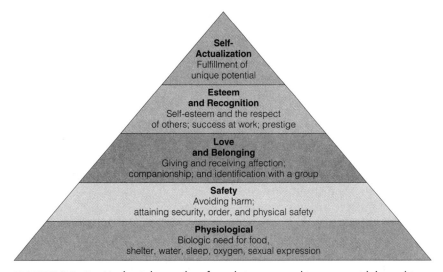

FIGURE 21–3 Maslow's hierarchy of needs is presented in a pyramidal graphic format. The size of each level represents its relative importance to the other needs in the hierarchy.
Source: Maslow, Abraham H.; Frager, Robert D.; Fadiman, James: *Motivation & Personality* 3/E © 1987. Adapted by permission of Pearson Education, Inc., Upper Saddle River, NJ.

safety and security. It is only after these needs are met that sociopsychological forces such as love and social belongingness, self-esteem, and self-actualization become prime motivators of behavior. If the oral health professional makes incorrect assumptions about the client's level of need, he or she may be ineffective. For example, if the client presents with a toothache, she is not going to be interested in improving her toothbrushing or diet until the pain is relieved. However, once the problem has been alleviated, the dental health professional might say: "Now that we've resolved your pain, I can help you try to prevent it from happening again. How does that sound?" The client may be more receptive at this point. Or the oral health professional may assume that the teenager has come to the office so that his teeth will look nice when, in reality, he is interested most in preventing bad breath. The only way that the dental professional can determine the patient's level of need is by engaging the client in conversation about himself and his needs and wishes.

The Health Belief Model

The health belief model was developed to help explain general preventive health behavior, but it is also useful for dentistry (Weinstein, Getz, Milgram, 1991). It states that people's beliefs about health determine their readiness to take action. To be ready to change the person must:

1. **Believe that she is susceptible to developing the condition.** The oral health care provider tries to convince the client that she has a dental condition that she doesn't know or believe she has. Questions such as "Why don't I feel anything then?" or "Why didn't my previous dentist tell me about this?" are clues to client skepticism. Using mirrors, radiographs, bleeding indices, pocket depths, and other visual aids helps clients discover problems for themselves and helps justify the existence of the condition.

2. **Believe that the condition is potentially serious.** Clients may also not understand the implications of the condition even if they believe they have it. They may say "everyone gets cavities" or "what's the difference, my teeth are going to fall out anyway." These are cues for the dental health professional to explain possible effects that will be meaningful to the client.

For example: "Did you know that cavities can lead to broken teeth and are preventable?" or "Did you know that gum disease can lead to heart infection?" People who come from a family of denture wearers may assume that edentulousness is inevitable. If this is the belief, where is the motivation to improve?

3. **Believe that preventive strategies are practical and the benefits outweigh the risks of inaction.** Clients may be concerned about their oral condition and its implications, but may believe that preventive management is unrealistic for them. Dental professionals unwittingly promote this barrier to action when they make unrealistic demands: "Now don't forget to brush three times a day for at least 3 minutes each time, and floss nightly for 5 minutes, and stay away from all snacks." With such directives it is no wonder that clients get discouraged and give up. Nondirective, client-centered counseling will prevent this from happening.

The counselor must skillfully elicit client information that answers two questions: First, is the client *willing*, and second, is the client *able* to enter into the change process? Determining client willingness to change involves understanding the client's values about oral health based on two factors: (1) the client's perceived need and knowledge of the oral health problem; and (2) whether the client has taken ownership of the problem.

If the client is willing to participate in the process of change then the second component of client readiness is determined—the client's ability to change. Weinstein and colleagues (1991) suggest ability is based on four factors: (1) the client's self-care orientation—whether the client is generally health conscious; (2) the client's internal or external locus of control—whether the client takes control of life's issues or believes other persons or factors will solve the problems; (3) social support systems in family and friends; and (4) absence of stress, anxiety, and chaos in one's life. Any or a combination of these factors can negatively impact the client's ability to change behavior, even if a client expresses willingness to change. Once the readiness assessment has been completed, the client's stage of change can be determined. A simplified method of determining client readiness is outlined in Figure 21–4.

Making Communication Effective

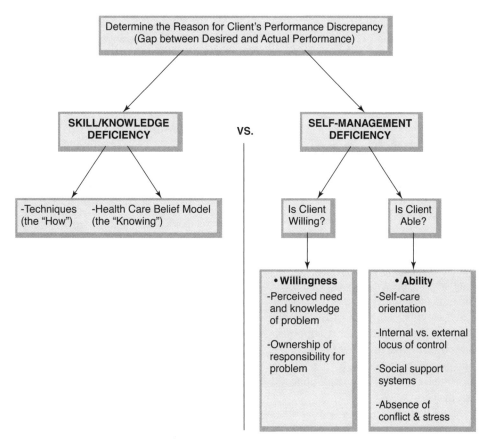

FIGURE 21–4 Assessing readiness.
Source: Adapted from *Oral Self-Care: Strategies for Preventive Dentistry* 3/E by Weinstein/Getz/Milgram
© 1991 by University of Washington, Seattle, WA.

The Stages of Change Model

Yet another model useful in dentistry to help determine and guide client motivation shows how readiness to change evolves through a series of phases or "stages of change" (Prochaska, DiClemente, 1992). The earliest is the precontemplation stage, where there is no intention to change behavior. Next is the contemplative stage, in which the client considers the change and is aware of reasons supporting change. In the next stage, the client takes early steps to change and institutes some modification of behavior. The final stage is the maintenance and relapse prevention stage, in which clients integrate the changes into their daily lives. Providing dietary information aids in the transition from the precontemplative to the contemplative stage, but does not result in behavioral change by itself. In the process of instituting change, clients may go through each step in the process several times before a stable change is achieved. Oral health care providers need to understand these stages to deal effectively with clients. Table 21–2 describes the stages of change model and shows how to deal effectively with clients at each stage of the process.

Motivational Interviewing—For Clients Ambivalent about or Not Ready for Change

This client-centered approach, borrowed from social psychology, evolved from treatment of medical patients including problem drinkers but has been adapted to a number of health care settings (Britt, Hudson, Blampied, 2004). The focus of motivational interviewing (MI) is helping clients explore and resolve their resistance or ambivalence to behavioral change using a systematic

TABLE 21-2 Stages of Change

Stage	Meaning	Implications
Precontemplation	No thought or intention to change	Provide balanced, meaningful information about issues, and leave alone for now
Contemplation	Plans to change in near future, but may be ambivalent	Help reinforce pros over cons
Readiness	Sincere desire to change	Provide specific information and guidance via nondirective counseling
Action	Has started to change	Reinforce new habits, help intervene in problem areas
Maintenance	Has put change in place	Positive reinforcement, give self-monitoring strategies
Relapse	Has neglected changes	Provide relapse prevention strategies *before* relapses occur indicate that these are normal

Source: Adapted from "Understanding Human Motivation," in *Primary Preventive Dentistry* 6/E by Christen/Katz © 2003 by Appleton and Lange, Stamford, CT.

technique (Emmons, Rollnick, 2001). The client does most of the talking while expressing his or her thoughts and feelings. Some of the clinical principles on which MI is based—such as expressing empathy, avoiding argumentation, managing resistance, and supporting self-efficacy—have been discussed earlier in the chapter. The MI systematic procedure and strategies are designed to increase the likelihood that the client will choose to make a behavioral change.

In its most simplified form using a brief intervention, MI involves four stages of suggested questioning to encourage decision making. Ask the client:

1. "How have things changed for you because of the high root caries rate," or "because of the adjustment to new dentures?"
2. "What will happen if your present behavior continues [e.g., choosing high-sugar foods as substitutes for regular meals]?"
3. "Weigh the pros and cons of possible behavior changes by writing them down."
4. "Where does that [pros and cons exercise] leave you now?"

Brief motivational interviewing was designed for use in a single 40-minute session in primary health care settings, with non-help-seeking problem drinkers (Britt et al., 2004). Studies are evaluating whether even briefer encounters of 5–10 minutes can be effective following the principles and goals of MI. The focused method is designed for health care practitioners who

have limited time with clients. MI has also been conducted by telephone in several studies.

Emmons and Rollnick suggest that concrete behavior change should not be the sole goal of counseling. The oral health care practitioner might also attempt to increase the client's readiness for change through the use of motivational interviewing.

In summary, clients are not always ready to change. Whether or not clients decide to accept counseling, it is our professional responsibility to:

- Alert them to the oral signs of poor eating habits.
- Educate them on the factors contributing to their oral condition.
- Help determine the barriers to improvement and help clients overcome them.
- Use motivational interviewing and guidance to help clients take responsibility for their own oral health.
- Document clients' improvements and barriers to improvement in their records.

THE NUTS AND BOLTS OF SUCCESSFUL COMMUNICATION

The Setting

Good communication takes place in a nonthreatening environment with few distractions. If the guidance must take place in the dental operatory, the client should be sitting upright in the chair. The tray can be used as a table to write and place visual aids such as mirror, models, and food diary. Threatening equipment (e.g., drill) should not be visible. Learning takes place during periods of moderate "anxiety," so people don't learn well if they are sleepy (e.g., lying back in the dental chair) or just before an oral surgical procedure.

The Attitude of the Dental Professional

The attitude of the oral health professional can also have a major impact on the success or failure of the communications. The oral health professional's interest in the client must be genuine. This interest or lack of it can be communicated even unconsciously to the client by facial expression and degree of attentiveness. Rapport is the mutual trust that develops between two people. Good rapport between the oral health professional and the client is the foundation for successful counseling. If the oral health professional is rushed or gives the impression that "this is what we do with all of our clients," the client may feel devalued, and this can undermine rapport. A raised eyebrow or a scowl can also undermine rapport as can showing disapproval and only half listening.

CONDUCTING THE SESSION: SIX STEPS TO SUCCESS

Effective communication is a two-way process. It involves a feedback loop where information is presented, perceived by the client, and fed back to the dental health professional to make sure it was heard. Miscommunication can occur at any point along the way. The next chapter details a stepwise process for actually conducting diet screening, education, and guidance. This section provides the essential underlying communication principles to make the diet component successful and meaningful.

1. Setting the Stage and Putting the Client at Ease Do not begin by asking the client "Would you like to have dietary counseling?" or "I would advise dietary counseling?" as this approach may be setting yourself up for a negative response from clients unused to such a service. For clients to embrace the diet component of dental care, they must first understand why diet screening is relevant to their particular dental problem.

Begin by determining why the client has come to the dental office (to determine where the client fits on Maslow's hierarchy of needs). Then explain the purpose

of the session from the perspective of why it is important for the client. For example, you might ask, "How did you happen to come to our office?" A response of "I have a toothache" versus "I heard that you give good family care" will result in very different next steps. You might ask, "Do you know what we're going to discuss at this visit?" The client may say, "Yeah, you're gonna tell me what I can't eat." The client's preconceived negative attitude will be a major barrier to success and must be dispelled. You might say: "Actually, we aren't going to tell you what to eat or not eat. You mentioned that you have a lot of decay. Today we're going to try to determine what is causing the decay and see if there are things that you can do to control it. How does that sound to you?" Asking the client to agree with the plan is an important strategy to elicit partnership. The client might even sigh with relief that this is not going to be yet another "dos and don'ts" session. This approach focuses on helping solve the problem rather than assign blame.

It is also important to begin by discussing topics that are comfortable to the client. People can be threatened when the dental health professional makes assumptions about the client's knowledge of his own condition. For example:

> Counselor: Your periodontal disease is severe so we need to get going on home care right away.
> Client: What do you mean? I didn't know I had periodontal disease.

This approach places the client on the defensive and can undermine rapport. The Johari window model (Figure 21–5) demonstrates how the initial approach can facilitate or undermine communications from the earliest stages.

2. Determining the "Why" of the Diet: The Interview The interview should be an open conversation between participants, not a cross-examination. The interviewer asks questions, the client responds, and the interviewer listens and follows up on the responses. The counselor must project the warmth, empathy, and respect needed to establish rapport.

The most practical and effective way to conduct the interview is to ask the client to describe a typical day. This approach allows the information to emerge in context, like a mental videotape. When the client recounts the day from earliest morning to bedtime, the

	Known to self	Not known to self
Known to others	I Area of free activity	II Blind area
Not known to others	III Avoided or hidden area	IV Area of unknown activity

In Quadrant I, "the Arena," both parties know the particular piece of information about the subject individual. Open communication is based on common assumptions and knowledge.

In Quadrant II, "the Façade," the client knows something about himself that the health professional is unaware of. The choice is up to the client whether or not to bring the information into the open (self-disclosure).

In Quadrant III, "the Blind Spot," the health professional is aware of something about the client that the client himself is unaware of. The issue is how the health professional can inform the client about his "blind spot" in a non-threatening manner.

Quadrant IV, "the Unknown," is an area unknown by either the client or the health professional. This is an important area in psychotherapy, but probably not relevant to dentistry.

FIGURE 21–5 Johari window.
Source: Wikipedia, http://en.wikipedia.org/wiki/Johari_window.

information is easily remembered, unlike with a list of isolated questions and answers. This also provides important insight into the client's lifestyle and values.

Ask Questions Appropriately

The wording of questions in interviews is as important as manner and tone of voice. A friendly approach communicates the desire to understand and help. The types of questions asked should require the client to talk 60–70% of the time (Holli, Calabrese, 1991). The two common types of questions are closed-ended and open-ended. Closed-ended questions require simple information such as "How old are you?" or "How many snacks do you have a day?" Open-ended questions invite exploration such as "What is a usual day like for you?" Each has its place. Certainly it wouldn't be worthwhile to say to a client "Tell me a little bit about your age." Nor would it be appropriate to say "Do you eat three meals a day?" (example of a leading question). In general, if you need specific facts, use closed-ended questions. If you want understanding, use open-ended questions. Leading questions lead the client to one answer over another, such as "You do eat breakfast, don't you?" These types of questions should be avoided. Table 21–3 compares the types of questions.

Be an Active, Reflective Listener

The art of listening is essential to good communication. By carefully listening to what a client is saying, essential issues may emerge that may assist the counselor to understand the client. The active listener hears what the client is saying, paraphrases (or reflects back) what the client has said, and picks up on statements that may need further probing or clarification. The active listener recognizes and addresses the feelings underlying clients' statement (Geboy, 1985). Active listening is useful in dentistry, as it:

- Allows the oral health professional to check understanding of the client's feelings to ensure accuracy of the message received.

TABLE 21-3   Types of Questions

Type of Question	Advantages	Disadvantages	Example
Closed-ended	• Gives interviewer control • Provides quick answers • Gives specific facts • Explains "what"	• Discourages exploration • Leads to possibly incomplete answers • Results in more questions	How much? How many? When, where, how often, do you?
Open-ended	• Gives patient control • Shows trust and interest • Elicits patient values and • Explains "why"	• Is more time consuming • Results in unneeded information	What about? Please tell me about, could you describe, how do you feel about . . . , attitudes
Leading	• None	• Shows interviewer biases • Forces simple answer	Why? Didn't you say, . . .

Source: Adapted from *Communication and Education Skills: The Dietitian's Guide* 2/E by Holli/Calabrese © 1991 by Lea & Febiger, Philadelphia, PA.

- Indicates caring by the oral health professional.
- Helps the client verbalize feelings.
- Encourages the client to continue talking.
- Effectively manages emotional arousal.
- Facilitates counselor–client rapport (Darby, Walsh, 2003; Geboy, 1985).

Example
Client: I don't know what to do about my teeth. I feel like giving up.
Counselor: You sound very frustrated. What have you been through before this visit?

Here the oral health care professional picks up on the client's frustration and encourages the client to discuss concerns.

Example
In recounting a typical day's food intake, Steven, age 12, said that he started his breakfast with a glass of fruit juice, and that he drank several other glasses of juice throughout the day. Because Steven's family consisted of nine brothers and sisters and they were receiving social assistance, we suspected that drinking large amounts of fruit juice may not have been economically feasible. By gentle probing ("What kind of juice do you drink Steven?") we found that he was drinking orange *drink* rather than orange juice, and it was diluted half-strength to make it go farther. Although feelings were not addressed in this case, accuracy of food intake could have been easily overlooked had the interviewer not been listening attentively.

The interviewer who is not actively listening may ignore or trivialize clients' expressed concerns:

Example
Client: I hate dentists.
Counselor: What do you usually have for breakfast?
Or
Client: I hate dentists.
Counselor: You shouldn't hate dentists; we're nice people.

Don't Cut Off the Client
Inexperienced interviewers are often so intent on thinking of the next question that they are not actively listening, and they cut off the client in midsentence. When this happens, most clients feel rebuffed and insulted, and will hesitate to speak freely any longer. Few will be bold enough to speak up and finish the sentence.

Cutting off the client conveys to the client that the interviewer isn't really listening to what is being said. In addition to undermining rapport, interrupting a client's train of thought may also produce incomplete and inaccurate information.

Example
Counselor: What do you usually have for breakfast?
Client: Coffee, juice, toast, um—
Counselor: And what about lunch?

The client would have continued to state that he also ate eggs and bacon, but when interrupted, he hesitated to continue. Common courtesy demands that we let the client finish answering the first question completely before asking a second, but more than just courtesy is at stake.

Maintain Eye Contact

The client's mannerisms and facial expressions provide insight into his or her personality, attitudes, and reactions and may belie the client's words. Eye-to-eye contact can provide feedback about a client's unspoken feelings. Discovering how and what the client really feels is an important goal.

Interviewers are often so concerned with their questions or details, that they pay little attention to the client's physical reactions and expressions. Yet, the client's facial expressions will indicate when we are talking down to her or over her head, or reaching her at the proper level, or making impractical suggestions.

The following is an example of a situation in which awareness of the client's facial expressions made the difference between success and failure.

During a dental visit, the dental student asked Danny (age 12) if he could possibly brush his teeth after lunch at school. Danny said he couldn't because he didn't have time. The dental student then started to write a note to Danny's teacher asking that he be given special permission to brush his teeth at lunchtime. While the dental student was busily writing, a look of despair came over Danny's face. The dental student's instructor instinctively reacted by saying to him, "Danny, you look very unhappy. What's the matter?" "I can't brush after lunch because the kids will laugh at me," he replied. So the instructor asked Danny how else he might solve the problem. Danny said he might try to rinse out his mouth after eating. The note to the teacher was discarded.

A month or so later Danny returned for a revisit smiling broadly. He took out of his pocket what appeared to be a pen, but when he pulled it apart, it was a toothbrush. On his own initiative he had found the cleverly disguised toothbrush in a local store and uses it at school without the fear of being ridiculed by his classmates (Palmer, 1972).

If the instructor had not been observing Danny's pained look and had not probed for the real problem (concern over peer acceptance), this session probably would have failed in its goal. As it turned out, the solution to the problem was realistically and successfully arrived at by the client himself with the help of the instructor who observed the client's response and promptly acted on it.

Avoid Passing Judgment (Verbal or Nonverbal)

Possibly the greatest barrier to effective counseling is judgmentalism by the dental professional. It is important to listen to whatever the client says without passing personal judgment. This can be extremely difficult since we all have opinions and are used to expressing them. Nevertheless, passing judgment on the client often results in mistrust and unwillingness of the client to open up further. The basis for any communication must be honesty and truthfulness. Clients can easily be encouraged to lie if they sense that they will be reprimanded for the truth. They will tell us what they think we want to hear rather than the truth.

Even the most subtle signs of judgment can destroy the rapport. Judgmentalism can be nonverbal (raised eyebrow, disgusted look) or verbal ("You had pizza for breakfast!").

Example:

A dental student and her client were developing a nice rapport until the child told the student that he had two candy bars and a soft drink for breakfast. At this, the dental student responded, "Two candy bars and a soft drink! Didn't you have anything else?" This remark indicated extreme disapproval of the breakfast. Furthermore, her question implied that not only was the meal unacceptable but it was inadequate as well.

People may react to this scolding in one of several ways:

- They may feel threatened and refuse to talk further except for "yes" and "no" answers.
- They may fabricate the type of lunch and dinner that they think the dental health professional would like to hear.
- They may become rebellious and make up a fictitious lunch and dinner that are twice as bad as the actual ones.

In any of these scenarios, rapport between client and dental health professional is undermined and the client may no longer feel free to be open and honest.

Positive judgment (approval) can be just as harmful at the earliest stages of the relationship because this still shows personal judgment by the dental health professional. For example, the dental health professional may express approval of the client's breakfast. However, what if the client skipped lunch? The chances are that he will be reticent to admit the truth, so he may resort to lying in an attempt to please again.

A more appropriate approach is to listen and respond nonjudgmentally by using response that merely paraphrases back to the client content that was heard (reflective response). For example: "OK, so you had no breakfast and had a candy bar for lunch; then what happened?" This response is nonthreatening to the client and encourages further honest responses. Acknowledge any statement with a nod, and encourage the client to go on. By doing this, the client appreciates that we are listening attentively and are interested in hearing more, but are not going to pass judgment.

Interestingly, once a relationship has been built, these rules can be relaxed to some extent because comments will be perceived as caring rather than critical.

3. Facilitating the Instructional Process

Give a man a fish and he eats for a day
Teach a man to fish and he eats for a lifetime
Chinese proverb

Make Learning Effective

As with interviewing, effective teaching is a skill that requires an understanding of how people learn. The adult learns by building on what he already knows. All new information is integrated into his existing knowledge.

Furthermore, information needs to be understood and remembered. Learning occurs best when as many senses as possible are involved. The more involved the client is in the educational process, the greater the learning.

People learn least well what they merely hear. Their minds can wander and they may be only half-listening. Furthermore, they must translate what they hear into concrete perception that can be inaccurate.

People learn better what they can also see. That is why pictures, charts, models, radiographs, or other visual aids are important. Visual aids help prevent misperceptions by ensuring that client and oral health care professional are seeing the same thing.

TABLE 21–4 How People Remember

People remember:
10% of what they read
20% of what they hear
30% of what they see
50% of what they see and hear
70% of what they say
90% of what they say and do

Source: Adapted from *Communication and Education Skills for Dietetics Professionals* 3/E by Holli/Calabrese © 1998 by Williams & Wilkins, Baltimore, MD.

People learn best when they actually participate because they are then totally involved. This is why clients need to be involved in their own plaque assessment and diet screening. When the client actively participates, behavioral change is more likely to occur. Table 21–4 shows how people remember.

Communicate on the Client's Level: Always Ask before You Tell

Because people learn by incorporating new ideas into their current knowledge base, it is important to determine what the client knows before providing information. A major common error in teaching is to provide information before determining what the client already knows. When this happens, one of two things may occur:

1. We may talk down to the client, thereby insulting his intelligence, boring him, and making him realize that we aren't interested enough in him to find out what he already knows.
2. We may talk "way over her head" and lose her completely. She will become confused and may be too embarrassed to admit it. Most people who find themselves in this situation are embarrassed to speak up and admit their ignorance.

The only way to determine what the client already knows about a specific topic is to ask in a nonthreatening manner. For example, "What is your understanding of what causes gum disease?" This allows the client to offer his understanding of the topic, and it gives the dental health professional a clear view of the client's level of knowledge. Never make assumptions about a client's specific oral health knowledge based on age, education, profession, or other stereotype (some

5-year-olds know the caries process from watching children's television, and some PhD candidates in physics think that caries result when "food sticks between your teeth and rots").

By determining a client's level of knowledge, the dental health professional can then provide additional information and clarification. This fosters rapport by indicating that the information is specifically relevant and personalized—not just something that we tell all our clients.

It is important to avoid using jargon that the client may not understand. Instead, provide a definition for each term that might be new to the client.

Also, it is the job of the teacher, not the student, to make sure that learning has taken place. Periodically the educator should monitor client understanding by asking open-ended questions such as "In your own words, what does what we just covered mean to you?" or "How would you explain to your mother what we went over today?" Unfortunately, all too often the exchange goes like this:

> Counselor: Do you understand what I told you
> about periodontal disease?
> Client: Yes.
> Counselor: Good.

In summary, the "always ask before you tell" rule is an important tool to facilitate optimal learning at all ages.

4. Assessing and Diagnosing the Problem The process of interviewing and educating the client should lead naturally to the client's ability to assess her own eating habits as she relates to general adequacy and oral health risk. The nondirective, client-centered philosophy is best served by having the client assess her own diet. The counselor can guide the client in the process but the client should conduct the self-assessment and determine the findings. This is an important concept because it gives the responsibility for judgment to the client and eliminates the need for judgment by the counselor that may put the client on the defensive. For example:

Wrong Way
> Counselor: Now we are going to evaluate your
> diet to see if you're missing anything and
> to see if what you're eating is causing your
> tooth decay.
> Client: There's nothing wrong with what I eat.
> I have been eating this way for as long as
> I can remember.

Better Way
> Counselor: Now that you understand the
> relationships between diet and oral
> health, why don't you look at your eating
> habits and see if you can rule out diet
> as a contributing factor in your dental
> situation.
> Client: This should be interesting. I never
> thought that my diet might have something
> to do with my dental problems.

5. Fostering Client Change When the client, with the counselor's assistance, has assessed the general adequacy and oral health risks of his diet, if the need for change is evident, the next step is to help the client make improvements (Lechky, 1995).

The successful oral health professional is sensitive to the client's feelings, and understands how the client's personal and environmental situation may affect attitudes and the ability to change. The unsuccessful oral health professional overlooks these essential personal factors and concentrates solely on the facts.

Have the Client Make All Decisions for Change

It is important to have the client make all decisions for change. When the oral health professional has guided the client through a process of understanding what he is doing and how it relates to the dental condition, the client should be able to make practical improvements based on what he has learned. For example, we would not say, "Don't you think you could have an apple instead of a candy bar?" Rather we would say, "Now that you understand how those hard candies can affect your teeth, can you think of ways that you can improve the situation?"

It is a great temptation to think for the client and to work out a solution for him. However, it is better to have the client develop strategies that may not be ideal but that he has chosen and can live with. Diet suggestions may seem perfect from a nutritional standpoint, but if they are unrealistic, they will end up in the wastebasket. This is why preprinted, nonpersonalized diet sheets should never be used as primary counseling materials.

Additionally, when people have committed (verbally or in writing) to a course of action (sometimes called contracting), there is much greater likelihood that they will follow through with promises.

Make Sure Changes Are Realistic

Some clients are so eager to improve that they commit themselves to changes that seem unrealistic. It is the oral health professional's job to maintain reality checks by saying things such as "Are you sure you want to try all of this at once?" It is important to make sure that patients do not commit to too much change at once (even when they are making the suggestions), as that sets them up for failure. When people try to do too much at once and fail, they often give up entirely. It is better to set modest, manageable, short-term goals that can be successful (Barker, 1994) (Figure 21–6). Success provides positive reinforcement and gives the client incentive to do more.

Overcome Resistance and Barriers to Change

The change process faces many potential barriers that can occur in any health and lifestyle guidance (Baranowski, Perry, Parcel, 1997; Ley, 1988; Perry, Lytle, Kelder, 1994). Understanding the factors that motivate individuals will help guide the process of overcoming or avoiding barriers to change. It is the dental health professional's responsibility to develop a climate in which the client can make realistic suggestions.

It is also important to avoid creating any situation that could cause the client to become antagonistic. The following are some potential causes of client resistance or negativity:

- The client perceives that she is going to be told what she is doing wrong.
- The client does not understand the purpose of the session.

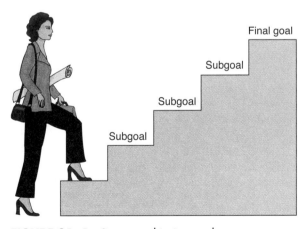

FIGURE 21-6   Steps to achieving goals.

- The dental health professional, by passing judgment, may have put the client in a situation that threatens her ego or deflates her self-esteem.
- The oral health professional may have bulldozed the client into making choices that she may not be truly motivated to follow.
- The dental health professional may create a conflict between what is therapeutically ideal and what is realistic by not being sufficiently aware of the client's life situation. This is avoided by having the client make her own decisions for changes.

Apply Strategies from Transactional Analysis

Transactional analysis (TA) is a useful way to understand how communications between people work and how to resolve conflicts when they occur. TA was developed by Berne (1973) and popularized in his book *I'm OK— You're OK*. Developed from the work of Freud, it showed that everyone has the potential at any time to behave from one of three inherent ego states: the parent (P), the adult (A), and the child (C). The child aspect of personality (C) is a collection of natural feelings developed before having developed the capacity to think rationally. The child (C) is emotional, irrational, and even magical. The parent (P) aspect of personality incorporates values from the adult world and forms a belief structure of social expectations and values used to be critical, prejudiced, and directive. The adult (A) ego state's primary role is to logically mediate between the two illogical ego states P and C. The A produces rational concepts and can think, analyze, and reconcile the P and the C (Curry, Jaffe, 1998). The ego states can be identified by voice, facial expression, posture, vocabulary, and gestures. Communication between people is really between ego states. For example, if you are speaking in ego state A, and expect a response in A but get it in P or C, the communication stops until one of the parties involved changes ego state to be complementary. This is called a cross transaction. This all may seem complicated, but actually is simple and useful. Here is an example:

a. Counselor: What did you have to eat this morning? (A)
   Client: I had a bowl of cereal, coffee, and orange juice. (A)

                    vs.

b. Counselor: What did you have to eat this morning? (A)

Client: If I tell you you'll just yell at me. (C)

vs.

c. Counselor: What did you have to eat this morning? (A)

Client: Aren't you pretty young to be trying to counsel me? (P)

In scenario *a*, the counselor asked a question and the client responded in a complementary fashion, unlike in scenarios *b* and *c* where the client acted either as a child or a parent rather than an adult. When this occurs, the counselor needs to probe for the reasons why the client is acting as he is and try to get him back to a more equal transaction. A reflective response is often a useful way to do this. For example, in scenario *b* the counselor might respond, "It appears that you have had bad experiences with people yelling at you; would you be willing to tell me about them?" Or in scenario *c*, the counselor might say "Yes I am young,

but I have knowledge and experience that I hope I can share with you if you are interested." Figure 21–7 shows examples of how the TA model can be most useful in dentistry.

6. Maintaining Change Change occurs slowly over time, and must be reassessed periodically and reinforced. If one approach isn't working, other strategies should be pursued. For example, the client may have decided to try artificial sweeteners in her coffee. However, she may have found the substitutes leave an aftertaste. The dental health professional may help by suggesting another sweetener or cutting back on the amount used. With each dental visit, the diet modifications should be reviewed along with home care strategies.

As self-management programs have evolved, emphasis has been placed on helping people modify the factors surrounding the target changes as well as their thoughts and beliefs about the changes. The dental professional can help the client maintain change by helping

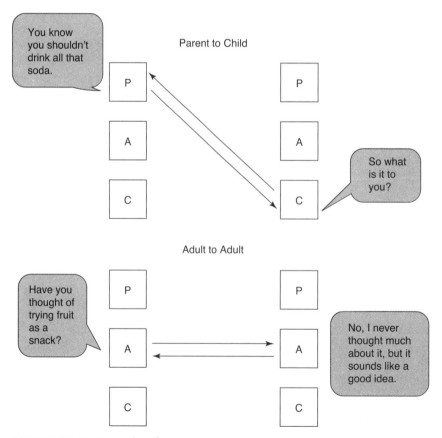

FIGURE 21–7 *Examples of transactions.*

TABLE 21–5 Helping Maintain Habits through Rewards and Lapse Rebounding

Rewards

Having family and friends help support change.

Using self-monitoring (e.g., food diary, disclosing tablets) to stay on track.

Giving rewards for staying on track (not food).

Lapse Rebounding

Encourage clients to avoid attributing lapses to lack of "will power" and to look for specific factors associated with the lapses.

Encourage clients to see lapses as single, reversible events rather than signs of total failure.

Encourage clients to learn from the experience so that they can avoid another lapse in motivation.

Source: From *Communication and Behavior Management in Dentistry* by Geboy © 1985 by Williams & Wilkins, Baltimore, MD.

her set up a reward and reinforcement system. It is also important to prepare clients for lapses in motivation; temporary lapses are common. Preparing clients in advance for lapses decreases the likelihood that they will give up in frustration. Table 21–5 lists ways to help clients reward follow-through and overcome temporary lapses.

TIPS FOR SUCCESSFUL COMMUNICATION AND GUIDANCE

The oral health care professional:

- Treats all clients with equal respect and dignity.
- Focuses on helping clients help themselves rather than correcting error and wrongdoing.
- Communicates well with clients by developing rapport with them and having a nonjudgmental approach that alleviates their fear of reprimand or disapproval.
- Personalizes the approach to the specific client's needs, current habits, and life situation.
- Provides clients with the information they need about their own oral condition rather than a "canned" presentation.
- Seeks out clients' opinions and wishes rather than trying to force personal opinions on them.
- Encourages clients to make the decisions for improvement themselves, and provides suggestions as potential options rather than directives.

Figure 21–8 summarizes the factors involved in effective communication.

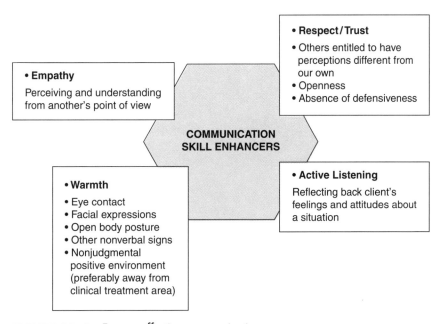

FIGURE 21–8 Factors affecting communication.

SUMMARY AND IMPLICATIONS FOR DENTISTRY

The dental health professional needs to be able to communicate effectively with clients to foster a successful collaboration that will promote good oral health. Poor communication can lead to misunderstanding, hostility, lack of follow-up with home care strategies, and even lawsuits.

Oral health care team members need to attend to their communications skills as carefully as they do their clinical skills. The best clinical dentistry can fail if the client doesn't maintain it. Role playing with colleagues or others who will be honest is one approach to hone communication skills. Communication is a learned skill that requires practice and can always be improved. The time spent improving communications skills will have a lifetime of value for both patient care and life in general.

QUESTIONS PATIENTS MIGHT ASK

Q. Why are you asking me about my diet? No dentist has ever asked me these questions before.

A. As we learn more about the importance of diet on oral health, it becomes more important not to overlook nutrition when we provide you with comprehensive oral health care.

Q. Why are you asking me about lifestyle, my past dental experiences, and the dental health of other family members?

A. I am trying to get an understanding of what kind of activities you engage in and where oral health falls on your list of priorities in your life. That way, I can help you with strategies that will fit into your unique lifestyle and therefore will work for you.

CASE STUDY

Mr. Bronsen is a 75-year-old retired farmer who has come to you for a new partial denture. He complains that "several of my teeth are sore around the roots." Your oral examination reveals moderate gingivitis and 7 new carious lesions on the root surfaces, primarily in molar areas. Mrs. Bronsen does most of the cooking, and Mr. Bronsen likes to snack on dried prunes throughout the day because he likes the taste and says they help his constipation.

Note the following scenarios:

1. Dentist: Mr. Bronsen, we're going to evaluate your diet to find out what you're doing wrong with your eating.
   Mr. Bronsen: There's nothin' wrong with my eating. I'm a farmer, and my wife cooks great.

2. Dentist: Oh, I'm sure she does but the first thing you'll have to do is eliminate all those prunes.
   Mr. Bronsen: But I need the prunes for my bowels.

Questions:
1. What error did the dentist make in scenario #1?
2. Why was the dentist's response inappropriate in scenario #2?
3. What is the best way to determine what Mr. Bronsen knows about his oral condition?
4. If, during the course of your session with Mr. Bronsen, he begins to look distracted and uneasy, what would be the most appropriate response?

REFERENCES

Baranowski T, Perry CL, Parcel GS: How individuals, environments, and health behavior interact: Social cognitive theory. In Glanz K, Lewis FM, Rimer B (eds): *Health Education and Health Behavior*. San Francisco: Jossey-Bass, 1997.

Barker T: Realistic dietary advice for patients. *Dent Update* 1994; 21(1):28–34.

Berne E: *Games People Play*. New York: Ballentine Books, 1973.

Britt E, Hudson S, Blampied N: Motivational interviewing in health settings: A review, Department of Psychology, Univ. of Canterbury, Christchurch, New Zealand. *Patient Education and Counseling* 2004; 53:147–55.

Christen AG, Katz CA: Understanding human motivation. In Harris NO, Garcia-Godoy F: *Primary Preventive Dentistry*, 6th ed. Stamford: Appleton and Lange, 2003.

Contento I, Balch GI, Bronner YL, Lytle LA, Maloney SK, Olson CM, et al.: The effectiveness of nutrition education and implications for nutrition education policy, programs, and research: A review of research. *J Nutr Educ* 1995; 36: 277–420.

Curry R, Jaffe A: *Nutrition Counseling and Communication Skills*. Philadelphia: W.B. Saunders, 2004.

Darby M, Walsh M: *Dental Hygiene Theory and Practice*. Philadelphia: W.B. Saunders, 1995.

Emmons KM, Rollnick S: Motivational interviewing in health care settings. Opportunities and limitations. [Review] [40 refs] *Am J Prev Med* 2001; 20(1):68–74.

Geboy MJ: *Communication and Behavior Management in Dentistry*. Baltimore: Williams & Wilkins, l985.

Holli B, Calabrese RJ: *Communication and Education Skills for Dietetics Professionals*, 3rd ed. Baltimore: Williams & Wilkins, 1998.

Holli BB, Calabrese RJ: *Communication and Education Skills: The Dietitian's Guide*, 2nd ed. Philadelphia: Lea & Febiger, l991.

Lechky O: Persuasion techniques can motivate patients to change eating behaviors. *Can Med Assoc J*, 1995; 152(4): 583–85.

Ley P: *Communicating with Patients*. London: Croom Helm, 1988.

Lytle-Trenkner LA, Kelder SH: *Nutrition Education and School Food Service Intervention as Components of Comprehensive School Health Education: Final Report to the American Cancer Society's Advisory Committee on Technology Transfer of Behavioral Research*. Atlanta: American Cancer Society, 1991.

Palmer C: The art of communication and counseling. In Nizel AE: *Nutrition in Preventive Dentistry*. Philadelphia: Science and Practice, 1972.

Perry CL, Lytle LA, Kelder SH: Teaching healthful eating habits. In Filer LJ, Lauer RM, Luepker RV (eds): *Prevention of Atherosclerosis and Hypertension Beginning in Youth*. Philadelphia: Lea & Febiger, 1994.

Prochaska JO, DiClemente CC, Norcross JC: In search of how people change. *Am Psychol* 1992; 47(9):1102–14.

Rogers C: *Client-Centered Therapy: Implications and Theory*. Boston: Houghton Mifflin, 1965.

Weinstein P, Getz T, Milgram P: *Oral Self-Care: Strategies for Preventive Dentistry*, 3rd ed. Seattle, WA: Continuing Dental Education, University of Washington, 1991.

Zeman FJ, Ney DM: Cultural factors in nutritional care. In Zeman FJ, Ney DM: *Applications in Medical Nutrition Therapy*, 2nd ed. Upper Saddle River, NJ: Merrill, 1988.

Chapter **22**

Principles of Diet Screening, Risk Assessment, and Guidance

Carole A. Palmer

OBJECTIVES

The student will be able to:

- Describe how diet screening and guidance can be integrated into dental practice.
- Discuss the concept of risk assessment as it applies to diet care.
- Detail a logical procedure for conducting diet screening, education, and guidance.
- List the steps to effective diet care and describe their underlying principles.
- Discuss appropriate strategies for helping motivate clients to improve dietary behaviors.
- Describe some of the common errors made in diet screening and guidance in dental practice.
- Discuss how to follow up and reevaluate initial diet care.

INTRODUCTION

As prior chapters show, diet and nutrition have many implications in oral health. Problems in the oral cavity can affect food intake and resulting nutritional status. Conversely, dietary factors can impact oral health directly or indirectly. For these reasons, the dental team needs to be able to recognize dietary concerns if they exist and provide appropriate guidance and referral. Diet risk assessment, guidance, and referral should be standard components of clinical dental care. Just as blood pressure is taken routinely as a screening tool in the dental office, dietary risk assessment should also be included as a component of total oral risk assessment. Since the dental team sees clients more often than physicians or dietitians do, dental team members are important "gatekeepers" for recognizing dietary risk and referring patients to dietitians and physicians for further care when indicated.

The American Dental Association and the American Dental Hygienists' Association both have position statements regarding nutrition that can be summarized as follows:

The role of the dental team regarding nutrition should be to:

- maintain current knowledge of nutrition recommendations.
- encourage dentists to effectively educate and counsel their patients about proper nutrition and oral health, including eating a well-balanced diet and limiting the number of between-meal snacks.
- work with school officials to ensure that school food services, including vending services and school stores, provide nutritious food selections.
- oppose targeting children in the promotion and advertisement of foods low in nutritional value and high in cariogenic carbohydrates. (Preventive Health Statement on Nutrition and Oral Health, 1996).

Despite the acknowledgment that risk assessment and counseling are important components of dental practice, one group of dentists admitted that few of them actually implemented these services in their practices. The primary reason for not doing so was a lack of confidence in their ability or that of their hygienists to conduct meaningful and appropriate diet risk assessment and counseling (Palmer, Dwyer, Clark, 1990).

To help rise above this problem, this chapter will provide a simple, stepwise procedure for integrating diet risk assessment and guidance into dental practice. We will offer an organized procedure to follow, and describe common pitfalls and how to avoid them. The accompanying CD-ROM/DVD demonstrates this risk assessment and counseling process, applying the counseling principles detailed in Chapter 21. It is important to practice this procedure (role play) to become comfortable with the process. With practice, diet risk assessment and guidance can become as second nature as any other routine dental procedure.

WHAT IS THE APPROPRIATE SCOPE OF DIET INTERVENTION IN DENTAL PRACTICE?

Nutritional versus Dietary Assessment

The type of diet interventions appropriate to dental practice are different from the nutritional services provided by a registered dietitian or other licensed nutritionist, but should be complementary. The role of the dental team is to conduct routine diet risk assessment. The assessment conducted in dental practice is a general qualitative assessment using reported diet to screen for risk (Boyd et al., 1998).

This process is *not* to be confused with true nutritional assessment. *Nutritional* assessment requires physiological, anthropometric, and biochemical analyses to determine actual nutritional status, and is beyond the scope of dental practice. *Diet* assessment involves assessing reported dietary intake in comparison to an accepted standard. If the initial screening shows a need for further assistance, then a more in-depth assessment or referral to a registered dietitian is indicated.

If the diet screening indicates, the dental team should provide dietary guidance to help clients improve general diet quality or dietary factors related to oral health. Clients with more complicated dietary issues related to underlying medical conditions need to be referred to a physician and registered dietitian.

Which Clients Need Diet Screening?

Diet care for dental clients may be at the level of true prevention or intervention. *Prevention* is proactive, and involves helping clients prevent problems from occurring. Examples would be:

- Information on diet and caries prevention for all age groups.

- Guidance to individuals who have a high risk of developing caries such as those with xerostomia.
- Diet guidance for clients about to receive dentures or have oral surgery or radiation therapy.

Intervention is reactive, and attempts to intervene to solve problems that already exist. Intervention would include providing guidance and making appropriate referrals. Examples would be clients with:

- Dental conditions in which diet likely plays a causative role (e.g., new or recurrent dental caries including root caries).
- Another oral condition in which diet may play a role such as oral lesions, impaired healing, or severe periodontal disease, unexplainable by local factors.
- A dental condition that could affect diet and eating ability such as oral surgery, oral cancer, dentures, xerostomia, malocclusion, or face/head trauma.
- A medical condition that can affect or be affected by nutrition and oral health (e.g., radiation therapy, immune-compromising conditions, diabetes mellitus, eating disorders, or physical disabilities).
- Lifestyle factors that may affect oral health and nutrition such as older people living alone or those on restrictive diets or having unusual eating habits.

Dietary risk factors are rarely evident clinically. It is usually not possible to detect a dietary problem solely by visual signs or by asking general questions. So it is a major mistake to assume that if there are no clinical signs of a problem, then there is no problem. Clinical signs are evident only in later stages of deficiency or toxicity when the condition is far advanced. For this reason, if observable clinical signs are used as the sole criterion for diagnosing nutritional problems, most will be missed (see Figure 22–1).

Another common mistake is to use client feedback exclusively to judge dietary status. For example, the clinician asks, "How are you eating, Mrs. Martin?" Mrs. Martin responds, "Just fine, thank you," and the clinician reports that Mrs. Martin's nutritional status is "fine." The error in this case is using subjective information (client's statement) as criteria for an objective judgment (diet status).

Thus, clinical signs or client responses cannot be relied on as determinants of dietary risk. Rather, all clients should be screened for dietary risk as a component of total risk in a systematic way to determine current status, contributing factors, and level of risk for developing future dental conditions (Hildebrand, 1995; Stoddard, 1995; Suddick, 1997; Tinanoff, 1995).

DIET SCREENING IN THE 21ST CENTURY: COMPUTERIZED DIET ASSESSMENT PROGRAMS

Computer-assisted diet assessment is used routinely by nutrition professionals to assess general nutrient adequacy of reported diets. Such programs can be useful

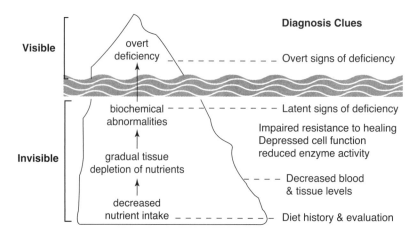

FIGURE 22-1 Progress of nutritional deficiency.

in the dental office because they can save time and provide greater potential accuracy than the approach just described; however, there are also significant limitations for dental use. For example, these programs usually do not address major issues specific to dentistry such as the cariogenic potential of dietary patterns. Furthermore, the findings of such assessments are open to misinterpretation. Such programs *cannot* assess nutritional status. The programs analyze the nutrient content of reported foods using pooled data on the average nutrient content of foods. Results rely on the accuracy and representativeness of the diet record provided. They will merely show how closely the client's reported food intake comes to general recommendations. They should *never* be used as sole justification for recommending supplements. A variety of sound computerized diet assessment tools is readily available.

The website http://www.mypyramid.gov has a diet assessment tool built in that is very user-friendly. Beware of companies that use computer-assisted diet assessments as thinly veiled tools for selling supplements and other dietary products.

A STEPWISE PROCESS FOR DIET RISK ASSESSMENT IN DENTAL PRACTICE: THE *S-O-A-P* METHOD

The following is a model stepwise procedure that can be adapted to meet the needs of the specific dental practice. Just as with other aspects of dental practice, to be meaningful the diet risk assessment and guidance should follow a standard procedure. Logically, the diet risk assessment would be done in conjunction with the dental history and examination, and would be followed by dietary guidance when indicated in conjunction with home care instruction. Many dental nutrition professionals have developed assessment forms of their own, similar in approach and goals. One example is in Table 22–1. Appendix B also includes several DRIs from the Institute of Medicine.

Ideally, a several-day food record should be sent to the client and returned, completed, to the dental appointment. However, practical experience has shown that this rarely occurs. Clients may neglect to complete the form, forget to bring it, or both. Therefore, a more practical approach is to take a modified diet history during the dental appointment.

A common approach to organized case note writing in medical practice is the *S-O-A-P* method. This stands for:

S = Subjective	That which the client reports, but the clinician does not directly observe. This includes the history and is the information that the client reports to you. The diet history and recall is often placed in this category.
O = Objective	That which can be observed or obtained clinically.
A = Assessment	Clinician's evaluation of the condition based on subjective and objective information. This is your synthesis of the above findings into a diagnosis.
P = Plan	The treatment plan that evolves from the above steps.

Using this approach leads to a logical, ordered approach that will be clinically meaningful to the patient as well.

Step 1 Subjective: Introduction and History

For many dental clients, diet assessment has not been a common part of past dental experiences, and they may ask why diet is being discussed. A meaningful introduction sets the stage for a productive session. It is important to personalize the explanation of the purpose of the diet screening and guidance to meet the individual client needs. Explain to clients that oral conditions such as dental caries and periodontal disease are infectious diseases with known causes that can be prevented.

Example:
"We want to provide you with the best dental service we can by treating the dental problems you have now, and also helping you prevent future problems. To do that, we need to make sure we don't miss any important factors. What you eat may or may not play a role in your oral condition, but we need to rule it out as a factor. Does that sound reasonable to you?"

This last question is important in that it solicits the client's understanding and agreement with the process and sets the stage for successful communication at the outset. If the client has any questions or reservations, the door is open for the client to voice

TABLE 22-1 Sample Diet Assessment Form

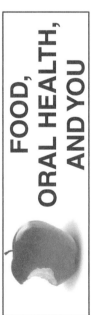

FOOD,
ORAL HEALTH,
AND YOU

What you eat can help or harm your mouth and teeth.

Good nutrition keeps the mouth healthy, helps heal wounds, helps fight gum disease, and helps prevent tooth decay.

This booklet will help you see how your oral health nutrition shapes up.

Promoting Good Nutrition

Please begin by answering the following:

Are you being treated for any nutrition-related condition?	Yes	No
Do you have any dental problems which affect your eating?	Yes	No
Have you changed your eating habits in the past 6 months?	Yes	No
Have you lost or gained more than 10 pounds **without trying** in the last 6 months?	Yes	No
Do you drink more that 3 alcoholic beverages daily?	Yes	No
Do you take vitamins or nutritional supplements? If yes, what type and how often?	Yes	No

If you answered Yes to any of the above, please explain:

What do you eat in a typical day . . .

Please list all of the foods (including snacks drinks), that you have on a USUAL weekday. Give your best guess as to amounts and times eaten.

Time of Day	Food/drink	Amount

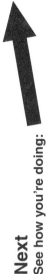

Next
See how you're doing:

- Using your typical intake from above, put a check in the appropriate pyramid box on the next page for each serving you ate from each group
  Example: a banana and a piece of toast would be one check in the fruit section and one check in the grain section.
- Be sure to use the appropriate serving sizes to check off the boxes correctly.
  Example: One cup of cooked broccoli counts as 2 vegetable servings.

How Does Your Diet Rate?

Put a check in the appropriate **Food Pyramid** box below for each serving you have daily and compare to the **minimums** recommended below

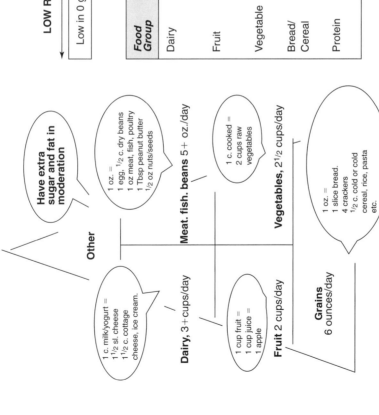

Have extra sugar and fat in moderation

Other

1 oz. =
1 egg, 1/2 c. dry beans
1 oz meat, fish, poultry
1 Tbsp peanut butter
1/2 oz nuts/seeds

Meat, fish, beans 5+ oz./day

1 c. cooked =
2 cups raw vegetables

Vegetables, 2 1/2 cups/day

1 c. milk/yogurt =
1 1/2 sl. cheese
1 1/2 c. cottage cheese, ice cream.

Dairy, 3+ cups/day

1 cup fruit =
1 cup juice =
1 apple

Fruit 2 cups/day

Grains
6 ounces/day

1 oz. =
1 slice bread.
4 crackers
1/2 c. cold or cold cereal, rice, pasta etc.

Record your general nutrition results on the next page

Results of your diet evaluation

IF YOU WERE BELOW THE LOWEST RECOMMENDED SERVINGS IN ANY OF THE FOOD PYRAMID GROUPS, YOU MAY BE AT NUTRITIONAL RISK.

PLOT YOUR RISK ON THE LINE BELOW:

LOW RISK	MEDIUM RISK	HIGH RISK
Low in 0 groups	Low in 1–2 groups	Low in 3+ groups

Food Group	Important Nutrients	Suggestions
Dairy	Protein, Calcium, Vitamin D	Have some yogurt or cheese for a snack. Put milk on your cereal.
Fruit	Vitamins A & C, Fiber	Add to cereal. Eat as a snack or instead of dessert.
Vegetable	Vitamins A & C, Fiber	Add to sandwiches or pasta. Have a salad with your meal.
Bread/ Cereal	B vitamins Fiber Carbohydrate	Snack on pretzels, popcorn, or crackers. Have rice with dinner.
Protein	Protein, Zinc, Iron, B vitamins	Have some peanut butter on your crackers. Add cheese to a salad.

Now check your risk
for developing **Tooth decay**

(continued)

TABLE 22-1 Sample Diet Assessment Form (Continued)

Your Dental Caries Risk

Frequently eating sugar-containing foods is a major risk factor for dental caries (tooth decay).

The longer and more frequently these foods stay in the mouth, the greater the risk of developing **tooth decay.**

Using your usual weekday again . .

Put a check (✓) in **Box 1** below for each food or beverage you had for dessert or between meals **(at least 20 minutes apart).**

Put the total in **Box 2** and multiply by the number in the box

Examples of types of decay-promoting foods	*Box 1* *Put a check for each decay-promoting food or beverage you eat daily*	*Box 2* *Multiply the number of checks in Box 1 by the risk number in the box below. Add up the numbers for your final risk score*
LIQUID Soft drinks, fruit drinks, cocoa, sugar & honey in drinks, non-dairy creamers, puddings, ice cream flavored or frozen yogurt, sherbet, jello, popsicles etc.		x 1 =
SOLID/STICKY Sweetened canned fruit, bananas, dried fruits, cake, cookies, pie & pastry, candy, sweet rolls, donuts, caramel, jelly/jam, marshmallow etc.		x 2 =
SLOWLY DISSOLVING Hard candy, breath mints, cough drips, antacid tablets		x 3 =

Figure total score and go to next page: TOTAL SCORE —————

Oral Health Results

Find out Your Caries Risk

Place your Dental Caries Risk Score on the *Caries Risk Line below.*

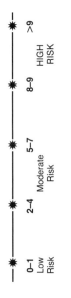

| 0–1 | 2–4 | 5–7 | 8–9 | >9 |
| Low Risk | Moderate Risk | | HIGH RISK | |

To lower your risk of caries, keep these points in mind:

* **Reduce** the frequency of between meal sweets.

* **Don't** sip contantly on sweetened beverages.

* **Do** use water or milk instead.

* **Avoid** using slowly dissolving items like hard candy, cough drops or breath mints.

* **Eat more** non-decay-promoting foods such as low-fat cheese, raw vegetables, crunchy fruits, popcorn, nuts, artificially sweetened beverages and natural spring waters.

Source: © Division of Nutrition and Preventive Dentistry, Department of General Dentistry, Tufts University School of Dental Medicine.

them. Notice, also, that phrasing the plan as a way to "rule out" any factors is much less threatening or intimidating than saying "we want to find out what you are eating that may be causing all this decay" (even though this is what you may mean). The concept of ruling out is generally more acceptable to the client because it does not imply wrongdoing on his part. Chapter 21 reviews the principles of good communication.

Understanding the Personal, Social, Medical, and Dental History (Why People Eat as They Do)

A common error made by those attempting to provide dietary guidance is to concentrate exclusively on what the client is eating and ignore the underlying reasons for existing eating habits (Brown, 1997). The reasons people eat what they do are just as important, if not more so, than the actual food eaten. Understanding the client and helping her make meaningful changes requires an understanding of the factors that influence the foods chosen as well as the foods themselves. Chapter 21 reviews the reasons underlying food habits. Few people make conscious diet choices based exclusively on the nutritional value of the food. More likely influences include timing, location, cost, availability, peer influence, medical condition, and dental condition. The clinician must determine these influences, so

that he or she can help facilitate changes that will be actionable within the client's lifestyle (Baer, Harris, 1997). The best way to accomplish this is to ask the client to describe a typical day's activities from the time she arises until she goes to bed. This will accomplish several goals:

- Provide essential information about the factors influencing food selection (lifestyle, peer influence, attitudes).
- Help facilitate the rapport needed to facilitate client interest and cooperation.
- Provide information about the client in a logical order and context that can be remembered easily from visit to visit.
- Provide a personalized focus.

A short list of important questions that target the major dietary risk factors of dental patients is shown in Table 22–2. This list is adapted from the Nutrition Screening Initiative's "DETERMINE Your Nutritional Health Checklist" (Saunders, 1995) (see Chapter 19), and is used as the first page of the Tufts diet screening form. These questions should be asked of the client during the initial discussion.

TABLE 22–2 Questions Indicating Major Risk Factors for Nutritional Problems

• Do you have any dental problems that affect your eating or appetite?	Yes _____	No _____
• Have you changed your eating habits in the past 6 months?	Yes _____	No _____
• Have you gained or lost more than 10 pounds without wanting to in the last 6 months?	Yes _____	No _____
• Do you eat fewer than 2 meals a day?	Yes _____	No _____
• Do you eliminate any food group totally from your diet? (dairy, fruit, vegetables, meat/fish/poultry, grains)	Yes _____	No _____
• Do you have a problem having enough money and help to get and prepare the food you need?	Yes _____	No _____
• Do you eat alone most of the time?	Yes _____	No _____
• Do you have more than 3 drinks of beer, wine, or other alcohol most days?	Yes _____	No _____
• Do you have a dry mouth most of the time?	Yes _____	No _____
• Do you use hard candy, breath mints, or cough drops on a daily basis?	Yes _____	No _____
	For any "Yes" responses, pursue further for details	

Determining the Client's Usual Dietary Intake (What People Are Eating)

An important step in diet risk assessment is determining the client's usual eating habits. In dental practice the major concerns are for patterns of eating (for cariogenic risk) and for overall diet adequacy. The ideal method for determining food intake is to ask clients to keep a record of their food intake for a period—the longer the better. Unfortunately, this is usually impractical in dental practice because they often forget to keep the record, or forget to bring it with them to the dental appointment. For these reasons, the 24-hour recall, which can be done on the spot, is the most useful tool for dental practice assuming that its limitations are recognized and appreciated. The 24-hour recall does *not* provide an accurate picture of nutrient consumption over time (it is just a snapshot of one day), so it *cannot* be used to determine true nutrient adequacy. People may eat more or less frequently on other days and usually eat differently on weekends. Thus, the 24-hour recall is usually combined with a "food frequency" cross-check to determine if the foods consumed in that one day reflect the usual eating pattern.

The 24-hour recall is done by asking clients to detail everything they ate and drank in a typical day, preferably the previous day (people can usually remember what they ate yesterday), with careful attention to eating times, portion sizes, preparation method, added items (sugar, butter), between-meal items, and nonfood items. Nonfood items may be particularly important, as clients often do not consider items such as breath mints and cough drops to be food and may neglect to report them. Because it is often difficult to determine portion sizes of foods consumed, it helps to provide examples of portion sizes to help clients judge their portions as accurately as possible. This recall approach is useful for dentistry because it can show usual eating patterns and habits, specifically:

- Frequency of eating
- Types of meals and snacks commonly consumed
- Use of cariogenic items in addition to foods such as cough drops and breath mints
- General pattern of food types consumed daily

Table 22–3 shows a typical 24-hour food recall format. Figure 22–2 provides handy ways to help clients estimate portion sizes.

TABLE 22–3 Food Record

Time	Food	Amount
7:00 AM	Coffee with sugar	1 cup—2 tsp
	English muffin with butter	2 tsp butter
12:00 PM	Canned chili with beans	1 cup
	Flour tortilla	2
	2% milk	1 cup
4:00 PM	Cola	12 fl oz
	Chips	2 oz bag
	Chocolate chip cookies	2
7:00 PM	Fried chicken	1 breast
	Mashed potatoes with gravy	1/2 cup potato, 2 Tbsp gravy
	Coleslaw	½ cup
	Sweetened tea	12 fl oz
	Chocolate cake with ice cream	1 slice (2 × 3 inches) cake, ½ cup ice cream
9:00 PM	Chocolate chip cookies	4
	Other:	
	Breath mints, multivitamin tablet	5x/day one/day

Step 2 Objective: The Clinical Examination

Just as the clinician carefully examines oral tissues and structures, performs caries charting, and records plaque scores, she should also be observing the clients' skin, eyes, mouth, and oral soft and hard tissue for signs of nutritional problems. Clinical observations provide important cues to the existence of nutritional problems. However, it is important to remember that clinical observations must be corroborated with the proper biochemical tests before true diagnosis is made. For example, cracks in the corners of the mouth (angular cheilosis) may indicate vitamin B-complex deficiency, but can also be caused by drooling from lack of vertical dimension or by fungal infections. Conversely, a lack of clinical signs does not necessarily indicate that no problem exists. Nutrient depletion or excess and biochemical changes cannot be seen, yet they are responsible for the majority of functional problems (e.g., reduced immunity, poor healing). Table 22–4 lists the clinical signs that may be indicators of nutritional problems. Table 22–5 shows an oral screening process.

Food Group	Portion equal to One Serving	Similar Portion Size
Grain	• 1/2 cup cooked cereal, pasta, or rice • 1 slice bread, 1/2 bagel or English muffin, 4 crackers • 1 pancake or waffle • 1 muffin	• small fist • large coffee lid, hockey puck, cassette tape • 4 inch CD • large egg
Vegetables	• 1 cup leafy greens • 1/2 cup cooked • 1 medium piece (carrot) • small potato	• large fist • small fist • computer mouse
Fruits	• 1 medium piece • 1/2 cup canned or chopped	• tennis ball • small fist
Meats & other proteins	• 3 oz cooked meat, poultry, fish • 1/2 cup cooked dry beans • 2 Tbsp peanut butter	• deck of cards or palm of the hand or large bar of soap • small fist • golf ball
Dairy products	• 1 cup milk, yogurt • 1 1/2 oz cheese • 1/2 cup ice cream • 1 oz cheese	• large fist • 6 dice • entire thumb
Fats and snacks	• 4 small cookies • 1 tsp margarine or butter • 1–2 oz snack foods	• 4 casino chips • thumb tip • handful

FIGURE 22–2 Food portion sizes.

Patient Education

Determine what the client already knows about his or her oral condition and its causes and prevention. Then fill in any knowledge gaps and correct erroneous information. Explain dietary factors that increase caries risk (simple sugars result in bacterial acid formation). Oral contact time is the most important factor and is associated with frequency of eating and the physical form of the carbohydrates. Explain that good general nutrition provides resistance to infection, and poor nutrition lowers resistance and retards healing. Use the client's own radiographs and diagrams wherever possible.

Step 3 Assessment: Diet and Risk Assessment

Having determined the client's lifestyle, diet pattern, and 24-hour recall, the next step is to work with the client to assess his or her diet for overall adequacy and cariogenic risk (Olendzki et al., 1999).

Assessing General Diet Adequacy (see Chapter 2)

To assess diet adequacy:

- Review or explain the relationship(s) between diet and oral health (e.g., bone health, support for healing, optimizing immunity, minimizing tissue response to periodontal infection) using graphics (radiograph, MyPyramid handout, etc.).
- Explain recommended diet guidelines (MyPyramid) and how it represents the foundation of a healthy diet.
- Have the client assess his diet by comparing it to the food pyramid recommendations (by hand or computer at http://www.mypyramid.gov). This can be done by having him categorize each food item in his typical day into the appropriate food group us an assessment tool. (If the client has provided more than one day, all days can be assessed and averaged.) For the Tufts assessment form, see Table 22–1. In the Tufts form, we have provided a

TABLE 22–4   Oral Manifestations of Nutrient Deficiencies and Systemic Disease

Oral Symptom	Possible Condition	Nutrition Considerations
Swollen or bleeding gums	Rule out vitamin C deficiency	Determine etiology: treat with diet and/or supplements
Cheliosis, angular stomatitis	Rule out riboflavin, B_6, iron deficiency Chemotherapeutic agents	Determine etiology: treat with diet and/or supplements
Glossitis	Rule out folate, riboflavin, niacin deficiency Chemotherapeutic agent	Determine etiology: treat with diet and/or supplements Modify diet as needed Palliative therapy
Inflamed, sore tongue	Rule out riboflavin, niacin, B_6, B_{12}, iron deficiency	Determine etiology: treat with diet and/or supplements Modify diet: avoid spicy or acidic foods, room temperature foods, nutrient-dense and energy-dense foods that are soft and moist
Xerostomia	Poorly controlled diabetes Sjögren's syndrome Rheumatoid arthritis Drug-induced HIV/AIDS Radiation therapy	Determine cause of poor glucose control; modify diet Modify diet to include moist foods, no added salt or spice, increase water intake both with meals and between meals, eat fewer retentive, fermentable carbohydrates
Changes in taste	Rule out vitamin A deficiency Uremia (metallic taste) Medications Aging	Determine etiology: treat with diet and/or supplements Modify diet to exclude foods that cause aversions, use nutrient-dense and energy-dense foods
Dysphagia	Rule out iron deficiency Chemotherapeutic agents Neurologic conditions (stroke, multiple sclerosis) Rheumatoid arthritis Developmental disorders	Determine etiology: treat with diet and/or supplements Modify diet to include thickened liquids and moist, flavorful foods either very warm or chilled
Candidiasis	HIV/AIDS Radiation therapy	Palliative treatment Modify diet: avoid spicy or acidic foods, room temperature foods, soft, moist, nutrient-dense and energy-dense foods
Stomatitis, mucositis	HIV/AIDS Chemotherapeutic agents	Palliative treatment Modify diet: avoid spicy or acidic foods, room temperature foods, soft, moist, nutrient-dense and energy-dense foods

sample food pyramid with spaces for numbers of portions consumed in each food group. Many people are unaware of what a standard portion size is. Additionally, over the years portions have increased in size. Figure 22–2 shows standard portions and how to demonstrate them to clients. Figure 22–3 shows how portions have increased over the years.

• Have the client compare his intake to the recommended number of servings to determine his food group status.

TABLE 22–5   Steps to Oral Health Screening

When conducting an oral screening, you need to not only talk to the patient, but touch and explore the mouth. The screening should consist of six steps.

1. Be sure to wear disposable gloves, even if the patient has no visible lesions. Active viruses can be present before a lesion develops. Gloves protect the examiner and the patient from the transmission of bacteria and viruses.
2. Examine the patient's face and neck.
3. Ask the patient to open and close his or her mouth and note any related discomfort.
4. Note any unusual swelling in the head and neck.
5. Bilaterally palpate the lymph nodes under the jaw, behind the ear, and down the neck (lateral to the thyroid anteriorly and the nape of the neck posteriorly).
6. Ask about swallowing or chewing problems, as these can be warning signs of oral health problems.

Yes or No	*If Yes, Nutritional Considerations*
Oral Soft Tissue	
1. Were there observable or palpable lumps on any oral soft tissue (gingivae and other oral structures)?	Avoid acidic, salty, spicy, hard, or crunchy food.
2. Was there apparent swelling of the gingivae or other oral tissue?	Eat cool, soft, or pureed foods and use a straw when possible.
3. Were white or red patches or lesions identified in the soft tissue assessment?	Explore hypersensitivity to food, toothpaste, mouthwash, or other possible allergens.
4. Did the patient complain of pain or bleeding of the gingivae or other oral tissue?	Screen for anemia due to folate, vitamin B_{12} or iron deficiency and borderline vitamin or mineral deficiencies, such as vitamin C.
Teeth	
5. Was there pus or exudate between the teeth and gums?	Modify diet consistency and form.
6. Were there any broken teeth?	Modify food form and review adequacy of intake; consider need for supplements.
7. Were there any teeth loose?	
8. Were there apparent decayed teeth?	Evaluate diet adequacy and possible cariogenicity.
9. Did the patient complain of tooth pain?	
10. If the patient had dentures, were they reported to fit properly?	
Miscellaneous	
11. Did the saliva have a thick and ropey consistency, as opposed to being thin and serous?	Encourage intake of fluids; evaluate for dysgeusia and dyspagia.
12. Did the patient complain of xerostomia and were there clinical signs of this condition?	Add sauces, gravy, and juices to meals and snacks. Avoid bananas and dry foods. Encourage the use of sugarless gum or candy.
13. Did the patient complain of burning tongue or changes in taste?	Screen for anemia, diabetes, candidiasis, or Sjogren's syndrome.
14. Were there reported changes in dietary intake that could be related to findings in the oral health screening?	Screen for drug-induced conditions. Evaluate adequacy of macronutrients in diet.

Source: Adapted with permission from Mobley CC, Saunders MI: Oral health screening guidelines for nondental health care providers. *J Am Diet Assoc* 1997; 97:S123–6.

MUFFIN

20 Years Ago   Today

210 calories   500 calories
1.5 ounces   4 ounces

Calorie Difference: 290 calories

FIGURE 22-3 Portion distortion.
Source: National Heart, Lung, and Blood Institute—Obesity Education Initiative, National Institutes of Health, U.S. Department of Health and Human Services. Photo: Clive Streeter © Dorling Kindersley.

- For any food groups in which the client consumes *less* than recommended amounts, ask whether or not this is common practice. If it is common, suggestions for improvements can be made (Table 22–6).
- The general adequacy of the diet can then be summarized and issues that need improvement noted.

Assessing the Cariogenic Risk of the Diet (see Chapter 13)

To assess cariogenic risk:

- Review or explain to the client the relationship between fermentable carbohydrates and caries risk.
- Explain the difference in cariogenic potential between retentive and nonretentive sweets and

TABLE 22-6 Diet Suggestions for Various Oral Conditions

Food Group	Dental Caries	Periodontal Disease	Dentures	Mucositis/Oral Lesions	Oral Impairment and Surgery
General	• Limit number of eating times • Avoid sticky or retentive foods	• Avoid soft, mushy foods	• Encourage chewing • Begin by chewing on molar area • Work up to biting	• Avoid hard, sharp, or acidic foods • Avoid temperature extremes	• Aim for soft foods, or blenderize foods if needed
Grains/cereals (6–11/day)	• Eat whole grains • Have popcorn for snacks • Avoid crackers, donuts, potato chips between meals	• Avoid popcorn • Eat whole grains, foods requiring chewing	• Begin with softer foods like hot cereal, pasta, soft whole grain bread • Work up to bagels, hard rolls	• Eat soft grains like warm cereals, pasta, rice, potato • Avoid hard crusts	• Eat hot cereals, rice, pasta, soft bread, soups with pasta and rice
Fruits (3–5/day) Fresh, frozen, canned, juices	• Eat fruits for dessert/snacks • Avoid dried fruits or fruit roll-ups • Don't sip slowly or often on fruit juices • Avoid fruit drinks	• Eat plenty of fruits high in vitamins C and carotene like citrus fruits (oranges, grapefruit), tomatoes, apricots, cantaloupe, fruit nectars, fruit juices	• Avoid biting into large raw fruits at first like apples • Begin with soft or canned fruits, juices • Cut whole fresh fruit into small pieces and chew with molars • Work up to biting with central incisors	Avoid acidic fruits like citrus fruits (lemon, lime, orange, grapefruit • Have bland fruits like banana, apricot, pear, • Eat fruit nectars rather than acidic fruit juices	Drink juices, eat blenderized and pureed fruits
Vegetables (2–4/day) Fresh, frozen,	• Eat all vegetables • Watch sweetened salad dressings	• Eat all vegetables but concentrate on	• Avoid biting into raw vegetables at first, like carrots	Have bland vegetables, avoid tomatoes and tomato juice	Eat pureed vegetables, drink vegetable juices

canned, juices, potatoes	• Have raw vegetables for snacks	fresh and frozen rather than canned mushy vegetables • Try vegetable juices	• Cut these into pieces and chew with molars • Begin with soft or canned vegetables and juices • Work up to biting with central incisors		
Protein (2+/day) Meat, fish, poultry, eggs, beans (lentils, etc.), tofu, nuts	• Eat any protein sources • Have nuts for snacks	Eat any protein sources Avoid nuts that can get stuck in sulcus	• Eat soft meats like hamburger, ground chicken, or chicken cut in small pieces; eggs; beans • Avoid nuts—may be difficult to chew	• Eat most protein sources • Avoid nuts—may irritate oral tissues	Drink eggnogs, liquid breakfast beverages, eat blenderized meats in broth
Dairy* (2–3+/day) Milk, cheese, ice cream, tofu, cottage cheese	Have milk in coffee, soup Eat cheese in sandwiches, casseroles, etc. Eat cheese for snacks	Have plenty to maintain oral bone health (See *Dental Caries* for other suggestions)	• Have plenty to maintain alveolar bone health • Eat cottage cheese, cheese sauces, drink milk in beverages and soups • Eat ice cream for dessert	Eat or drink all dairy products; see *Dental Caries*	Have milk-based beverages with ice cream added, cheese soups, tofu or cottage cheese blended with milk, ice cream in sodas
Sweets/fats Oil, margarine, butter, salad dressing, candy, sweet desserts, soda pop	• Avoid slowly dissolving candies • Have sweets as dessert only • Avoid constant sipping on sweet beverages (soda, sports drinks)	See *Dental Caries* to prevent root caries	• Go light on these as they can be filling and take the place of more nutritious foods • Avoid hard candies that may crack dentures • Avoid sticky sweets, which may be hard to clean off • For partially dentate, see *Dental Caries* column	• Go light on these as they can be filling and take the place of more nutritious foods	As tolerated, have ice cream, sherbet, sorbet for dessert
Other	• Drink flavored club soda or diet soda • Chew sugar-free gum	See *Dental Caries* to encourage oral clearance	• Eat casseroles, lasagna, and other soft combination foods to boost nutrients		• Eat most foods pureed (more palatable than canned liquid supplements) • Eat pureed baby foods (be careful of psychological implications)

Note: See appropriate chapters for more detail on each of these conditions.

*Aim for low fat unless increased calories are indicated.

the importance of oral contact time and frequency of eating as a risk factor in cariogenicity. (The reaction of plaque bacterial enzymes with fermentable carbohydrates forms acid within about 20 seconds and continues forming for at least 20 minutes with each eating period.) Reinforce to the client that the pattern of eating is the most important factor in cariogenic risk. Between-meal eating increases risk; carbohydrates eaten at mealtimes are not of concern.)

- Have the client determine the number of usual daily fermentable carbohydrate exposures between meals, and whether items were potentially orally retentive (liquid/solid/slowly dissolving).
- Have the client add up the number of daily exposures to fermentable carbohydrates. On the Tufts form, clients multiply each fermentable carbohydrate exposure by a weighted score to determine potential cariogenic risk (Table 22–1). (Note that the Tufts form is not a scientific score, but rather an educational tool to highlight the relative risks of various types and usage patterns of cariogenic foods.)
- Have the client record his self-assessment of cariogenic risk.

At this point in the process, subjective and objective data have been gathered and assessed, and the contributing factors to the oral condition have been determined. The client should be able to summarize the findings of his self-assessment including general diet quality and cariogenic potential, as well as food habits that may be contributing to less than ideal food choices.

Sample Dialogue:
Counselor: So, Mrs. Jones, what did you find out from your self-evaluation?
Client: I found out that I'm eating too many decay-promoting sweets like hard candies and coffee with sugar, and not enough of some of the healthier foods.
Counselor: Like what?
Client: Dairy products and fruits. I don't eat any dairy products because they make me sick.

Step 4 Plan: Problem Management

Once the screening process is complete, having determined the dental problems and conducted the diet risk assessment, the clinician and the client together should

be able to pinpoint any dietary risk factors, and develop the management plan. Figure 22–4 provides a flow diagram of the decision tree for this process.

The diet risk assessment screening may have determined that the client's diet is excellent and apparently not contributory to any dental problem. In this case, reinforce the client's good habits and make sure that he understands why his habits are consistent with good general and oral health. This is important, as people change their dietary habits periodically, and new patterns may increase oral risk.

More likely, there may be areas of the diet that clearly need improvement, so further diet guidance or referral is indicated. If the problem is with cariogenic potential or poor food choices with no particular underlying medical condition, the dental team should be confident to provide guidance. If the client has underlying medical conditions (e.g., heart disease, diabetes) along with dietary concerns, he should be referred to his physician and registered dietitian for further evaluation and care.

If improvements are indicated, the clinician and the client should work together to develop improvements that will be practical and appropriate. The Tufts screening form provides suggestions for food group improvements. The client should make his own suggestions for improvements with the assistance of the dental professional. Improvements should not be general, but should be specific to the issue of concern. Table 22–6 shows some examples of appropriate suggestions for various oral conditions. Chapter 13 provides suggestions for reducing the cariogenic potential of the diet. Chapter 19 provides suggestions for improving the diet of elderly clients.

Sample Dialogue:
Counselor: So Mrs. Jones, is there anything you can do about this to improve?
Client: I need to get rid of all the hard candies that I eat between meals. I'll drink water instead or maybe suck on artificially sweetened hard candies. I am going to try to stop drinking so much sweetened coffee. I can plan to have coffee just at mealtimes.
Counselor: Is that realistic?
Client: Absolutely.
Counselor: And what about the other foods?
Client: I can easily drink orange juice with my breakfast. I just never thought about it.

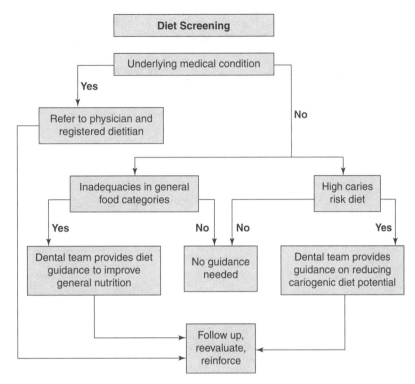

FIGURE 22–4 Decision tree.

Counselor: How about the calcium problem?

Client: Well, milk makes me sick, so I don't know.

Counselor: What other options might you consider? (Let the client identify and make the choices.) Have you tried the lactose-free milks in the supermarket? You might find that they are fine.

Client: No, I've never tried them, but I will and I'll let you know.

Summary and Closure

Before terminating the session, it is important to summarize the session with regard to:

- Client understanding of the causes and prevention of his or her oral condition.
- The results of the diet self-assessment.
- Reasonable strategies for improvement and commitment to improvement.

Ask clients to confirm existing behaviors that support good oral health. (What are they already doing that is beneficial?) Have clients prioritize possible changes. Encourage clients to state this in action statements.

Sample Dialogue:

Counselor: So Mrs. Jones, what does all of this mean to you?

Client: Well, now I know why I am getting all of this new decay.

Counselor: Why?

Client: Because my mouth is dry and I have been using too many candies and things to wet it. Also, because my brushing isn't as good as it should be.

Counselor: What about the rest of your eating?

Client: Well, I'm not eating nearly as much fruit or dairy products as I should have.

Counselor: What about the changes you've suggested for yourself? Do you really think you can make them?

Client: Oh sure, no problem; they're not big changes.

TABLE 22–7 Tufts University School of Dental Medicine Prescription for Promoting Good Oral Health

Recommended Changes in Oral Home Care Methods and Materials	Recommended Changes in Eating Habits
1. *Brushing:* Type of brush: Specific suggestions (technique, timing):	1. Have *more* of these nutritious foods: _____ _____ _____
2. *Flossing:* Type of floss: Specific suggestions (technique, timing):	2. Reduce the decay-promoting potential of your diet by: • reducing the number of times you eat _____ • changing the times you eat _____ • substituting _____ for more decay-promoting foods such as etc.:
3. *Supplemental Home Care Aids* (stimudents, denture brush, proxabrush, fluoride rinses, desensitizing agents)	_____ _____ _____
Type: Directions for use:	_____ Signature of student
Type: Directions for use	_____ Signature of instructor
Type: Directions for use:	_____ Date

Source: © Division of Nutrition and Preventive Dentistry, Department of General Dentistry, Tufts University School of Dental Medicine.

It is important to provide the client with a written summary of the session to reinforce important points and document the plan. Table 22–7 shows a sample take-home form for the client.

Follow-Up and Reevaluation

Follow-up and reinforcement are essential. At the next appointment, monitor client progress (e.g., "How are you doing with the diet changes?" "Any problems?"). Have the client complete another food record. Compare it with the original, reinforce improvements, clarify misconceptions, and revisit any unmanageable original plans. Table 22–8 summarizes this entire process.

AVOIDING PITFALLS IN DEALING WITH DIET

The following are common errors that are easily avoided, but can have a major impact on the success or failure of the diet guidance session.

• *Always* explain the relevance of diet and nutrition to the client's specific problem. *Don't* begin with a statement like "This is what we do with all our clients." People want care that is focused on their particular needs, not a canned presentation.
• *Don't* begin with the assumption that changes have to be made. Let the client come to that conclusion if warranted.
• *Don't* start making recommendations early in the assessment before all the needed information has been collected and assessed. The statement "cut down on sweets" has little meaning until after clients are shown which of their specific food habits may be dentally risky.
• *Make sure* that clients compare their food intake to the correct standardized portion sizes. *Don't* forget that the standardized portion sizes used for evaluation are not always the same as what the client considers a portion to be. A serving of steak to a teenager may be four to five times larger than the 4 oz standard portion.

TABLE 22-8 Nutrition Guidance for Oral Health Promotion: An Outline

Step 1 Subjective: Introduction and History (explain the *reason* for counseling)
Example: "Usually we deal with the *effects* of dental caries (decay) or periodontal disease (gums and bone) by technical procedures. We also need to find the *causes* of your problems to *prevent* rather than have to treat future ones. Diet and nutrition play important roles in these conditions. We would like to rule out diet and nutrition as factors in your situation."

The Personal History (the "why" of the diet)
Ask the client to describe a typical day's activities. This will:
• Provide essential history information and the factors influencing food selection (lifestyle, peer influence, attitudes).
• Facilitate the development of the rapport needed to help maximize client cooperation.

Food Intake (the "what" of the diet)
Obtain a representative food intake pattern by asking the client to keep a food diary (minimum one day, optimum one week, preferably including a weekend). A one-day record can be recorded on the Diet Screening Scorecard.

Step 2 Objective: The Clinical Examination
Clinical Observation:
Have an organized plan to carefully scan the head and neck for abnormal appearances that might be related to medical, dental, or nutritional problems.

Education about the Role of Nutrition in the Etiology and Prevention of Dental Diseases
• Determine what the client already knows about his or her oral condition and its causes and prevention.
• Fill in any knowledge gaps and correct erroneous information:
  • *Caries*: Explain the interaction of tooth, plaque, and sugar.
    Bacteria + Diet Carbohydrates = Acid + *Enamel* → demineralization + decay
  • *Periodontal Disease*: Plaque Bacteria → Toxins
    Toxins + Tissue + Bone → Infection
    Infection → Inflammation, bleeding, bone loss
    Dietary factors: Simple sugars encourage bacteria growth.
    Systemic nutrition factors: Good nutrition provides resistance to infection.
    Poor nutrition lowers resistance and retards healing.
  • *Edentulous Client*: Plaque + Gums → Infection, bleeding, soreness
    Good diet ensures tissue strength against infection and denture stress.
    Poor diet can undermine tissue resistance.

Step 3 Assessment: Diet and Risk Assessment
General Diet Adequacy
• Review the importance of an adequate diet for oral tissue health.
• Have the client categorize a typical day of foods from the food record into appropriate groups on the diet screening form.
• Have the client determine the adequacy of the diet by comparing his or her intake with the amounts recommended.
• Have the client record food group scores on the summary page.

Cariogenic Potential of the Diet (if applicable)
• Have the client circle in red all desserts and snacks on the food record sweetened with sugar.
• Explain the difference in cariogenic potential between retentive and nonretentive sweets and the importance of frequency of eating as an important factor in cariogenicity. (The reaction of bacterial enzymes [in the plaque] with sugar change sugar to acid within 20 *seconds* and continue forming for at least 20 *minutes* with each eating period.)
• Have the client categorize each sweet eaten at the end of or between meals as liquid, solid, or slowly dissolving.
• Multiply each exposure by the appropriate number in the box.
• Add numbers to determine a cariogenic potential score.
• Have the client record his or her score on the summary sheet.

(continued)

TABLE 22–8   Nutrition Guidance for Oral Health Promotion: An Outline (Continued)

Problem Diagnosis (findings)

Have the client review his or her general diet and cariogenic potential scores to summarize self-assessment findings. Information includes:
* General diet adequacy
* Cariogenic risk
* Reasons for diet pattern

Step 4 Plan: Problem Management (if indicated)

Have the client suggest his or her own improvements to:
* Improve diet quality.
* Reduce cariogenic potential.

Summary and Closure

Have the client summarize the session in terms of:
* Knowledge about the causes and prevention of his or her oral condition.
* Results on diet self-assessment.
* Reasonable strategies and commitment for improvement.

Follow-Up and Reevaluation (if improvements were indicated)

* A few weeks after initial diet assessment and guidance, have the client complete another food record.
* Compare it with the original document. Note improvements and clarify misconceptions.
* Monitor client progress chairside ("How are you doing with the diet changes?" "Any problems?").

Note: Results of diet screening should be documented in the client record along with other oral health data.
Source: © Carole A. Palmer, Tufts University School of Dental Medicine, 2001.

* *Always* have the client do her own assessment with your guidance. *Don't* take over and do the assessment yourself.
* *Guide* the client to make her own decisions for changes (with your assistance). *Don't* make suggestions until the client indicates that she needs assistance. Otherwise there is no way to tell if the client sees the changes as reasonable and practical. Have the client summarize and agree that the plan is workable because it helps ensure follow-through by the client.

PULLING IT ALL TOGETHER: DOCUMENTING DIET CARE IN THE CLIENT'S RECORD

Always document the results of diet screening and guidance in the client's record along with other oral health data. Again, the S-O-A-P method provides a well-organized structure for the report. A sample case report written in this style is shown in Table 22–9.

SUMMARY AND IMPLICATIONS FOR DENTISTRY

Diet screening, assessment, and guidance can and should be an integral component of the care process for dental clients. It is just as important to attend to diet issues as to fluoride or home care, as all can be major roles in oral health or disease. All clients should be screened for dietary risk factors. Those who exhibit some aspect of risk should receive personalized guidance or referral depending on the extent of the problem. Dietary guidance needs to be specific to the client's individual situation. No two clients are alike, and none have exactly the same eating habits. The process of diet care must be logical and organized, and the client needs to be committed to and actively involved in the process. Suggestions for improvement are based on the needs determined by the diet screening. All decisions for change must be made by the client under the guidance of the dental team, as this will help ensure commitment and compliance.

TABLE 22–9   Sample Case Note Using the S-O-A-P Method

Soap Format	*Case Writeup*
(S) Subjective	
Family history and lifestyle: family dental history, daily routine, activities, family situation	Joan Asher is a 26-year-old mother of a 2-year-old, and is 5 months pregnant with her second child. Mrs. Asher came for a dental checkup and complained that her gums are sore. She has avoided dental care for the most part because of bad dental experiences she had as a child.
	Joan lives in the town of Southgate, with her husband and two dogs. She has lived in Southgate all of her life, as has her husband. She is very active, although she has had to curtail her running since she became pregnant. She works as an accountant, and is fortunate to be able to work at home when she needs to.
Medical history: including medications, reported symptoms	Her medical history is unremarkable. She is in good health and takes no medications. She does take aspirin on occasion for a headache, but has stopped that during her pregnancy. She is being followed by her obstetrician and by a registered dietitian for her diet. She doesn't like milk and has avoided it for most of her adult years. However, she says that she has been following the dietitian's recommendations and is trying to increase her calcium intake and stop her habit of snacking on breath mints. Her weight has progressed at the recommended level.
Eating habits and patterns: frequency of eating, where, with whom	
Past dental history: frequency of *dental visits, past problems*	Her dental history indicates that she has been somewhat lax in her dental visits but is trying to improve to set a good example for the children. She brushes her teeth once a day in the morning with baking soda. She does this because it gives a "good mouth feel" and it feels like it is cleaning her teeth well. She uses a hard bristle brush for the same reason. She has had a lot of "cavities" in the past and would like to make sure her children don't have the same dental problems.
Home care habits: brushing, flossing, other aids, fluoride, frequency	
	She does not believe that the water supply in Southgate is fluoridated, but the family does not drink tap water most of the time.
	She is particularly concerned that her children get good dental care. Her 2 year-old has seen a dentist only once, when he fell out of the chair and broke a tooth. She is concerned that he may have some dental problems because sometimes he won't eat and points to his mouth to try to tell her that it hurts.
(O) Objective	
Clinical signs: observe skin, eyes, tongue, etc.	Clinical observations reveal no abnormal findings. Mrs. Asher has 6 new carious lesions around existing amalgams. She also has moderate to severe periodontal disease. Her plaque-free score is 52% plaque-free.
Oral condition: plaque score, gingival condition, dentate status, decayed, missing, or filled teeth (DMFT), etc.	
Medical and laboratory reports	

(continued)

TABLE 22–9   Sample Case Note Using the S-O-A-P Method (Continued)

Soap Format	*Case Writeup*
(A) Assessment *Dietary status:* results of diet evaluation *Dental summary:* diagnosis, *rampant caries, mild periodontitis* *Preventive dental issues:* poor plaque core, lack of topical or *systemic fluoride, no flossing* *Medical implications:* diabetes, xerostomia	Her general diet appears to be adequate in all food groups as she is following dietary recommendations of a registered dietitian. She is using low-lactose milk to make sure that she gets sufficient calcium. She has tried to cut down on the breath mints that she was using often, but still uses 2–3 a day. She also snacks frequently on cookies 2–3 times/day. Our assessment is that Mrs. Asher has active caries and periodontaldisease due to her frequent snacking, poor oral hygiene, and lack of fluoride.
(P) Plan (treatment plan based on above) *Dental treatment:* extractions, dentures, restorations, periodontal therapy *Preventive care:* home care, flossing, fluoride, salivary stimulation *Dietary guidance:* to improve overall diet, to reduce caries risk	Mrs. Asher has agreed to be more diligent with her oral care both for herself and as a role model for her children. She will start using a soft bristle brush—she thought the hard bristle brush was more effective previously. She will also start using fluoridated tooth paste. She does not wish to drink the fluoridated tap water, so the fluoridated dentifrice is especially important. She will also use an oral fluoride rinse once daily. Mrs. Asher agreed to eliminate all of the breath mints and cookies, now that she understands the implications of these in her oral condition. She will use artificially sweetened breath mints if she feels the need for mints, and will have a piece of low-fat cheese if she needs a snack. In summary, Mrs. Asher is eager to get her own mouth under control and to do what she can to avoid dental problems for her children. Therefore, she is very receptive at this point to preventive guidance.

QUESTIONS PATIENTS MIGHT ASK

Q. Why are you asking me about my diet in general? I thought that you were only interested in sugar because it caused cavities.

A. Your overall diet is important because good nutrition is necessary for the health of the oral cavity— your gums, teeth, tongue, palate, and so on. Poor nutrition can affect oral healing and can decrease your resistance to oral infections like periodontal disease.

Q. Why are you not focusing primarily on the sugar in candy and soda? I've always heard that these were the most dentally damaging things we eat.

A. Actually, any sugars that you eat can contribute to dental caries, not just candy and soda. The most important factor is how often you eat or how long you sip sugary foods. For this reason, sodas are high on the risky list. However, juices can be just as dentally harmful if you sip them often.

Q. Why are you concerned only with what I eat between meals and not at meals?

A. The pH (acidity) is always going to occur at mealtimes due to all of the mealtime carbohydrates you eat, so the effects of added carbohydrates are insignificant. On the other hand, between meals, the acidity is usually gone until you have a fermentable carbohydrate to start it up again.

Q. Why don't you just recommend vitamins?

A. Vitamins are only part of the picture. Proteins and other nutrients needed for oral health do not come from vitamins alone. A good diet is an important habit for life. Vitamins are only an add-on.

CASE STUDY

Emelio Gonzalez is a 17-year-old, medically healthy, male high school junior. He has lived all his life in Boston with his family (mother, father, older sister, younger sister) in a two-family house they share with his grandmother. Emelio is a good student who especially enjoys sports. He plays baseball and football on the high school varsity team. He also works at Burger King on weekends when he doesn't have a sports event.

Emelio's medical history is unremarkable. He is in good health and has no diagnosed medical problems. He is 5 feet 10 inches tall, weighs 180 pounds, and is very active. He is not on any special diets, and his eating habits are erratic due to his busy school, sports, and work schedule. He uses chewing tobacco and chewing gum two or three times a week, especially during sports activities. He is very concerned about how his girlfriend feels about his appearance.

Emelio has a family dental history of early tooth loss and intermittent dental care. He brushes once a day on the run, usually in the morning before he leaves the house. He uses an electric toothbrush and Crest toothpaste. He never flosses. He visits the dentist once every 3 or 4 years, or when he gets a toothache. He has all his teeth but his third molars, which were extracted as a result of severe caries. His gingival examination shows generalized moderate gingivitis and new rampant caries. His plaque score is 66% plaque-free.

24-Hour Diet Recall

Breakfast (if he eats—sometimes he will not have any breakfast)

2 breakfast pastries (PopTarts)
1 glass of orange juice (individual bottle)
Snack
Pastry from vending machine at school
1 can cola
Lunch (school lunch)
Cheeseburger with bun
1 order of French fries
1 candy bar or ice cream bar
1 can cola
Snack (usually before practice)
2 power bars
1 can cola (12 oz)
Dinner (usually not until 9 PM; eats leftovers)
2 cups white rice
1 cup black beans
2–3 chicken breasts
1 can cola
Bedtime
Large dish of chocolate ice cream
1 can cola

Questions:

1. How would you help motivate Emelio to improve his oral hygiene habits?
2. Which approach is most likely to motivate Emelio to reduce his use of chewing tobacco?
3. Which are the primary dietary cariogenic risk factors?
4. According to the Stephan Curve, what would happen to the plaque pH if Emelio ate a piece of cheese after drinking his cola?
5. Which is the *most important* dietary factor in predicting caries in general?

REFERENCES

Baer M, Harris AB: Pediatric nutrition asssessment: Identifying children at risk. *J Am Dietet Assoc* 1997; 97(10 Suppl 2): s107–s15.
Boyd LD, Dwyer DJ, Palmer CA: *Nutrition and Oral Health: Guidelines for Nutrition Intervention in the Dental Office.* Boston: Tufts University School of Dental Medicine, Frances Stern Nutrition Center/New England Medical Center Hospital, 1998.

Brown JP: Indicators for caries management from the client history. *J Dent Educ* 1997; 61(11):855–60.
Hildebrand G: Caries risk assessment and prevention for adults. *J Dent Educ* 1995; 59(10):972–79.
Mobley CC, Saunders MJ: Oral health screening guidelines for nondental health care providers. *J Am Dietet Assoc* 1997; 97(10 Suppl 2):s123–s26.
Olendzki B, Hurley T, Hebert JR, Ellis S, Merriam PA, Luippold R, et al.: Comparing food intake using the dietary risk assessment with multiple 24-hour dietary recalls and

the 7-day dietary recall. *J Am Dietet Assoc* 1999; 99(11): 1433–39.

Palmer C, Dwyer JT, Clark RE: Expert opinions on nutrition in clinical dentistry. *J Den Educ* 1990; 54:612–18.

Preventive Health Statement on Nutrition and Oral Health: American Dental Association, 1996:682. Retrieved from http://www.ada.org/prof/resources/positions/doc_policies.pdf.

Saunders MJ: Incorporating the Nutrition Screening Initiative into the dental practice. *Special Care Dent* 1995; 15:26–37.

Stoddard JW: Caries risk assessment used as a determinant for caries management and prevention. *J Dent Educ* 1995; 59(10):957–61.

Suddick RP: Caries activity estimates and implications: Insights into risk versus activity. *J Dent Educ* 1997; 61(11): 876–84.

Tinanoff N: Critique of evolving methods for caries risk assessment. *J Dent Educ* 1995; 59(10):980–85.

Chapter 23

Nutrition Resources for Dental Practice

Karen Schroeder Kassel

OBJECTIVES

The student will be able to:

- Discuss how to locate community nutrition resources.
- Describe how to evaluate the credibility of nutrition sources on the Internet.
- List where to go for sound nutrition resource materials.

INTRODUCTION

A middle-aged woman who lives alone and has no desire to cook; an elderly man who has difficulty preparing his own meals; a young mother who struggles to afford groceries—each of these clients can be helped with a simple referral to the appropriate nutrition professional or social service program. Health care professionals need to be aware of the abundance of nutrition-related information and services available. These include registered dietitians (RDs); federal, state, and local community services; websites; and pamphlets, books, and other printed educational materials. This chapter reviews the various types of nutrition resources available and provides tips on selecting sources of sound nutrition information to use in dental practice.

SCREENING TOOLS

Nutrition professionals have developed a variety of useful diet screening forms for use in dental settings (see Chapter 22). The Nutrition Screening Initiative (NSI) discussed in Chapter 19 is a joint project of the American Academy of Family Physicians, the American Dietetic Association, and 25 national health, aging, and medical organizations, and is designed to increase nutrition screening and intervention for older Americans. The NSI "DETERMINE Your Nutritional Health Checklist" can be self-administered or administered by health professionals or nonprofessionals as a "quick check" for warning signs of poor nutritional status. Steps to help correct possible warning signs are outlined in the "Strong and Healthy" handout, also available from NSI. Copies of screening forms, as well as instructions for use and details on appropriate referrals based on the screening results, can be ordered from NSI.

REFERRING FOR NUTRITION SERVICES

Referral to a Registered Dietitian

Clients who express nutrition concerns during their dental appointments or who may need nutrition counseling for any reason should be referred to the appropriate qualified professional, a registered dietitian (RD). The letters *RD* after a person's name signify that he or she has completed academic and experience requirements established by the Commission on Dietetic Registration, the credentialing agency for the American Dietetic Association. These requirements include a minimum of a bachelor's degree granted by a U.S. regionally accredited college or university and an approved preprofessional training program, successful completion of a national credentialing examination, and continuing professional education. The RD is skilled in nutritional assessment and counseling for clients with nutrition-related conditions (e.g., obesity, diabetes, hypertension, heart disease, food allergy, cancer, kidney disease, eating disorders, and liver disease).

It is important to direct clients to legitimate nutrition professionals, as unqualified "nutritionists" may advocate unhealthful and often unsafe dietary practices. In an effort to curtail the activities of unqualified nutrition providers, most states now require that all nutrition service providers be licensed in the state in which they work, in addition to maintaining national registration. To help clinicians and clients find local RDs, the American Dietetic Association offers a national "Find the Dietitian" service (Table 23–1). Hospitals, wellness centers, and universities often offer nutrition counseling by RDs as well.

Insurance Issues

Many people are hesitant to seek out nutrition services because they are unsure if their insurance plans will cover such care. However, many insurance providers will cover two or more visits to a dietitian per year. Since coverage can vary greatly among providers and terms are often changing, it is important to check with individual insurance companies to find out the terms of coverage, including the correct referral process. Often a referral from a primary care physician is necessary for proper reimbursement.

Community Resources

Dental professionals should also be aware of their clients' level of food security. Single-parent families, children, and elderly people who do not have the resources to meet their daily nutrient needs are among those who would benefit from referral to one of the many social programs designed to provide food, access to food, nutrition education, and/or support to specific population groups. Programs designed for women and children are outlined in Table 23–2, those targeted to adults and families are listed in Table 23–3, and those for elderly clients are shown in Table 23–4.

TABLE 23-1   Annotated Resources for Patient Education Materials

Organizations	*Resources*
Nutrition and Oral Health	
American Dental Association	The Diet and Oral Health section of A–Z Health Topics provides a brief overview of sound nutrition practices. Special attention is given to the effects of soft drinks.
211 East Chicago Avenue	
Chicago, IL 60611-2678	
(312) 440-2500	Dudley the dinosaur animations are available for kids in Grades K–3.
1-800-947-4746	One focuses on healthful snacking.
http://www.ada.org/public/topics/diet.asp	
National Institute of Dental and Craniofacial Research	"Snack Smart for Healthy Teeth!" brochure teaches kids how to cut down on sugary snacks, how cavities form, and how to choose tooth-friendly snacks. Other publications focus on oral health and hygiene.
National Institutes of Health	
Bethesda, MA 20892-2190	
(301) 496-4261	
http://www.nidcr.nih.gov/	
e-mail: nidcrinfo@mail.nih.gov	
Nutrition Screening Initiative	Training materials and forms to be used by caregivers to screen older adults for dental, dietary, medical, and psychosocial problems.
1010 Wisconsin Avenue N.W.	
Suite 800	Printable and interactive versions of the "DETERMINE" checklist and "Strong and Healthy" handout.
Washington, DC 20007	
http://www.aafp.org/nsi.xml	
General Nutrition	
American Dietetic Association	A wide selection of patient education materials available on basic nutrition topics including snacking, following vegetarian diets, decreasing sodium, increasing calcium, learning about sports nutrition, and understanding food labels.
120 South Riverside Plaza, Suite 2000	
Chicago, IL 60606-6995	
1-800-877-1600	
http://www.eatright.org	Scientific position papers on various issues are posted on the website or available for ordering.
Center for Nutrition Policy and Promotion	The USDA Center on Nutrition Policy and Promotion is the source for copies of the *Food Guide Pyramid*, the *Food Guide Pyramid for Young Children*, the *Dietary Guidelines for Americans*, and the *Healthy Eating Index*, and much more. Most publications can be downloaded from their website and the rest are available by mail.
3101 Park Center Drive, Room 1034	
Alexandria, VA 22302-1594	
(703) 305-7600	
http://www.usda.gov/cnpp/	
Consumer Information Center	Consumer-oriented pamphlets include "Snack Smart for Healthy Teeth!" and "Revealing Trans Fats." Recipes, food safety, health insurance, and dietary supplements are some of the other topics covered here. Pamphlets can be downloaded and printed for educational use at no charge. You can also order print copies for free or a small fee.
Federal Citizen Information Center	
Pueblo, CO 81009	
1-888-878-3256	
http://www.pueblo.gsa.gov/	
Food and Drug Administration	This is the place to find information on foodborne illness, biotechnology, food labeling, health claims, and dietary supplements.
Office of Consumer Affairs	
Department of Health and Human Services	
5600 Fishers Lane (HFE-88), Room 1685	
Rockville, MD 20857-0001	
Consumer Hotline: 1-888-463-6332	
http://www.fda.gov	

(continued)

TABLE 23-1 Annotated Resources for Patient Education Materials (Continued)

Organizations	*Resources*
International Food Information Council Foundation 1100 Connecticut Avenue N.W. Suite 430 Washington, DC 20036 (202) 296-6540 http://www.ific.org e-mail: foodinfo@ific.org	Offers thorough and well-designed brochures, fact sheets, and posters on topics such as food allergies, food ingredients, biotechnology, pesticides, fat replacers, and artificial sweeteners, as well as general nutrition information.
The National Dairy Council (http://www.nationaldairycouncil.org) Most states have a branch.	The National Dairy Council offers a variety of excellent nutrition education materials. The website provides links to all state affiliates. Limited numbers of educational resources are provided free to educators. Both professional and lay resources are available.
U.S. Department of Agriculture Food and Nutrition Information Center Agricultural Research Service, USDA National Agricultural Library, Room 105 10301 Baltimore Avenue Beltsville, MD 20705-2351 (301) 504-5719 http://www.nal.usda.gov/fnic/	The Food and Nutrition Information Center has several resource guides, including "Resource List on Food Allergies and Intolerances" and "Food Composition List for Professionals." This site also covers topics of consumer interest, such as dietary supplements and dietary guidelines.
Special Dietary Needs **American Cancer Society** 1599 Clifton Road N.E. Atlanta, GA 30329 1-800-ACS-2345 http://www.cancer.org	Clear, readable information about the connection between diet and cancer, including dietary guidelines, risk factors, prevention guidelines, answers to commonly asked questions, and balanced information about alternative and complementary therapies. Materials are available for both professionals and laypersons.
American Diabetes Association National Call Center 1701 North Beauregard Street Alexandria, VA 22311 1-800-342-2383	Information on professional resources such as position statements, nutrition recommendations for diabetes, and a large selection of patient education materials. The "Virtual Grocery Store" guides visitors through shopping, stocking the pantry, and preparing quick and healthful meals.
American Heart Association 7272 Greenville Avenue Dallas, TX 75231 1-800-AHA-USA-1 http://www.americanheart.org/	Extensive information about nutrition and heart disease available from the AHA's website and by mail. The importance of physical activity and other healthful behaviors are discussed as well.
American Institute for Cancer Research 1759 R Street N.W. Washington, DC 20009 1-800-843-8114 http://www.aicr.org	The *Health and Nutrition Resource Catalogue* lists a variety of materials dealing with nutrition and the prevention of cancer. The AICR disseminates information about new research on the connection between diet and cancer, as well as updates on such "hot" nutrition topics as antioxidants and phytochemicals.
The Food Allergy & Anaphylaxis Network 11781 Lee Jackson Highway, Suite 160 Fairfax, VA 22033-3309 1-800-929-4040 http://www.foodallergy.org e-mail: faan@foodallergy.org	This volunteer organization distributes information and debunks misconceptions about food allergies. The materials offer clear explanations of allergy testing, anaphylactic reactions, and the difference between food allergy and food intolerance. Regularly issued "Special Allergy Alerts" updating those with food allergies to product recalls and warnings are offered by e-mail.

National Cancer Institute

Office of Cancer Communications
31 Center Drive, MSC 2580
Building 31, Room 10A-29
Bethesda, MD 20892-2580
1-800-4-CANCER
http://www.cancer.gov
e-mail: cancergovstaff@mail.nih.gov

Many publications are offered that focus on cancer prevention and treatment for both patients and health professionals. Spanish language versions are available from the Institute as well.

National Heart, Lung, and Blood Institute Information Center

P.O. Box 30105
Bethesda, MD 20824-0105
1-800-575-WELL
http://www.nhlbi.nih.gov/
e-mail: nhlbiinfo@nhlbi.nih.gov

The NHLBI is a good source of information on diets to prevent and control cardiac disease, hypertension, cholesterol, diabetes, overweight, and physical activity. Many of the materials are available in Spanish. Special collections of resources focus on African Americans, Latinos/Latinas, and women.

OncoLink

Sponsor: University of Pennsylvania
http://cancer.med.upenn.edu/

This award-winning website supplies information ranging in complexity from simple tips for cancer patients to scholarly journal articles.

Osteoporosis and Related Bone Disease National Resource Center

2 AMS Circle
Bethesda, MD 20892-3676
1-800-624-BONE
http://www.osteo.org
e-mail: osteoinfo@osteo.org

This is a clearinghouse for osteoporosis information for both professionals and laypersons. Bibliographies and fact sheets are available on topics such as eating disorders and bone density, alcohol and osteoporosis, and osteoporosis research in Asian, Hispanic, and African American populations, as well as in men.

Vegetarian Resource Group

P.O. Box 1463
Baltimore, MD 21203
(410) 366-8343
http://www.vrg.org
E-mail: vrg@vrg.org

Produces practical, scientifically valid fact sheets, brochures, and books that can help clarify the sometimes confusing area of vegetarian nutrition. Publications cover meeting iron needs, eating out, and meatless eating for seniors, children, and pregnant women. Several articles are available in Spanish.

To find local programs for older Americans, a nationwide directory assistance service for seniors called the Eldercare Locator is available (1-800-677-1116, or http://www.eldercare.gov/Eldercare/Public/Home.asp). The Eldercare Locator can provide the names and contact information of organizations within a desired location anywhere in the country that offer a variety of services including meals, home care transportation, recreation, and social activities. In addition, each state has an agency on aging that provides similar information and resources. Local programs typically found in most communities include soup kitchens, food pantries, and shelters. To find such a facility in your local area, contact the local department of health or a religious organization in the community.

NUTRITION IN CYBERSPACE

The Internet is the electronic network that connects millions of computers worldwide. The number of people logging on is growing explosively. In 1998, 54 million people sought health information online and in 2002, this number more than doubled to 110 million (Akerkar, Bichile, 2004). For health care consumers, the Internet is an easy way to educate oneself on diseases, drugs, lifestyle modifications, and more.

The Internet is changing the relationship between health care providers and their clients. Such simple access to volumes of information is likely to improve consumers' sense of control, as well as their ability to participate actively in health care decisions. People can go online to research specific conditions and treatments

TABLE 23–2 Community Nutrition Resources for Women and Children

Resource	Eligibility	Benefits	More Information
Special Supplemental Food Program for Women, Infants, and Children (WIC)	Low-income pregnant and postpartum women and children (5 years old) who are at risk for poor nutrition	Nutrition assessment Nutrition education Vouchers for nutrient-dense foods (e.g., milk, infant formula, eggs, beans, cheese, peanut butter, fruit juice)	http://www.fns.usda.gov/wic/
Commodity Supplemental Food Program (CSFP)	Low-income pregnant and postpartum women and children (6 years old) Low-income adults over 60	Nutrition education Supplemental foods	http://www.fns.usda.gov/fdd/programs/csfp/
School Lunch Program	All children at participating schools and child care institutions (some children will qualify for free or reduced-price meals)	Nutritious lunch Education about nutritious food habits	http://www.fns.usda.gov/cnd/Lunch/
Special Milk Program	Children at schools not participating in other federal meal service programs	Milk	http://www.fns.usda.gov/cnd/milk/
School Breakfast Program	All children at participating schools and child care institutions (some children will qualify for free or reduced price meals)	Nutritious breakfast	http://www.fns.usda.gov/cnd/breakfast/
Child and Adult Care Food Program	Children and adults receiving day care	Cash reimbursements Commodities	http://www.fns.usda.gov/cnd/care/cacfp/cacfphome.htm
Summer Food Service Program	Children ≤ 18 years old attending schools, recreation centers, or camps during the summertime Children > 18 years who have a disability and are attending a school program for people who are disabled	Funds Commodities for breakfast, lunch, and snacks	http://www.fns.usda.gov/cnd/summer/

or to join support groups. Indeed, among consumers who research health issues online, 70% say that the information they find has influenced their treatment decisions. (Akerkar, Bichile, 2004). However, the enormity of the information online can be overwhelming to some patients. Therefore, it is essential that health practitioners be skilled in Internet use (Hart, Henwood, Wyatt, 2004). This includes guiding patients to the best information and

TABLE 23–3   Community Nutrition Resources for Adults and Families

Resource	Eligibility	Benefits	More Information
Food Stamp Program	Low-income families, people, who are elderly and disabled	Coupons and Electronic Benefits Transfer (EBT) cards that can be used to purchase eligible food in participating food stores	http://www.fns.usda.gov/fsp/
Temporary Emergency Food Assistance Program (TEFAP)	Low-income households	Commodities, such as egg mix, canned beans, canned pork, peanut butter, raisins, butter, flour, and cornmeal	http://www.fns.usda.gov/fdd/programs/tefap/

TABLE 23–4   Community Nutrition Resources for Senior Citizens

Resource	Eligibility	Benefits	More Information
Congregate Meals	Seniors, 60+, and their spouse, regardless of age	Group meal once a day, usually lunch, Monday through Friday; some offer meals on the weekend, too Nutritious meal Social interaction Some centers also include other services, including transportation to and from the center, information and referral for health and social services counseling, nutrition education, shopping assistance, and recreation	Agency on Aging
Home-Delivered Meals	Seniors, 60+ years old living in the program's service area Unable to prepare meals for themselves, usually people who are frail or homebound, or people with disabilities	Nutritious meals delivered to the home daily, usually midday, Monday through Friday (cold supper bags and weekend frozen meals are available in some areas)	Agency on Aging Local hospital
Child and Adult Care Food Program	Children to age 12 Elderly (age 60+) Individuals with disabilities who participate in a nonprofit, licensed, or approved day care program	Centers receive federal funds for 2 meals, and 1 snack per participant per day plus one additional meal or snack if the child or adult is in attendance for 8 hours or longer	Public or private not-for-private day care centers

steering them away from the rest. Exactly how to do this is explained in the next section.

Evaluating Nutrition Resources: The Internet Dilemma

Although clients may feel empowered, using the Internet as a source of health information has its drawbacks. One is the sheer quantity of information available. The second challenge is the variability in the quality of material available online. Because anyone with the necessary computer capabilities can post a website, consumers and health care providers alike need to exercise caution when retrieving information from the Web. Although Internet tools such as search engines, indices, and directories filter through information and bring it to the monitor quickly, most are not equipped to assess accuracy and validity (Jadad, Gagliardi, 1998).

The Food and Drug Administration offers some guidelines for locating legitimate websites (Larkin, 1996).

1. *Determine who maintains the site*. Those that are run by government agencies (.gov) or universities (.edu) are usually the most reliable. Sites maintained by private practitioners or commercial organizations may be trying to promote their business or cause and therefore may be one-sided in their presentation of material, as well as their links to other sites.
2. *Check credentials*. It is also important to know who is responsible for the day-to-day content of the site. Is there an editorial board, and do the members have recognized credentials? There should be a way to contact the writers, either via e-mail or telephone, to get additional information.
3. *Check out the quality of the links*. It is important for a site to acknowledge that it is not the exclusive voice in its area of expertise and to offer the reader links for further exploration. The quality of links is important. Just as anyone can create a website, any Webmaster can link his or her site to another without the knowledge or permission of the other site. Therefore, although quality links add depth to a website, they alone do not verify the accuracy and reliability of the original site.

4. *Note the frequency of updates*. Ideally, health and nutrition sites should be updated weekly or monthly to provide the most up-to-date material.
5. *Beware of fees*. If charges are involved, be sure that the information is not offered somewhere else for free and that what you are getting is truly worth the money.

Gateways to Nutrition on the Web

Finding a reliable gateway site can significantly reduce the amount of both time and frustration spent looking for information online. The sites listed below are all maintained by owners with nutrition credentials who prescreen the links to select accurate, useful resources.

Arbor Nutrition Guide

http://www.arborcom.com

This exceedingly thorough collection of annotated nutrition links for health care professionals is well maintained and frequently updated by Australian physician Tony Helman.

The Blonz Guide

http://www.blonz.com

Syndicated columnist Ed Blonz tends to this thorough collection of links to nutrition websites.

Healthfinder

http://www.healthfinder.gov/

This site collects health information from a variety of reputable government and professional sources. You can search on a specific topic, or browse the Nutrition section in the Prevention & Wellness section of the Health Library.

This ratings and review guide features close to 400 nutrition sites linked and ranked for accuracy, content, and usability. Visitors can search by key words or browse by topic or audience category.

SUMMARY AND IMPLICATIONS FOR DENTISTRY

Dental professionals treat more people more often than any other health care provider. Because they are highly respected for their knowledge of general health as well as oral health, they may be asked for information or resources on diet and nutrition. The dental professional is not expected to be an expert on nutrition, but he or she should be a resource person for sound nutrition information and services, and be able to steer clients away from unsound practices and products. Dental professionals should become familiar with nutrition services provided in their communities, so that they can refer clients when needed. By becoming aware of local resources (e.g., websites, nutrition service agencies, RDs), they can help clients locate meaningful resources and help foster good nutrition practices.

REFERENCES

Akerkar SM, Bichile LS: Health information on the Internet: Patient empowerment or patient deceit? *Indian J Med Sci.* 2004; 58:321–26.

D'Alessandro D, Huth L: Evaluation health information on the Internet. Virtual Children's Hospital. Retrieved January 24, 2005, from http://www.vh.org/pediatric/patient/pediatrics/cqqa/internethealth.html.

Hart A, Henwood F, Wyatt S: The role of the Internet in patient-practitioner relationships: Findings from a qualitative research study. *J Med Internet Res* 2004; 30:e36.

Jadad AR, Gagliardi A: Rating health information on the Internet: Navigating to knowledge or to babel? *JAMA* 1998; 279:611–14.

Larkin M: Health information on-line. *FDA Consumer* June, 1996.

Appendix A

Answers to Case Study Questions

CHAPTER 3

ENERGY BALANCE AND WEIGHT CONTROL

Questions

1. **Calculate her current BMI and her BMI 6 months ago. How would you classify Ms. Brody's weight 6 months ago? How would you classify her weight now?**
   BMI 6 months ago: 20.8 (normal). Current BMI: 16.6 (underweight).

2. **What is Ms. Brody's healthy weight range according to the DRIs?**
   A healthy weight range for Ms. Brody is between 110 and 150 lb (DRIs).

3. **Is she at risk for any diseases or disorders?**
   Because she is an underweight Caucasian female who does not exercise, and is lactose intolerant (limits some dairy consumption—a good source of calcium) she is at risk for osteopenia and osteoporosis. Because of her low weight, she may be at risk for amenorrhea, which will further increase her risk for osteopenia and osteoporosis. Since she is a vegetarian who reports reduced appetite, she may be at risk for anemia (diet may be low in iron).

4. **What are her most significant nutrition issues?**
   She is not consuming adequate amounts of energy—she is 978.5 calories too low.

5. **What may be contributing to her weight loss? Given the rapid rate of weight loss, what kinds of tissue were most likely lost?**
   Decreased appetite leading to decreased energy intake and weight loss. Her weight loss of 25 lb over 6 months has placed her in the underweight category. If there are considerable amounts of sugar alcohols in the gum she is chewing, that could be contributing to her diarrhea. In addition, her consumption of cheese with lactose intolerance may also cause diarrhea. Diarrhea may lead to fluid and electrolyte losses. She is not consuming enough protein to meet the RDA (0.8 g/kg) nor is she consuming enough calories, which is probably contributing to her loss in lean mass, fatigue, lack of energy, and weakness.

6. **What nutrition and oral health recommendations would you make for Ms. Brody?**
   Due to the rapidity of her weight loss, a combination of lean mass (higher percentage), fat, and fluid were probably lost. Diarrhea is likely contributing to her fluid loss. Prozac (fluoxetine) may decrease appetite, leading to decreased energy consumption, which may lead to weight loss.

   Mrs. Brody should:
   - See a physician.
   - Discuss medication side effects with psychiatrist.
   - See a registered dietitian for personalized diet guidance.
   - Gradually increase calorie intake to at least 2,278 calories.
     - Increase protein intake: educate her about non-meat protein sources: nuts, seeds, nut butters, beans, soy, soy milk, soy yogurt, seitan, texturized vegetable protein, eggs.
     - Try tofu (a meat substitute high in calcium) or soy-based products fortified with calcium (which will also be a source of protein).
     - Try an oral nutritional supplement such as Ensure or Boost.
   - Take a multivitamin, calcium supplements (600 mg 2x a day), and an iron supplement (at a separate time from the calcium supplement).
   - Try to eat at least 3 balanced meals with snacks in between.
   - Try stress management to decrease stress level.
   - Get more weight bearing exercise to build up bones (prevent osteoporosis) and increase lean muscle tissue.

- Drink at least eight, 8 fl oz glasses of water a day to ensure adequate hydration.
- Chew less sugar-free gum—the sugar alcohols may be contributing to diarrhea.
- Use a soft bristle tooth brush to avoid enamel and gingival abrasion.

CHAPTER 4

CARBOHYDRATES, DIABETES, AND ASSOCIATED HEALTH CONDITIONS

Case Study #1

Questions

1. **What problem does this child probably have?**

   Lactose intolerance: When lactose exceeds lactase activity, excess lactose is not broken down to glucose and galactose, but accumulates in the intestines where it is fermented by bacteria, producing flatulence, cramps, diarrhea, and abdominal pain.

2. **Why would you suspect this problem in an immigrant from Mexico?**

   Lactose is common in many ethnic groups other than whites of northern European ancestry. The prevalence can be as high as 70 to 90% in Asians, Native Americans, Indians, Jews, Mexicans, blacks, Italians, and Greeks.

3. **What special dietary considerations should be emphasized to promote adequate growth and dental health?**

   The mother would be advised to provide the child with a lactose-free or lactose-restricted diet, depending on the child's level of lactase activity. Since lactose is found in dairy products, eliminating all foods containing lactose can lead to dietary deficiencies. To promote adequate growth and dental health, it is important to provide the child with nondairy dietary sources of calcium. It is possible that the child may need a calcium and/or vitamin D supplement as well. There are strategies for consuming lactose-containing foods that may help prevent dietary deficiencies:
   - Space intake throughout the day.
   - Take lactose-containing foods with meals to delay emptying of the stomach.
   - Whole milk is sometimes better tolerated than skim milk.

- Aged cheese and yogurt with active cultures have decreased lactose.
- Add lactase to milk to break down lactose.
- Milk, ice cream, and cottage cheese treated with lactase are available in some areas.
- Take lactase tablets with food.

Case Study #2

Questions

1. **What issues would you discuss as possible reasons for this patient's health problems?**

   Many of the patient's health issues are related to diet. It appears that the patient is eating a low-fiber diet since many of the patient's gastrointestinal disturbances and oral health issues may be lessened with a high-fiber diet. Because the patient lacks knowledge of what a high-fiber diet is, which is apparent through his diet history, it may be that the majority of the carbohydrate in the patient's diet is in a digestible form, sugar or starch. Dental decay and periodontal problems occur when acids are produced because of the fermentation of these carbohydrates by bacteria. Dietary fiber, on the other hand, cannot be digested by human enzymes, and therefore is not fermented in the mouth. Constipation and diverticulitis are also aggravated by a low-fiber diet.

2. **How would you explain to this patient the benefits of a high-fiber diet?**

   There are many benefits to a high-fiber diet, particularly since this patient appears to have many health problems that could be alleviated, or at least improved, with an increase in fiber in the diet. High-fiber diets can:
   - Relieve constipation. Most healthy adults can usually achieve more normal GI transit time by consuming more insoluble fiber for as little as 2 days.
   - Relieve symptoms of uncomplicated diverticulitis and may also help prevent the condition.
   - Help lower cholesterol levels. Moderately increasing intake of fibrous foods may lead to small decreases in blood cholesterol levels that may significantly lessen cardiovascular risk over a long period.
   - Decrease risk of dental caries. Fibrous foods stimulate the flow of saliva, which helps wash

away sugar from teeth and contains materials that promote remineralization of eroded tooth enamel to a certain extent.

3. **What are some practical recommendations for increasing the intake of complex carbohydrates in the diet?**

Gradual changes in the patient's diet are most likely to last and will give the body time to adjust to the increase in fiber that can be found in many complex carbohydrates. First, the patient should try eating 5 servings of fruits and vegetables per day since many varieties of these foods contain fiber. Second, the patient should eat 6 to11 servings of bread, rice, grains, cereals, and pasta each day. It may also be beneficial for the patient to eat a variety of grain products, such as wheat, oats, rice, corn, or rye. If the patient eats few beans and starchy vegetables he may try the following: add black beans or lentils to soups, kidney beans or garbanzo beans to salads, hummus made from chickpeas in sandwiches, and starchy vegetables and beans to entrees like chili.

CHAPTER 5

PROTEIN FOR SYSTEMIC AND ORAL HEALTH: MEETING NEEDS IN A MULTICULTURAL WORLD

Questions

1. **What are the risks associated with Joanne's eating pattern?**

Although the woman has lost weight since initiation of the vegan diet, her weight remains within normal limits for her height. However, since her diet is limited, it is important to monitor her for weight loss. Despite that she is near her ideal body weight, the patient's diet does put her at nutritional risk since it is very restrictive. Vegans rely solely on foods that are of plant origin. Therefore, it is possible that she is not meeting all of her protein needs.

2. **Are all vegetarians at risk for protein deficiency?**

Not all vegetarians are necessarily at risk for protein deficiency. Vegans are at the highest risk since the foods they eat are exclusively of plant origin. Of particular risk are vegans, such as pregnant or lactating women, whose bodies need more protein,

but whose food intake may be too low to supply the necessary essential amino acids. Although other vegetarians have a plant-based diet, some also eat certain foods of animal origin, which may decrease their risk for protein deficiency:

- Semivegetarian: avoids only certain kinds of meat, fish, or poultry
- Lacto-ovovegetarian: avoids eating animal flesh but does use dairy products and eggs
- Lactovegetarian: avoids eating animal flesh and eggs, but does use dairy products

3. **How could Joanne get adequate protein in her diet while remaining vegan?**

It is important that she receives the essential amino acids in her diet. It isn't important that she receives the amino acids from one individual food, but that she fulfills her needs from everything eaten during the day so that her body can continue normal protein synthesis. Therefore, it is essential that she eats foods that are complementary— foods that when eaten together provide the essential amino acids, but individually would not. The proteins in plant foods have unique limiting amino acids (amino acids they are lacking). Typically, the essential amino acids in legumes (starchy beans, peas, and lentils) and in grains complement each other. Also, legumes and nuts or seeds usually complement each other. For example, corn is low in the amino acid lysine, whereas many beans contain adequate amounts of it. On the other hand, beans are limited in methionine, which corn contains. Therefore, by eating both of these foods in the same day she could consume adequate amounts of both amino acids, plus other amino acids contained in the foods.

4. **Do you have any oral health concerns about Joanne?**

Because she is at risk for protein deficiency, there are some possible oral health concerns. A deficiency in protein has been implicated in osteoporosis of the supporting bone that surrounds teeth. A lack of protein can also impair local tissue healing and may lead to problems with gingivitis. Furthermore, many nutrient deficiencies, including protein deficiency, can affect the tongue. Symptoms may include burning, swelling, and ulceration of the papillae. All of these oral health conditions should be looked for during an examination of a patient at risk for protein deficiency.

5. **What would you tell Joanne regarding her plans to raise her future children as vegans?**

Joanne needs to speak to her child's pediatrician about her plans to raise her children as vegans. The children's diets will need to be designed very carefully with special attention to nutrient quality and quantity. The pediatrician may recommend appropriate supplements and will monitor the children's growth to help ensure that the diet meets their developmental needs.

CHAPTER 6
LIPIDS IN HEALTH AND DISEASE
Questions

1. **What other factors besides dietary fat and cholesterol might be contributing to this patient's elevated blood cholesterol level?**

This patient has a family history of high cholesterol and heart disease. In addition, she is clinically obese and is unable to exercise due to her arthritis. All of these factors combined with a diet high in saturated fat may increase her risk for heart disease. A diet high in fiber (particularly soluble fiber) may help lower cholesterol levels.

2. **Help the patient identify sources of saturated fat in her diet.**

Sources of saturated fat in her diet include the half & half, whole milk, butter, mayonnaise, cheddar cheese, ice cream, and shortening or lard used to fry the chicken.

3. **What substitutions might you recommend for high-fat, saturated-fat foods?**

Recommendations:
- Gradual shift from whole milk to 1% or skim milk.
- Try a soft margarine free of trans fatty acids instead of butter.
- Try light or fat-free mayonnaise.
- Suggest broiling or grilling chicken instead of frying it.
- Try low-fat or fat-free frozen yogurt or nonfat ice cream.

4. **What is meant by "heart healthy" fats, and what foods are high in these fats?**

"Heart healthy" fats refer to specific fatty acids that do not lead to atherosclerosis and may even help lower the risk of heart disease.

Monounsaturated fats reduce plasma triglycerides and very low density lipoproteins (VLDL), both of which are risk factors for cardiovascular disease. MUFAs also increase high density lipoprotein (HDL) levels resulting in a protective effect against heart disease. It has little effect on total blood cholesterol levels, though. Foods high in MUFAs include olive oil, canola oil, peanuts and peanut oil, pecans, almonds, and avocados.

Polyunsaturated fats (PUFA) are considered essential fatty acids since our body is not able to make them. They significantly lower total cholesterol as well as low density lipoprotein (LDL) levels. However, they do not increase HDL levels. Omega-3 fatty acids can be found in cold-water marine fish (salmon and mackerel), some plant oils (soybean and canola oils) and leafy vegetables.

CHAPTER 8
THE MINERALS AND MINERALIZATION
Questions

1. **What are normal levels for hemoglobin and hematocrit? What is your interpretation?**

Normal hemoglobin (HbB) is 12 to 5g/dL. Normal hematocrit (Hct) for women is 34 to 44%. Morgan appears to be anemic.

2. **What are some reasons that teenage girls are especially at risk for iron-deficiency anemia? What factors apply to Morgan?**

Factors include eating too little food in general and too few iron sources in particular. This, in addition to the iron losses that occur monthly, can lead to anemia. In Morgan's case, most of her food choices are poor sources of iron. Her heavy bleeding exacerbates the problem.

3. **Why is fatigue a common symptom of anemia?**

Fatigue results when insufficient oxygen is carried in blood as a result of reductions in iron-dependent hemoglobin.

4. **An iron supplement, ferrous sulfate, was pre-scribed for Morgan. Could a high-iron diet achieve the same results?**

An iron supplement is an easier way of obtaining the iron needed. The iron could be obtained from food, but it would require a major change in diet to increase the iron content.

5. **In her health class at school, Morgan learned that some foods are good sources of heme iron. What is meant by heme iron? What foods supply heme iron? What are such foods in Morgan's typical day? What other foods in her current diet are good sources of nonheme iron?**

Heme iron is found in animal products, especially red meats. Good food sources are liver, steak, and so on. Morgan eats few sources of heme iron other than chicken and fish, which are not the best sources. Nonheme iron is found in vegetable foods such as whole grains and fortified cereals.

6. **What nutrients enhance or interfere with iron absorption? With Morgan, plan revised meal patterns and menu structures for a typical day to improve the food combinations at meals and snacks.**

Enhance: vitamin C, growth, heme iron, gastric acidity

Interfere: lack of stomach acid, coffee, calcium, phytates,

Breakfast: enriched cereal with banana, orange juice, skim milk

Lunch: school lunch, with meat, vegetable, salad, milk, dessert

Snack: peanut butter on crackers

Dinner: same as before

Bedtime: enriched cereal and skim milk

CHAPTER 9

VITAMINS TODAY

Questions

1. **What is the most likely cause of this executive's oral condition?**

Vitamin C deficiency is the most likely cause.

2. **What are the red dots on the patient's hard palate, arms, and chest?**

The dots are from petecchiae, resulting from vitamin C deficiency.

3. **Why would the gingiva bleed profusely upon provocation?**

Connective tissue defects allowed blood to effuse into the tissues from the blood vessels.

4. **What underlying mechanism caused these signs?**

Ascorbic acid deficiency results in defective collagen formation. The collagen formed has weak cross linkages, and results in friable tissues. Blood can then diffuse through capillary walls into surrounding tissue.

5. **What diet suggestions would you make?**

- See a registered dietitian for the vitamin therapy needed to correct the deficiency and develop a better long-term diet plan.
- Have some good vitamin C sources daily such as juice, tomato on sandwiches, fresh fruit, or any other approach acceptable to the patient. If all vitamin C sources are rejected, suggest a daily multivitamin supplement.

CHAPTER 10

DIETARY SUPPLEMENTS

Questions

1. **What would you say to Altagracia about her supplement usage?**

Tell her that although her goal of improving health is praiseworthy, like anything else, some level of supplementation may be appropriate and some may not or may even be harmful.

For a woman her age the major nutrients of concern are calcium/vitamin D and folic acid if she is planning to become pregnant. She is not taking any folic acid, which is important if she is planning to become pregnant.

2. **What issues are of concern regarding her supplement usage?**

Several of the supplements she is taking are in doses higher than the UL (upper level of intake). These are vitamins A, B_6, and C. Vitamin A in particular can be teratogenic to a developing fetus in high levels. There may be risks in using some of the herbals as well. Ginkgo biloba can counteract the antihypertensive effects of the thiazide diuretic she is taking and can increase her blood pressure.

3. **What recommendations would you make to her?**

If she wants to take supplements, she should take a once-daily type of multivitamin/mineral at the level of no higher than 100x the DRI for the included nutrients.

She should try to take a supplement that contains folate as well. Her calcium supplement should contain vitamin D, and should not be from bone meal or oyster shell due to the risk of contamination of these "natural" types of supplements. A pharmacy or name-brand pure source like calcium carbonate or calcium citrate malate is a safer choice.

CHAPTER 11

NUTRITIONAL AND ORAL IMPLICATIONS OF COMMON CHRONIC HEALTH CONDITIONS: HYPERTENSION, OSTEOPOROSIS, AND IMMUNE-COMPROMISING CONDITIONS

Case Study #1

Questions

1. **What aspects of this patient make you feel that a consultation with his physician is necessary?**
   - His high blood pressure reading of 170/105
   - The symptoms of thirst and frequent urination, which may indicate undiagnosed diabetes mellitus
   - His alcohol consumption; he may need referral to an addiction specialist

2. **What dietary recommendations might you make to this patient?**
   - Smaller, lean cuts of red meat
   - Increased poultry and fish
   - Smaller food portions to help with weight loss
   - Three to 4 servings per day of non-fat or low-fat dairy
   - Five or more servings of fruits and vegetables per day
   - Reduced alcohol intake

3. **What is the dental professional's role in assisting this patient with tobacco cessation?**

The patient is interested in quitting smoking, so now is the time to provide him with information on local support groups and assess his nicotine dependence to determine if a nicotine replacement is needed. Stress long-term success is improved if he starts attending a support group and formulates a quit plan before setting a quit date. Provide encouragement and support at subsequent appointments.

4. **What concerns do you have for this patient regarding his healing response to initial periodontal therapy?**

It would be ideal to get the blood pressure under better control, begin tobacco cessation, and determine whether he has diabetes before beginning initial periodontal therapy.

Case Study #2

Questions

1. **What are the potential side effects of radiation therapy? How do these side effects affect the oral cavity?**

Some potential side effects of radiation therapy include xerostomia, increased risk of root caries, decreased vascular blood supply to oral cavity, increased risk of infection, decreased appetite, and decreased sense of taste.

2. **What factors may have contributed to Rose Jackson's extensive caries problem?**

Several factors may have contributed to Rose Jackson's extensive caries problem including the consumption of high-sugar foods, decreased saliva production, and a lack of dental home care.

3. **How does cancer affect nutritional status? What is the *most important nutritional* issue?**

The most important nutritional issue in this case would be to maintain weight because cancer is associated with an increased need for energy and protein while most patients experience a lack of desire to eat.

4. **What would your dental care plan be to ameliorate her current dental problem and prevent future problems?**

The dental care plan would include oral hygiene instruction, artificial saliva, and an oral anesthetic to overcome the painful mucositis that prevents Rose from brushing her teeth and gums properly.

5. What should the nutrition care rationale be?

The nutrition care rationale would be a high calorie, high protein diet via small, frequent meals throughout the day. Rose would probably not be able to tolerate large amounts of food at one sitting, so the recommendation would be to eat as many meals as often as she wanted. A nutritional supplement (e.g., Ensure, Boost, Carnation Instant Breakfast, etc.) would also be appropriate in this situation, as it would serve as a concentrated source of calories and protein.

6. How should the dental and nutrition care be coordinated?

The dental care plan would involve decreasing the cariogenicity of the nutrition care plan. Suggestions would include stimulating the production of saliva by suggesting chewing sugarless gum, rinsing with water after eating, and emphasizing the importance of oral home care.

Case Study #3
Questions

1. Why is a consultation with the patient's physician necessary?

- His rapid, unexplained weight loss
- To get more information about what medications will be used in the short- and long-term treatment for this patient
- To let the physician know the dental health status of the patient and discuss prevention of oral health problems

2. What general dietary recommendations would you make to this patient?

First, ask if the patient has seen a registered dietitian (RD) to get some individualized dietary advice. If he is under the care of an RD, then you can offer support for his recommendations. If not, this might be something to discuss with the physician. In the meantime, respect the patient's choice to become a vegetarian, but encourage him to choose high-calorie, high-protein foods:

- Encourage dairy foods, which are good sources of protein along with soy and legumes combined with grains.
- Give suggestions to increase calories such as adding margarine, gravies, sour cream, cream, or whipped cream to favorite foods.

- Encourage frequent small meals and snacks.
- Advise him to eat solid foods before liquids at meals.

These are just a few of the possible suggestions.

3. What are some of the potential oral side effects of his treatment protocol?

The major potential side effects of chemotherapy, total body irradiation, and bone marrow transplant include nausea, vomiting, mucositis, candidiasis, and anorexia.

4. What is the role of the dental office in the patient's treatment?

The dental professional needs to consult with the physician to find out when treatment can be safely performed. Perform all necessary dental treatment stressing the importance of thorough and meticulous home care techniques in the prevention of mucositis and caries.

The patient can be instructed on the selection of mild toothpaste and oral rinses. If xerostomia is identified as a potential side effect of treatment, fluoride trays can be made to protect the patient from root caries. Ascertain if the treatment protocol includes use of chlorhexidine mouthrinse to prevent mucositis and oral antifungal agents to prevent candidiasis. The physician and dentist need to be in communication so that the dental office knows when it is appropriate to provide maintenance and follow-up care.

CHAPTER 12
NUTRITION IN THE GROWTH AND DEVELOPMENT OF ORAL STRUCTURES
Questions

1. Is Martha's diet nutritionally adequate? Why or why not?

No. Her diet is deficient in all food groups, but particularly dairy products, and fruits and vegetables. Empty-calorie sweets provide significant calories to the detriment of important nutrients.

2. Are there any diet-related dental or oral problems?

Gum bleeding may be caused by vitamin C deficiency, or it could be merely a result of poor oral hygiene. The high sugar content of the diet and the erratic nature of her eating may have contributed to her new carious lesions.

3. **Are there any risks to Martha or her baby if she becomes pregnant?**

If Martha is not consuming sufficient folic acid sources before her pregnancy, the risk of neural tube disorders in her fetus is increased. The lack of calcium puts her bone health at risk, since her requirement is increased with pregnancy. Nutrient deficiencies, if they are severe enough, can affect epithelial tissue development, ameloblastic activity, and tooth calcification in the baby.

Oral bacteria are transferred from mother to child, so Martha needs to improve her oral hygiene habits to minimize the transfer of cariogenic bacteria to the baby after birth.

4. **What would be appropriate nutritional and dental suggestions for Martha?**
   - Increase vegetable consumption.
   - Try some new fruits, or try water-packed canned fruits and juices.
   - Increase the consumption of dairy products (have milk instead of soda).
   - Take prenatal multivitamin mineral supplement with folic acid.
   - Try to eat more balanced meals.
   - Eat breakfast in the morning before leaving for work.
   - Drink more water.
   - Improve oral hygiene habits.

CHAPTER 13

DIET, NUTRITION, AND TEETH

Questions

1. **What characteristics of Julia's diet are possibly contributing to her oral disease?**
   - Frequent and prolonged intake of beverages that contain a high percentage of fermentable carbohydrate
   - Skipping meals and replacing them with sugar- or starch-processed foods
   - Avoiding chewy foods like fruits, vegetables, and grains that might increase salivary production
   - Possible low intake of cariogenic foods that might buffer the oral acidic environment

2. **List and explain the key issues to consider in how these dietary variables are interacting with the infectious agents responsible for caries activity.**
   - The diet plays a role in the production of saliva.
   - Cariostatic food in the diet can interfere with bacterial activity.
   - Sources and forms of fermentable carbohydrates can promote caries activity.
   - Dietary patterns can either prolong or moderate bacterial activity.

3. **What changes can Julia make in her diet to alter the course of her future risk for caries and at the same time improve her general health status?**
   - Replace fermentable carbohydrate beverages with noncaloric beverages or beverages high in proteins (dairy based).
   - Plan meals that:
     1. meet nutrient requirements and replace consumption of starchy or sugary snacks
     2. include unprocessed whole grains, fruits, and vegetables that promote saliva production
     3. include foods from all food groups but are nutrient dense so as to promote weight management
   - Space eating occasions to achieve and enhance a neutral oral pH the majority of the time.

CHAPTER 14

NUTRITION AND THE PERIODONTIUM

Questions

1. **What are the nutritional concerns with this patient? How might they affect her periodontal treatment?**
   - lack of appetite
   - rapid and unwanted weight loss
   - avoidance of dairy products
   - excessive use of antacids

   The loss of lean body mass may result in mild to moderate protein malnutrition, as well as generally suboptimal intakes of all nutrients need for maintenance of health. The ones specific to periodontal health would include the protein, B vitamins, calcium, vitamin A, D, magnesium, copper, boron, zinc, and iron.

2. **Do you feel a consultation with her physician is indicated? Why or why not?**

A consultation with her physician would be helpful to:

- determine if her serum albumin levels have decreased which would help in diagnosing malnutrition
- ask if the patient can take an alternate medication for her heartburn besides antacids
- ask if the MD has recommendations for other calcium supplements
- find out what kind of nutritional advice she was given and whether the physician felt referral to a registered dietitian was indicated
- see if the physician feels that the patient can tolerate the periodontal treatment that is planned

3. **What dietary recommendations would you make for this patient?**

This patient ideally should be seen by a registered dietitian for an individualized nutrition plan. If that is not an option, we want to get this patient repleted prior to treatment so suggestions for a high-calorie, high-protein diet should be recommended. Suggestions might include:

- Eating frequent small meals and snacks
- Eating milkshakes, pudding, cottage cheese, yogurt, and ice cream
- Adding cheese, margarine, sour cream, cream cheese, and whipped cream to foods
- Eating all solid foods prior to liquids to prevent feeling prematurely full
- Encouraging her to go to congregate meal sites to meet others and have a nutritious meal without having to cook
- Finding out what her favorite foods are and encouraging frequent intake
- Taking a daily multivitamin/mineral supplement

CHAPTER 15

NUTRITIONAL CONCERNS FOR THE DENTALLY COMPROMISED PATIENT: ORAL SURGERY, ORTHODONTICS, DENTURES, DYSPHAGIA, TEMPOROMANDIBULAR DISORDERS

Questions

1. **Is Margaret's diet nutritionally adequate? Why or why not?**

No, her diet does not meet the food guide pyramid guidelines for fruits, vegetables, protein sources, or dairy products. As a result, she is most likely not obtaining sufficient vitamins and minerals.

2. **Might there be a relationship between Margaret's diet and any of her general health problems? If so, what?**

Yes, low intake of fruits, vegetables, and high-fiber grain products translates into low intake of dietary fiber. Weight loss can occur from low-calorie intake or limited variety of foods. Low fiber intake can be a major contributor to constipation. In addition, the calcium carbonate can cause constipation as well. Her diet is not nutrient dense. Her diet is high in fat and sodium from the processed foods, which increases her risk of heart disease.

3. **How might her oral condition affect her diet?**

Her dentures are poorly fitting, making it difficult for her to chew or bite. Thus, she prefers soft foods and avoids eating anything hard. The result is a soft diet with little fiber. She also avoids foods that might be too difficult to chew. The more limited the diet, the greater the risk of deficiencies. Weight loss could also be a problem.

4. **How might her diet affect her oral condition?**

If limited intake of fruits and vegetables results in vitamin or mineral deficiencies, the result can be friable oral soft tissues such as under Margaret's denture. Poor diet can also affect tissue healing ability. If she snacks frequently throughout the day on retentive carbohydrates, this pattern can contribute to an increased caries risk.

5. **What would be appropriate nutritional and preventive dental suggestions for Margaret?**

- Encourage Margaret to have her dentures fixed.
- Encourage her to take her dentures out at night.
- Promote oral health: brush teeth after meals, use a soft bristle toothbrush, clean tissues under dentures regularly, use dental floss, use fluoridated toothpaste, and regular dental visits.
- Increase consumption of fruits and vegetables (if she finds them too hard to cut into bite-sized pieces, recommend canned products).

- Limit sugar intake by replacing calorie-dense meal choices with nutrient-dense foods (replace doughnuts with whole wheat toast and sugar-free preserves).

CHAPTER 17

NUTRITION IN PREGNANCY, INFANCY, AND CHILDHOOD

Questions

1. **What are the important differences between breast milk and cow's milk?**

   Cow's milk has more protein, calcium, and phosphorus and can be harmful for human babies. Breast milk is designed for humans. It has all the nutrients needed for the first few months and provides immunity to the infant as well.

2. **Is there a problem with letting Emily drink breast milk rather than weaning her to cow's milk?**

   Breast milk is the optimal food for the first year of life. Iron deficiency and low calcium intake is a problem among toddlers. Adequate iron is provided up until 4 to 6 months of age in the breast-fed infant but there is need for supplementation after that point. Vitamin D is found in cow's milk and it is very important in the calcification process of bones and teeth. Bottle feeding or breastfeeding over 1 year of age may be associated with early childhood caries (ECC).

3. **What are the potential hazards of allowing Emily to sip on apple juice and eat honey-flavored toasted oats cereal over a long period?**

   Juice sipped constantly in a "sippy cup" can be a major contributor to dental caries in addition to the sticky cereal sitting on her teeth. High juice intake has been linked to short stature and obesity.

4. **What suggestions could you make to Catherine regarding Emily's diet?**

   Allow Emily to make her own food choices. A child needs a variety of food and nutrients to grow properly. Limiting her diet to vegetarian choices could cause her to have stunted growth. Place 3/4 water and 1/4 fruit juice in the sippy cup

to limit the amount of juice that she is consuming all day.

CHAPTER 18

ORAL HEALTH NUTRITION AND DIETARY CONSIDERATIONS IN ADOLESCENCE AND ADULTHOOD

Questions

1. **What are the effects of Andrew's beverage consumption?**

   Andrew's significant regular carbonated beverage consumption is affecting both oral and systemic health. Frequent exposure to sugar has provided bacteria with a substrate for acid production and plaque development resulting in rampant caries and periodontitis. Sugar from regular carbonated beverages contributes 50 to 80% of Andrew's total energy intake; such beverages do not contain accompanying nutrients.

2. **How appropriate is Andrew's calorie intake?**

   Andrew's energy intake is appropriate for his size and activity level as evidenced by weight maintenance within normal limits. To maintain an appropriate energy intake, he has limited intake of nutrient dense foods. This is confirmed by pyramid and nutrient analysis of the 3-day diet record. Andrew's diet places him at risk for limited tissue healing, compromised immune function, and chronic disease.

3. **What would be appropriate dietary recommendations for Andrew?**

   Appropriate dietary recommendations for Andrew include:
   - Consume three meals and one to three defined snacks.
   - Select foods from all food groups. Strategies for incorporating individual foods into a meal plan depend on food preferences.
   - Switch to sugar-free beverages (coffee, tea, diet carbonated beverages, water) for between-meal consumption.
   - Consume a daily multivitamin/mineral supplement until diet is consistent with the food guide pyramid.

CHAPTER 19

THE OLDER DENTAL PATIENT

Questions

1. **What are Mrs. Murphy's oral problems?**

   Intraoral exam and nutritional history suggest that this patient may suffer from xerostomia secondary to her medication use. As is the case with this person, to relieve the dryness associated with xerostomia, individuals often let hard candy dissolve in their mouths to stimulate salivary flow. This practice is deleterious to oral health since the teeth, which are already vulnerable to decay, are being constantly bathed in sugar, increasing the potential for decay and periodontal disease

2. **What are her nutritional problems?**

   The patient may be at high risk for malnutrition based solely on her social history. The fact that she recently lost her spouse, has been prescribed Prozac, has limited family in the area, and reports missing meals and a lack of desire to cook for herself are all warning signs that should be addressed with patient.

   The patient's diet is currently too high in carbohydrates and too low in fruits and vegetables and protein. This may be due to the ill-fitting upper denture as pastas and breads tend to be more easily eaten by individuals with poorly fitting dentures, and the most difficult foods to chew are fruits and some forms of meat.

3. **How would you manage Mrs. Murphy's oral and nutritional problems?**

   Assuming that her medication cannot be altered, a more appropriate approach to treat xerostomia is to use sugarless gum, sugar-free candies, saliva substitutes, and salivary stimulants if the xerostomia is severe. Since this patient has not been to the dentist in 3 years and now has a high caries rate, it is important to educate her on the importance of regular dental visits to maintain the health of her remaining teeth as well as to ensure the proper fit of her dentures. Although the denture reline will help with the patient's chief complaint of an ill-fitting upper denture, xerostomia may also play a role in the lack of denture retention. It is important to educate the patient about the relationship of dry mouth and denture retention both to increase the patient's motivation to treat the xerostomic symp-

toms and to ensure that the patient has realistic expectations regarding the outcome of the reline.

It is also important to discuss any changes in food selection based on her ability to chew and to develop strategies for expanding her selections, for example, choosing bananas instead of apples to increase her fruit intake. The dietary history should be retaken after completion of the reline to ensure that a more balanced diet has been achieved.

CHAPTER 20

ORAL AND NUTRITIONAL CONCERNS FOR PEOPLE WITH SPECIAL HEALTH CARE NEEDS

Questions

1. **Is a baby food/pureed diet appropriate for this child? Why or why not? What dental risks are associated with this type of diet?**

   Yes, a pureed diet is appropriate because children with special health care needs, particularly cerebral palsy, experience delayed feeding development. Modifying foods to increase calorie and protein intake may be necessary to meet the individual's needs. Also, the texture and consistency of foods and liquids should be adjusted according to the oral motor capabilities of each individual.

   Children with cerebral palsy commonly have poor oral motor control, which may result in poor chewing and swallowing ability, excessive drooling, and/or tongue thrust. People on this diet are at increased risk for dental caries due to the prolonged exposure of their teeth to the pureed, cariogenic foods.

2. **Identify three common nutritional problems seen in individuals with special health care needs**

   Three common nutritional problems seen in people with special health care needs include inadequate calorie intake, mastication problems, and dysphagia.

3. **How does prolonged bottle feeding affect oral health?**

   Prolonged bottle feeding or delayed weaning is common in children and infants with special health care needs because of oral motor problems. This increases the child's risk for early childhood caries (also known as baby bottle tooth decay) due to the extensive contact between the teeth and sweetened (cariogenic) beverages. Suggest substituting water in the bottle instead of sugary drinks such as juices and milk.

4. **Discuss the oral consequences of anticonvulsant medications such as Dilantin.**
   Anticonvulsant medications such as Dilantin (phenytoin) may cause gingival overgrowth, which can impair tooth eruption, chewing and appearance. Calcium channel blockers and cyclosporine may also cause overgrowth of the gums. Many drugs cause low saliva (xerostomia). Because saliva helps wash away food debris, a dry mouth increases risk of dental decay. Proper oral hygiene and antimicrobial rinses are recommended to help prevent gum infections and dental decay.

CHAPTER 21

EFFECTIVE COMMUNICATION IN DENTAL PRACTICE

Questions

1. **What error did the dentist make in scenario #1?**
   In scenario #1, the dentist put Mr. Bronsen on the defensive. The most appropriate introduction would have been to say "We need to be sure not to overlook any factors that might be involved in your dental problem. One of the factors we would like to rule out is diet."

2. **Why was the dentist's response inappropriate in scenario #2?**
   In scenario #2, this was an inappropriate approach by the dentist because:
   - A diet assessment was not done, so a recommendation was made without a proper diagnosis.
   - Mr. Bronsen was placed on the defensive by being told, unilaterally, what to do.
   - The reason that prunes might contribute to his dental problem was not explained to him.
   - He was not given enough information to make an appropriate decision himself.

3. **What is the best way to determine what Mr. Bronsen knows about his oral condition?**
   The best way to find out what Mr. Bronsen knows about his oral condition is to ask him in a non-threatening manner what he knows or has been told about his dental condition.

An example might be: "Mr. Bronsen, what did your previous dentist tell you about what is happening with your teeth and gums?"

4. **If, during the course of your session with Mr. Bronsen, he begins to look distracted and uneasy, what would be the most appropriate response?**
   The most appropriate response would be to tell him what you are observing and ask him if there is a problem. For example, "You seem to be a bit uncomfortable, Mr. Bronsen. Is there something wrong?" This gives him the opportunity to share his feelings. He might say, "No, nothing is wrong. I am just tired." Or he might say, "Well, I don't know if I can do all the things you are asking me to do." Whatever the response, the counselor now has an understanding of what is happening and can respond appropriately.

CHAPTER 22

PRINCIPLES OF DIET SCREENING, RISK ASSESSMENT, AND GUIDANCE

Questions

1. **How would you help motivate Emelio to improve his oral hygiene habits?**
   Use his interest in his appearance for his girlfriend as the basis for your guidance.

2. **Which approach is most likely to motivate Emelio to reduce his use of chewing tobacco?**
   Since Emelio is a teenager, interested in being attractive, the best approach would probably to focus upon the aesthetic aspects of chewing tobacco—the fact that it will contribute to tooth staining and bad breath.

3. **Which are the primary dietary cariogenic risk factors?**
   The between-meal snacks and sodas are the major risk factors for Emelio.

4. **According to the Stephan Curve, what would happen to the plaque pH if Emelio ate a piece of cheese after having his cola snack?**
   The cheese would facilitate the pH return to neutral faster than if cheese were not eaten.

5. **Which is the *most important* dietary factor in predicting caries in general?**
   The oral contact time of fermentable carbohydrates is the most important factor.

Appendix B

Dietary Reference Intakes (DRI) Tables

TABLE B–1 Dietary Reference Intake (DRI): Recommended Intake for Individuals, Vitamins

Life Stage Group	Vit A (µg/d)a	Vit C (mg/d)	Vit D (µg/d)b,c	Vit E (mg/d)d	Vit K (µg/d)	Thiamin (mg/d)	Riboflavin (mg/d)	Niacin (mg/d)e	Vit B_6 (mg/d)	Folate (µg/d)f	Vit B_{12} (µg/d)	Pantothenic Acid (mg/d)	Biotin (µg/d)	Choline (mg/d)g
Infants														
0–6 mo	400*	40*	5*	4*	2.0*	0.2*	0.3*	2*	0.1*	65*	0.4*	1.7*	5*	125*
7–12 mo	500*	50*	5*	5*	2.5*	0.3*	0.4*	4*	0.3*	80*	0.5*	1.8*	6*	150*
Children														
1–3 y	300	15	5*	6	30*	0.5	0.5	6	0.5	150	0.9	2*	8*	200*
4–8 y	400	25	5*	7	55*	0.6	0.6	8	0.6	200	1.2	3*	12*	250*
Males														
9–13 y	600	45	5*	11	60*	0.9	0.9	12	1.0	300	1.8	4*	20*	375*
14–18 y	900	75	5*	15	75*	1.2	1.3	16	1.3	400	2.4	5*	25*	550*
19–30 y	900	90	5*	15	120*	1.2	1.3	16	1.3	400	2.4	5*	30*	550*
31–50 y	900	90	5*	15	120*	1.2	1.3	16	1.3	400	2.4	5*	30*	550*
51–70 y	900	90	10*	15	120*	1.2	1.3	16	1.7	400	2.4i	5*	30*	550*
>70 y	900	90	15*	15	120*	1.2	1.3	16	1.7	400	2.4i	5*	30*	550*
Females														
9–13 y	600	45	5*	11	60*	0.9	0.9	12	1.0	300	1.8	4*	20*	375*
14–18 y	700	65	5*	15	75*	1.0	1.0	14	1.2	400j	2.4	5*	25*	400*
19–30 y	700	75	5*	15	90*	1.1	1.1	14	1.3	400j	2.4	5*	30*	425*
31–50 y	700	75	5*	15	90*	1.1	1.1	14	1.3	400j	2.4	5*	30*	425*
51–70 y	700	75	10*	15	90*	1.1	1.1	14	1.5	400	2.4h	5*	30*	425*
>70 y	700	75	15*	15	90*	1.1	1.1	14	1.5	400	2.4h	5*	30*	425*
Pregnancy														
14–18 y	750	80	5*	15	75*	1.4	1.4	18	1.9	600j	2.6	6*	30*	450*
19–30 y	770	85	5*	15	90*	1.4	1.4	18	1.9	600j	2.6	6*	30*	450*
31–50 y	770	85	5*	15	90*	1.4	1.4	18	1.9	600j	2.6	6*	30*	450*

(continued)

TABLE B–1 Dietary Reference Intake (DRIs): Recommended Intake for Individuals, Vitamins (Continued)

Lactation													
14–18 y	1,200	115	5*	19	75*	1.4	1.6	17	2.0	500	2.8	7*	35*	550*
19–30 y	1,300	120	5*	19	90*	1.4	1.6	17	2.0	500	2.8	7*	35*	550*
31–50 y	1,300	120	5*	19	90*	1.4	1.6	17	2.0	500	2.8	7*	35*	550*

Note: This table (taken from the DRI reports, see www.nap.edu) presents Recommended Dietary Allowances (RDAs) in **bold type** and Adequate Intakes (AIs) in ordinary type followed by an asterisk (*). RDAs and AIs may both be used as goals for individual intake. RDAs are set to meet the needs of almost all (97 to 98 percent) individuals in a group. For healthy breastfed infants, the AI is the mean intake. The AI for other life stage and gender groups is believed to cover needs of all individuals in the group, but lack of data or uncertainty in the data prevent being able to specify with confidence the percentage of individuals covered by this intake.

[a]As retinol activity equivalents (RAEs), 1 RAE = 1 μg retinol, 12 μg β-carotene, 24 μg α-carotene or 24 μg β-cryptoxanthin. The RAE for dietary provitamin A carotenoids is twofold greater than retinol equivalents (RE), whereas the RAE for preformed vitamin A is the same as RE.

[b]As cholecalciferol, 1 μg cholecalciferol = 40 IU vitamin D.

[c]In the absence of adequate exposure to sunlight.

[d]As α-tocopherol, α-tocopherol includes *RRR*-α-tocopherol, the only form of α-tocopherol that occurs naturally in foods, and the 2*R*-stereoisomeric forms of α-tocopherol (*RRR*-, *RSR*-, *RRS*-, and *RSS*-α-tocopherol) that occur in fortified foods and supplements. It does not include the 2*S*-stereoisomeric forms of α-tocopherol (*SRR*-, *SSR*-, *SRS*-, and *SSS*-α-tocopherol), found in fortified foods and supplements.

[e]As niacin equivalents (NE). 1mg of niacin = 60 mg of tryptophan; 0–6 months = preformed niacin (not NE).

[f]As dietary folate equivalents (DFE). 1 DFE = 1 μg food folate = 0.6 μg of folic acid from fortified food or as a supplement consumed with food = 0.5 μg of a supplement taken on an empty stomach.

[g]Although AIs have been set for choline, there are few data to assess whether a dietary supply of choline is needed at all stages of the life cycle, and it may be that the choline requirement can be met by endogenous synthesis at some of these stages.

[h]Because 10 to 30 percent of older people may malabsorb food-bond B_{12}, it is advisable for those older tha 50 years to meet their RDA mainly by consuming foods fortified with B_{12} or a supplement containing B_{12}.

[i]In view of evidence linking folate intake with neutral tube defects in the fetus, it is recommended that all women capable of becoming pregnant consume 400 μg from supplement or fortified foods in addition to intake of food folate from a varied diet.

[j]It is assumed that women will continue consuming 400 μg from supplements or fortified food until their pregnancy is confirmed and they enter prenatal care, which ordinarily occurs after the end of the periconceptional period—the critical time for formation of the neutral tube.

Source: Reprinted with permission from *Dietary Reference Intakes for Water, Potassium, Sodium, Chloride, and Sulfate.* Copyright © 2004 by the National Academy of Sciences. Courtesy of the National Academy Press, Washington, D.C.

TABLE B–2 Dietary Reference Intakes (DRIs): Recommended Intakes for Individuals, Elements

Life Stage Group	Calcium (mg/d)	Chromium (µg/d)	Copper (µg/d)	Fluoride (mg/d)	Iodine (µg/d)	Iron (mg/d)	Magnesium (mg/d)	Manganese (mg/d)	Molybdenum (µg/d)	Phosphorus (mg/d)	Selenium (µg/d)	Zinc (mg/d)	Potassium (g/d)	Sodium (g/d)	Chloride (g/d)
Infants															
0–6 mo	210*	0.2*	200*	0.01*	110*	0.27*	30*	0.003*	2*	100*	15*	2*	0.4*	0.12*	0.18*
7–12 mo	270*	5.5*	220*	0.5*	130*	11	75*	0.6*	3*	275*	20*	3	0.7*	0.37*	0.57*
Children															
1–3 y	500*	11*	340	0.7*	90	7	80	1.2*	17	460	20	3	3.0*	1.0*	1.5*
4–8 y	800*	15*	440	1*	90	10	130	1.5*	22	500	30	5	3.8*	1.2*	1.9*
Males															
9–13 y	1,300*	25*	700	2*	120	8	240	1.9*	34	1,250	40	8	4.5*	1.5*	2.3*
14–18 y	1,300*	35*	890	3*	150	11	410	2.2*	43	1,250	55	11	4.7*	1.5*	2.3*
19–30 y	1,000*	35*	900	4*	150	8	400	2.3*	45	700	55	11	4.7*	1.5*	2.3*
31–50 y	1,000*	35*	900	4*	150	8	420	2.3*	45	700	55	11	4.7*	1.5*	2.3*
51–70 y	1,200*	30*	900	4*	150	8	420	2.3*	45	700	55	11	4.7*	1.3*	2.0*
>70 y	1,200*	30*	900	4*	150	8	420	2.3*	45	700	55	11	4.7*	1.2*	1.8*
Females															
9–13 y	1,300*	21*	700	2*	120	8	240	1.6*	34	1,250	40	8	4.5*	1.5*	2.3*
14–18 y	1,300*	24*	890	3*	150	15	360	1.6*	43	1,250	55	9	4.7*	1.5*	2.3*
19–30 y	1,000*	25*	900	3*	150	18	310	1.8*	45	700	55	8	4.7*	1.5*	2.3*
31–50 y	1,000*	25*	900	3*	150	18	320	1.8*	45	700	55	8	4.7*	1.5*	2.3*
51–70 y	1,200*	20*	900	3*	150	8	320	1.8*	45	700	55	8	4.7*	1.3*	2.0*
>70 y	1,200*	20*	900	3*	150	8	320	1.8*	45	700	55	8	4.7*	1.2*	1.8*
Pregnancy															
14–18 y	1,300*	29*	1,000	3*	220	27	400	2.0*	50	1,250	60	12	4.7*	1.5*	2.3*
19–30 y	1,000*	30*	1,000	3*	220	27	350	2.0*	50	700	60	11	4.7*	1.5*	2.3*
31–50 y	1,000*	30*	1,000	3*	220	27	360	2.0*	50	700	60	11	4.7*	1.5*	2.3*
Lactation															
14–18 y	1,300*	44*	1,300	3*	290	10	360	2.6*	50	1,250	70	13	5.1*	1.5*	2.3*
19–30 y	1,000*	45*	1,300	3*	290	9	310	2.6*	50	700	70	12	5.1*	1.5*	2.3*
31–50 y	1,000*	45*	1,300	3*	290	9	320	2.6*	50	700	70	12	5.1*	1.5*	2.3*

Note: This table presents Recommended Dietary Allowances (RDAs) in **bold type** and Adequate Intakes (AIs) in ordinary type followed by an asterisk (*). RDAs and AIs may both be used as goals for individual intake. RDAs are set to meet the needs of almost all (97 to 98 percent) individuals in a group. For healthy breastfed infants, the AI is the mean intake. The AI for other life stage and gender groups is believed to cover needs of all individuals in the group, but lack of data or uncertainly in the data prevent being able to specify with confidence the percentage of individuals covered by this intake.

Source: Reprinted with permission from *Dietary Reference Intakes for Water, Potassium, Sodium, Chloride, and Sulfate.* Copyright © 2004 by the National Academy of Sciences. Courtesy of the National Academy Press, Washington, D.C.

TABLE B-3 Dietary Reference Intake (DRIs): Tolerable Upper Intake Levels (UL[a]), Vitamins

Life Stage Group	Vitamin A (µg/d)[b]	Vitamin C (mg/d)	Vitamin D (µg/d)	Vitamin E (mg/d)[c,d]	Vitamin K	Thiamin	Ribo-flavin	Niacin (mg/d)[d]	Vitamin B_6 (mg/d)	Folate (µg/d)[d]	Vitamin B_{12}	Pantothenic Acid	Biotin	Choline (g/d)	Carotenoids[e]
Infants															
0–6 mo	600	ND[f]	25	ND	ND	ND	ND	ND	ND	ND	ND	ND	ND	ND	ND
7–12 mo	600	ND	25	ND	ND	ND	ND	ND	ND	ND	ND	ND	ND	ND	ND
Children															
1–3 y	600	400	50	200	ND	ND	ND	10	30	300	ND	ND	ND	1.0	ND
4–8 y	900	650	50	300	ND	ND	ND	15	40	400	ND	ND	ND	1.0	ND
Males, Females															
9–13 y	1,700	1,200	50	600	ND	ND	ND	20	60	600	ND	ND	ND	2.0	ND
14–18 y	2,800	1,800	50	800	ND	ND	ND	30	80	800	ND	ND	ND	3.0	ND
19–70 y	3,000	2,000	50	1,000	ND	ND	ND	35	100	1,000	ND	ND	ND	3.5	ND
>70 y	3,000	2,000	50	1,000	ND	ND	ND	35	100	1,000	ND	ND	ND	3.5	ND
Pregnancy															
14–18 y	2,800	1,800	50	800	ND	ND	ND	30	80	800	ND	ND	ND	3.0	ND
19–50 y	3,000	2,000	50	1,000	ND	ND	ND	35	100	1,000	ND	ND	ND	3.5	ND
Lactation															
14–18 y	2,800	1,800	50	800	ND	ND	ND	30	80	800	ND	ND	ND	3.0	ND
19–50 y	3,000	2,000	50	1,000	ND	ND	ND	35	100	1,000	ND	ND	ND	3.5	ND

[a] UL = The maximum level of daily nutrient intake is likely to pose no risk of adverse effects. Unless otherwise specified, the UL represents total intake from food, water, and supplements. Due to lack of suitable data. ULs could not be established for Vitamin K, thiamin, riboflavin, vitamin B_{12}, pantothenic acid, biotin, carotenoids. In the absence of ULs, extra caution may be warranted in consuming levels above recommended intakes.

[b] As preformed vitamin A only.

[c] As α-tocopherol; applies to any form of supplemental α-tocopherol.

[d] The ULs for vitamin E, niacin, and folate apply to synthetic forms obtained from supplements, fortified foods, or a combination of the two.

[e] β-Carotene supplements are advised only to serve as a provitamin A source for individuals at risk of vitamin A deficiency.

[f] ND = Not determined due to lack of data of adverse effects in this age group and concern with regard to lack of ability to handle excess amounts. Source of intake should be from food only to prevent high levels of intake.

Source: Reprinted with permission from *Dietary Reference Intakes for Water, Potassium, Sodium, Chloride, and Sulfate.* Copyright © 2004 by the National Academy of Sciences. Courtesy of the National Academy Press, Washington, D.C.

TABLE B–4 Dietary Reference Intakes (DRIs): Tolerable Upper Intake Levels (UL[a]), Elements

Life Stage Group	Arsenic[b]	Boron (mg/d)	Calcium (g/d)	Chromium	Copper (μg/d)	Fluoride (mg/d)	Iodine (μg/d)	Iron (mg/d)	Magnesium (mg/d)	Manganese (mg/d)	Molybdenum (μg/d)	Nickel (mg/d)	Phosphorus (g/d)	Potassium	Selenium (μg/d)	Silicon[d]	Sulfate	Vanadium (mg/d)[e]	Zinc (mg/d)	Sodium (g/d)	Chloride (g/d)
Infants																					
0–6 mo	ND[f]	ND	ND	ND	ND	0.7	ND	40	ND	ND	ND	ND	ND	ND	45	ND	ND	ND	4	ND	ND
7–12 mo	ND	ND	ND	ND	ND	0.9	ND	40	ND	ND	ND	ND	ND	ND	60	ND	ND	ND	5	ND	ND
Children																					
1–3 y	ND	3	2.5	ND	1,000	1.3	200	40	65	2	300	0.2	3	ND	90	ND	ND	ND	7	1.5	2.3
4–8 y	ND	6	2.5	ND	3,000	2.2	300	40	110	3	600	0.3	3	ND	150	ND	ND	ND	12	1.9	2.9
Males, Females																					
9–13 y	ND	11	2.5	ND	5,000	10	600	40	350	6	1,100	0.6	4	ND	280	ND	ND	ND	23	2.2	3.4
14–18 y	ND	17	2.5	ND	8,000	10	900	45	350	9	1,700	1.0	4	ND	400	ND	ND	ND	34	2.3	3.6
19–70 y	ND	20	2.5	ND	10,000	10	1,100	45	350	11	2,000	1.0	4	ND	400	ND	ND	1.8	40	2.3	3.6
>70 y	ND	20	2.5	ND	10,000	10	1,100	45	350	11	2,000	1.0	3	ND	400	ND	ND	1.8	40	2.3	3.6
Pregnancy																					
14–18 y	ND	17	2.5	ND	8,000	10	900	45	350	9	1,700	1.0	3.5	ND	400	ND	ND	ND	34	2.3	3.6
19–50 y	ND	20	2.5	ND	10,000	10	1,100	45	350	11	2,000	1.0	3.5	ND	400	ND	ND	ND	40	2.3	3.6
Lactation																					
14–18 y	ND	17	2.5	ND	8,000	10	900	45	350	9	1,700	1.0	4	ND	400	ND	ND	ND	34	2.3	3.6
19–50 y	ND	20	2.5	ND	10,000	10	1,100	45	350	11	2,000	1.0	4	ND	400	ND	ND	ND	40	2.3	3.6

[a] UL = The maximum level of daily nutrient intake that is likely to pose no risk of adverse effects. Unless otherwise specified, the UL represents total intake from food, water, and supplements. Due to lack of suitable data, ULs could not be established for arsenic, chromium, silicon, potassium, and sulfate. In the absence of ULs, extra caution may be warranted in consuming levels above recommended intakes.

[b] Although the UL was not determined for arsenic, there is no justification for adding arsenic to food or supplements.

[c] The ULs for magnesium represent intake from a pharmacological agent only and do not include intake from food and water.

[d] Although silicon has not been shown to cause adverse effects in humans, there is no justification for adding silicon to supplements.

[e] Although vanadium in food has not been shown to cause adverse effects in humans, there is no justification for adding vanadium to food and vanadium supplements should be used with caution. The UL is based on adverse effects in laboratory animals and this data could be used to set a UL for adults but not children and adolescents.

[f] ND = Not determinabe due to lack of data of adverse effects in this age group and concern with regard to lack of ability to handle excess amounts. Source of intake should be from food only to prevent high levels of intake.

Source: Reprinted with permission from *Dietary Reference Intakes for Water, Potassium, Sodium, Chloride, and Sulfate.* Copyright © 2004 by the National Academy of Sciences. Courtesy of the National Academy Press, Washington, D.C.

TABLE B-5 Dietary Reference Intakes (DRIs): Estimated Energy Requirements (EER) for Men and Women 30 Years of Age[a]

Height (m [in])	PAL[b]	Weight for BMI[c] of 18.5 kg/m² (kg/[lb])	Weight for BMI of 24.99 kg/m² (kg/[lb])	EER, Men[d] (kcal/day)		EER, Women[d] (kcal/day)	
				BMI of 18.5 kg/m²	BMI of 24.99 kg/m²	BMI of 18.5 kg/m²	BMI of 24.99 kg/m²
1.50 (59)	Sedentary	41.6 (92)	56.2 (124)	1,848	2,080	1,625	1,762
	Low active			2,009	2,267	1,803	1,956
	Active			2,215	2,506	2,025	2,198
	Very active			2,554	2,898	2,291	2,489
1.65 (65)	Sedentary	50.4 (111)	68.0 (150)	2,068	2,349	1,816	1,982
	Low active			2,254	2,556	2,016	2,202
	Active			2,490	2,842	2,267	2,477
	Very active			2,880	3,296	2,567	2,807
1.80 (71)	Sedentary	59.9 (132)	81.0 (178)	2,301	2,635	2,015	2,211
	Low active			2,513	2,884	2,239	2,459
	Active			2,782	3,200	2,519	2,769
	Very active			3,225	3,720	2,855	3,141

[a] For each year below 30, add 7 kcal/day for women and 10 kcal/day for men. For each year above 30, subtract 7 kcal/day for women and 10 kcal/day for men.
[b] PAL = physical activity level.
[c] BMI = body mass index.
[d] Derived from the following regression equations based on doubly labeled water data:
   Adult man: EER = $662 - 9.53 \times$ age (y) + PA $\times$ ($15.91 \times$ wt [kg] + $539.6 \times$ ht [m])
   Adult woman: EER = $354 - 6.91 \times$ age (y) + PA $\times$ ($9.36 \times$ wt [kg] + $726 \times$ ht [m])
Where PA refers to coefficient for PAL

PAL = total energy expenditure + basal energy expenditure

PA = 1.0 if PAL $\geq 1.0 < 1.4$ (sedentary)

PA = 1.12 if PAL $\geq 1.4 < 1.6$ (low active)

PA = 1.27 if PAL $\geq 1.6 < 1.9$ (active)

PA = 1.45 if PAL $\geq 1.9 < 2.5$ (very active)

TABLE B–6A   Dietary Reference Intakes (DRIs): Recommended Intakes for Individuals, Macronutrients

Life Stage Group	Total Water[a] (L/d)	Carbohydrate (g/d)	Total Fiber (g/d)	Fat (g/d)	Linoleic Acid (g/d)	α-Linolenic Acid (g/d)	Protein[b] (g/d)
Infants							
0–6 mo	0.7*	60*	ND	31*	4.4*	0.5*	9.1*
7–12 mo	0.8*	95*	ND	30*	4.6*	0.5*	**11.0**[c]
Children							
1–3 y	1.3*	**130**	19*	ND	7*	0.7*	**13**
4–8 y	1.7*	**130**	25*	ND	10*	0.9*	**19**
Males							
9–13 y	2.4*	**130**	31*	ND	12*	1.2*	**34**
14–18 y	3.3*	**130**	38*	ND	16*	1.6*	**52**
19–30 y	3.7*	**130**	38*	ND	17*	1.6*	**56**
31–50 y	3.7*	**130**	38*	ND	17*	1.6*	**56**
51–70 y	3.7*	**130**	30*	ND	14*	1.6*	**56**
>70 y	3.7*	**130**	30*	ND	14*	1.6*	**56**
Females							
9–13 y	2.1*	**130**	26*	ND	10*	1.0*	**34**
14–18 y	2.3*	**130**	26*	ND	11*	1.1*	**46**
19–30 y	2.7*	**130**	25*	ND	12*	1.1*	**46**
31–50 y	2.7*	**130**	25*	ND	12*	1.1*	**46**
51–70 y	2.7*	**130**	21*	ND	11*	1.1*	**46**
>70 y	2.7*	**130**	21*	ND	11*	1.1*	**46**
Pregenancy							
14–18 y	3.0*	**175**	28*	ND	13*	1.4*	**71**
19–30 y	3.0*	**175**	28*	ND	13*	1.4*	**71**
31–50 y	3.0*	**175**	28*	ND	13*	1.4*	**71**
Lactation							
14–18 y	3.8*	**210**	29*	ND	13*	1.3*	**71**
19–30 y	3.8*	**210**	29*	ND	13*	1.3*	**71**
31–50 y	3.8*	**210**	29*	ND	13*	1.3*	**71**

Note: This table presents Recommended Dietary Allowances (RDAs) in **bold** type and Adequate Intakes (AIs) in ordinary type followed by an asterisk (*). RDAs and AIs may both be used as goals for individual intake. RDAs are set to meet the needs of almost all (97 to 98 percent) individual in a group. For healthy infants fed human milk, the AI is the mean intake. The AI for other life stage and gender groups is believed to cover the needs of all individuals in the group, but lack of data or uncertainty in the data prevent being able to specify with confidence the percentage of individual covered by this intake.

[a] *Total* water includes all water contained in food, beverages, and drinking water.

[b] Based on 0.8g/kg body weight for the reference body weight.

[c] Change from 13.5 in prepublication copy due to calculation error.

TABLE B–6B   Dietary Reference Intakes (DRIs): Acceptable Macronutrient Distribution Ranges

	Range (percent of energy)		
Macronutrient	*Children, 1–3y*	*Children, 4–18y*	*Adults*
Fat	30–40	25–35	20–35
n-6 polyunsaturated fatty acids[a] (linoleic acid)	5–10	5–10	5–10
n-3 polyunsaturated fatty acids[a] (α-linoleic acid)	0.6–1.2	0.6–1.2	0.6–1.2
Carbohydrate	45–65	45–65	45–65
Protein	5–20	10–30	10–35

[a] Approximately 10% of the total can come from longer-chain *n*-3 or *n*-6 fatty acids.

TABLE B–6C   Dietary Reference Intakes (DRIs): Additional Macronutrient Recommendations

Macronutrient	*Recommendation*
Dietary cholesterol	As low as possible while consuming a nutritionally adequate diet
Trans fatty acids	As low as possible while consuming a nutritionally adequate diet
Saturated fatty acids	As low as possible while consuming a nutritionally adequate diet
Added sugars	Limit to no more than 25% of total energy

Source: Tables B–6A, B, and C reprinted with permission from *Dietary Reference Intakes for Energy, Carbohydrate, Fiber, Fat, Fatty Acids, Cholesterol, Protein, and Amino Acids (Macronutrients).* Copyright © 2002 by the National Academy of Sciences. Courtesy of the National Academy Press, Washington, D.C.

TABLE B–7 Dietary Reference Intakes (DRIs): Estimated Average Requirements for Groups

Life Stage Group	CHO (g/d)	Protein (g/d)[a]	Vit A (µg/d)[b]	Vit C (mg/d)	Vit E (mg/d)[c]	Thiamin (mg/d)	Riboflavin (mg/d)	Niacin (mg/d)[d]	Vit B_6 (mg/d)	Folate (µg/d)[e]	Vit B_{12} (µg/d)	Copper (µg/d)	Iodine (µg/d)	Iron (mg/d)	Magnesium (mg/d)	Molybdenum (µg/d)	Phosphorus (mg/d)	Selenium (µg/d)	Zinc (mg/d)
Infants																			
7–12 mo		9*												6.9					2.5
Children																			
1–3 y	100	11	210	13	5	0.4	0.4	5	0.4	120	0.7	260	65	3.0	65	13	380	17	2.5
4–8 y	100	15	275	22	6	0.5	0.5	6	0.5	160	1.0	340	65	4.1	110	17	405	23	4.0
Males																			
9–13 y	100	27	445	39	9	0.7	0.8	9	0.8	250	1.5	540	73	5.9	200	26	1,055	35	7.0
14–18 y	100	44	630	63	12	1.0	1.1	12	1.1	330	2.0	685	95	7.7	340	33	1,055	45	8.5
19–30 y	100	46	625	75	12	1.0	1.1	12	1.1	320	2.0	700	95	6	330	34	580	45	9.4
31–50 y	100	46	625	75	12	1.0	1.1	12	1.1	320	2.0	700	95	6	350	34	580	45	9.4
51–70 y	100	46	625	75	12	1.0	1.1	12	1.4	320	2.0	700	95	6	350	34	580	45	9.4
>70 y	100	46	625	75	12	1.0	1.1	12	1.4	320	2.0	700	95	6	350	34	580	45	9.4
Females																			
9–13 y	100	28	420	39	9	0.7	0.8	9	0.8	250	1.5	540	73	5.7	200	26	1,055	35	7.0
14–18 y	100	38	485	56	12	0.9	0.9	11	1.0	330	2.0	685	95	7.9	300	33	1,055	45	7.3
19–30 y	100	38	500	60	12	0.9	0.9	11	1.1	320	2.0	700	95	8.1	255	34	580	45	6.8
31–50 y	100	38	500	60	12	0.9	0.9	11	1.1	320	2.0	700	95	8.1	265	34	580	45	6.8
51–70 y	100	38	500	60	12	0.9	0.9	11	1.3	320	2.0	700	95	5	265	34	580	45	6.8
>70 y	100	38	500	60	12	0.9	0.9	11	1.3	320	2.0	700	95	5	265	34	580	45	6.8
Pregnancy																			
14–18 y	135	50	530	66	12	1.2	1.2	14	1.6	520	2.2	785	160	23	335	40	1,055	49	10.5
19–30 y	135	50	550	70	12	1.2	1.2	14	1.6	520	2.2	800	160	22	290	40	580	49	9.5
31–50 y	135	50	550	70	12	1.2	1.2	14	1.6	520	2.2	800	160	22	300	40	580	49	9.5
Lactation																			
14–18 y	160	60	885	96	16	1.2	1.3	13	1.7	450	2.4	985	209	7	300	35	1,055	59	10.9
19–30 y	160	60	900	100	16	1.2	1.3	13	1.7	450	2.4	1,000	209	6.5	255	36	580	59	10.4
31–50 y	160	60	900	100	16	1.2	1.3	13	1.7	450	2.4	1,000	209	6.5	265	36	580	59	10.4

Note: This table presents Estimated Average Requirements (EARs), which serve two purposes: for assessing adequacy of population intakes, and as the basis for calculating Recommended Dietary Allowance (RDAs) for individuals for those nutrients. EARs have not been established for vitamin D, vitamin K, pantothenic acid, biotin, choline, calcium, chromium, fluoride, manganese, or other nutrients not yet evaluated via the DRI process.

[a] For individual at reference weight (Table 1–1).

[b] As retinol activity equivalents (RAFs). 1 RAE = 1 µg retinol, 12 µg β-carotene, 24 µg α-carotene, or 24 µg β-cryptoxanthin. The RAE for dietary provitamin A carotenoids is two-fold greater than retinol equivalents (RE), whereas the RAE for preformed vitamin A is the same as RE.

[c] As α-tocopherol, α-Tocopherol includes *RRR*-α-tocopherol, the only form of α-tocopherol that occurs naturally in foods, and the 2*R*-stereoisomeric forms of α-tocopherol (*RRR*-, *RSR*-, *RRS*-, and *RSS*-α-tocopherol) that occur in fortified foods and supplements. It does not include the 2*S*-stereoisomeric forms of α-tocopherol (*SRR*-, *SSR*-, *SRS*-, and *SSS*-α-tocopherol), also found in fortified foods and supplements.

[d] As niacin equivalents (NE). 1 mg of niacin = 60 mg of tryptophan.

[e] As dietary folate equivalents (DFE). 1 DFE = 1 µg food folate = 0.6 µg of folic acid from fortified food or as a supplement consumed with food = 0.5 µg of a supplement taken on an empty stomach.

*indicates change from prepublication copy due to calculation error.

Source: Copyright © 2002 by the National Academy of Sciences. All Rights Reserved.

Appendix C

Sample Diet Assessment Form

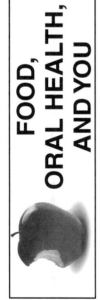

FOOD, ORAL HEALTH, AND YOU

What you eat can help or harm your mouth and teeth.

Good nutrition keeps the mouth healthy, helps heal wounds, helps fight gum disease, and helps prevent tooth decay.

This booklet will help you see how your oral health nutrition shapes up.

Promoting Good Nutrition

Please begin by answering the following:

Are you being treated for any nutrition-related condition?	Yes	No
Do you have any dental problems which affect your eating?	Yes	No
Have you changed your eating habits in the past 6 months?	Yes	No
Have you lost or gained more than 10 pounds **without trying** in the last 6 months?	Yes	No
Do you drink more that 3 alcoholic beverages daily?	Yes	No
Do you take vitamins or nutritional supplements? If yes, what type and how often?	Yes	No

If you answered Yes to any of the above, please explain:

What do you eat in a typical day . . .

Please list all of the foods (including snacks drinks), that you have on a USUAL weekday. Give your best guess as to amounts and times eaten.

Time of Day	Food/drink	Amount

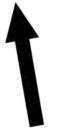

Next
See how you're doing:

- Using your typical intake from above, put a check in the appropriate pyramid box on the next page for each serving you ate from each group
  Example: a banana and a piece of toast would be one check in the fruit section and one check in the grain section.
- Be sure to use the appropriate serving sizes to check off the boxes correctly.
  Example: One cup of cooked broccoli counts as 2 vegetable servings.

How Does Your Diet Rate?

Put a check in the appropriate **Food Pyramid** box below for each serving you have daily and compare to the **minimums** recommended below

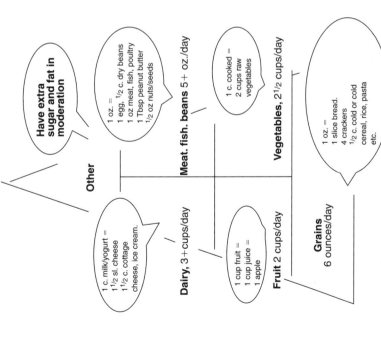

Have extra sugar and fat in moderation

Other

1 oz. =
1 egg, 1/2 c. dry beans
1 oz meat, fish, poultry
1 Tbsp peanut butter
1/2 oz nuts/seeds

Meat. fish. beans 5+ oz./day

1 c. cooked =
2 cups raw vegetables

Vegetables, 2 1/2 cups/day

1 c. milk/yogurt =
1 1/2 sl. cheese
1 1/2 c. cottage cheese, ice cream.

Dairy, 3+ cups/day

1 cup fruit =
1 cup juice =
1 apple

Fruit 2 cups/day

1 oz. =
1 slice bread.
4 crackers
1/2 c. cold or cold cereal, rice, pasta etc.

Grains
6 ounces/day

Record your general nutrition results on the next page

Results of your diet evaluation

IF YOU WERE BELOW THE LOWEST RECOMMENDED SERVINGS IN ANY OF THE FOOD PYRAMID GROUPS, YOU MAY BE AT NUTRITIONAL RISK.

PLOT YOUR RISK ON THE LINE BELOW:

LOW RISK   **MEDIUM RISK**   **HIGH RISK**

| Low in 0 groups | Low in 1–2 groups | Low in 3+ groups |

Food Group	Important Nutrients	Suggestions
Dairy	Protein, Calcium, Vitamin D	Have some yogurt or cheese for a snack. Put milk on your cereal.
Fruit	Vitamins A & C, F ber	Add to cereal. Eat as a snack or instead of dessert.
Vegetable	Vitamins A & C, Fiber	Add to sandwiches or pasta. Have a salad with your meal.
Bread/ Cereal	B vitamins Fiber Carbohydrate	Snack on pretzels, popcorn, or crackers. Have rice with dinner.
Protein	Protein, Zinc, Iron, B vitamins	Have some peanut butter on your crackers. Add cheese to a salad.

Now check your risk
for developing **Tooth decay**

(continued)

485

Sample Diet Assessment Form (Continued)

Your Dental Caries Risk

Frequently eating sugar-containing foods is a major risk factor for dental caries (tooth decay).

The longer and more frequently these foods stay in the mouth, the greater the risk of developing **tooth decay.**

Using your usual weekday again . .

Put a check (✓) in **Box 1** below for each food or beverage you had for dessert or between meals **(at least 20 minutes apart).**

Put the total in **Box 2** and multiply by the number in the box

Examples of types of decay-promoting foods	Box 1 *Put a check for each decay-promoting food or beverage you eat daily*	Box 2 *Multiply the number of checks in Box 1 by the risk number in the box below. Add up the numbers for your final risk score*
LIQUID Soft drinks, fruit drinks, cocoa, sugar & honey in drinks, non-dairy creamers, puddings, ice cream flavored or frozen yogurt, sherbet, jello, popsicles etc.		x 1 =
SOLID/STICKY Sweetened canned fruit, bananas, dried fruits, cake, cookies, pie & pastry, candy, sweet rolls, donuts, caramel, jelly/jam, marshmallow etc.		x 2 =
SLOWLY DISSOLVING Hard candy, breath mints, cough drips, antacid tablets		x 3 =

Figure total score and go to next page: TOTAL SCORE _____

Oral Health Results

Find out Your Caries Risk

Place your Dental Caries Risk Score on the

Caries Risk Line below.

*	*	*	*	*
0–1	2–4	5–7	8–9	>9
Low Risk	Moderate Risk		HIGH RISK	

To lower your risk of caries, keep these points in mind:

- **Reduce** the frequency of between meal sweets.

- **Don't** sip contantly on sweetened beverages.

- **Do** use water or milk instead.

- **Avoid** using slowly dissolving items like hard candy, cough drops or breath mints.

- **Eat more** non-decay-promoting foods such as low-fat cheese, raw vegetables, crunchy fruits, popcorn, nuts, artificially sweetened beverages and natural spring waters.

Source: © Division of Nutrition and Preventive Dentistry, Department of General Dentistry, Tufts University School of Dental Medicine.

Index